P9-ARZ-640

THE ENCYCLOPEDIA OF

ADOPTION

THE ENCYCLOPEDIA OF

ADOPTION

Third Edition

Christine Adamec
Laurie C. Miller, M.D.

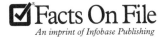

An imprint of Infobase Publishing

The Encyclopedia of Adoption, Third Edition

Copyright © 2007, 2000, 1992 by Christine Adamec and Laurie C. Miller, M.D.

Facts On File, Inc.
An imprint of Infobase Publishing
132 West 31st Street
New York NY 10001

Library of Congress Cataloging-in-Publication Data

Adamec, Christine A., 1949-
The encyclopedia of adoption / Christine Adamec, Laurie C. Miller.—3rd ed.
p. cm.
Includes bibliographical references and index.
ISBN 0-8160-6329-X (alk. paper)
1. Adoption—United States—Encyclopedias. I. Miller, Laurie C. II. Title.
HV875.55.A28 2007
362.7340973—dc22   2005055514

You can find Facts On File on the World Wide Web at http://www.factsonfile.com

Text and cover design by Cathy Rincon

Printed in the United States of America

VB Hermitage 10 9 8 7 6 5 4 3 2 1

This book is printed on acid-free paper.

CONTENTS

FOREWORD

Adoption is a constantly evolving institution that changes to fit the perceived needs of children who need families, whether they are healthy newborns, children in foster care, children from other countries, or children of all ages with special needs. In addition to the "triad" members of adopted children, adoptive parents, and birthparents, there are many others who are actively involved in adoptions. State and federal legislators enact new laws or rewrite old laws to fulfill new needs or to manage newly recognized problems. Sometimes new laws are made in order to correct unanticipated problems that old laws created, as with the Adoption and Safe Families Act (ASFA). This federal law was written because the earlier federal law, the Adoption Assistance and Child Welfare Act of 1980, had the unanticipated consequence of keeping abused and neglected children in foster care indefinitely rather than returning them to their parents or placing them for adoption with relatives or nonrelatives. ASFA restored the needs of children as the paramount concern, as we discuss in the entry on ASFA.

States also change their adoption laws to reflect current needs of adults; for example, many states have changed their laws on issues related to adopted adults who are searching for their birthparents, providing increased access to adoption records compared to past years. We discuss these changes in our search overview.

Medical issues related to adoption also change with time. Physicians, particularly pediatricians, assist children and their adoptive parents with a variety of medical issues. With increasing numbers of international adoptions, more doctors are becoming aware of medical problems that do not commonly occur in the United States or Canada but which are common in children adopted from other countries, such as intestinal parasitic infections and tuberculosis, entries that we cover in this new edition. In fact, a new specialty, adoption medicine, has been created to deal with such problems, and we have added an entry on adoption medicine to the third edition.

Researchers seek to study and uncover the reasons behind medical and psychiatric issues related to adoption. However, they are often hamstrung by issues of confidentiality and the great expense of large and long-term studies and, as a result, must frequently consider a population at a single point in time, which may not reflect the ongoing status of study subjects. For example, adopted children who are evaluated as adolescents might show very different results if they were evaluated again by researchers as adults. Birthmothers who may be depressed or anxious about a recent adoptive placement are not necessarily clinically depressed or anxious for life (although they may be). As a result, research studies need to be considered in context and we discuss this issue further in our new entry on research and problems that need to be considered, as well as in our revised entry on adoption studies.

Social workers and therapists work to assist children who have been affected by past problems of abuse or with current issues with which they struggle. However, sometimes because of old and outdated information, mental health professionals perceive adoption itself as inherently pathological, failing to see problems that may have occurred either before the child's adoption or subsequent to the adoption, and that are unrelated to the child's adopted status. They may also be unaware of new research on adopted children, which reflect that although some children are troubled, many do well with their adoptive families. These are issues that we cover in our updated entry on psychiatric problems of adopted persons.

In this new edition of *The Encyclopedia of Adoption,* we have updated many former entries, and we have also added a great deal of new information. New and/or revised overview entries are now included on abuse, foster care, international adoption, the medical problems of internationally adopted children, search issues for birthparents or adopted adults, and transracial adoption. In addition, we have included a new overview entry on prenatal exposures, discussing exposures to alcohol, drugs, and tobacco, all of which can have profound effects on the developing fetus and later on the child.

We have also heavily revised the entry on bonding and attachment and have added a new entry on attachment disorder, a serious problem of concern to many adoptive parents as well as to professionals, such as physicians and therapists. We also discuss abuse and neglect, and the long-term effects on young children. It is important to note that although abuse and neglect take a terrible toll on many children, some children have overcome the effects of these early life problems. We cover this topic in our new entry on resilience.

Many people are interested in medical issues, and as a result we have updated all the earlier entries on medical topics and have added some major new medical topics, including new entries on anemia, assisted reproductive technology, early intervention programs for young children, eating disorders, *Helicobacter pylori,* the human immunodeficiency virus (HIV), infectious diseases, intestinal parasitic infections, language delay, paternity testing, pediatricians, rickets, sensory integration disorder, sleep disorders in newly adopted children, syphilis, and tuberculosis.

Adoption is also a legal entity, and there are important legal issues that are of interest to people who wish to understand adoption. We have added new entries related to the law, such as the adoption subsidy for parents who adopt children from foster care, the Child Citizenship Act of 2000, and a new entry on fraud in adoption. In addition, we have added appendixes on state laws on the placement of children with relatives for adoption (Appendix 4) and state laws on the involuntary termination of parental rights (Appendix 5).

The international adoption scene is one that is constantly shifting, and we have worked hard to accommodate the great interest in this topic. We have added a new entry on Guatemala, currently the third most popular country for Americans adopting children from other countries, after China and Russia. We have also completely updated our entries on adoptions from China, India, Romania, Russia, and South Korea.

Because of the strong interest in adopted adults and/or birthparents seeking to locate each other, we have completely revised the entry on search, making it an overview entry, and we have heavily revised the entries on open records, mutual consent registries, sealed records, and search and consent laws. In addition, we have added Appendix 7 listing state laws on who may obtain identifying information and/or the original birth certificate of the adopted person.

Some other updated topics include: abandonment, abuse, adjustment, advertising and promotion, alcoholism and adopted persons, attitudes about adoption, birthfathers, birthmothers, Canada, costs to adopt, developmental disabilities, disruption/dissolution, Down syndrome, drug abuse, early puberty, employment benefits, explaining adoption, fetal alcohol syndrome, foster parent adoption, genetic predispositions, grandparent adoptions, hepatitis, immunizations, independent adoption, infertility, inheritance, intelligence, international adoption, the Interstate Compact on Adoption and Medical Assistance, kinship care, military members and adoption, neglect, open records, orphanages, photolistings, preparing a child for adoption, psychiatric problems of adopted persons, sealed records, search and consent laws, sexual abuse, special needs, statistics, surrogacy arrangements, teachers and adopted children, termination of parental rights, and videotapes.

It is important to point out that many adoption topics are closely linked, and as a result, we have provided extensive cross-references with many entries to assist readers seeking more information. For example, the subject of abuse is linked to foster care, since many abused children enter the foster care system. The topic of abuse itself is also linked to entries on such topics as abandonment, neglect, and sexual abuse.

In the case of international adoption, we have cross-referenced our overview entry on this topic to other entries on adoption from China, Guatemala, India, Russia, South Korea, Latin American adoptions, and eastern European adoptions, as well as to our overview entry on the medical problems of internationally adopted children.

Readers interested in the adoption of children by their relatives will wish to read our revised overview entry on kinship care as well as other revised entries, such as on grandparent adoption.

Individuals who have adopted or are interested in adopting a child may wish to read our revised entries on adoptive parents, birthfathers, and birthmothers, as well as our updated entries on the so-called baby shortage, costs to adopt, employment benefits, hospitals' treatment of birthmothers, income tax benefits for adoptive parents, independent adoption, infant adoption, open adoption and transracial adoption. Readers interested in genetic issues will wish to read our completely revised entry on genetic predispositions, as well as our revised entry on intelligence. Readers who are interested in other options to expand a family besides adoption will wish to read our entries on assisted reproductive technologies, infertility, and surrogacy arrangements.

To conclude, the institution of adoption will continue to shift and change to meet the needs of children, while reflecting social and cultural practices and beliefs. One thing does not change, however, and that is that children throughout the world will need parents. We hope that many people will step up to this rewarding task.

We also hope that the extensive information that we provide in this volume will give readers insight to how adoption works in the lives of many people who are affected by it, and they will find this volume to be useful and thought-provoking.

PREFACE

by Christine Adamec

Adoption is a life-changing experience for the key participants, including the adopted child, the birthparents, and the adoptive parents. There are also many others who are affected less directly, such as siblings, grandparents, and other relatives, as well as professionals, including teachers and physicians. Nearly everyone knows someone who was adopted, who adopted a child, or who placed a child for adoption, or "all of the above"—although sometimes this information is withheld from others.

There is both pain and joy with adoption. The birthparent suffers the pain of the loss of the biological child, while infertile individuals must cope with the pain of the unrealized dream of a biological child. Adopted children must face their loss, which is that the families who are raising them are not the families of their birth. Even in the case when the adoptive parents are clearly wonderful parents and the birthparents would equally clearly have provided very poor parenting to the child, there is still often a feeling of loss and "what if" among adopted children. If all children could be reared by their biological parents, adoption would be unnecessary, but it is unlikely that day will come. If it did, I personally would rejoice, since the main purpose of adoption is to provide good families for children who need them.

There is also joy in adoption, which continues to bring hope and love to many thousands of children and their families worldwide. Rather than condemning children to a life with birthparents who are unable or unwilling to care for them, children can instead be raised by individuals who are ready and eager to be parents. The birthparents can feel assured that their children are with parents who love and care for them, and for the adoptive parents, the child is a precious joy.

Sometimes birthparents willingly choose adoption for their children, and in other cases, the choice is made for them by others, whether the dysfunction that led them to be abusive or neglectful parents is due to alcoholism, drug addiction, mental illness or other problems, or a combination of problems. New families are then formed when former foster children join their families as legally adopted children. Some children travel thousands of miles to live with their "forever families," adopted from orphanages and foster care in other countries. International adoption has become an increasingly important part of adoption as a whole.

Yet there is still often a great deal of confusion about whether adoptive families are "as good as" biological families, which was probably a key impetus behind the past policy of returning foster children to abusive homes, again and again. (The Adoption and Safe Families Act has improved that situation considerably.)

In addition, most research studies concentrate on pathology, such as alcoholism, drug abuse, psychiatric problems, and so forth. Few studies seek to identify what is healthy about adoptive children and their families, and some researchers seem amazed that so many adoptive families and adopted children function even moderately well.

This should not be a surprising finding, however, given that most adoptive parents intensely desired to adopt their children, were usually thoroughly screened before they were allowed to adopt them, and actively seek to be good parents. Sometimes they try too hard and worry too much, and some adoptive parents take their children to a therapist for minor emotional problems. Of course, a good therapist will advise parents when the problem is a normal childhood issue.

At the same time, sometimes adopted children do have serious emotional problems, and denying that they exist, and hoping that they will magically go away, is a harmful strategy for the child. It can be difficult, although it is possible, to find a therapist who acknowledges that the fact of adoption may cause pain to adopted children, while at the same time the therapist realizes adoption itself is not the sole explanation for every emotional disorder of a person who happens to be adopted. We explore these issues in the entries of *The Encyclopedia of Adoption, Third Edition.*

It is also important to consider how adopted children might have developed had they *not* been adopted: if the sexually abused six-year-old girl remained with her abusive family, what would have been her likely outcome? Or what of the single mother who desires to make an adoption plan and she is talked out of it—or the single mother who wishes to parent her child and is talked *into* an unwanted adoption? What would be the outcomes in these alternative cases? Such events profoundly affect and shape the lives of the birthmother and the child and, when the child is adopted, the adopting parents, as well.

To a certain extent, there are some answers. It is known that children who remain with abusive parents have a worse outcome than children who are adopted. It is known that children who remain in foster care for years and who "age out" of the system as adults usually have worse outcomes than children adopted as infants or small children.

Yet most studies do not compare the outcome of adopted children to the likely outcome had they not been adopted, largely because such studies are difficult to perform because of confidentiality. Instead, researchers often compare adopted children directly to nonadopted children, who have not been exposed prenatally to toxic substances, have not lived in deprived circumstances, have not been beaten or starved, and instead who came directly home from the hospital with Mom and

Dad. As a result, it is not surprising that sometimes adopted children do not fare as well as children born to the family, in many different measures. Instead, what is surprising is that so often, adopted and nonadopted children are very close in terms of positive outcomes.

When adopted children have serious problems, it is often the events that preceded the adoption which are the primary contributors to the child's problems, whether they are prenatal exposures to alcohol and illegal drugs, genetic predispositions to psychiatric problems, the experience of abuse and/or neglect, and other factors that may have profound effects on children. Yet, despite even the most severe neglect or abuse, some children are resilient, and being adopted is one means to allow them to transcend these problems.

This does not mean that adoptive parents themselves are without flaws. Sometimes adoptive parents know far too little about adoption in general or about the particular child they wish to adopt, even when information is readily available. They may assume that love will conquer all problems, which is not a good working premise. They may change the name of an older child and urge her to forget everything that happened to her before today, assuming that she can or should.

There are many mistakes that adoptive parents can and do make; however, from my observations based on studying adoption for nearly 20 years and speaking to hundreds of adoptive parents, most do their best, and when they have problems, they seek help from others who are more experienced, including other adoptive parents, physicians, and therapists.

However, it should also be mentioned that perhaps once a year, the media report on an adoptive parent who has abused or even killed a child. These rare and shocking circumstances happen and they are real, but the overwhelming majority of adoptive parents are loving and caring people.

A major problem is that more adoptive parents are needed. Hundreds of thousands of children in foster care and in orphanages worldwide need adoptive families now. They do not know or care about rules and regulations or why they must stay in an orphanage or in a series of foster homes. They only know they want a family to love them. Yet in some cases, they do *not* know they need a family to care for them, in the same way that a child who is nearsighted does not know she needs glasses until glasses are placed in front of her, and suddenly everything is acutely clear.

Similarly, some older children have never known the love of a family, and it is an alien concept. When they experience it, however, the transformation to the life of the child can be truly amazing. No one attains a perfect life with adoption, but the changes in opportunities and emotional fulfillment can be staggering.

In this book, Dr. Miller and I have attempted to seek out as much of the current research we could identify that might be salient and interesting to readers who want to know more about adoption, whether they seek information on one specific topic or are intrigued by many different topics related to adoption. We have included many new medical topics, such as new entries on attachment disorders, hepatitis, prenatal exposures, rickets, and many other topics that readers may find useful.

We could not hope to include every study and every possible aspect of adoption within one volume, but we have provided an extensive breadth of subjects as well as a detailed bibliography for those who wish to learn even more. *The Encyclopedia of Adoption* also provides appendixes with listings of organizations related to adoption, including private and governmental organizations.

This book is meant for the general reader, and we hope that it will also interest the adoption expert. As a result, jargon has been kept to a minimum, or, when the use of jargon has been necessary, clear explanations on what these terms mean and what they imply are provided.

We hope this new edition of *The Encyclopedia of Adoption* will not only enlighten readers but may also inspire them to look further into this subject, even to launch a study or investigation on some aspect of adoption that needs further exploration. In my view, adoption is a very complicated, imperfect, and yet wonderful institution. Learning about adoption further advances the knowledge and understanding among those who are directly affected by adoption—adopted individuals, birthparents, and adoptive parents—as well as those within our society who set the standards for adoption and the federal and state lawmakers who make the rules that we live by. The children are worth every effort that we all can make. They are our future.

—Christine Adamec

PREFACE

by Laurie C. Miller, M.D.

Biology dictates that all children need loving and attentive adult care in order to thrive. Yet untold numbers of children throughout the world cannot be cared for by their parents. Poverty, immaturity, lack of emotional resources, substance abuse, mental or physical illness, and death may all prevent parents from caring for their children. In recent decades, death from infection with the human immunodeficiency virus (HIV) has plagued millions of families globally, leaving more than 15 million children without parents. Some children without families live on the streets in cities throughout the world, others are trafficked as prostitutes or virtual slaves, while still others are consigned to orphanages or other institutions. In America, more than 500,000 children who cannot be cared for by their parents reside in foster care, too many of them moving from one home to another throughout their childhoods. Some of these children are adopted, while tens of thousands urgently need families.

Adoption is the legal means by which a child permanently joins a family. An astonishing one in five Americans is directly touched by adoption, according to a survey conducted by the Evan B. Donaldson Institute in 1997. Our friends, coworkers, relatives, and close family members are themselves adopted or are connected to adoption in some other way. They may be birthparents, birth siblings, birth grandparents, or other relatives. They may be adoptive parents, grandparents, aunts, uncles, cousins, siblings, friends, and neighbors. In recognition of the far-reaching nature of adoption, Adam Pertman aptly subtitled his recent book *Adoption Nation* "How the Adoption Revolution is Transforming America."

Although the Donaldson survey found that 90 percent of Americans viewed adoption positively and 95 percent agreed it serves a useful purpose, some responses were not so favorable. Half of the respondents stated that adoption is not quite as good as having one's own child, 25 percent said it is sometimes harder to love an adopted child, and nearly 33 percent doubted that children could love adoptive parents as much as they could love birthparents.

This attitude reflects our Western cultural bias about adoption. In other parts of the world, for example, the Pacific Islands, adoption is considered a particularly revered form of family. In Tahiti, 25–40 percent of all children are adopted, and families hope, as quoted by author Elizabeth Bartholet, "to establish between parents and natural children relationships which coincide as nearly as possible with those between parents and adopted children."

However, in other nations, misconceptions about adoption abound. In some countries, adoption is considered a shameful secret, or an act to be spurned. Occasionally, popular opinion becomes aroused when sensational, shocking, and false stories appear that children are adopted by rich Westerners to be used as servants.

In the United States and other countries, adoption practice has been tainted at times by charges of baby-selling, "false advertising," and massively inflated costs. Clearly, for the benefit of children in need of families, and all parties involved, adoption practice wherever it occurs must be held to the highest ethical standards.

Regardless of difficulties, adoption goes on, driven by the desire of adoptive parents for children to love and by the recognition of the need of children for families. Parents choose to adopt for many reasons—best summarized by the Persian poet Kahlil Gibran: "Your children are not your children—they are the sons and daughters of life's longing for itself." Adoptive parents can be married or single, heterosexual, gay, or lesbian, young or old, fertile or infertile, first-time or experienced parents. They share a willingness to jump through endless hoops to get a child—sometimes even involving laws of other countries, exotic diseases, and travel to unfamiliar places. The desire to adopt does not discriminate—it can strike almost any adult, and one adoption may not be enough to satisfy the urge!

All child development experts agree that children need families. Experiments conducted by Harry Harlow and others demonstrate convincingly that young primates need responsive parenting in order to grow and thrive. For children whose own families cannot care for them, adoption provides a positive alternative, allowing many children to grow up healthy, happy, and loved.

Surprisingly, there are few definitive statistics about domestic adoption. However, statistics are readily available about international adoption through the Department of State. International adoption has increased dramatically in the past 10 years, from 8,195 in 1994 to 22,728 children in 2005.

Many of these adoptions are "visible," that is, children who are placed with ethnically and racially different parents. The rise in these visible placements has greatly increased awareness about adoption. Indeed, Pertman writes, "Across the United States today, it is getting increasingly difficult to find a playground without at least one little girl from China, being watched lovingly by a white mother or father." In some parts of the country, every school, every grade, and every classroom has internationally adopted children. Indeed, an adoptive father recently told me of his delight when the anticipated difficulties of a search for an "adoption-friendly" day care for his Russian-born son quickly vanished. In the first day-care center he visited, there were three international adoptees out of the five children in his son's age group.

The most common countries of origin for international adoptees have been China, Russia, Guatemala, Korea, and Ukraine, which together account for 82 percent of the 167,174 children placed with American parents in the past 10 years. Parents in other nations, including Canada, Spain, England, Italy, France, Australia, New Zealand, and Scandinavian countries also adopt children from abroad.

Until recently, adopted children and families have been ignored by physicians, except for those with research interests in the field, or those whose clinical practices brought them into proximity with many adopted individuals. Over the past several years, a burgeoning interest in adopted children has arisen among pediatricians, triggered in part by the visibility and urgent medical issues of the increasing number of internationally adopted children arriving in the United States.

Some of these issues are related to medical problems specific to the country of origin, including "exotic" infectious diseases such as malaria or intestinal parasites. However, more commonly, the issues reflect the suboptimal care of the children in early life, including prenatal exposures (drugs and alcohol), malnutrition, micronutrient deficiencies, toxic environmental exposures (lead), and most importantly, emotional and physical neglect.

Recognition of these problems in international adoptees has also increased the awareness of the medical needs of American children residing in foster care—a group with specialized health-care issues which for too long has been sadly neglected for the most part by the medical community. Pediatricians are recognizing the need for these children to have a "medical home" during their time in foster care and the need for continuity of care for those who are later adopted. In 2000 the American Academy of Pediatrics formally recognized a Section of Adoption and Foster Care, a group of pediatricians interested in promoting the care of foster and adopted children.

This long overdue step places adopted and foster children on the national pediatric agenda for health policies. Among the many issues confronting the Section are the development of appropriate diagnostic codes for necessary medical care of foster and adopted children (necessary for insurance, billing, and reimbursement), support of legislation (such as the Adoption and Safe Families Act, or ASFA), which expedites adoptions, improved coordination of care and medical record keeping for foster children, compliance with medical provisions contained within the Hague Convention on Intercountry Adoption, promotion of high-quality research on health and developmental issues for adoptees, and many other activities devoted to serving the best interests of these children.

Research on adoption has expanded as awareness of the special issues of this population has become more widespread. For many years, researchers took advantage of adoption as a natural "experiment" to test hypotheses about nature and nurture. Such investigations yielded valuable information about genetic and environmental contributions to behavior, health, and mental and physical disorders. Although this important work continues, in recent years the focus of adoption research has expanded to address the health and well-being of adoptive children and families, and the factors which promote favorable outcomes. Research by Joyce Maguire Pavao and others has improved understanding of "normative crises" in adoptive families, shedding light on normal, expected stages of adjustment for children and parents. Such research is directly applicable to the lives of adopted children and families and may aid professionals who deal with these individuals in their daily practice.

This book provides an overview of many of the issues faced by adoptive families, adopted children, birthparents, foster children, and adoption professionals. It contains valuable information for high school and college students as well as professionals—teachers, therapists, physicians—who encounter people touched by adoption in their work. Christine Adamec and I have assembled a compendium of detailed information, references, and resources. This book will be a useful guide to those with long and close familiarity with adoption, or to anyone new to this fascinating and wonderful world.

It is worth noting that the United Nations Declaration on the Rights of the Child addresses the needs of children without parental care. The United States is the only UN member state to have signed this document but not ratified it, as of June 2005. (UN member Somalia has neither signed nor ratified the convention.) The Declaration asserts that all children are entitled to "grow up in a family environment, in an atmosphere of happiness, love and understanding." Sadly, this goal is a long way from being achieved. Untold thousands of children reside in institutional care throughout the world. In many countries, domestic adoption programs are virtually nonexistent.

In our own country, too many children languish in foster care and despite changes to laws to facilitate their adoption, large numbers are caught in "legal limbo" which while admirably attempting to preserve the rights of their birthparents does so at the expense of freeing the child for adoption. Some would-be adoptive parents are dissuaded from pursuing adoption due to perceived legal complexities and the fear of the birthmother "changing her mind"—a statistically unlikely event, despite the noisy publicity about the few episodes that do occur. Although progress has been made in facilitating, supporting, and expediting adoption, much more remains to be done. All must remember the urgency of the mission to provide loving and permanent homes for *all* children in need. As the Chilean poet Gabriela Mistral wrote:

> Many things we need can wait.
> The child cannot.
> Now is the time his bones are being formed,
> his blood is being made,
> his mind is being developed.
> To him we cannot say, "tomorrow,"
> His name is "today."

Sources

U.S. Department of State. Bureau of Consular Affairs, Travel.State.Gov. Available online. URL: http://travel.state.gov/family/adoption/adoption_485.html. Downloaded June 15, 2005.

Bartholet, E. *Family Bonds: Adoption, Infertility, and the New World of Child Production.* Boston: Beacon Press, 1993.

Donner, W. W. "Sharing and compassion: Fosterage in Polynesian society," *Journal of Comparative Family Studies* 30, no. 4 (1999): 703.

Evan B. Donaldson Adoption Institute. *Benchmark Adoption Survey: Report on Findings.* New York: Evan B. Donaldson Adoption Institute, 1997.

Harlow, H. F., and S. J. Suomi. "Nature of love—simplified," *American Psychology* 25 (1970): 161–168.

Miller, L. C. *The Handbook of International Adoption Medicine.* New York: Oxford University Press, 2005.

Pavao, J. M. *The Family of Adoption.* Boston: Beacon Press, 1998.

Pertman, A. *Adoption Nation: How the Adoption Revolution Is Transforming America.* New York: Basic Books, 2000.

ACKNOWLEDGMENTS

Without the assistance of many talented and knowledgeable professionals, this interdisciplinary compendium of sociological, psychological, psychiatric, legal, and medical information would not have been possible. We owe a great debt of gratitude to many people.

First, we would like to thank the many dedicated researchers who have so carefully studied the numerous complex aspects of adoption and the topics related or important to the field of adoption. Some of them have spent years of their lives dedicated to uncovering information that has helped and will continue to help adopted individuals, adoptive parents, birthparents, and the wide variety of adoption professionals who seek to assist the entire triad. We are convinced that their professional studies, books, and magazine features deserve to be read in their entirety by many people. We hope that readers of this volume will be encouraged to explore more freely many of the materials we have only begun to tap. We hope our book will encourage many readers in their further studies and analyses of the fascinating topic of adoption.

There are also many people we would like to thank individually. Our thanks to the following people: Robin Hilborn, publisher of Family Helper in Ontario, Canada (www.familyhelper.net); Joe Kroll, executive director of the North American Council on Adoptable Children in St. Paul, Minnesota; and Liz Oppenheim, director of interstate affairs, American Public Human Services Administration, Washington, D.C. Thanks also to Aaron Britvan, an adoption attorney in Woodbury, New York.

Although we deeply appreciate the assistance of these individuals, as well as the assistance of many others, we alone are responsible for any errors of fact or interpretation or for any inadvertent omissions.

Christine Adamec would like to thank, above all people, her husband and best friend, John M. Adamec Jr. His unflagging conviction of the importance of this topic and his total support have been immeasurable.

She would also like to thank reference librarians Marie Mercer of the DeGroodt Public Library in Palm Bay, Florida, and Mary Jordan at the Central Library Facility in Cocoa, Florida, for their extensive assistance in locating books and journal articles needed to update this edition.

Dr. Miller offers her grateful appreciation to colleagues Wilma Chan, Linda Tirella, and Kathleen Comfort Salas for their enormous contributions to the International Adoption Clinic in Boston, Massachusetts. Their passion and compassion for adopted children and their families is inspiring to all. Many thanks also to her husband, David Sherman, for his encouragement and support of this and many other projects.

INTRODUCTION
A BRIEF HISTORY OF ADOPTION

by Christine Adamec

Adoption, the lawful transfer of parental obligations and rights, is not solely a practice of the 20th century but is a very old and constantly evolving institution. Societies have formally sanctioned the adoption of children, or closely similar arrangements, for more than 4,000 years, since the Babylonian Code of Hammurabi in 2285 B.C.—and probably before recorded history. Adoption is also mentioned in the Hindu Laws of Manu, written about 200 B.C. Perhaps the earliest known adoption is mentioned in the Bible, which describes the adoption of Moses by the Pharaoh's daughter.

The ancient Romans supported and codified adoption in their laws; in fact, Julius Caesar continued his dynasty by adopting his nephew Octavian, who became Caesar Augustus. The ancient Greeks, Egyptians, Assyrians, Germans, Japanese, and many other societies all practiced some form of adoption.

Adoption satisfied religious requirements in some cases; for example, in the Shinto religion, ancestral worship and the performance of certain religious rituals were perceived as necessary and important reasons for the institution of adoption. Adopted individuals could still carry on the family lineage and rituals when the family did not have biological children.

Despite a disparity of motivations in cultures worldwide for institutionalizing adoption formally or informally, the common denominator among them all was that adoption functionally satisfied the needs of society or the family.

Although the adopted person usually benefited from the adoption, such benefit was peripheral and was generally a happy accident. This underlying societal view sharply contrasts with views toward adoption today, when the needs and interests of the child are usually considered the primary reason and purpose for adoption as an institution. This is not to say that the benefits of adoption to society are not important. For example, many individuals believe that orphanage-raised children may be less effective as adults than are adopted children.

Today, most cultures worldwide provide for children needing families, although they may not provide the legal family membership that is inherent in adoption.

Most Western societies (with the exception of England) base their adoption laws on the original Roman code or the later Napoleonic code. Most experts agree that U.S. adoption law has combined aspects of Roman law with its own U.S. adaptations.

Adoption is a far newer institution in Europe, which has followed the lead of the United States. The first adoption law in England was the Adoption of Children Act of 1926. The Swedes enacted their first Adoption Act in 1917, and in 1959, adopted children in Sweden became full-fledged family members by law. Modern adoption laws came into being in West Germany in 1977.

It is critically important to understand that adoption laws and practices should be evaluated based on their functionality and the existing conditions of the time rather than on our contemporary values only. How adoption was and is now perceived in society and how adoption was and is now actually practiced has depended on a myriad of factors: social, economic, and political conditions; societal attitudes toward orphans and deprived children; out-of-wedlock births; minimum standards of parenting; views on parental rights and children's rights; views on the importance of property and inheritance, as well as other issues in the social order; the perception of the overriding importance of blood ties; and religious and moral values. This essay will only be able to touch on key issues within several periods in past history and in modern times.

Historical Adoption Practices

Babylonian adoption laws stated, "If a man has taken a young child from his waters to sonship and has reared him up no one has any claim against the nursling."

There are also biblical references to adoption; for example, Moses' mother, in an attempt to save her child from death by the Pharaoh's decree, placed him in a reed basket at the edge of the Nile River. Found by the Pharaoh's daughter, Moses was later formally adopted by her. (His birthmother served as his nurse during Moses' infancy.)

The ancient Romans practiced two types of adoptions: "adrogatio" (or "adrogation") and "adoptio" (or "adoption"). Adrogation usually referred to the adoption of an adult male, who became the legal heir of the adopter.

Adrogation was fairly common in ancient Rome, according to author John Boswell. Its purpose was to enable a childless man to ensure the continuity of his family name and also to provide someone to carry out religious rituals and memorials after his death.

In contrast, adoption was the process by which a minor child became a legal heir and dependent of the adoptive parent, with the agreement of his or her biological father. According to the law at that time, and based on the Laws of the Twelve Tables (mid-500s B.C.) the birthfather would perhaps sell his son up to three times and his daughter or granddaughter once, after which he could not reclaim the children. Unquestioned family allegiance was expected whether the person was adopted as a child or an adult.

The "paterfamilias" (male family head) had great power and could literally condemn his children to death. He could also sell them or abandon them (apparently girl children were more likely to be abandoned) with no negative social or legal consequences accruing to such acts.

In Roman law, only men were allowed to adopt until A.D. 291. Thereafter, women were allowed in special circumstances to adopt, for example, in the event of the loss of a biological child.

It is unclear whether the ancient Hebrews recognized adoption, although some experts have contended that St. Paul referred to adoptions among Hebrews in his writings, while other experts contend that his examples referred to adoptions among the Romans or Galatians.

Laws slowly changed and evolved. Under the reign of Byzantine emperor Justinian (A.D. 527–565), the adoptive parents, the person to be adopted, and the head of the birth family all were required to formally appear before a magistrate in order for an adoption to be legally recognized (a precursor of the "consent" aspect of Western law).

Some societies attached military significance to the act of adoption; for example, in ancient Germany, military ceremonies occurred at the point of adoption, with weapons placed in the hands of the adopted person. In ancient France, the adopted person swore to defend the adoptive family.

The English law of inheritance, with its heavy emphasis on bloodlines, became prominent in the Western world, and little or no provisions were made for a family name to "live on" through adopted children.

The concept of primogeniture—a practice whereby the eldest son would inherit the family property and, in turn, his eldest son would inherit from him—was core to the English, Germans, and other Europeans.

According to law professor C. M. A. McCauliff, "There could be no question of adoption in England so long as the heir at law held sway. The notion of any heir outside a natural orderly succession was repugnant to English society."

Legitimation, an issue of concern for centuries, was seen as a particularly important issue to the Christian church. In A.D. 335, Emperor Constantine, a Christian, ordered that children born to unmarried parents who later married would automatically become legitimate children. This legitimation law was ultimately abolished in 1235 in England, after which legitimation was to be determined by a jury on a case by case basis.

Legitimation was especially important in England because it was bound up in inheritance and rights. Since there was no legal way to adopt a child, legitimation was the only route for a child born out of wedlock to be considered an heir.

Children who needed parents were cared for by relatives, friends, or others who "took pity on them." Or they fended for themselves, living as thieves, prostitutes, or beggars. Abandoned children were also at risk of being kidnapped by individuals who would put out their eyes or cut off their feet, mutilating them so they could be more effectively used as beggars.

It is also important to remember that the Black Death claimed the lives of many thousands of people in the 14th century. Thus survival was the primary goal at that time, and many people could only afford to care for children related to them. Consequently, many children who were orphaned quickly died.

The Elizabethan Poor Law of 1601 formally provided for poor people in England, requiring parents either to care for their children or indenture them to others. This law was also the basis for the local systems of public charity in the colonies that later became the United States. Local overseers of the poor provided local relief for orphans. Although there were people in Europe who wished to legally tie children to their families through adoption, there were no provisions for such status to be attained.

In some areas, the situation for unwed mothers and their infants became very desperate.

C. M. A. McCauliff described a horrifying practice of unscrupulous "baby farmers," partially quoting the *Report of the Select Committee on the Protection of Infant Life:*

In Victorian England, unwed mothers were practically forced to give up their babies, who were then sent to baby-farming houses where they were fed "a mixture of laudanum, lime, cornflour, water, milk and washing powder . . . with rare exceptions they all of them die in a very short time."

According to author Diana Dewar, baby farmers took out insurance policies on children's lives and ensured their rapid demise so they could collect payments. These people also reassured unsuspecting single mothers that their children would be placed with loving families; however, many baby farmers would subsequently sell the children to the highest bidders.

Not everyone was indifferent to the plight of the children, and some individuals decided to take action. Nineteenth-century British social reformer Thomas Coram, horrified by the sight of abandoned dead babies in the streets, started a foundling hospital. Handel, the famous composer, donated all the royalties for his work *Messiah* to the hospital.

Because people in Britain could not adopt children and have parental rights and obligations transferred to them (as adoptive parents), many children who were orphaned or whose parents could not care for them were placed in foster homes or almshouses.

The concept of *parens patriae,* wherein the government acts as a parent, enabled the government to take such actions. This aspect of British common law has been incorporated into U.S. law and is part of U.S. child protection statutes and of the Indian Child Welfare Act, allowing the state to remove children from abusive or neglectful families.

The concept of the dominance of parental rights prevailed prior to the establishment of adoption and child protection statutes. Many 19th-century individuals in Britain (as well as in other countries) who were otherwise interested in fostering children were fearful of doing so because they could be subjected to blackmail threats from birthparents demanding money in exchange for allowing the foster parents to rear the child. (Recall, if you will, the attempt at blackmail by Eliza Doolittle's father present in the movie *My Fair Lady* for an example of practices common at the time or read *Oliver Twist* by Charles Dickens to gain a feel for the hopelessness and helplessness of children during this era.)

In addition, unscrupulous relatives could reclaim the child and literally sell him to tramps, prostitutes, or anyone. It must be remembered that children were not revered or protected as they are now by statute and were often conceptualized as property rather than persons. Yet many kind individuals would have eagerly adopted children had that legal option been available and had they been assured that the integrity of their family would not be disrupted by birthparents or others.

It was not until 1851 that the first modern adoption statute worthy of the name was passed, and it was in the state of Massachusetts: "An Act to Provide for the Adoption of Children." Adoptions were, however, taking place with regularity in Texas, Louisiana, and other localities long before 1851. Although most law in the United States is based on British common law, the United States was the pioneer in modern adoption. When the English passed their first adoption laws in 1926, they based them on U.S. adoption laws, specifically New York adoption laws.

Prior to the Massachusetts adoption statute, no judicial review or court appearance was required to adopt a child. As a result, it was considered to be the first modern adoption law that formally (and, by today's standards, very minimally) took into account the interests of the child. It is interesting to note that the adoption statute in Massachusetts was barely noticed by the press, and few, if any, people envisioned the impact of this statute on other states or noted that Massachusetts was a pacesetter in adoption law.

The institution of adoption cannot be fully discussed without also providing a brief historical overview of the institutions of foster care, or "placing out," as well as the institution of the group home, also known as the almshouse, "poor house," and orphanage.

To date, the argument continues, not just in the United States but worldwide, as to whether institutional care or foster care is preferable for children who cannot remain with their birthparents and who need temporary care. This essay will also include a brief overview of these institutions.

Orphaned Children and Adoption in the United States

Informal adoptions were the norm in the colonial days of early America, long before the passage of the Massachusetts law.

Governor Sir William Phips of Massachusetts was allegedly the first recorded adoptive father in the original thirteen colonies. He adopted a child in 1693. The word *adoption* appeared in Governor Phips's will, as well as in the act of the colonial legislature that allowed for the legal name change of the son.

In fact, it was fairly common for colonial legislatures to pass special bills recognizing the adoption of a child. Some historians have hypothesized that legislators became weary of passing so many bills for individual cases, bills that increased to such a great extent they bottlenecked other legislation. As a result, the legislators may have eased their legislative load by legalizing what was already common.

Laws prior to the 1851 Massachusetts adoption law, for example, in Texas (1850) and Mississippi (1846), have not been considered adoption laws by experts because such laws simply enabled individuals to leave their estates to nonrelatives in a similar manner in which property deeds were registered.

The groundwork for a philosophy favoring adoption had been laid well ahead of this time by Thomas Jefferson, who detested the concept of primogeniture and dedicated time during his early political career as a member of the Virginia House of Delegates to eliminate primogeniture in Virginia, ultimately succeeding in 1783. It is interesting to note that some British parents, still shackled by the bonds of primogeniture, sent their second or later-born sons to Virginia subsequent to Virginia's lifting of primogeniture.

Another status granted to children during the colonial era of the United States was that of godchild, and often the godchild did assume the name of the godparent. In addition, godchildren frequently inherited from godparents, although such an inheritance had to be stipulated in the will of the godparent.

According to Kawashima, one man left his estate to his wife and ordered that after her death the property would be left to a goddaughter, "except for one cow, which was given to the other goddaughter."

In his 1694 will, New Yorker William Moncom bequeathed half his property to his godson, and the other half was divided among his three children.

Some colonists informally fostered orphaned children, treating them as adopted children. These early "foster families" frequently developed great affection for the children, and in some cases, the children inherited property when the "master" died; for example, as early as 1769, William Russell of Georgia provided a dowry of 300 pounds to Anna Hunter, a child who resided with him, to be paid "on the day of her marriage or when she became of age."

Another key problem of the period was that illegitimacy was seen as evil and a shocking rip in the fabric of socially acceptable behavior and norms. Many people believed that if they solved the problem of the out-of-wedlock mother and child by arranging for another family to raise the child, they were condoning her "sin" and "making it easy" for her. Instead, it was believed she should be forced to raise her child, whether she wanted to or not, an opinion that continues to be held by some individuals today.

The effect on the child of pressuring the mother into parenting (or seeing the child reside in an orphanage and contributing money toward the child's support) was not of concern to society at large because the child was illegitimate and many people presumed the child was probably "bad," too. The severe shunning that Hester Prynne faced in the book *The Scarlet Letter* gives an idea of the prevalent view toward women who bore children out of wedlock and their children.

In later years, states began to create laws requiring investigations of the prospective adoptive parents. Michigan's 1891 statute was the first to order such an investigation (the precursor to today's home study) to further protect the child.

However, it should be noted that child protection laws were not passed until many years after the adoption statutes of Massachusetts and other states were legislated. It was not until an incident occurred in 1874 in New York City, in which Mary Ellen Wilson was severely beaten and abused by her parents, that any type of formal action was taken to protect children.

Outraged neighbors were unable to convince anyone to intervene to help Mary Ellen. Finally, the New York Society for the Prevention of Cruelty to Animals intervened to protect children, and the New York Society for the Prevention of Cruelty to Children, the first organization in the world to pro-tect children from abuse, was subsequently formed in 1874.

The Rise and Fall of the Almshouse

In the 19th and early 20th centuries, not only unwed parents but poor people in general were often regarded with disdain and contempt. "Outdoor relief" was the early precursor to today's Temporary Aid to Needy Families (TANF) and referred to cash or items such as food that were given to people who remained in their home rather than residing in an institution. Such relief was administered by the town or county in most cases; for example, the towns generally administered outdoor relief in New England, and the system of overseers was first introduced in Boston in 1691. In other areas of the country, the county managed outdoor relief.

In addition to almshouses or outdoor relief, there were also two other methods of dealing with the poor: one was literally selling the poor, and the other was selling their labor. According to historian Michael B. Katz, the labor of the individual was literally auctioned off to the highest bidder in a form of slavery of the poor. Understandably, many people considered such practices to be unfair and inhumane. Children were also routinely apprenticed or indentured to families, some of whom were kind, some of whom were not.

There were also numerous problems of settlement (determining which town or city was financially responsible for poor individuals) in the 19th century and early 20th century. Sometimes overseers of the poor actually transported poverty-stricken individuals to other towns to avoid a financial liability.

Some social reformers believed outdoor relief was bad for the character of the individual and could ultimately encourage a class of individuals dependent on public welfare. In addition, outdoor relief was perceived as bad for children, the mentally ill, and other categories of helpless individuals. Outdoor relief has always cost much less than institutionalization; however, social reformers believed that almshouses and later other institutions, such as orphanages, would be far better for the individuals as well as for society.

As a result, the rise of the almshouse (poorhouse) began in the mid-18th century. Yet although the almshouse was seen as the ultimate answer for indigent people by social reformers of the day, outdoor relief continued on throughout the almshouse era; for example, at the height of the almshouse era in 1880, there were an estimated 89,909 individuals residing in almshouses in New York, contrasted to 70,667 individuals receiving outdoor relief.

Supporters of almshouses stated that individuals would no longer be auctioned off nor would they receive outdoor relief and be allowed to be indolent. The settlement problem would be solved because the institutions would be county-run. It was also believed the almshouse would be a place where better character would be ingrained and where individuals would not wish to stay too long.

The almshouse social experiment, initially running an almost parallel course in England, was not the ideal solution envisioned by early social reformers such as Josiah Quincy, author of the Quincy Report in 1821, or by Douglas Yates, author of the Yates Report of 1824. Many children suffered greatly, and too many died.

Infants were particularly at risk, primarily because they had to be breast-fed before the advent of safe formulas for infants. Wet nurses sometimes were used to breast-feed babies, although this solution was often unsatisfactory, due to unsanitary conditions and other problems.

According to author Homer Folks, 514 infants were nursed in a New York City almshouse in 1849, and of these, 280 died. "Boarding out" of infants with foster parents was begun again in 1871. (It had previously been a policy, then was discontinued.) Said Folks, "It was so successful in reducing the death rate that in 1900 and 1901 it was extended to include all foundlings coming directly under the care of New York."

When the child was weaned from the breast, he or she was usually returned to the almshouse, despite any affection and love that may have developed between the foster mother and the child.

Although the goal of those who recommended almshouses was the creation and maintenance of clean and safe facilities, almshouses were far more often crowded and disease-ridden institutions, rampant with dangerous and then-fatal diseases such as cholera or pneumonia as well as numerous chronic diseases. Nor were they safe: some almshouses housed juvenile delinquents and seriously mentally ill individuals (and the indigent elderly) in the same facility that held the children of paupers.

The children were often not educated, nor were they sent to public schools because of the fear they would spread contagious diseases to the other children. As a result, they could neither read nor write nor were they trained for any trade, perpetuating the horrors of poverty into their adulthood.

Concerned citizens and child advocates became vocally opposed to almshouses in the mid-1800s when a variety of reports were written condemning almshouses. In 1856, a state Senate committee in New York issued a denunciation of the almshouse system. In 1857, commissioners of the poor in Charleston, South Carolina, described dismal conditions at an almshouse, which was "swarming with vermin." In addition, although almshouses had been perceived as a means to encourage idle individuals to work, often people living in almshouses could not find employment, either because of youth or infirmity or because of a lack of available jobs.

As a result, although the almshouses had initially been created because of concerned citizens' strong convictions that they would be far preferable to outdoor relief, the reality did not resemble the dream.

Finally, by the end of the 1800s, many almshouses were no longer operating, and children who could not remain with their parents were instead housed in orphanages or placed with foster families. Institutions were created to care for the mentally ill, aged, and juvenile offenders, thus separating the many categories of the poor that had formerly been housed together.

Several states led a movement away from almshouses and toward placing children in orphanages or with families; for example, in 1883, Ohio passed a law banning children over age three in almshouses, unless they were separated from indigent adults. Ohio dropped the age limit allowed in almshouses to one year in 1898.

According to the 1880 census, there were 7,770 children in almshouses throughout the United

States. Author Homer Folks estimated the number to have declined to about 5,000 by 1890.

It is important to note that some prominent politicians and child welfare experts today are calling for a return to orphanages to care for the increasing numbers of abandoned, neglected, or abused infants and children born to drug-addicted mothers. Proponents of modern-day orphanages insist that such facilities are not or would not be Dickensian scourges but instead would be clean and safe homes. Of course, it could also be argued that 19th-century orphanage advocates clearly envisioned clean and safe facilities and did not wish for children to suffer from a lack of bonding to parental figures or from a failure to thrive.

In the 19th century and early 20th century, orphaned children or the children of poverty-stricken parents were often "put out" or apprenticed, often to childless couples.

If a family died and there were no living relatives or persons named in a will who would care for the child, then the court was required to bind them out to a responsible person.

Children who were indentured did not usually assume the name of the masters nor were they given any legal rights or inheritance rights. In addition, the responsibility of the master usually ended when the child reached adulthood and was given $50, a Bible, and two suits of clothes. Children were not legally protected from abuse or overwork at the hands of the master, either.

Indenture was later decried by many as a form of slavery, although this practice persisted for some years even after the abolition of slavery.

The indenture system ultimately fell out of favor by the early 1900s, at about the same time that society decided against housing children and adults together in almshouses. Wrote Homer Folks, "The bound child has often been alluded to as typifying loneliness, neglect, overwork, and a consciousness of being held in low esteem."

Placing Out: The Orphan Train

Experts estimate over 10,000 homeless children roamed the streets of New York City in the mid-1800s, living on the ill-gotten gains from crimes they committed. Police reports in New York City in 1852 revealed that in 11 wards, 2,000 homeless girls ages eight to 16 were arrested for theft. Things only got worse: According to author Francis Lane in his 1932 doctoral dissertation for the Catholic University of America in Washington, D.C., there were 5,880 commitments of female children for vagrancy in 1860.

Part of the problem was that there was almost no need for "honest labor" of children in the large cities, which was why the children had turned to dishonest labor. (This was prior to the child labor movement, and at this time, everyone worked.) Large numbers of immigrants streamed into the major cities of the Northeast, such as New York City, between 1847 and 1860.

There was insufficient demand for the labor of this huge influx of adults, let alone children. At the same time, the midwestern and western farmers suffered a severe labor shortage.

Social reformers such as Charles Loring Brace, founder of the New York Children's Aid Society, saw almshouses and indenture as the problem, not the solution, and Brace initiated the Orphan Train movement in the mid-1850s. Brace believed that sending children to distant families would solve two problems: the family's desire for a child and the child's need for a family.

An estimated 150,000 children from the Northeast traveled to the Midwest, West, and South to foster or adoptive homes from 1854 until the movement ended in about 1929, when the Great Depression hit the entire United States very hard, especially farmers. (Some of these children were not placed by the New York Children's Aid Society, Brace's organization, but were actually indentured by other agencies.)

From 1854 to 1929, these homeless children were placed on trains and taken to rural sites concentrated in the Midwest and West in search of rural homes where the children could live and work. The children ranged from as young as about one year old to age 16 or 17.

Limited follow-ups of the children revealed that then, as now, the children who adapted the most readily were usually the younger children, and the older teenagers faced the greatest difficulty in adjusting to a radically different environment.

Most of the children were poor, and some had been involved in minor or serious infractions of the law. Many also had siblings and were separated from them for life as a result of the move. Yet most of the children (including two later governors—Andrew Burke of North Dakota and John Brady of the Alaska Territory—and other prominent citizens) made successful new lives for themselves, leaving behind them severe poverty and desolation.

Brace was initially supported in his movement by organizations within the Catholic Church and other groups. The Sisters of Charity of St. Vincent de Paul and the New York Foundling Hospital, for example, were both actively involved in the Orphan Train movement. The movement was also known as the "Placing Out" program and preceded adoption as we know it today. (It is unknown how many of the children received de facto family membership.)

The children left the train at each stop and were chosen or not chosen by people who came to the station to see them. The children were "put up" on platforms for all to see, which is supposedly the source of the phrase "put up for adoption."

Critics questioned whether all the homeless children Brace sent off on the orphan trains were really without parents or relatives and challenged whether or not sufficient checking and safeguards were made of parental rights. Notice to birthparents was not required, and consequently, there were parents who might (and did) object to their children being "placed out."

In addition, most of the homeless children were from Jewish or Catholic immigrant parents, yet large numbers were placed by Brace in Protestant homes. Laws were subsequently created in many states, including New York, that mandated or strongly suggested religious matching, so that children of Catholic parents would be placed only with Catholic adoptive parents, Jews with Jews and so forth.

Critics also said Brace made insufficient investigations of the foster or adoptive homes and little follow-up or documentation. In Brace's defense, communications and transportation systems of his era had little resemblance to our society today: he could not just pick up the phone and contact someone in the Midwest nor could he send or receive fax messages or e-mail.

Modern Adoption

Adoption in the early 20th century was very different from adoption in the United States in the 21st century. Most adoptions were still informal rather than legal, and adoption agencies did not become prominent until after World War II. Indeed, the first professional conference on adoption was held by the Child Welfare League of America in 1955. (The Child Welfare League of America was formed in 1921 and was first led by C. C. Carstens, former director of the Massachusetts Society for the Prevention of Cruelty to Children.)

Many would-be adoptive parents could see no benefit to a legal adoption other than to provide for an inheritance, and there were no state or federal legal requirements to adopt or formally foster a child whom they were rearing. Children needing parents were primarily cared for through orphanages ("orphan asylums") or by foster parents.

Confidentiality of the identities of the birthparents and adoptive parents was not commonly practiced, babies and children were bought and sold, and the whole concept of adoption was questioned by many as to whether or not it served a social good. Unwed mothers routinely advertised their children for sale in newspapers, and there was little or no protection for the children.

The economic climate of the early 1930s must also be taken into account: the Great Depression had forcibly ejected numerous people from their only means of livelihood, and poverty was rampant.

Society at large continued to view children born out of wedlock as liabilities, and the word *illegitimate* was often placed on birth certificates. The phrase *strangers of the blood* was used commonly to connote children raised by other than their biological parents or to connote the people who reared them. The word *bastard* was a value-laden insult against children born to unwed parents and was used with great effect.

Sometimes the birth certificate of a person born out of wedlock was a different color. Social reformers such as Edna Gladney of Texas believed labeling children from birth as "illegitimate" was a form of name-calling that was horrendously unfair to innocent children, often haunting them for life. She successfully fought to have references to illegitimacy removed from birth certificates in Texas in 1933. Said Edna Gladney in 1933, "There is no such thing as an illegitimate child. There are only illegitimate parents."

Unaware that moral values are received by children via parenting, child welfare experts and prospective parents worried a great deal about eugenics and genetics and whether or not the "illegitimate" child would or could ever turn out to be all right.

Still, lawful adoptions did occur and were sanctioned by the state in which the adoptive parents resided. Some states required a social investigation of the adopting parents, but many did not. Many adoptions were arranged by the parties themselves (birthparents and adopting parents); others were arranged by physicians, attorneys, and other intermediaries.

According to a 1927 analysis by Boston researcher Ida Parker of 810 adoptions, about two-thirds of the adoptions in Massachusetts had not been arranged by agencies but were instead independent adoptions.

When adopted, infants were not placed immediately in adoptive homes but were held back for months, primarily because society at large believed it was important to ensure they were not "defective children." At this time, children born out of wedlock were still regarded as potentially abnormal and hence the great caution.

In addition, many individuals continued to believe that women should care for their infants, whether they wanted to or not. Five states, Maryland, Minnesota, North Carolina, Ohio, and South Carolina, actually passed laws requiring birthmothers to parent their infants for a minimum of three to six months.

Another change was the institution of confidential adoptions. States began to pass laws requiring the sealing of the birth certificates of adopted children in the 1930s. The basis of the emphasis on confidentiality or anonymity and privacy was not only to protect the privacy rights of the adopted child, birthmother, and adoptive family from the prying and curious eyes of outsiders but also to stress that the adoptive family would completely assume the parental rights and obligations in regard to the child. In World War II, a heightened interest in confidentiality resulted from the need for married women who were pregnant outside their marriage to be able to be guaranteed privacy. The U.S. Children's Bureau at that time saw this confidentiality as part of their role as feminists.

An element of protection for the security of the family is inherent in these laws as well in that the birthparents might intrude or make later monetary or other demands on the adoptive parents or the adopted child if their identities were known.

The majority of states have retained confidentiality in adoptions today, although some groups actively seek to open all identifying adoption information. These groups, most notably the Adoptees' Liberty Movement Association (ALMA), state that the rights of the adopted adult should be of primary concern. This group believes an adopted adult's desire for information from the original birth record should take precedence over a birthparent's desire to withhold such information or to retain his or her privacy. They do not, however, believe a birthparent has a corresponding automatic right to the new amended birth record with identifying information about the adoptive parents and adopted child.

A variety of important social reforms occurred in the 1930s. By 1913, 20 states had passed laws authorizing pensions for indigent women, primarily widows. Historian Michael Katz says these laws were used as a basis for the Aid to Dependent Children portion of the 1935 Economic Security Act, itself a basis for today's Temporary Aid to Needy Families (TANF).

Child labor laws were passed, limiting the use of children in the factories. Interestingly enough, the removal of children from the workplace, along with theories of child psychology by popular psychologists such as G. Stanley Hall, led to an even greater enhancement of the value of the child. According to Katz, "A seismic shift in the perceived value of children underlay the new child psychology." As a result, by the late 1930s, adopting a child for his or her labor was no longer seen as a valid or acceptable motive. The shift to wanting to adopt a child because of a desire to become a loving parent had begun.

Starting in about the 1950s, society began to accept and broadly sanction the idea of adopting infants, and infant adoptions flourished until the 1970s. In 1951, an estimated 70 percent of the children adopted in 21 states were under the age of one year. Unwed mothers were urged or pressured to choose adoption over single parenthood.

Prospective adoptive parents did not need to wait many years before being able to adopt infants, and the system appeared to be in approximate equilibrium insofar as the number of infants needing families and the number of couples desiring to adopt infants was roughly equivalent.

From about the 1950s to the 1970s, most adoption agencies and adoption intermediaries, such as attorneys or physicians, concentrated on placing healthy white infants with adoptive families. The number of nonrelative adoptions increased from about 33,800 nationwide in 1951 to 89,200 in 1970.

During this period, there still existed strong social disapproval of premarital or extramarital sex and out-of-wedlock pregnancies. Unmarried pregnant women were often expected to keep the impending birth a secret and either wait out their pregnancies at a maternity home or visit a "sick aunt" until the child was born. Illegitimacy was a stigma and a problem: there was even a National Council on Illegitimacy.

It should be mentioned that, in all these changes and activities, primary concern by society overall centered on white people, and few provisions were made for black orphans and orphans of other racial or ethnic minorities until the late 19th century. These minorities usually raised such children within the extended family or community, and children born out of wedlock were not as stigmatized in their social groups.

However, the Colonial Orphan Asylum, founded in 1836, was the first orphanage for black children and the predecessor of the Harlem-Dowling children's service agency in New York City, which still exists today.

Authors Patricia Turner-Hogan and Sau-Fong Siu said some black children were placed in almshouses and were indentured; however, the social welfare available to poor black children was limited and often even more harshly administered than the dismal situation faced by the white children of the time.

Black children were generally excluded from the mainstream charities as part of a general pattern of racial discrimination, a pattern that persisted until the landmark U.S. Supreme Court decision of *Brown v. Board of Education* in 1954. As a result, blacks began to develop their own child welfare. Not until the 1960s and the civil rights movement did blacks become prominent in child welfare services. To this date, black children are overrepresented in foster care, and they are often the last to be adopted.

Some blacks continue to believe the child welfare system is not sufficiently responsive to the needs of blacks and other minority children and adults.

There is also great controversy and debate today over whether or not whites should be allowed to adopt black or biracial children in transracial adoptions. Opponents argue that insufficient efforts are made to recruit African-American adoptive parents. Supporters of transracial adoptions contend that carefully screened white parents are far superior to long-term (and often a succession of several) foster care arrangements for black and biracial children. Assisted by advocates and researchers such as Elizabeth Bartholet, Senator Metzenbaum made a historic breakthrough with his legislation banning racial discrimination in adoption—the Multiethnic Placement Act.

In the 1970s, the emphasis on adoption began to shift again as social reformers became very alarmed at the burgeoning numbers of children living in private or group foster homes, usually for their entire childhoods. Policymakers became concerned about the rising costs of maintaining thousands of children in foster homes. Studies indicate as many as 500,000 children were living in publicly supported foster homes in 1975.

Some studies revealed that many foster children went in and out of numerous placements, and researchers concluded this instability was very bad for children. There was also an apparent unwitting federal disincentive to place children in adoptive families. If the children remained in foster care, their foster families would receive monthly payments, the child would remain eligible for Medicaid, and the state would also receive federal funds. If the child was adopted, the adoptive family would usually become fully responsible for all costs associated with the child, and Medicaid benefits would end. (Some states, such as New York, offered their own state subsidy to adoptive parents.) Congress also passed legislation giving tax credits to adoptive parents.

Social workers, foster parents, and others made a call for what came to be known in the 1980s as "permanency": to either return the children to their original families ("reunification") or, if that was not possible, to sever parental rights so the child could be adopted. (Other alternatives included placing the child in a group home or institution or allowing the child to remain in foster care.)

The culmination of this concern was the Adoption Assistance and Child Welfare Act of 1980, a federal law that mandates a judicial review of the status of a foster child after 18 months in foster care.

Child advocates later charged that, because of indifference on the part of the Department of Health and Human Services and Congress, the law was not monitored adequately or properly enforced. One result to this inadequacy was the passage of the Adoption and Safe Families Act of 1997.

Still, the 1980 act did result in the adoption of many children who would not otherwise have been adopted, and it is hoped that many more families will be identified for the children who still wait for families and that such children can be pried loose from the bureaucratic quagmires where they are entrapped.

Another impetus to the adoption of children with special needs has been the continuance of Medicaid coverage in some cases. (Children placed through public agencies are the primary beneficiaries.) Adoption subsidies have also been created to provide monthly payments for some families who adopt some children with special needs, again, mostly children from public agencies. These legislative and legal actions were taken to encourage the adoption of foster children.

The concept that an older child could be successfully adopted and thrive in an adoptive family was a novel idea to many social workers and most of the general public in the late 1970s and early 1980s. (The emphasis and successful experience of child welfare experts in the early 20th century with the adoption of older children had been ignored or forgotten by most.)

It should be noted that, as more children are adopted at an older age, it is possible that increasing numbers of these children and their families will need some help with child or family adjustment. Whether the children will exhibit behavior problems because they were adopted or because of damage that occurred prior to the adoption is a matter of intense debate and a likely subject for further study.

Another development was the change in contraceptive use and effectiveness, particularly the variety of contraceptive choices and especially the increased use of the birth control pill, which enabled women to have more control in avoiding pregnancies.

It became increasingly acceptable for single women and even young girls to engage in premarital sexual intercourse with the result that some number of them would become pregnant, bear, and rear children.

This change in attitude became so pervasive in society that whereas adoption was earlier considered the presumed solution for a pregnant single woman, many individuals in the 1970s and to date began to believe that single parenting was a far preferable answer to adoption for both the mother and her child.

Yet some women continue to choose to adopt children from the United States and other countries. Most adoption agencies today pride themselves on seeking families for children more than on finding children for prospective parents. It must also be noted, however, that adoption agencies arrange an estimated half of all infant adoptions of children born in the United States today while the remaining 50 percent of infant adoptions are arranged or facilitated by private intermediaries.

Home studies (also known as parent preparation or preadoptive counseling) of adopting parents are always required prior to any adoptive placement, while home studies may not be initiated until after placement of the child in an independent arrangement. States license agencies to make adoptive placements, and agencies in turn are responsible to society for their work. In some states, private, licensed social workers may do the home study.

In addition, counseling of the adopting parents and birthparents occurs with far more frequency in agency adoptions than in independent adoptions, which leads to the primary criticism leveled by agency practitioners against independent adoptions. There appear to be an increasing number of independent intermediaries today who require or urge counseling prior to an adoptive placement, both in response to this criticism and also out of a desire to do better adoption work.

One change that has taken place over the past decade is that many professionals have begun to argue that "open adoptions" (disclosure of the identities of birthparents and adoptive parents to each other) should be standard practice. Supporters of open adoptions frequently cite adoptions that occurred in the early 20th century and prior to the institution of confidentiality, sealing of birth records, and so forth.

Some professionals believe open adoptions are more "humane" for adoption triad members, arguing, for example, that adults who seek to locate their birthparents will not have difficulty when the adoptions are open because they will know the identity of their birthparents.

Other professionals have responded to competitive pressures from lawyers and other adoption intermediaries who offer open adoptions and have begun to offer open adoptions or "semi-open" adoptions. Most adoption agencies and intermediaries continue to arrange adoptions with choices, such as the birthmother choosing the religion of the adopting couple, with the majority retaining the confidentiality aspect. (Open adoption is discussed at greater length within the text of this book.)

In addition, most agencies seek genetic and medical information from birthparents so this information can be provided to adopting parents who need this information to provide optimal appropriate care for the child and to help the child attain his or her full potential. Upon reaching adulthood, the adoptive parents will pass on the information to the adopted person, who can then plan for necessary preventive and other medical care for himself or herself and any offspring.

Another change that has taken place is in the area of birthfathers' rights. Prior to *Stanley v. Illinois* in 1972, no consideration was given to the desires of a birthfather not married to a child's birthmother. If the birthmother chose adoption for "her" child, then the adoption could go forth.

After the *Stanley* decision and several other subsequent U.S. Supreme Court decisions, states passed a variety of laws designed to protect the paternal rights of the birthfather. Today, a crazy quilt of laws nationwide provide for what actions, if any, must be taken by the state to obtain consent from the birthfather.

The sometimes overlapping and conflicting rights of the adoptive parents, birthparents, adopted person, and relatives will undoubtedly continue to be debated, legislated, and fought in court battles nationwide as states and the federal government struggle to achieve an equitable balance for all parties.

Changes and Trends through the Twenty-first Century

Adoption is an evolving institution and one which, it is hoped, fits the needs of the children who need families, whether they are infants or older children and whether they are children from orphanages in other countries, foster care in the United States, or are in the hospital just days after birth. Past trends included a movement toward more open adoptions as well as more information provided to birthparents about adoptive parents in domestic adoptions.

Early in the 21st century, several emerging trends seem evident, including an increased emphasis on adoption as one good option for many children in the foster care system in the United States; a continued and very high interest in the adoption of children from other countries; and a trend toward states providing more information for adopted adults who seek identifying information and/or an original birth certificate so that they can search for their birthparents. In addition, some states provide identifying information to birthparents and sometimes to birth siblings.

A further trend is that, much more so than in past years, people interested in adoption actively use the Internet. Prospective adoptive parents use the Internet to locate information on how to adopt as well as on how to rear children they have adopted, and they seek information on how to resolve any problems that may arise. They use the Internet to communicate with other adoptive parents, who recommend magazine articles to read, sometimes providing links to the actual articles, as well as recommending books to read. Adopted adults and birthparents use the Internet to help them access information that will simplify their search and also find others who are facing the same struggles and concerns as they are experiencing. The Internet can be a very positive tool, such as its use to help agencies recruit families for waiting children, although sometimes the Internet is misused or abused.

The Adoption of Children in Foster Care

With the passage of the Adoption and Safe Families Act (ASFA) in 1997 and the subsequent implementation of its provisions, the primary emphasis in protective services shifted to what the *child* needed, rather than on what the abusive or neglectful parent wanted or needed. In recent past years, many children entered the foster care system as infants or toddlers and remained "in the system"—or they entered and left in a revolving door fashion—until they reached the age of 18. Since ASFA was passed, the number of children adopted from foster care has nearly doubled to about 50,000 children a year.

Federal requirements based on ASFA mandate child protection services either to release children back to their parents, place them with relatives, or terminate parental rights within a reasonable period. This requirement to promote adoption has caused states to change their own laws and also to actively seek out adoptive parents. It is shocking and probably unbelievable, but in past years, even when a parent severely abused a child or caused a child's death or the death of a child's other parent, sometimes social workers left other children in the home if the parent had not yet abused those particular children, because the law did not allow them to remove the other children unless they were directly abused. Today, states have provisions

to terminate parental rights in such circumstances. (See the entry on termination of parental rights as well as Appendix V for more information on state laws on termination of parental rights.)

In addition, in past years, women or girls who were raped or suffered incest and, as a result, conceived a child, sometimes had to get permission from the rapist to place the baby for adoption. In some cases, the rapist refused permission and actively blocked the adoption. Many states now have laws that automatically terminate the parental rights of the father in these circumstances, such that the mother, if she continues the pregnancy, can choose adoption if she wishes.

In the past, judges, social workers, and other professionals who decided the fate of abused and neglected children felt very sympathetic to the children's parents who were alcoholics, drug addicts, mentally ill, or had other problems that led to the abuse or neglect of the child. These individuals felt that the parents should not be punished for the huge problems with which they struggled, and they were extremely reluctant to terminate parental rights because of the emphasis on the "blood ties" of the parent to the child. The concept of "family preservation" guided many decisions about the placement of the child. Ultimately, however, the law was changed at the federal level because of a growing realization that the people who were truly being punished by the failure to sever parental rights were the children. Children who remained in these difficult environments often grew up to exhibit the same problems as their parents.

At long last, adoption is now perceived as a viable alternative for children whose parents will not or cannot resolve their problems within several years.

Although the change to the law and the paradigm shift to adoption was a positive one for children, insufficient numbers of Americans seek to adopt foster children and insufficient numbers serve as foster parents. This continues to be a problem. Prospective adoptive parents may be fearful that most of the children in foster care are physically or mentally ill or developmentally delayed, although this is usually not the case. It is true that some foster children have suffered severe abuse or neglect in the past, but many children are resilient and can overcome their past painful histories. However, some children are less resilient. Parents who adopt foster children need to realize that problems may occur as the child grows up and sometimes adolescence can be a rocky road for the former foster child.

The Adoption of Children from Other Countries

Many people who wish to adopt have chosen to adopt children from other countries, in far greater numbers than in past years. For example, in 2005, 22,728 children from other countries were adopted by parents in the United States. The largest portion of this figure, nearly a third of all international adoptions, was children adopted from China, or 7,044 children, followed by 5,865 adopted from Russia. Since 1995 when a total of 8,987 children were adopted from all countries outside the United States, international adoptions have more than doubled.

As long as China, Russia, and other countries around the globe continue to allow adoptions, it is likely that this trend of international adoptions will continue, although the numbers of children who are adopted from other countries by Americans will probably plateau by 2010 or 2015. The youngest baby boomers, born in 1964, will age further, and the numbers who are seeking to adopt children—whether it is because they are infertile or they are humanitarians or a combination of both reasons—will eventually abate. Unfortunately, it is unlikely that the tens of thousands of children in orphanages worldwide will decrease. Perhaps some families will choose to adopt a second and a third child, but many will not. It is also possible that, as the numbers of adoptive parents decline, adoption fees may decrease, but it is too soon to predict this eventuality.

More Information for Adopted Adults Who Search for Birthparents

It is unclear how many adopted adults are actively searching for their birthparents, but it is apparent that searching is a popular activity among many.

Some adopted adults and birthparents have lobbied states to change their laws so that it will become easier for them to obtain identifying information about the other party. In general, the laws are more favorable toward adopted adults than toward birthparents.

In past years, nearly all states banned the release of adoption records and/or the sealed birth certificate of a person adopted in the United States, but some states have revised this position and provide increased opportunities for adopted adults to obtain information. For example, in 2004, New Hampshire passed a law which allowed for the release of the original birth certificate on the request of the adopted adult. Interestingly, some states, such as Montana and Nebraska, will provide identifying information to adopted adults if they are Native Americans who need the information to prove they are valid members of a tribe.

Other states, including Delaware, Hawaii, Indiana, Minnesota, Mississippi, Nebraska, Ohio, and Washington, have passed laws that allow adopted adults access to identifying information and/or the original birth certificate unless the birthparents have filed a specific request with the state that the information be withheld. Since most birthparents probably do not realize that they would need to take this action to prevent the release of information, or they may be reluctant to do so, then it seems likely more adopted adults will be able to access the information they seek.

Some states have passed laws that offer increased access to adopted individuals who are born after a certain date. For example, in Michigan, if the adoption was finalized before September 12, 1980, identifying information will only be released to adopted adults if both birthparents have consented in writing to the release. After that date, however, the identifying information will be provided automatically unless the birthparents have specifically denied consent. Other states have enacted similar laws that depend on when the adoption occurred, such as Montana, Ohio, Vermont, and Washington. This appears to be a trend.

Whether the actual reunion between the adopted adult and the birthparent will be a happy one is no certainty. Some adopted adults and birthparents report very positive experiences while others are more mixed, and in a few cases, the individuals do not develop a good rapport or do not even speak to each other. However, many adopted adults say that they would rather have a chance at obtaining the information, even at the risk of being rebuffed.

The Internet

The explosion of the use of the Internet has also meant an explosion of information on adoption, and many research studies and reports and even medical journal articles that were inaccessible in the past to the general public can now be read by adopted adults, adoptive parents, and birthparents as well as others. Information on state laws, ways to adopt children, and methods of searching are also readily available.

However, information obtained through the Internet can be a double-edged sword. On the one hand, it can be liberating to locate information quickly and may save the user considerable time and money. On the other hand, sometimes information on the Internet is either wrong or outdated. Worse, the Internet is increasingly used by some individuals to defraud others, whether their victims wish to adopt children, seek a birthparent, or obtain other types of information that relate to adoption.

Many individuals are far too willing to trust strangers with their private information such as their social security number, credit card number, or home address, letting down their guard because the other person promises them whatever it is that they most want. For this reason, we have added entries on fraud in adoption and on the Internet to this new edition of the book.

It is also important to note that some people seem to think that the Internet will provide all the answers that they need, so that they can feel confident in the choices they make. However, this is not necessarily true. For example, if a family is considering adopting a child, they may use the Internet to choose an excellent adoption agency, they may find a great deal of information about the circumstances of other children similar to the child they may adopt, and they may receive information about the particular child by e-mail.

Yet the Internet still cannot erase all uncertainty. The sickly and/or abused child may grow up healthy and strong while the hearty baby may develop serious problems later. Adoption has always been, and continues to be, a leap of faith for the adoptive parent (and adopted child and the birthparents), because what will happen may be predicted by others, but it cannot absolutely be known. There is no perfect set of information that can be attained and there are no guarantees.

What will be the next new or few trends on adoption, other than what are described here? It is hard to know. However, whatever changes to laws and whatever trends may occur, when there is a choice about what to do, several key points should always be sincerely considered: Will this change help children now? Is it likely to help them to grow up to be healthy adults, or at least, healthier than they might otherwise be? And also, does this seem to be the best solution for many children or for an individual child?

In the past, orphanages and then the Orphan Train were considered the best answer to these questions, and more recently, international adoption and the adoption of foster children are modern answers. As long as we keep asking the questions, and the answers are at least a qualified "yes," then we may make some mistakes, but we are also much more likely to be on the right track.

Ben-Or, Joseph. "The Law of Adoption in the United States: Its Massachusetts Origins and the Statute of 1851," *New England History & Genealogical Registry* 130 (1976): 259–272.

Bohman, Michael, and Soren Sigvardsson. "Outcome in Adoption: Lessons from Longitudinal Studies," in *The Psychology of Adoption.* New York: Oxford University Press, 1990.

Boswell, John. *The Kindness of Strangers: The Abandonment of Children in Western Europe from Late Antiquity to the Renaissance.* New York: Pantheon Books, 1988.

Brace, C. L. *The Best Method of Disposing of Our Pauper and Vagrant Children.* New York: Wynkoop, Hallenbeck & Thomas, 1859.

Brosnan, John Francis. "The Law of Adoption," *Columbia Law Review* 22 (1922): 322–335.

Carp, E. Wayne. *Family Matters: Secrecy and Disclosure in the History of Adoption.* Cambridge, Mass.: Harvard University Press, 1998.

———. *Adoption in America: Historical Perspectives.* Ann Arbor: University of Michigan Press, 2004.

Cole, Elizabeth S., and Kathryn S. Donley. "History, Values, and Placement Policy Issues in Adoption," in *The Psychology of Adoption*. New York: Oxford University Press, 1990.

Costin, Lela B. "The Historical Context of Child Welfare," in *A Handbook of Child Welfare: Context, Knowledge, and Practice*. New York: Free Press, 1985.

Dewar, Diana. *Orphans of the Living: A Study of Bastardy*. London: Hutchinson, 1968.

Folks, Homer. *The Care of Destitute, Neglected, and Delinquent Children*. New York: Macmillan, 1902.

Howe, Ruth-Arlene W. "Adoption Practice, Issues, and Laws," *Family Law Quarterly* 17 (Summer 1983): 173–197.

Huard, Leo Albert. "The Law of Adoption: Ancient and Modern," *Vanderbilt Law Review* 9 (1956): 743–763.

Katz, Michael B. *In the Shadow of the Poorhouse: A Social History of Welfare in America*. New York: Basic Books, 1986.

Kawashima, Yasuhide. "Adoption in Early America," *Journal of Family Law* 20, no. 4 (August 1982): 677–696.

Lane, Francis E. *American Charities and the Child of the Immigrant*. New York: Arno Press, 1974.

McCauliff, C. M. A. "The First English Adoption Law and Its American Precursors," *Seton Hall Law Review* 16 (Summer/Fall 1986): 656–677.

Parker, Ida R. *"Fit and Proper"?: A Study of Legal Adoption in Massachusetts*. Boston: Church Home Society, 1927.

Pelton, Leroy. "The Institution of Adoption: Its Sources and Perpetuation," in *Infertility and Adoption: A Guide for Social Work Practice*. New York: Haworth Press, 1988.

Piester, Ruby Lee. *For The Love of a Child*. Austin, Tex.: Eakin Press, 1987.

Rothman, David J., and Sheila M. Rothman, eds. *The Origins of Adoption*. New York: Garland Publishing, 1987.

Turner-Hogan, Patricia, and Sau-Fong Siu. "Minority Children and the Child Welfare System: An Historical Perspective," *Social Work* 33 (November–December 1988): 493–498.

Wheeler, Leslie. "The Orphan Trains," *American History Illustrated* 18 (December 1983): 12–23.

Zainaldin, Jamil S. "The Emergence of a Modern American Family Law: Child Custody, Adoption, and the Courts, 1796–1851," *Northwestern University Law Review* 73, no. 6 (1979): 1,038–1,045.

ENTRIES A–Z

abandonment   The desertion of an infant or a child by a parent, or other adult with legal custody of the child, who has made no provisions for reasonable child care or has no apparent intention to return and resume care of the child. Abandonment is a form of child NEGLECT. A child may be considered abandoned if left alone or with siblings who are minors or with nonrelated and unsuitable individuals.

Abandonment can be more dangerous than physical abuse. If the abandoned child is an infant or small child who is unable to obtain food and/or shelter, and if the child's basic survival needs are not identified and then met, abandonment leads to serious health problems up to and including death.

Researchers who studied infants who were killed or left to die in North Carolina from 1985 to 2000 said, "The risk of homicide on the first day of life (neonaticide) is 10 times greater than the rate during any other time of life." According to the researchers, who reported on their findings in a 2003 issue of the *Journal of the American Medical Association,* 34 newborns were killed or abandoned in North Carolina by their parents, which was a rate of 2.1 per 100,000 newborns per year.

No one knows how many children in the United States are abandoned nationwide, although about 31,000 babies were abandoned in hospitals in 1998, according to the Administration for Children & Families.

Parental Reasons for Abandonment

In the United States, often the primary problem of the biological parent who abandoned a child is alcohol or drug abuse-related. Some abandoning parents have psychiatric disorders. Some of these parents may be aware that adoption is an option for their child but may not wish to identify themselves or deal with social workers or attorneys. Other parents know little or nothing about adoption.

Some people who abandon infants are teenagers fearful of their parents learning of the birth. Some research has indicated that a small number of abandoning parents are married women, based on limited data reported in the 2003 study of abandoned newborns in North Carolina, reported in the *Journal of the American Medical Association.*

Consequences to the Parent Who Commits Child Abandonment in the United States

In the United States, if the deserting parent does not return home or contact the child or if the parent fails to provide any support for the child for an extended period, the state may seek to terminate the individual's parental rights and place the child with an adoptive family. The parent may also be prosecuted, unless the abandonment was performed according to a state "safe haven" law as described below.

Before parental rights can be terminated, a social worker must prove to the court of appropriate jurisdiction that an abandonment has occurred. States vary on what proof is required before parental rights may be terminated. (See TERMINATION OF PARENTAL RIGHTS.) Under the provisions of the federal ADOPTION AND SAFE FAMILIES ACT, if neither parent and no relatives make a claim on the infant within the course of about a year after placement into a foster home, the court may opt to terminate the birthparents' parental rights so that the child may be adopted.

"Safe Haven" Laws on Infant Abandonment

Most states in the United States have passed laws that allow for the abandonment of newborn or young infants to particular facilities that operate around-the-clock, such as firehouses or hospital emergency rooms. These laws were passed in reaction to reports of women leaving their new-born infants to die in dumpsters and other unsafe locations. Texas was the first state to pass a safe haven law in 1999. States that have *not* passed such laws as of 2005 include Alaska, Hawaii, Nebraska, and Vermont.

State laws vary on the age of the baby who may be abandoned in this manner, and most states limit the law to newborns or babies up to 30 days old.

In these cases, the abandonment of the infant is not a criminal act and may be performed anonymously. One exception to this exclusion from anonymity and prosecution would be if the infant was abused prior to the abandonment.

Proponents of safe haven laws believe that these laws will save babies who would otherwise have lost their lives due to abandonment. However, others worry that when a child is abandoned, no background or genetic information is gathered, which is information that could be provided to adoptive parents. They also fear that safe haven laws make abandonment an option that would not otherwise have been chosen by the parent. In addition, they are concerned about the protection of fathers' rights, since most states do not have a provision addressing fathers' parental rights.

Supporters of the safe haven laws say that if a child dies from an abandonment that occurs outside of safe haven laws, then the genetic history and the fathers' rights are irrelevant, since there is no child. They also see safe haven laws as important for child protection. Further research is needed on the impact of these laws.

Older Children Who Are Abandoned

Infants are not the only children who are abandoned: children of all ages are abandoned by their parents. Older children are sometimes abandoned when the parent believes he or she cannot care or provide for the child or when the parent is overcome by personal problems, alcoholism, drug abuse, financial difficulties, or a combination of these problems.

Homeless families with children may attempt to live out of their cars or makeshift shelters. Such living arrangements may be considered to be neglect or, if the parent leaves the child alone in such circumstances for an extended period, abandonment. If a child abuse worker is notified, the children may be taken from the parents by a state or county social worker and placed in a certified state foster home until and unless the parents provide adequate shelter or their parental rights are terminated.

Child Abandonment in Other countries

Thousands of children in countries outside the United States are abandoned every year, usually by their mothers, and some of them are placed in ORPHANAGES. People from the United States and abroad adopt many children from other countries who need families, but despite this fact, large numbers of children continue to spend their entire childhoods in institutions until they are turned out to make room for younger homeless children.

Birthmothers from other countries who abandon their children do so primarily because of cultural factors or because they are destitute, powerless, or they are lacking in support and options and see no hope for a chance to parent their children. Drug or alcohol abuse may contribute to child abandonment, as in the United States. Birthmothers may or may not have other children. They may have been rejected by their parents or by the father of the baby. In eastern Europe, some birthmothers were themselves raised in orphanages after abandonment.

In some countries, such as China, many parents may be actively discouraged from having more than one child. If the first child is a female, parents may abandon the child in the hopes that their second child is male, since males hold a higher status than females in this culture. Often it is the second daughter in the family who is abandoned in China.

In some cases, the birthmother from another country may be legally prohibited from voluntarily signing a consent to adoption. Abandoning her child at an orphanage or hospital may be the only route that allows the child to be placed in an orphanage and hopefully later in an adoptive home. However, many birthmothers who cannot care for their children, particularly in eastern Europe, voluntarily and legally choose adoption rather than abandonment.

See also ABUSE.

Child Welfare League of America. "Baby Abandonment: Fact Sheet," http://www.cwla.org/programs/baby/faq. htm, downloaded on March 1, 2005.

Herman-Giddens, Marcia E., et al. "Newborns Killed or Left to Die by a Parent: A Population-Based Study," *Journal of the American Medical Association* 289, no. 11 (March 19, 2003): 1,425–1,429.

National Clearinghouse on Child Abuse and Neglect Information, National Adoption Information Clearinghouse. "Infant Safe Haven Laws: Summary of State Laws," Statutes Series 2004, http://naic.acf.hhs.gov/general/legal/statute/safehaven.pdf, downloaded on March 21, 2005.

abuse   Physical, sexual, or long-lasting emotional harm to a child. NEGLECT is also a form of child abuse, as is ABANDONMENT, which is a form of neglect. Abuse may cause severe injuries or even death, although many forms of abuse are more insidious and do not cause long-term injuries or fatalities. More children who are part of the foster care system in the United States have experienced neglect rather than physical abuse; however, many have suffered from both abuse and neglect.

Some parents have purposely withheld food from their children of all ages for long periods, to the point that they became malnourished and extremely undersized for their age, and in some cases, the children die of starvation and/or dehydration. One mother force-fed her child large quantities of salt because the child stole a few cookies. The toddler died of sodium overdose. Other parents have shaken an infant so violently that brain hemorrhage and death have resulted.

An estimated 1,500 children died of abuse or neglect in 2003 in the United States, according to the Administration for Children, Youth and Families in their annual report on child maltreatment. Most children who died (79 percent) were younger than four years old. Male infants under age one year had a higher fatality rate than girls, or 18 deaths per 1,000 for boys and 14 deaths per 1,000 among girls. Some children have died from neglect because they were too young to obtain food, shelter, or clothing for themselves without assistance from others and they were also too young or unable to ask others for help.

Considering Forms of Abuse

All forms of abuse and neglect are difficult for the child, but how they cope with their maltreatment in later life (if they are able to cope) varies depending on the child's age, level of RESILIENCE, and other factors, such as the presence of a positive parental figure in the child's early life.

Physical abuse   Physical abuse involves harm to a child, ranging from the harm caused by slapping the child to injuries that the child incurred from actual torture. Physical abuse may cause short-term or long-term harm to the child's body, depending on the nature of the abuse and the frequency, as well as the child's age. Each state has its own definition of physical abuse (as well as of sexual abuse, neglect, and other forms of abuse).

Sexual abuse   Sexual abuse can range from an individual inappropriately touching the child in the genital areas to forcing the child to touch another's genitals to compelling a child to engage in full sexual intercourse. Adults have attempted intercourse with children as young as tiny infants with dire results.

See also SEXUAL ABUSE, CHILDHOOD.

Emotional abuse   Emotional abuse can be difficult to define and varies according to state laws. In general, it refers to nonphysical actions that cause extreme stress to the child. Some examples of emotional abuse may include telling the child constantly that she is evil or no one wants her or she should die. Locking a child in a closet for several hours constitutes emotional abuse.

Neglect   Neglect is a form of child abuse. Neglectful parents may leave children alone for extended periods when they are very young or may otherwise fail to meet the normal needs of the child. For instance, a young child may be expected by the parent to supervise an infant—social workers report that children as young as two or three have been left alone to watch an infant sibling.

Medical neglect is another form of neglect and it refers to the parent or caregiver's failure to provide needed medical treatment for a sick child. In the most extreme case, medical neglect can lead to the child's death.

Abandonment   Abandonment, which is included under the category of neglect, refers to a parent or caretaker leaving a child alone for an extended period and with no apparent intention to return. Abandonment can be fatal to an infant or small child, with no means to care for themselves and no way to seek help from others.

Risk Factors for Infant Maltreatment

Babies in some circumstances face an increased risk of suffering from abuse and neglect. For example, a study of about 189,000 children in Florida in 1996 revealed five key factors causing infants to be at greatest risk of maltreatment. These factors included the following:

- The child has three or more siblings.
- The family or child receives Medicaid.
- The mother is unmarried.
- The baby was born with low birth weight.
- The mother smoked during her pregnancy.

According to the researchers, who reported their findings in a 2004 issue of *Child Abuse and Neglect,* mothers and babies with four (or all five) of these risk factors had maltreatment rates that were seven times greater than average for the population.

Federal and State Actions on Behalf of Abused Children

The initial key legislation affecting how states should deal with child abuse and neglect is the Child Abuse Prevention and Treatment Act (CAPTA), which was first enacted in 1974. CAPTA has gone through several amendments through the years, and the most recent amendment and reauthorization was the Keeping Children and Families Safe Act of 2003.

Under CAPTA, the federal government provides funds to states to investigate allegations of child abuse and it also funds research projects on topics related to abuse and neglect. The federal government funds the National Clearinghouse on Child Abuse and Neglect and established the Office on Child Abuse and Neglect.

Statistics on Child Abuse and Neglect

The federal Children's Bureau of the Administration on Children, Youth and Families collects and analyzes data on child abuse and neglect, amassed from the individual states. The National Child Abuse and Neglect Data System (NCANDS) is the reporting system of this statistical information. The first NCANDS report used data from 1990, and each year thereafter an annual report was released.

According to the annual report by NCANDS on child maltreatment, released in 2005 and based on children who were abused and neglected in 2003, about three million children in the United States were *reported* as victims. However, not all cases were substantiated. Of about 1.6 million investigations in 2003, about 420,000 cases were substantiated. The rate of substantiated victimization has declined somewhat in recent years, from 13.4 children per 1,000 in 1990 to 12.3 children per 1,000 in 2002.

Note: A lack of substantiation does not automatically mean that no abuse or neglect occurred. It may mean that the social worker was unable to confirm that abuse or neglect occurred, rather than that an allegation was unfounded.

Most children who were abused or neglected in 2003 experienced neglect (61 percent). About 19 percent of the children were physically abused and 10 percent were sexually abused. (Some states have additional categories of abuse and neglect.)

Age of child In the 2003 child maltreatment data from the federal government, infants and small children ages newborn to three years suffered the greatest rates of victimization of all ages, or 16.4 per 1,000 children.

Sex of victim Boys are slightly more likely to be abused than girls. However, when it comes to sexual abuse, the broad majority of reported victims are female.

Race and ethnicity The abuse rates for Pacific Islander (21.4 children per 1,000), American Indian or Alaska Native (21.3 per 1,000), and African-American children (20.4 per 1,000) were double the rate among Hispanic (9.9 per 1,000) and White children (11.0 per 1,000).

Perpetrators of abuse and neglect Parents represented most of the perpetrators of abuse and neglect in 2002, or 84 percent. In the case of children who were sexually abused only, however, parents were usually *not* the perpetrators, and they represented only 2.7 percent of the total.

In looking at gender alone and considering all forms of abuse and neglect, female perpetrators were responsible for about 58 percent of all abuse in 2003, compared to 42 percent committed by males.

Study on Foster Children in Care for One Year

Researchers on the National Survey of Child and Adolescent Well-Being Research Group performed a federal study on foster children and provided detailed information in 2003 based on their analysis of data on 727 children who remained in foster care 12 months after the initial sampling. The children

TYPE OF PAST ABUSE PRIOR TO PLACEMENT, IN FOSTER CHILDREN IN ONE YEAR IN FOSTER CARE (OYFC) STUDY

Type of Abuse/Neglect	Total Weighted Percentage
Physical	10
Sexual	8
Emotional	7
Neglect (failure to provide)	33
Neglect (failure to supervise)	27
Abandonment	7
Other	8

Source: Adapted from U.S. Department of Health and Human Services, Administration for Children, Youth and Families (November 2003). *National Survey of Child and Adolescent Well-Being: One Year in Foster Care Report.* Washington, D.C.

ranged in age from one year to older than 10 years (the oldest child was age 15), and they were about evenly split between females (49 percent) and males (51 percent).

Many children (41 percent) had experienced more than one form of past abuse, although 4 percent had not been abused. (Sometimes children are placed in foster care because of domestic violence situations between their parents or because of their own medical or mental health problems.) See the

TYPE OF ABUSE PRIOR TO PLACEMENT, BY AGE, IN PERCENT IN THE FOSTER CHILDREN IN ONE YEAR IN FOSTER CARE (OYFC) STUDY

Type of Abuse/Neglect	Age of Child				
	1–2	3–5	6–10	11+	Total
Physical	26	12	36	25	100
Sexual	2	15	45	39	100
Emotional	17	14	39	31	100
Neglect (failure to provide)	33	19	25	24	100
Neglect (failure to supervise)	18	20	38	24	100
Abandonment	18	16	31	35	100
Other	56	4	11	30	100

* Percentages are rounded.
Source: Adapted from U.S. Department of Health and Human Services, Administration for Children, Youth and Families (November 2003). *National Survey of Child and Adolescent Well-Being: One Year in Foster Care Report.* Washington, D.C.

MOST SERIOUS TYPES OF PAST ABUSE, RECORDED ABUSE CATEGORIES IN THE FOSTER CHILDREN IN ONE YEAR IN FOSTER CARE (OYFC) STUDY

Type of Abuse/Neglect	Percent
Physical	10
Sexual	8
Neglect (failure to provide)	36
Neglect (failure to supervise)	37
Other	9

Source: Adapted from U.S. Department of Health and Human Services, Administration for Children, Youth and Families (November 2003). *National Survey of Child and Adolescent Well-Being: One Year in Foster Care Report.* Washington, D.C.

tables for the number of main abuse types and the percentage of children who suffered.

The researchers considered the types of maltreatment that the child experienced *before* placement into foster care. As can be seen from the tables, neglect was the largest category of abuse for the children, including 33 percent of the children whose parents or caretakers had failed to provide food, clothing, shelter, or other needs and 27 percent whose parents had failed to supervise them, leaving them alone for long periods unattended.

The type of abuse also varied depending on the age of the child. For example, only 2 percent of children ages 1–2 were sexually abused, while abuse rates increased to 15 percent for children ages

MAIN ABUSE TYPES EXPERIENCED BY FOSTER CHILDREN FROM THE ONE YEAR IN FOSTER CARE (OYFC) STUDY

Number of Main Abuse Type	Percent
None	4
Physical Abuse	6
Sexual Abuse	3
Failure to Provide	17
Failure to Supervise	27
Combination of Two	32
Combination of Three	8
Combination of Four	1

Source: Adapted from U.S. Department of Health and Human Services, Administration for Children, Youth and Families (November 2003). *National Survey of Child and Adolescent Well-Being: One Year in Foster Care Report.* Washington, D.C.

3–5 years and 45 percent for children ages 6–10. Sexual abuse declined to about 39 percent for children ages 11 and older.

For the youngest children, ages 1–2, the largest category of abuse was neglect (failure to provide) at 33 percent, followed by physical abuse (26 percent).

Many children experienced more than one form of abuse or neglect; however, when the most serious category was considered among all the children, the largest percentages of children suffered from neglect.

Do Adoptive Parents Ever Abuse Children?

Experts believe that the rate of abuse among adoptive parents is extremely low; however, some cases have been reported prominently in the media. According to Richard Barth, in his essay in *Adoption Policy and Special Needs Children* in 1997, abuse occurs in about 1 percent of adoptive families.

This low rate of abuse may be due to the fact that adoptive parents intensely desired to become parents, and they were also screened before they were able to adopt a child. The home study process almost invariably includes a complete report from one's physician. A person with a serious problem, such as drug abuse or alcohol abuse, is likely to be detected. Individuals with a history of abuse or violence or a criminal history would also not be allowed to adopt a child. However, rarely, some individuals who should not have been approved to adopt do receive such an approval.

In several high-profile cases, adoptive parents alleged to have abused (or in some cases, proven to have abused) their internationally adopted children defended themselves by suggesting that their child suffered from reactive attachment disorder and had caused his own injuries.

Placements with Relatives

Sometimes abused children are removed from their homes and placed with grandparents or in other KINSHIP CARE arrangements. This may be a good idea in many cases, but in other cases it could be very problematic because the extended family may have problems similar to the abusers' problems, such as substance abuse.

Attorney Howard A. Davidson, director of the American Bar Association Center on Children and the Law, advises caution with this approach of placing foster children with extended relatives. In an article for *Trial*, he wrote, "In recent years, federal and state laws and child welfare agency practices have reflected a preference for placement of abused, neglected, or abandoned children with extended family members rather than in foster homes with strangers. This 'kinship care' preference must be cautiously applied. Prospective homes, whether temporary or permanent, should be screened for safety and suitability. This should include screening the criminal records of adults in the home."

Determining Abuse

Abusive parents are typically reported to police officers or to the state social service department by neighbors, relatives, teachers, physicians, and others. When an allegation of abuse or neglect is made, a social worker is generally assigned to investigate and either substantiate or refute the allegations, if possible. The abuse, if it occurred, may have happened only one time, but it is far more likely that it has been recurrent over a period of months or years. Often, abuse is not detected until a child enters kindergarten or first grade because abusive parents often keep their children out of sight. Some abusive parents continue to hide abuse by using the option of homeschooling their children, although certainly most homeschoolers are not abusive.

If a social worker or investigator determines that abuse or neglect has occurred to a child and further determines that abuse was caused by a parent, relative, or other person with whom the child lives (such as an unmarried mother's boyfriend), the child is usually removed from the home and placed with other relatives or in a state-approved foster home or group home.

The child will not be returned to the home unless and until it is determined by social workers, and the court also concurs, that the parent or other person living in the home has been rehabilitated from the problem leading to the abuse or neglect, whether it was alcohol or drug use, the emotional or mental problems of the abuser, or some other cause. In some cases, the person causing the abuse, such as a friend or relative of the mother, must leave the home in order for the child to return home. However, follow-up visits may occur to ensure that the abusive person has not returned to the home.

In some cases, it may be difficult for investigators to determine whether or not abuse has actually occurred, especially if injuries have healed over time, or theoretically could have been caused by an accident. Investigators and physicians look for a pattern of "accidents" and also consider the type of injury that results from the alleged accident; for example, an injury incurred from a fall may be very different from an injury incurred by a parent violently jerking a child's arm. A small child who has periodically "fallen" into scalding water or has wounds or lacerations that probably would not be the natural result of childhood mishaps should be checked as a potential abuse victim.

Witnesses to the abuse are extremely helpful, although many people may be reluctant or fearful of testifying against a violent person. Physician reports, such as from a hospital emergency room, may be used to help substantiate abuse.

In cases of severe abuse or when the social worker determines that it is unlikely the abusive parent can successfully raise the child in a healthy nonabusive atmosphere, the child will be permanently removed from the home, and parental rights will be terminated in a court of law. The child will then be in need of an adoptive family if authorities believe it is in the best interest of the child to be adopted. In many cases, children are adopted by their foster parents.

Some children are so damaged physically and/or psychologically by abuse that it is difficult and sometimes impossible to meet the child's needs. Consequently the child may be better off living in a group home or even in a psychiatric treatment setting. It has been speculated that many adults who are currently in prison were once abused children.

Abuse and Neglect and Adolescent Parents

Findings are mixed on whether adolescent single parents are more abusive or neglectful than other single parents, and some researchers say that it cannot and should not be presumed that a child is at greater risk from an adolescent mother than an older mother; however, there are factors that could theoretically predispose an adolescent to abuse her child.

For example, according to the *Encyclopedia of Child Abuse*, infants who are born prematurely and are of low birth weight may be at risk for abuse.

Such infants are "more restless, distractible, unresponsive and demanding than the average child. Child-specific factors when combined with a parent who is inexperienced or easily frustrated greatly increase the risk of abuse." Teenagers also have a high rate of low birth weight infants.

Children from Orphanages and Abuse

Families who adopt children from other countries, particularly children older than two or three years, should realize that sometimes children are abused and neglected in orphanages. Some children from other countries are placed in orphanages because of abuse and neglect in the birth home. As in the United States, this may result in termination of parental rights.

Adults who adopt children from other countries should be prepared to accept that children who have lived in overseas orphanages have, at the least, suffered from neglect, although conditions in orphanages vary greatly. The children may have been abused by adults or by other children in the orphanage. As a result, they may experience many of the same emotional problems as foster children adopted in the United States.

When Adoption Is Planned for an Abused Child

If social workers are making an adoption plan for an abused child in foster care, ethical social workers will brief the adopting parents completely in a nonidentifying way (not revealing the names of the child's parents and/or abusers) about the child's abusive treatment or the conditions of neglect under which the child has lived. However, social workers are often not fully aware of the extent of the abuse and in some cases may not even know that past abuse has occurred. (The child may have been removed from the home for the reasons of overt abandonment or neglect rather than physical or sexual abuse.)

Abused children may also suffer physical handicaps resulting from their abuse, and these handicaps should be fully disclosed to prospective adoptive parents. Such handicaps may make it more difficult to locate a suitable adoptive family.

The effects of abuse may be long-term, even when the abused child was only an infant or toddler at the time of the abuse. Psychologists have found that love cannot always overcome the emotional and psychological effects of severe abuse and the internalized feelings of anger and guilt experienced even by very young children. However, in general, children adopted at younger ages (under age three) appear to be more resilient than older children who have been living in an institution for many years or all of their lives.

Adoptive Parents of Abused Children

Abused children may "act out" their anger and aggression on adoptive parents and siblings. They may also behave in sexually precocious ways, based on what they have learned as "normal" behavior from their parents or the persons who sexually abused them. Adults who adopt sexually abused children must be very sensitive to this problem in their child's past and comfortable with their own sexuality. Social workers report that children who are sexually abused are the hardest children to fit successfully into adoptive families.

When parents adopt abused children, they should realize the child may need therapy immediately or in 10 years. It is also possible that he or she could blossom in the adoptive home and never require counseling; however, adoptive parents should be open to the need for treatment. One precaution: not all counseling is competent—or needed. As a result, counselors should be chosen carefully and therapists who pathologize all adopted children should be avoided, lest they create a problem that was not present. (See THERAPY AND THERAPISTS.)

Many parents and adoption professionals agree that adoptive parent support groups can be very helpful to parents adopting older children if other members of the group have themselves adopted older children or children with SPECIAL NEEDS, but it is very difficult to find appropriate groups.

Gregory C. Keck, Ph.D., and Regina M. Kupecky, L.S.W., authors of *Adopting the Hurt Child: Hope for Families with Special-Needs Kids*, say that positive indicators of real changes in the abused child are: "abbreviated, although perhaps intense, retreats to old behavior; faster recovery time after the retreat; decreased frequency of retreats" and "child's acknowledgment of his responsibility for the retreat without blaming others."

They state, "Once these four features listed above are witnessed over a period of time, we can assume that the child's growth and development have been activated from an earlier dormant state. Subsequently, all other change is made with less resistance, reduced turmoil, and little complication. Getting 'unstuck' is the key to adjusting to a new life, and once this happens, the child will most likely continue to grow into a more integrated individual."

Wrongful Adoption

In some instances, social workers have failed to alert adopting parents to known severe problems that children faced in their past lives, and adoptive parents have successfully sued the state or agency for the withholding of information and the subsequent WRONGFUL ADOPTION. Adoptive parents have generally argued in such cases that they would not have adopted the child had they known about these problems or that they would have obtained therapy and treatment for the child had they been informed.

Abused Children Who Grow Up

Abuse causes severe consequences in many who were abused. Adults abused as children are more likely to become substance abusers and to commit suicide. Some studies indicate that a large proportion of women who are prostitutes were abused as children. (This does not, however, mean that children who are abused usually become prostitutes.) However, some children have a RESILIENCE that enables them to cope in later life, despite their early adverse experiences.

See also ADOPTION AND SAFE FAMILIES ACT; CHILDREN'S RIGHTS; FOSTER CARE; FOSTER PARENT.

Administration for Children, Youth and Families, Department of Health and Human Services. *Child Maltreatment 2003.* Washington, D.C.: 2005.

Administration for Children, Youth and Families. *National Survey of Child and Adolescent Well-Being: One Year in Foster Care Report.* Washington, D.C.: November 2003.

Avery, Rosemary J., ed. *Adoption Policy and Special Needs Children.* Westport, Conn.: Auburn House, 1997.

Davidson, Howard A. "Protecting America's Children: A Challenge," *Trial* 35 (January 1999): 22.

Clark, Robin B., Judith Freeman Clark, and Christine Adamec. *The Encyclopedia of Child Abuse.* New York: Facts On File, 2001.

Keck, Gregory C., and Regina Kupecky. *Adopting the Hurt Child: Hope for Families with Special-Needs Kids.* Colorado Springs, Colo.: Pinon Press, 1998.

Wu, S. S., et al. "Risk Factors for Infant Maltreatment: A Population-Based Study," *Child Abuse and Neglect* 28, no. 12 (2004): 1,253–1,264.

academic progress When used in references to adopted children, this term generally refers to school achievements of children under age 18.

Children who were adopted as infants can expect to achieve at a normal rate commensurate with their intelligence.

Children who are adopted as older children, especially children who have already begun school and were foster children, will often struggle with academic achievement, primarily because much energy is spent adjusting to the new family and learning the daily ways of this family as well as what is acceptable and what is unacceptable behavior.

It is also possible that a newly adopted child's grade may rapidly improve if he or she feels very positive about the adoption; however, this should not be expected, and poor grades should not be considered by the family as an indication they have failed.

If the older child enters the adoptive family after the school year has already begun and must change schools, this adds to the adjustments the child must make.

Adoptive parents need to understand that teachers, like other members of society, may have negative and outdated views about adoption; consequently, a behavioral problem could be magnified in the teacher's eyes because it is blamed on adoption. In turn, the child perceives the teacher has a negative attitude, although she or he probably does not know the reason why, and may misbehave even more, resulting in a continuing cycle of problems. Parents must be very active and work hard to identify the details, not always assuming the teacher is right and the child is wrong or vice versa.

See also ADJUSTMENT; EARLY INTERVENTION; SCHOOL; SPECIAL NEEDS ADOPTION; TEACHERS AND ADOPTED CHILDREN.

acting out Negative behavior such as stealing, lying, constant whining, and other behavioral problems. If the child was adopted, often these dis-ciplinary problems can be directly or indirectly tied to unhappy experiences that occurred while the child lived in an abusive or neglectful home, faced many foster care placements, or endured other psychological hardships.

Even children as young as two years old who are adopted into a new family can be expected to exhibit behavioral problems because it is difficult for them to adjust to new routines, loss of former security figures, and new parents.

Social workers expect most older children will act out to some extent, and parents must learn how to gain the child's trust while at the same time setting appropriate disciplinary limits. Often, spanking and harsh words are the least effective forms of discipline because severe physical or verbal abuse may have been the reason for the initial development of negative behavior. If children receive a response only when they misbehave, they will learn that negative behavior is a good way to gain attention.

Adoptive parents can learn techniques of positive reinforcement, "time-out" (sending the child to his or her room), and other methods of discipline from social workers and also from other adoptive parents; for example, one adoptive mother of an older child was dismayed that her daughter kept stealing items from her jewelry box. Other adoptive parents with similar experiences advised the mother to put a lock on her bedroom door. Although she considered this solution to be very radical, everything else she'd tried had failed, so the mother tried this technique, and the stealing stopped. Years later, her daughter thanked her for removing the temptation and making it impossible to steal.

Some adopted children born in other countries may initially gorge themselves or hoard food, dismaying the rest of the family, but such behavior is understandably based on previous circumstances. The child may have experienced starvation or extreme hunger and consequently must gradually learn that food will always be provided, and he or she need not stockpile food for hard times ahead.

Many newly adopted older children are not grateful they have been adopted and may evince resentment, anger, or distrust of adoptive parents until it becomes clear that the adoption is regarded as permanent by the parents. Until the adopted child feels confident and secure, he or she will test parents. (In fact, even after the child is secure, the normal testing that all children exhibit will continue.)

Acting out may be a temporary serious problem, although all children, adopted or born into their families, have times when they misbehave, especially when they are tired, ill, or upset.

If acting out continues and the parents feel unable to cope with the child, they may need to seek professional help. Researchers have discovered that adoptions may actually disrupt if adoptive parents believe the older child's behavior is not improving and the acting out continues without abeyance.

See also DISRUPTION; OLDER CHILD.

adjustment The process by which adopted children and adoptive parents relate to and accept one another in their respective child-parent roles. (Readers should refer to ADULT ADOPTED PERSONS for questions relating to the lifelong psychological adjustment of adopted persons.) It should be noted that adjustment is an ongoing process for parents as children grow older and become more independent: it is not a one-time achievement. An adoptive parent support group composed of other families who have also adopted children of about the same age can be a tremendous help to a new adoptive family.

As the child grows up, questions about adoption are common and are often related to the child's age and stage of development; for example, young children are usually accepting of positive explanations about adoption, while older children and especially adolescents may not perceive their adoption in the positive way parents may wish. It is also true that all children go through problems as they grow, and sometimes it is not clear whether children have difficulties because they were adopted or because they are adolescents. Some mental health or other professionals may incorrectly ascribe the child's difficulties to his or her adoptive status. The term *normative crises* has been suggested to describe the expected challenges and difficulties that many adopted children and their families experience as part of normal adjustment after adoption.

A variety of parenting books have been written for adoptive parents. *Parenting Your Adopted Child: A Positive Approach to Building a Family* (McGraw-Hill,

2004) by Andrew Adesman, M.D., offers parenting advice for different stages of the child's life. *Adopting the Older Child* (Harvard Common Press, 1979) by Claudia Jewett was specifically written for parents choosing to adopt older children rather than infants. *Parenting the Hurt Child: Helping Adoptive Families Heal and Grow* (Pinon Press, 2002) by Gregory Keck and Regina Kupecky discusses issues helpful to parents who have adopted abused children. Another useful book is *Adopting the Hurt Child: Hope for Families with Special-Needs Kids: A Guide for Parents and Professionals* (Navpress Publishing Group, 1998) by Gregory Keck and Regina Kupecky.

Adjustment Directly after an Adoption

Despite the age of the child, after a child new to the family is adopted, it takes time for all parties to begin to feel comfortable with one another and accepting of each other. How much time is needed varies greatly depending on circumstances. The older child adopted from another country may need more time than a newborn infant to adjust to a family, because of major cultural and language differences in the older child. A child adopted from foster care may adjust rapidly to the family or it may take months or longer for the family and the child to adjust to each other's needs and expectations.

Experts agree that adjustment is generally the easiest and most rapid when a child is an infant and when the prospective parents are well-prepared for the child and have seriously considered adoption issues, such as their own INFERTILITY and their feelings about the birthparents. They should also realize there will be a need to communicate about adoption issues with the child they hope to adopt. This communication, at the child's level of understanding, is vital once the child is old enough to understand, and the parents should be willing to be candid about adoption as the child grows up. (See EXPLAINING ADOPTION.)

One reason why all states do not instantly "finalize" an adoption is to ensure that a sufficient time period has passed that has enabled the adoptive parents and the child to adjust to each other. As a result, most adoptions are not finalized for at least six months.

After the adoption of older children, the child and parents usually go through several stages of adjustment. Initially, there is often a "honeymoon period" that may last for days, weeks, or even months. During this time, the child strives mightily to behave in a perfect way and please the adoptive parents. Adopting parents may shower the child with gifts and wish to throw away a child's old and well-worn stuffed animal. This would be a serious mistake, because the item may be the only element of continuity the child knows, and it is very important for him to retain it until he feels ready to discard it.

A testing phase may come next, when the child misbehaves on purpose to see if the adopting parents will continue to parent him, despite his behavior. Although it may strain their patience, most adoptive parents do survive this period. Finally, the child assimilates into the family, not overstressing the family but making reasonable demands on it.

Some adoptive parents experience a post-adoption depression. This is comparable in some ways to postpartum depression, although it is less understood and even less well recognized. Parents are often secretive if they experience such a depression, as they feel ashamed that the carefully planned and long-awaited arrival of the child brings negative feelings, rather than the joy that was anticipated.

The parents may feel unsure and insecure about disciplining an older child, and some children are adept at turning on the tears to manipulate their new mom and dad. Most parents and children must feel their way along until they feel truly comfortable with each other. To reach that point may take months or as long as a year or more, depending on the family.

If the child is an older child from another country or has serious disabilities, both the child and the adoptive parents will need extra time to adjust. The parents cannot expect the child to learn English overnight nor should parents expect themselves to know automatically and immediately how to cope if their child has special needs.

The parents of children with SPECIAL NEEDS must also learn about resources available in the community so that they can assist their children with specific conditions or problems.

Older children appear to fare better in families with more than one child, and studies reveal they adjust the most rapidly in large families.

Although on the surface this may seem contradictory, in that it would appear difficult for parents of large families to provide much attention to an additional child, what often happens is that the children already in the home assist the adopting parents in welcoming the child and helping the child fit in to the family.

Studies also reveal that people who already have children are favored by social service agencies as prospective parents for older children. The theory is that families with existing children understand child rearing and are not seeking a perfect child.

Extended Family and Community Resources Can Help

Another factor in adjustment is the attitudes of the family and friends. Studies of new adoptive mothers indicate that many feel adoption is not accepted, at least initially, by their family and peers; thus it would appear that much more work needs to be done to educate the general public about adoption.

See also ADOLESCENT ADOPTED PERSONS; ATTITUDES ABOUT ADOPTION; EXPLAINING ADOPTION; PREPARING A CHILD FOR ADOPTION; SIBLINGS.

Adesman, Andrew, M.D., and Christine Adamec. *Parenting the Adopted Child: A Positive Approach to Building a Family.* New York: McGraw-Hill, 2004.
Hopkins-Best, Mary. *Toddler Adoption: A Weaver's Craft.* Indianapolis, Ind.: Perspectives Press, 1998.
Register, Cheri. *"Are Those Kids Yours?": American Families with Children Adopted from Other Countries.* New York: Free Press, 1990.

adolescent adopted persons Adopted children ranging in age from the onset of puberty through about age 17 or 18.

Adolescence is a tumultuous period for many children, and nonadopted children as well as adopted children may face many conflicts during this time of physical and emotional changes. Research on adopted adolescents offer very mixed findings on the level of adjustment or lack of adjustment within this group. Some researchers have identified numerous problem areas while others insist that much research is biased because the researchers find what they are looking for: problems. One very large study of adopted adolescents was performed by the Search Institute in 1994. Adopted adolescents were compared to their non-adopted siblings and to peers. In the broad majority of cases, the adopted adolescents were as well-adjusted as the other groups.

Whether researchers believe adolescence is more difficult for adopted teenagers than non-adopted adolescents, one finding seems consistent: many researchers report that even among adopted adolescents who are troubled, the wide majority of them find stability in adulthood.

Some researchers who have studied populations of psychiatric patients have reported a disproportionate number of adopted teenagers. Other researchers insist such samples are biased and contend that studies of adopted adolescents should be drawn from the general population and compared with nonadopted adolescents who are also drawn from the population at large.

Some researchers agree that the teen years can be stressful for any child but contend they may be particularly stressful for an adopted child because of the identity issues that must be faced during this period. Many adolescents are tempted to believe that they *must* be adopted, otherwise how could they have come from such "hopeless" parents? When children know they are adopted, they argue, this information may intensify fantasies about birthparents.

However, researchers Janet Hoopes and Leslie Stein found no evidence indicating that adopted adolescents have a more difficult adolescence than do nonadopted adolescents.

See IDENTITY.

Societal Attitudes

Sometimes it is very difficult for a teenager to admit to others that he or she was adopted because peers may feel it is heartless to "give away" a baby and some express the opinion that abortion is more humane than adoption if the subject of a pregnant peer is brought up.

As a result, the child may be ashamed or embarrassed about the fact of having been adopted. Sometimes the family's attendance in an adoptive parent support group can help, particularly if the adolescent can meet other adopted teenagers.

A child's age at the time of adoption should be taken into account when considering the impact of adoption. In the past, nearly all adopted persons were adopted as infants; however, increasing numbers of children with SPECIAL NEEDS today are adopted over the age of eight.

The majority of children adopted as older children were abused or neglected by their birthparents or stepparents and subsequently placed in FOSTER CARE for at least a year. As a result, they may bring to the adoptive home many emotional and psychological problems they must resolve.

Studies by Barth, Festinger, and others have also revealed that the older the child was at the time of the adoption, the greater the probability the adoption will be at least initially troubled or even disrupted; however, children adopted as adolescents may also develop a strong rapport with their adoptive parents and resolve the earlier conflicts life placed on their young shoulders. (See DISRUPTION.)

As a result, when considering adopted adolescents, it is critically important to determine both the age of the adopted child at the time of adoption and the quality of nurturing care prior to the placement. It would be unreasonable to include adolescents adopted at birth in a study with adolescents adopted at age 14 and to then presume any valid conclusions could be drawn.

See RESEARCH, PROBLEMS WITH.

Unrealistic Societal Attitudes

Adopted adolescents must also contend with a variety of unrealistic, negative, and often erroneous ideas that society at large holds about adoption, for example, that the child should be grateful about the adoption, particularly if he or she was adopted from outside the United States.

It is usually presumed by society that the child's birthparents were poverty-stricken and of a lower socioeconomic status than the adoptive parents and, consequently, many people believe that the adopted person should be thankful he or she was "saved" from a less positive situation. This idea can cause conflict in the adopted adolescent, because few teenagers feel a constant gratitude for their parents—adoptive or biological.

Transracially Adopted Adolescents

Adolescents whose appearance is greatly different from their adoptive parents may experience a crisis during adolescence; for example, black children adopted by white parents may experience particular questions of identity. However, studies to date indicate that transracial adoption generally works very well.

A study by Ruth G. McRoy and Louis Zurcher on transracially and "inracially" adopted teenagers was described in their book, *Transracial and Inracial Adoptees: The Adolescent Years.*

According to the authors, it was primarily the "quality of parenting" that was critical to the child's adjustment rather than whether the adoption was transracial or inracial. Most of the adoptive parents studied by the researchers were able to successfully handle the challenges of transracial adoption; however, they conceded that some parents do not succeed as well.

They also noted that adopted adolescents in transracial adoptions who were raised in integrated neighborhoods had a more flexible racial perception than those who were raised in all-white neighborhoods.

Said the authors, "Adoptees in those contexts seemed to acknowledge their black background not only on a cognitive level but also on an affective level. Their parents instilled in these adoptees positive feelings about their racial background. They tended to desire contact with other black children and their families."

It is also clear from studies of children adopted transracially that these adoptions have good results.

See also ADULT ADOPTED PERSONS; "CHOSEN CHILD"; PSYCHIATRIC PROBLEMS OF ADOPTED PERSONS; TRANSRACIAL ADOPTION.

Feigelman, William, and Arnold Silverman. *Chosen Children: New Patterns in Adoptive Relationships.* New York: Praeger, 1983.

Krementz, Jill. *How It Feels to Be Adopted.* New York: Knopf, 1988.

McRoy, Ruth G., and Louis Z. Zurcher Jr. *Transracial and Inracial Adoptees: The Adolescent Years.* Springfield, Ill.: Thomas, 1983.

Sharma, Anu R., Matthew McGue, and Peter L. Benson. "The Emotional and Behavioral Adjustment of United States Adopted Adolescents: Part II Age at Adoption," *Children and Youth Services Review* 18 (January 1996): 101–114.

adolescent birthmothers   See BIRTHMOTHER.

adopted-away/adopted-in   Two terms often used to identify adopted persons in legal matters, usually in regard to INHERITANCE questions. "Adopted-away" refers to a child in reference to the family of the birthmother; an "adopted-in" child is one who has entered a family via adoption. Adoption practitioners find these terms to be negative and prefer to avoid them altogether.

"adoptee" v. "adopted person"   "Adoptee" is sometimes considered to be the less acceptable substitute label for the words "adopted person," "adopted adult," "adopted child," or "adopted teenager." (In many cases, the word *adopted* is an unnecessary descriptive adjunct, as in a newspaper article describing a public figure and his two daughters and "adopted son.")

See also ATTITUDES ABOUT ADOPTION.

adoption   The act of lawfully assuming the parental rights and responsibilities of another person, usually a child under the age of 18. A legal adoption imposes the same rights and responsibilities on an adoptive parent as are imposed on and assumed by a parent when the child is born to the family. Adoption grants social, emotional, and legal family membership to the person who is adopted.

An old and inappropriate definition of adoption is "to raise someone else's child," and in some minds, this definition may still prevail. Yet it mistakenly implies the concept of ownership, and people cannot own other people, including children. Instead, parents are responsible for their children, unless they choose to end that responsibility or the state decides to end the responsibility.

The birthparent cannot sever the genetic inheritance; however, she or he can terminate parental rights by transferring them to another family, or the court may opt to terminate parental rights and transfer them to another family who adopts the child.

The act of adoption generally includes a HOME STUDY, or family study, evaluation, and counseling of the prospective adoptive parents, either before or after placement. The study is usually performed by a licensed social worker or individual serving in a caseworker capacity. This home study and the recommendations of the social worker are provided to the JUDGE at the time of FINALIZATION of the legal completion of the adoption.

The judge will then approve or disapprove the request for adoption. If approved, the adoption is valid thenceforth. The adopted child has all the rights of children born to a family, and the birthparents' parental rights and obligations are permanently severed by law.

The original birth certificate is usually "sealed" (see SEALED RECORDS), and a new birth certificate is prepared with the adoptive parents listed as parents.

If the birthparents wish to revoke their consent to the adoption, they must petition the court for a legal hearing and provide compelling reasons why the finalized adoption should be invalidated. Very few adoptions are invalidated after finalization.

See also ADOPTIVE PARENTS; BIRTHMOTHER; BIRTHFATHER; INHERITANCE.

adoption agencies Organizations that screen prospective adoptive parents and that place children with approved adoptive families. Most adoption agencies are nonprofit organizations. The size of agencies varies greatly, ranging from agencies with a small staff placing 10 children a year to large facilities that place hundreds of children per year. Agencies are usually staffed by social workers who have a degree in social work or a helping profession, such as psychology or counseling.

Agencies vary according to the types of children they place. Some agencies concentrate on placing mostly healthy newborns, while others primarily place older children or children with special needs. Some agencies concentrate on U.S.-born children while others specialize in international adoption.

Licensing of Agencies

Agencies that make adoptive placements must be licensed by the state in which they practice. Agencies that place children in other states usually work with another agency in that state and through the INTERSTATE COMPACT ON THE PLACEMENT OF CHILDREN, which is a sort of treaty between the states that governs interstate adoption. A small number of agencies are licensed by more than one state to make direct adoptive placements in a state other than the one in which they are based.

Agencies that place children from other countries must also comply with the laws of those countries. In addition, the provisions for the enforcement of the HAGUE CONVENTION ON INTERCOUNTRY ADOPTION, which are being finalized as of this writing, require compliance. The Hague Convention is a treaty between countries that governs how children should be placed for adoption.

Sectarian and Nonsectarian Agencies

Agencies under the auspices of a particular religious faith are called sectarian agencies. Such agencies may concentrate on serving individuals of a particular faith or group of faiths. Some sectarian agencies serve persons of all faiths and allow adoptive parents of other faiths to apply to adopt a child.

Agencies operated under nonreligiously affiliated auspices that do not restrict applications from prospective adoptive parents based on their religious preference are called nonsectarian agencies. Although questions may be asked about the applicants' background and current religious participation, membership in a specific religious group is not required as a criterion for adopting.

Public adoption agencies managed by the state or county government are nonsectarian, as are many private adoption agencies. Public agencies place children in foster care for adoption when the parental rights of their biological parents have been terminated.

Agency Criteria for Adopting Parents

Most adoption agencies believe strongly that their mission is to find loving families for "their" children, rather than to find babies and children for families. They may have criteria limiting the applications for healthy infants to only infertile couples. They may also have other criteria, such as those wishing to adopt healthy infants must be under a certain age, be married a certain number of years (if married), and so on. They may require that couples wishing to adopt be willing to engage in an OPEN ADOPTION or to meet with a pregnant woman considering them as parents for her child.

If the agency is placing children from other countries, they must also consider requirements of those countries; for example, some countries are opposed to children being placed with single people or with gay or lesbian parents. Some countries have more restrictive (or looser) age restrictions than many agencies in the United States place on prospective parents for children born in the United States.

Assistance to Pregnant Women Considering Adoption

Pregnant women considering adoption are almost always in a period of crisis. The woman may have been abandoned by a man she thought loved her, or she may have been shunned by her own parents. In addition, she may have difficulty meeting her basic needs of survival, including food and shelter. The birthfather may feel that he and the birthmother are too young and immature to marry and raise a child. (Some birthparents are married. See MARRIED BIRTHPARENTS.)

The agency may assist a pregnant woman in the United States by finding her a place to live, showing her how to apply for public assistance, including MEDICAID, and providing extensive supportive services so desperately needed. In addition, they will help her find a physician who can provide her much-needed prenatal care. Agencies may also assist pregnant women in other countries who are considering adoption for their babies; however, most children placed from other countries reside in orphanages before their adoption.

Most agencies engaged in adoption work in the United States provide counseling to pregnant women and mothers considering placing their infants or older children for adoption. Their goal is to ensure that the birthparents make a good parenting plan for their child and for themselves and that, if adoption is chosen, they will be as comfortable as possible with it.

Agencies also offer counseling and assistance to birthfathers and the parents of birthmothers and birthfathers.

Assistance to Prospective Adoptive Parents

Adoption agencies provide counseling to prospective adoptive parents and perform an evaluation of their potential parental fitness in a process called the HOME STUDY or family study.

When prospective parents are applying to adopt an infant, many social workers try to ensure that the family has worked through most of their feelings of grief related to infertility. They want parents to consider adoption their first choice now, rather than a poor "second-best" option.

Many adoptive parents have been through extensive infertility treatments, which were painful, both physically and emotionally. Some prospective parents have suffered the loss of one or more miscarriages. By the time they come to the adoption agency, they may still be distraught, and the social worker helps them work through trauma connected with their infertility.

Adoption Résumés

Some agencies encourage the adopting parents to write a nonidentifying RÉSUMÉ describing why the family wants to adopt, what the family's hobbies and interests are, and other facts. In some cases, the woman may select several résumés and then meet the families, choosing the one she prefers. A pregnant woman or a birthmother considering adoption will review these résumés and select the family she wants for her child.

Assistance to Older Children

Agencies placing older children and children with special needs provide counseling to the child(ren), prepare the child for adoption, explain adoption, introduce the prospective parents to the child, and serve as a child advocate if there are any questions or problems subsequent to placement.

Children with Special Needs

Virtually all agencies place children with special needs, and the definition of special needs varies drastically from agency to agency. One agency may consider any child over the age of two as having special needs, because that agency rarely receives children over that age. In addition, newborn infants and older children with birth defects and/or other problems are also considered to have special needs. Sibling groups are often considered to have special needs because it is generally harder to find a family for two or more children than for one child.

Children who are black and biracial are often considered to have special needs, even when they are healthy, because their number apparently exceeds the number of people available to adopt them. The reason for this "surplus" is complex and much-disputed. The National Association of Black

Social Workers has alleged that insufficient numbers of black parents have been recruited and contends that many more black adoptive parents could be identified. Others contend that the problem is in public or private agencies that discourage TRANSRACIAL ADOPTION despite laws designed to prevent racial considerations, such as the MULTIETHNIC PLACEMENT ACT.

Agency criteria for individuals wishing to adopt a child with special needs are usually relaxed in the sense of age limits, number of children already in the home, and other criteria in effect for people who want to adopt healthy white infants. As a result, a person who already has three children may be considered as a prospective parent for an older child or a child with special needs although he or she often would not be considered as a candidate to adopt a healthy infant. The reason for this is that it is easier for agencies to find families for infants than for older children.

Long-term Postplacement Services

Many agencies will provide counseling to adopted persons, adoptive parents, and birthparents for years after the adoption. If the adopted adult wishes information about birthparents, the agency will usually provide assistance within the limits of their agency policies and the laws of the state.

Fees to Agencies

Adoption agency fees vary considerably from agency to agency for several reasons. Those agencies with religious auspices, such as Catholic Social Services, Jewish Family Services, LDS (Latter-day Saints) Social Services, and similar agencies, may receive partial funding from the members of their respective religious groups, and consequently, they are able to charge less than agencies that receive no outside funding.

Other agencies are nonsectarian but they receive a portion of their funding from charitable, fund-raising organizations, such as the United Way. The balance of their funding comes from the money paid by adoption applicants.

Many adoption agencies, however, rely solely on the fees that are paid by prospective adoptive parents. These fees must cover expenses related to the pregnant women themselves (for example, shelter provided to them or money paid for food or medical bills), counseling services to adoptive parents, salaries of social workers, and office expenses, such as rent, heat, lights, and phone.

Agencies may charge a flat rate or a percentage of gross income or have some other means of computing the adoption fee; for example, they may charge a flat rate for the home study and add on the cost of the prenatal care and hospital bill as well as charge for postplacement fees. Some agencies charge on a sliding scale, with less affluent prospective parents paying a lower fee than more affluent individuals.

See also AUTOBIOGRAPHY; INFANT ADOPTION; "OPENNESS"; SOCIAL WORKERS.

Adoption and Foster Care Analysis Reporting System (AFCARS) A system that reports the number of children in the foster-care system. States are required to provide statistical data to the Department of Health and Human Services.

See also FOSTER CARE; STATISTICS.

Adoption and Safe Families Act (ASFA) Signed into law by President Bill Clinton, the Adoption and Safe Families Act (ASFA) of 1997 was enacted by Congress in an attempt to correct problems inherent in the foster care system that deterred the adoption of children in foster care. Many of these problems had stemmed from unforeseen consequences of an earlier bill, the ADOPTION ASSISTANCE AND CHILD WELFARE ACT OF 1980. As a direct result of ASFA, many more children were freed for adoption and many more were and are adopted. Since the passage of ASFA, the numbers of children adopted from foster care each year have more than doubled, to about 50,000 per year nationwide, as in fiscal year 2003.

Problems with the Old Law

One key problem with the Adoption Assistance and Child Welfare Act was its emphasis on the principles of FAMILY PRESERVATION. At times, child protection agencies felt compelled to return a child to abusive or neglectful parents who had not resolved their problems that led to the abuse or neglect (such as alcoholism, drug abuse, and emotional or serious psychiatric problems). As a result, adoption became a secondary or tertiary goal, while reunification with parents became the primary or sole goal.

The underlying idea of family preservation was that parenting classes and various support programs would enable the parents to overcome their problems that resulted in the abuse and neglect of their children, and thus would help them become effective parents. However, many parents were unable and/or unwilling to resolve their underlying problems. Consequently, their children eventually returned to foster care, often in a revolving-door fashion. Many children were in and out of foster care for years and sometimes for their entire childhoods, entering foster care as infants or small children and leaving as young adults. The impact of extended and/or frequent stays in the foster-care system greatly affected many children, often in a negative way. (See FOSTER CARE.)

Another problem was that the number of children in the foster-care system ballooned subsequent to the passage of the Adoption Assistance and Child Welfare Act, in part because of greatly increased public awareness about abuse. In addition, the length of time children spent in the system was much greater than in past years, largely because of the heavy emphasis on solving parental problems that led to the removal of the child from the home. The only number that seemed to decline was the number of children who were adopted.

It should be noted that in some cases, family preservation worked well. In many cases, however, it was a failure, and many children remained in the foster care system (or were in and out of the system) until they "aged out" as young adults.

As Howard A. Davidson wrote in a 1999 issue of *Trial,* "Too many caseworkers have misapplied principles of family preservation or reunification. The result: Children are maintained in or returned to hellish living environments where they suffer further severe, sometimes lethal, harm. . . . Too much deference to parental rights has sometimes led child welfare agencies and courts to delay resolving cases, giving unfit parents inordinately long periods of time to remedy their various 'problems.' In these cases, children spend critical childhood years in limbo, sometimes in unsafe foster homes, and many of them come away from the experience emotionally scarred by the instability of multiple temporary placements."

Implementation of ASFA

In the past, states received funds for foster children and there was little financial incentive for states to terminate parental rights and place children for adoption, which may have further increased the retention of children in foster care. To reverse this trend and encourage adoptions, ASFA authorized additional funds as bonus payments to motivate states to increase the numbers of adoptions. Many states responded to the new incentives.

There were other philosophical changes with ASFA. Marcia Robinson Lowry, executive director of Children's Rights in New York City, says in *Children and Youth Services Review,* "ASFA rejects linking the 'best interests of the child' standard to a bias in favor of family reunification, specifically decreeing that a child's health and safety are 'paramount,' including when decisions are made about the removal or return of a child from or to the home of a biological parent."

The law requires that a PERMANENCY PLANNING hearing be held within 12 months after the child enters foster care and every 12 months thereafter. If a court rules that reasonable efforts to reunite the child with his or her parents are not required, then a permanency planning hearing must be held within 30 days. Most states have incorporated this requirement into state law. A permanency planning hearing will decide whether the child should be returned to the parent, adopted by a nonrelative (or in some cases, by a relative), placed as a foster child with a relative (KINSHIP CARE), or placed under a legal guardianship arrangement or another planned permanent living arrangement. In fiscal year 2003, about half (55 percent) of the children who left foster care returned to their parents.

Termination of Parental Rights Under ASFA

The ASFA requires states to terminate parental rights and find an adoptive family if a child has been in foster care for 15 months or longer of the past 22 months. Prior to the passage of the law, if a parent severely abused a child or even murdered that child, another child in the family could be returned from foster care to that parent by a judge. Subsequent to ASFA, terminations were also allowed if a parent assaulted or killed another child in the family or if a child was determined to be an abandoned infant, according to state law.

The major goal of ASFA is to move children more quickly out of foster care back to their own homes or into adoptive homes. This goal appears to have been met, although some critics believe that even more children in the foster care system should be adopted.

Note that there are exceptions in ASFA to the requirements to terminate parental rights. These three exceptions include:

- If the child is being cared for by a relative
- If a state agency has documented that terminating parental rights would not be in the child's best interests
- If the state has not provided the family with the services they need so that the child could return safely home

Some Children Still Remain in Foster Care

Despite the laudable goals of ASFA, many children remain in foster care for years. Even among many children whose parents' rights were terminated, and who are eligible to be adopted, they remain in foster care. One probable reason why many children remain in foster care is that prospective adoptive parents usually seek to adopt infants or toddlers, and they are not interested in adopting older children.

According to a General Accounting Office (GAO) report in 2003, all 43 states that responded to their survey said they did not have enough adoptive homes for children with special needs. Thirty-nine states said that this problem was a moderate, great, or very great hindrance to finding permanent homes for children. (Most children in foster care are considered to have one or more special needs, whether due to age, being a member of a sibling group, being a minority member, and so forth. The GAO estimates that 85 percent of foster children who were adopted in 2000 had one or more special needs.) It is possible that a more active and/or national recruitment campaign for adoptive parents would be effective, although this is unknown. At present, each state manages its own adoptive parent recruitment programs.

Says Robinson Lowry, "The current reality is that children in foster care in this country are not achieving the positive outcomes that Congress intended ASFA to produce. The goals of the legislation will not be met, and children will continue to be denied the benefits that Congress intended for them, unless and until minimum national standards are developed and made enforceable."

See also FOSTER CARE; FOSTER PARENT ADOPTION; TERMINATION OF PARENTAL RIGHTS.

Adoption and Foster Care Analysis and Reporting System (AFCARS). The AFCARS Report: Preliminary FY 2003 Estimates as of April 2005," U.S. Department of Health and Human Services, Administration for Children and Families, Administration on Children, Youth and Families, Children's Bureau. Available online. URL: http://www.acf.hhs.gov/programs/cb/publications/afcars/report10.pdf, downloaded on July 17, 2005.

Ashby, Cornelia M., Director, Education, Workforce, and Income Security Issues. *Foster Care: States Focusing on Finding Permanent Homes for Children, But Long-Standing Barriers Remain.* Testimony before the Subcommittee on Human Resources Committee on Ways and Means, House of Representatives. Washington, D.C.: General Accounting Office, April 8, 2003, GAO-03-626T.

Boyd Rauber, Denise, ed. *Making Sense of the ASFA Regulations: A Roadmap for Effective Implementation.* Washington, D.C.: American Bar Association, 2001.

Davidson, Howard A. "Protecting America's Children: A Challenge," *Trial* 35 (January 1999): 22.

Robinson Lowry, Marcia. "Putting Teeth into ASFA: The Need for Statutory Minimum Standards," *Children and Youth Services Review* 26 (2004): 1,021–1,031.

Adoption Assistance and Child Welfare Act of 1980

Public law 96-272, passed by Congress in 1980. This act was passed to correct or alleviate problems in the foster care system and to promote permanency rather than multiple foster placements. Another goal of the act was to encourage social workers to work toward reunification of the family and to avoid long-term foster care for the children, if possible. If the child could not be returned to the family, another plan was to be sought: long-term foster care, adoption, or some other resolution. The act established the ADOPTION SUBSIDY through which SPECIAL NEEDS ADOPTIONS are partially subsidized by the federal government.

The act also provided federal funds and required states to create adoption subsidy programs. In past years, many children with special needs were not adopted because adoptive parents could not afford the extensive medical bills. This problem has increased in recent years. Because of problems with the Adoption Assistance and Child Welfare Act, such as children remaining in foster care for years, Congress passed the Adoption and Safe Families Act in 1997.

See also WAITING CHILDREN.

adoption benefits   See EMPLOYEE BENEFITS FOR ADOPTION; INSURANCE; PARENTAL LEAVE.

adoption circle   Refers to the key parties involved in an adoption: the adopted individual, the birthparents, and the adoptive parents, as well as birthgrandparents, adoptive grandparents, siblings, and others. A similar concept is more frequently expressed as an ADOPTION TRIAD or ADOPTION TRIANGLE.

adoption medicine   Medical specialty of physicians who specialize in treating adopted children, especially those from other countries. People in the United States and Canada (as well as many families in Europe) adopt thousands of children from other countries each year, including many countries in which the children may have illnesses that are not common or familiar to many physicians in the adoptive parents' country. Furthermore, many of these children reside in institutional care prior to adoption, predisposing them to certain conditions. As a result, some physicians have developed specialty clinics or they provide expertise in addition to their regular practices to families who are considering adopting children from other countries or who have already adopted them.

Preadoption Assistance

Some families seek help with evaluating the health of a particular child their agency has told them they may adopt. Photographs are usually provided to the prospective parents. In some cases, usually from Russia or Kazakhstan, a VIDEOTAPE of the child is available. In addition, medical information provided by physicians in the child's country can be translated so that the adoption medicine expert can have both written and visual information to aid in the evaluation that they provide the prospective adoptive parents.

The physician may be able to detect indicators of FETAL ALCOHOL SYNDROME or other DEVELOPMENTAL DISABILITIES as well as apparent medical problems, such as RICKETS, malnutrition, and other health problems.

Even though a preadoptive evaluation of a child using videotapes, photos, and translated medical records cannot screen for all potential medical and emotional problems, it is one step that may flag key issues that would otherwise go unnoticed until after the child was adopted.

Most physicians who perform a preadoptive evaluation will not advise a prospective parent that they should or should not adopt a particular child, but instead they will offer their professional medical opinion on the health of the child. Some parents feel they can deal with serious medical problems while others do not, and thus the decision to adopt is a personal family matter. However, some physicians may discourage families if the child appears to have profound disabilities or multiple risk factors for future difficulties.

Adopting the Child

If the family decides to adopt a child, in most cases they will travel to the other country, where they will meet the child and take required legal actions, including going to a foreign court. Many families request additional medical input after first meeting the child.

When the Child Comes Home

After a child is newly adopted, the parent may wish to have the child evaluated by an adoption medicine expert because this physician will be more likely than most doctors to look for medical problems that are common in other countries or result from institutionalization, such as intestinal parasites or malnutrition. The adoption medicine expert should be seen within about two to three weeks after arrival in the country, unless the child is ill. In most cases, the child can subsequently receive treatment from his or her family doctor or pediatrician, with follow-ups to the adoption medicine expert as needed.

To identify an adoption medicine expert, contact the American Academy of Pediatrics or go to the

Web site at: http://www.aap.org/sections/adoption/
adopt-states/adoption-map.html.

See also INTERNATIONAL ADOPTION; MEDICAL
PROBLEMS OF INTERNATIONALLY ADOPTED CHILDREN.

Miller, Laurie C., M.D. *The Handbook of International Adoption Medicine: A Guide for Physicians, Parents, and
Providers.* New York: Oxford University Press, 2005.

adoption studies   Clinical research that uses
adopted children, adolescents, or adults as subjects.
Sir Francis Galton was the first researcher to undertake adoption studies, in about 1876, and many
researchers since then have undertaken such studies. Galton also introduced the use of twin studies
to determine the impact of heredity on individuals
versus that of environment. The largest adoption
studies, based on the adoption records of thousands
of subjects, have been performed in Europe, particularly in Denmark and Sweden. Often the results of
these studies are extrapolated to adopted individuals in the United States.

The advantage of adoption studies is that they can
help to illustrate the impact of both environment and
heredity on a variety of issues. (See also GENETIC PRE-
DISPOSITIONS.) They may also provide helpful information for adopted adults and adoptive parents.

The disadvantage is that sometimes there are
biases that are not perceived by the researchers
themselves, such as including a population of children adopted as infants along with children
adopted at much older ages, and using the results
of this diverse population to make sweeping gen-
eralizations to all adopted individuals. This is of
particular concern because children adopted later
in their lives have often been abused or neglected,
and these issues may have resulted in problems for
the child, rather than the adoptive status. (See
RESEARCH, PROBLEMS WITH.)

As a result, any time an adoption study is consulted, it is important to review whether the age
and past abuse and/or neglect status of the subjects
at the time of the adoption were noted. It is also
advisable to look at the percentage of children or
adults in the study who were about the same age
at placement and how the subjects were recruited
to participate in the research study (for example,
all were clients at mental health facilities, or all
were students in the same school).

Some researchers have mounted longitudinal
(long-term) studies of adopted individuals; for
example, the Colorado Adoption Study conducted
in-depth evaluations of adopted individuals every
few years starting in early childhood. Rita Simon
and Howard Altstein also conducted longitudinal
studies of children placed in TRANSRACIAL ADOP-
TIONS, but because such studies are expensive and
it is difficult to stay in touch with subjects over
many years, most researchers study their subjects
at a single point in time.

Adoption studies are often used to attempt to
differentiate the effects of heredity and environment. If traits of adopted children are similar to
their birthparents, then these may be seen as inherited traits. If they are more similar to the adoptive
family, this may be seen as an environmental effect.
For example, some studies have shown that children of alcoholic birthparents have a greater risk for
developing alcoholism than children whose birthparents were not alcoholic, thus this propensity is
perceived as an inherited risk. In contrast, some
studies have shown that children adopted by obese
parents are more likely to be obese than children
adopted by thin parents. This is attributed to an
environmental effect, that is, parents who overeat
and who overfeed their children.

There are several potential difficulties with
these types of studies. Sometimes adoptive families experience problems unrelated to the adoption which may contribute to difficulties for the
child, including divorce, illness, and other traumas. These events must be accounted for when
assessing outcomes. Moreover, some critics have
suggested that factors involved in matching children to specific families deserve careful scrutiny.
For example, children whose biological background contains a particular problem may be
intentionally placed with an adoptive family that
shares this problem, making it difficult to differentiate environmental versus genetic influences.
Furthermore, studies which relate characteristics
of adopted children to their birthparents may be
misleading: the accuracy of information about the
birthparents may be incomplete or outdated if it
was collected at the time of the adoptive placement and is only available by a retrospective
review of records.

Notably, most adoption studies consider traits that are usually considered unfavorable, such as alcoholism, drug abuse, obesity, and psychiatric problems. The problem with this research slant is that some people tend to believe that most adopted people are at risk for negative traits; however, adopted children may also inherit positive traits from their birthparents, such as athletic ability or musical or artistic talents.

David Howe said in *Patterns of Adoption*, "The choice of behaviours by scientists is often that which also concerns policy makers and practitioners: education, mental health and antisocial behavior. To this extent, the knowledge produced about adopted children's development appears a little unbalanced, concentrating mainly on the disturbed and the deviant. More 'normal' behaviours receive less attention. Thus, a digest of behavioural genetic research that might interest adoption workers needs to be read with this distortion in mind. By association, one can have the feeling that because these scientists write a lot about schizophrenia or crime using adoption as one of their 'natural experiments,' then adoptions themselves are beset with these behaviours. This, of course, is not the case."

The comparison groups used in adoption studies are important to consider when assessing research outcomes. Adopted individuals are generally compared with nonadopted persons in a clinical or a general population. Sometimes adopted adults or children are compared to adopted but unrelated siblings in the adoptive family or to children born to the adoptive parents.

Few adopted children are compared to their biological siblings who remained with their birthparents; however, some studies *have* compared such children, and in most cases the adopted children fared better in many areas.

These findings are described in *Patterns of Adoption*, which discussed a study of children adopted as infants compared to their nonadopted siblings who remained with the birthparents.

The author stated, "Adopted children achieve higher IQ scores, lower rates of criminal behaviour and fewer psychiatric admissions than their non-adopted counterparts. [Their siblings who remained in the biological family.] Whatever genetic risk factors adopted children bring with them, the interactional qualities generated by their more advantaged adoptive families acts as a developmental protective factor." Clearly, adoptive families may provide enriched environments which support the development of innate abilities and talents of adopted children.

A study reported in the *Journal of the American Medical Association* in 2005 used the statistical technique of meta-analysis to extract data from over 100 studies on behavioral problems of a total of about 3,000 children adopted from other countries compared with similar studies of about 2,000 domestically adopted children in the United States as well as to nonadopted children. They found that most international adoptees were well-adjusted although they were referred to psychiatric services more frequently than the nonadopted subjects. They also found that the international adoptees had fewer behavioral problems than the domestic adoptees; however, the age at the time of adoption among the domestic adoptees was unknown, so this finding needs further exploration, since children adopted at older ages and/or from foster care often have experienced abuse or neglect, and this troubled past may explain the child's propensity toward behavioral problems.

Howe, David. *Patterns of Adoption: Nature, Nurture and Psychosocial Development*. Oxford: Blackwell Science, 1998.

Juffer, Femmie, and Marinus H. van Ijzendoorn. "Behavior Problems and Mental Health Referrals of International Adoptees," *Journal of the American Medical Association* 293, no. 20 (May 25, 2005): 2,501–2,515.

Miller, Laurie. "International Adoption, Behavior, and Mental Health," *Journal of the American Medical Association* 293, no. 20 (May 25, 2005): 2,533–2,535.

adoption subsidy Monthly check paid to adoptive parents on behalf of a child adopted from the foster care system. The eligibility for the subsidy lies with the child rather than with the adoptive parents, and the child must have been removed from families that either received or would have met the criteria for the former Aid to Families with Dependent Children (AFDC) program, now called the Temporary Aid to Needy Families (TANF) program. The children must also have special needs. (Most children in the foster care system are defined as children with special needs by virtue of their age, race, the need to be placed with siblings, or other qualifiers.) In fiscal year 2001, 39,135 children in the United States received an adoption subsidy.

Major adoptive parent groups, such as the North American Council on Adoptable Children in St. Paul, Minnesota, have long supported the adoption subsidy as an important means to aid parents who have adopted children from foster care.

The ADOPTION ASSISTANCE AND CHILD WELFARE ACT OF 1980 was the initial enabling legislation that authorized federal subsidies on the behalf of adopted foster children. Prior to that time, only some states offered subsidies to encourage adoption. Today all states offer subsidy programs as a result of federal legislation. Some children receive both federal and additional state-funded subsidies, depending on the state.

According to a 2005 report from the U.S. Department of Health and Human Services on adoption subsidies, less than $400,000 was spent on adoption subsidies in 1981 and this amount increased to $1.3 billion in fiscal year 2002. Subsidy expenses are expected to reach about $2.5 billion by fiscal year 2008.

Determining Eligibility

In most cases, a determination is made of the child's eligibility prior to the time of adoption, and a written adoption assistance agreement is drawn up between the adopting parents and the state or other public agency with legal custody of the child.

In some cases, adoptive parents have sought a subsidy for their child months or years after the adoption has been finalized, based on new information about the child or serious medical problems that have occurred, as well as a major negative change in the family's financial status. States vary in how such situations are handled. Some adoptive parents have sued and prevailed while others have not.

Children with special needs who are adopted under the federal program are also eligible for MEDICAID. The Medicaid card is automatically issued by the state in which the child resides with the adoptive parents. In the past, when children were adopted from other states or moved with their adoptive families to other states, the "sending" state issued the Medicaid card; however, many providers refused to accept an out-of-state card. As a result, the rules were changed.

Statistics on Adoption Subsidies

The results of a study analyzing state statistics on subsidies was provided in the 2005 report from the Department of Health and Human Services, based on data from the Adoption and Foster Care Analysis Reporting System, or AFCARS. The study found that 88 percent of the foster children adopted in fiscal year 2001 received a subsidy, and the median subsidy was $444 per month. (A median is not the same as an average. A median is the middle point, in which half are below and half are above the median amount.)

States vary considerably in their median adoption subsidies, ranging from highs of $856 in Iowa and $741 in the District of Columbia to lows of $171 in Indiana and $174 in Puerto Rico. States were also ranked in order of their median monthly payment amounts. States such as Missouri and Idaho both received rankings of 38 because they paid the same median amount in adoption subsidies. (See Table I.)

The percent of children who were adopted from foster care in fiscal year 2001 and the percent who received a subsidy also varied considerably from state to state. For example, in some states, nearly all children adopted from foster care received a subsidy, as with Minnesota (99.3 percent), Maine (99.2 percent), and Wisconsin (99.2 percent). In other states, less than half of the foster children who were adopted received a subsidy, as with Connecticut (16.4 percent), Georgia (48.3 percent), and Alabama (46.8 percent). See Table II for a state-by-state breakdown of the percentage of children adopted from foster care who received an adoption subsidy.

The study also found that the following groups of children were affected by the subsidy:

- Children adopted by their foster parents were more likely to receive subsidies than other groups.

- Children over age six were more likely to receive a subsidy.

- Hispanic children and children adopted by Hispanic mothers received lower subsidies, although the researchers did not speculate on the reasons for this difference.

TABLE I: MEDIAN MONTHLY ADOPTION SUBSIDY AMOUNT, BY STATE, FISCAL YEAR 2001

State	Number of Children with Subsidy	Amount in Dollars	State Ranking
Alabama	111	$241	39
Alaska	271	$650	4
Arizona	687	$479	18
Arkansas	262	$425	23
California	8,982	$441	20
Colorado	515	$510	15
Connecticut	73	$659	3
Delaware	112	$479	18
District of Columbia	130	$741	2
Florida	1,123	$300	37
Georgia	412	$411	24
Hawaii	216	$529	12
Idaho	104	$275	38
Illinois	3,917	$410	25
Indiana *	294	$171	41
Iowa	504	$856	1
Kansas	295	$400	29
Kentucky	364	$600	6
Louisiana	428	$353	35
Maine	341	$650	4
Maryland	796	$543	11
Massachusetts	644	$471	19
Michigan	2,868	$591	7
Minnesota	561	$427	22
Mississippi *	—	—	—
Missouri	1,052	$275	38
Montana	248	$408	26
Nebraska	201	$527	13
Nevada *	—	—	—
New Hampshire	79	$552	9
New Jersey	899	$437	21
New Mexico *	135	$503	16
New York *	—	—	—
North Carolina	1,170	$365	32
North Dakota	91	$402	28
Ohio	2,116	$500	17
Oklahoma	899	$360	33
Oregon	1,038	$400	29
Pennsylvania	1,368	$510	15
Rhode Island	265	$407	27
South Carolina	364	$359	34
South Dakota	63	$390	31
Tennessee	517	$402	28
Texas	1,681	$516	14
Utah	266	$300	37

State	Number of Children with Subsidy	Amount in Dollars	State Ranking
Vermont	99	$549	10
Virginia	424	$344	36
Washington	1,107	$572	8
West Virginia	277	$400	29
Wisconsin	696	$639	5
Wyoming	39	$399	30
Puerto Rico	31	$174	40

* These states had missing or invalid subsidy amount data for more than 30 percent of their cases.

Source: Adapted from Office of the Assistant Secretary for Planning and Evaluation, *Understanding Adoption Subsidies: An Analysis of AFCARS Data.* U.S. Department of Health and Human Services, Washington, D.C., 2005, A-14, A-15, A-16.

- Children adopted by single females received higher subsidies than children adopted by married couples.
- Children who waited longer from the point of the termination of parental rights (greater than 18 months) received a greater monthly subsidy than children who were adopted more quickly.

Deferred Subsidies

Deferred (delayed and which may never be implemented) subsidy agreements are offered for a small number of some foster children who are adopted, should the needs of the child or the family warrant a subsidy. Overall, less than 1 percent of children receive deferred subsidies.

Changes in Subsidies

Adoption subsidy payments may change or may stop altogether, depending on circumstances. Federal subsidies end when the child is 18 unless he or she is physically or mentally handicapped, in which case, at state option, payments may continue until the child is 21. The subsidy payment will end if the adoptive parents are no longer supporting or are no longer legally responsible to support the child or if the parents (or the child) die.

TABLE II: PROPORTION OF CHILDREN ADOPTED FROM FOSTER CARE WHO RECEIVED SUBSIDY ASSISTANCE, BY STATE, FY 2001

State	Number of Adopted Children	Percent Receiving Any Subsidy	Percent Receiving No Subsidy
Alabama	237	46.8	53.2
Alaska	278	97.5	2.5
Arizona	938	94.3	5.7
Arkansas	361	89.2	10.8
California	9,822	91.5	8.5
Colorado	596	92.1	7.9
Connecticut	444	16.4	83.6
Delaware	115	97.4	2.6
District of Columbia	227	57.3	42.7
Florida	1,748	64.2	35.8
Georgia	896	48.3	51.7
Hawaii	260	83.1	16.9
Idaho	123	84.6	15.4
Illinois	4,079	96.2	3.8
Indiana	867	51.8	48.2
Iowa	659	76.5	23.5
Kansas	423	72.8	27.2
Kentucky	571	70.8	29.2
Louisiana	470	91.1	8.9
Maine	363	99.2	0.8
Maryland	812	98.4	1.6
Massachusetts	721	89.3	10.7
Michigan	2,975	96.4	3.6
Minnesota	565	99.3	0.7
Mississippi	264	81.4	18.6
Missouri	1,091	96.4	3.6
Montana	275	90.2	9.8
Nebraska	292	68.8	31.2
Nevada	243	94.7	5.3
New Hampshire	95	88.4	11.6
New Jersey	1,025	90.1	9.9
New Mexico	369	89.4	10.6
New York	3,888	97.9	2.1
North Carolina	1,298	94.2	5.8
North Dakota	145	62.8	37.2
Ohio	2,225	96.0	4.0
Oklahoma	955	99.5	0.5
Oregon	1,071	99.0	1.0
Pennsylvania	1,525	90.2	9.8
Rhode Island	267	99.6	0.4
South Carolina	364	100	0.0
South Dakota	97	64.9	35.1
Tennessee	638	81.2	18.8
Texas	2,317	72.6	27.4
Utah	348	77.3	22.7
Vermont	116	85.3	14.7
Virginia	493	95.5	4.5
Washington	1,203	97.7	2.3
West Virginia	362	91.7	8.3
Wisconsin	753	99.2	0.8
Wyoming	46	93.5	6.5
Puerto Rico	250	13.2	86.8
Total	50,565	88.1	11.9

Source: Adapted from Office of the Assistant Secretary for Planning and Evaluation, *Understanding Adoption Subsidies: An Analysis of AFCARS Data.* U.S. Department of Health and Human Services, Washington, D.C., 2005, A-8, A-9.

Subsidies Facilitate Adoptions, and the Lack of Subsidies May Predict Problems

Often the existence of a subsidy may mean the difference between children being adopted or remaining in foster care. (This is why Congress, responding to child advocacy groups, created legislation enabling subsidies.)

Researcher Richard Barth found that the receipt of adoption subsidies was a positive element in the success of the adoption of a child with SPECIAL NEEDS.

Families with high-risk placements disrupted less often when the family received a subsidy. Perhaps the subsidy eased the financial burden for the family that succeeded, and the lack of one added to the problems of the families who were denied subsidies or who received inadequate subsidies.

Authors L. Anne Babb and Rita Laws of *Adopting and Advocating for the Special Needs Child: A Guide for Parents and Professionals* say that sometimes there are "roadblocks" to receiving an adoption subsidy. For example, social workers may fail to inform families about adoption subsidies or they may not know how to manage the application process. They may also view such payments as "charity" and thus discourage adoptive parents from applying for them.

In one study, described in *After Adoption: The Needs of Adopted Youth,* the researchers found risk factors in predicting behavioral problems in the child. One risk factor lay with families who needed services that were not offered in the subsidy agreement that the families had made with the state agency.

Babb and Laws say that there are three major forms of subsidies: the basic rate, the specialized rate, and the state-funded subsidy. The basic rate is the lowest rate and the most common rate. It is usually lower than the monthly rate paid to a foster parent. The specialized rate is for children with severe special needs; specialized rates may vary from state to state; and states may also have subcategories of specialized rates. The state-funded rate is for children who are in state custody, but for some reason they do not qualify for the other two forms of subsidy.

Babb, L. Anne, and Rita Laws. *Adopting and Advocating for the Special Needs Child: A Guide for Parents and Professionals.* Westport, Conn.: Bergin & Garvey, 1997.

Barth, Richard P., and Marianne Berry. *Adoption & Disruption: Rates, Risks, and Responses.* New York: Aldine De Groyter, 1988.

Howard, Jeanne A., and Susan Livingston Smith. *After Adoption: The Needs of Adopted Youth.* Washington, D.C.: CWLA Press, 2003.

Office of the Assistant Secretary for Planning and Evaluation. *Understanding Adoption Subsidies: An Analysis of AFCARS Data.* U.S. Department of Health and Human Services, Washington, D.C., 2005.

Wiedemeier Bower, Jeanette, and Rita Laws. *Support for Families of Children with Special Needs: A Policy Analysis of Adoption Subsidy Programs in the United States.* St. Paul, Minn.: North American Council on Adoptable Children, July 2002.

adoption triad   Concept describing the genetic and/or legal relationship of the birthparents, adoptive parents, and adopted child to each other. Those who support the concept of a "triad" rather than a "triangle" or a "circle" believe that the triad concept is more clear because it does not connote a tightly knit relationship.

Rather than being at opposite ends, as in a triangle, or facing each other, as in a circle, the triad describes the major parties to the adoption but does not presume there will be a continuing relationship between the birthparents and the adopted person (although such a relationship could theoretically develop as in the case of an OPEN ADOPTION).

adoption triangle   Similar concept to the ADOPTION CIRCLE; refers to the adopted person, birthparents, and adoptive parents as three points on the triangle and the three parties most involved in an adoption. It is considered a negative phrase by many adoption professionals.

See also ADOPTION TRIAD.

adoptive parents   People who lawfully adopt children. (This entry concentrates on nonrelative adoptions. See GRANDPARENT ADOPTIONS or RELATIVE ADOPTIONS for information on those topics.) They may adopt children who are infants, older children, or adolescents. Rarely, adults adopt other adults, for purposes of inheritance and/or the personal affection they have in an informal parent–child-like relationship.

Adoptive parents may adopt children of the same race or of another race. Some adoptive parents adopt children from their own country, while others adopt children from other countries. Some adoptive parents are infertile, while others already have one or more biological children. Some do not know if they are fertile because they have never sought to create a pregnancy, as with some single adoptive parents. One common denominator of nearly all adoptive parents is that they hope to become loving parents to the child(ren) they adopt.

Age of Adoptive Parents

Most individuals who seek to adopt infants range in age from their late 20s to their early 40s. Some agencies have an upper age limit and will not accept applicants older than age 45 (or some other age cutoff).

Nearly half of the parents who adopted children from foster care in fiscal year 2001 were ages 30–39 years: 47.9 percent of mothers and 44.1 percent of fathers. (See table for characteristics of adoptive families who adopted foster children.)

It should be noted, however, that adoptive parents who adopt internationally may be older than those who adopt infants domestically. Age guidelines may be less strict among some countries because so many children in orphanages urgently need parents. Another reason some countries allow older individuals to adopt is a differing cultural attitude toward age. In some countries, people are esteemed because they have more life experience.

Thus, if the health of the adoptive applicants is good, they may be able to adopt children beyond the age of 50 years. Other countries, however, have age guidelines that are as strict as or even stricter than U.S. adoption agencies have for infants born in the United States.

As with other limiting criteria, however, age limits are often relaxed when a child is considered to fall into a special needs category by virtue of the child's race or ethnicity, age, sibling group membership, disability, or another category that is considered a special needs category. In addition, if the adoptive parents have been the foster parents to the child, age restrictions are usually relaxed as well.

Marital Status

Most adoptive parents are married couples; for example, data on children adopted from foster care in fiscal year 2001 revealed that two-thirds (66.8 percent) of the adoptive families were married couples. (See table.) The next largest percentage of adoptive parents is single females, or a total of 29.6 percent. The percentage of married couple adoptive parents is probably higher among adoptions arranged independently and through private adoption agencies. However, single people also adopt independently and through private (nongovernmental) adoption agencies.

If singles are openly gay or lesbian they may adopt in most states, with the exception of Florida, while in other states, adoption may be prohibitive or difficult. (See GAYS AND LESBIANS ADOPTING CHILDREN.) It is unknown as of this writing what impact the legal marriages of gays and lesbians, such as in Massachusetts, will have on the adoption of children.

Preadoptive Relationship with the Child

In the majority of cases of children adopted from foster care, the adoptive parents had a prior relationship with the child. (See table.) Most adoptive parents (52.3 percent of the total) were the child's foster parents, followed by the child's relatives (21.1 percent). Only in 15.3 percent of the cases was there no prior relationship with the child. This is in stark contrast to adoptions of children *not* in the foster care system, in which case at least half of all adopted children are adopted by nonrelatives with no prior relationship with the children.

Education

According to the National Center for Health Statistics, in 1999, of women ages 22–44 at the time of interview who had ever adopted, about 33 percent were college graduates or higher. Another 27 percent had some college although no degree. Thus, the majority (60 percent) were either college graduates or had some college education. About 24 percent of the adoptive mothers were high school graduates.

Income Level

Income data were not available for all the women in the National Center for Health Statistics report in 1999, but of the data available, more than half (about 55 percent) of the married adoptive mothers ages 22–44 were at an income level of 300 percent or more above the poverty level. Only 15 percent were at the 0–149 percent poverty level.

Parents who adopt their foster children generally are blue-collar or working-class, primarily because most foster parents tend to fall into these categories. Increasingly, relatives are being encouraged to adopt children in the foster-care system. This population of parents is older and has fewer financial resources than the nonrelated family adopting foster care children. Fees involved in adopting a former foster child are usually nonexistent, and subsidies may be available to those parents who adopt children with special needs from the public child welfare system.

In contrast, adoptive parents who adopt infants through adoption agencies or with the assistance of attorneys in the United States, as well as those who adopt children internationally, are primarily middle-class individuals, largely because of the significant expenses involved in adopting outside the foster care system.

Foster Parent Status

Some adoptive parents were previously foster parents to the children they subsequently adopted. In many states, the majority of the children adopted through the state social services department were adopted by their foster parents. (See FOSTER PARENT ADOPTION.) In such cases, when the court terminated parental rights, the foster parents requested permission to adopt the child. Such placements are often called foster/adopt placements.

Studies by Richard Barth and other researchers have revealed that foster parent adoptions of children from the public child welfare system disrupt at a lower rate than "new" adoptions, and

**CHARACTERISTICS OF FAMILIES WHO ADOPTED CHILDREN FROM FOSTER CARE,
BY AGE GROUPS OF CHILDREN, FISCAL YEAR 2001**

	Age 0–5		Age 6–12		Age 13–17		Total	
	Number	Percent	Number	Percent	Number	Percent	Number	Percent
Number of adopted children	24,415	48.2	21,569	42.5	4,719	9.3	50,703	100.0
Adoptive family structure								
Married couple	16,289	71.7	12,041	62.4	2,446	59.8	30,776	66.8
Unmarried couple	354	1.6	245	1.3	37	0.9	636	1.4
Single female	5,794	25.5	6,460	33.5	1,405	34.3	13,659	29.6
Single male	275	1.2	546	2.8	205	5.0	1,026	2.2
Total	22,712	100.0	19,292	100.0	4,093	100.0	46,097	100.0
Preadoptive parent-child relationship								
Foster parent	13,730	56.3	10,534	48.9	2,237	47.4	26,501	52.3
Stepparent	57	0.2	47	0.2	13	0.3	117	0.2
Other relative	4,579	18.8	5,034	23.4	1,100	23.3	10,713	21.1
Nonrelative	3,847	15.8	3,248	15.1	655	13.9	7,750	15.3
Adoptive mother's age								
18–29	10,626	51.6	4,592	26.5	82	2.3	15,300	36.8
30–39	8,024	38.9	9,678	55.8	2,231	61.5	19,933	47.9
40 and older	1,954	9.5	3,078	17.7	1,314	36.2	6,346	15.3
Total	20,604	100.0	17,348	100.0	3,627	100.0	41,579	100.0
Adoptive father's age								
18–29	5,309	34.1	1,750	13.1	32	1.2	7,091	22.3
30–39	6,058	38.9	6,850	51.2	1,083	39.2	13,991	44.1
40 and older	4,225	27.1	4,784	35.7	1,646	59.6	10,655	33.6
Total	15,592	100.0	13,384	100.0	2,761	100.0	31,737	100.0
Child same race/ethnicity as adoptive parents								
Yes	14,483	91.3	11,710	93.9	2,595	96.0	28,788	92.8
No	1,378	8.7	758	6.1	107	4.0	2,243	7.2
Total	15,861	100.0	12,468	100.0	2,702	100.0	31,031	100.0

Notes:
1. Numbers in categories may not add to the total number of adopted children due to missing data.
2. More than one preadoptive parent-child relationship could be specified for a child, therefore the denominator for each category is based on the number of responses for that category.
3. A child was considered the same race as adoptive parents if the child was classified as white, African-American, Hispanic, or "other," and at least one parent was classified the same. "Other" includes American Indians, Asians, Native Hawaiians, and children with more than one race designation. The percentage of transracial adoptions reported here may be lower than that reported elsewhere due to differences in how this variable is calculated.
Source: Adapted from Office of the Assistant Secretary for Planning and Evaluation, *Understanding Adoption Subsidies: An Analysis of AFCARS Data*. U.S. Department of Health and Human Services, Washington, D.C., 2005, pages 3–7.

various states have begun instituting programs to train people who wish to become foster parents about adoption as well, sometimes combining classes for adoptive and foster parents. (See DISRUPTION/DISSOLUTION.)

A possible reason for this success is that foster parents have had ongoing in-service training opportunities and also ongoing social work post-placement support. Adoptive parents who were not foster parents receive counseling and assistance to the point of finalization, when services stop.

See POST-LEGAL ADOPTIVE SERVICES.

Infertility

Infertility is a prerequisite to apply to many adoption agencies placing babies born in the United States, but it is generally not a requirement for families adopting children from other countries. When infertility is a prerequisite, the applicant may be required to provide medical proof of infertility.

Many adoptive parents have a primary infertility, which means they are childless and have never borne a child. Others have a secondary infertility, which means they have had one or more children but are now infertile.

When infertility is an issue of concern to the agency, the social worker seeks to determine if the couple has successfully resolved most of their conflicts and anxieties about their infertility so they will be able to fully accept an adopted child.

Fertility or infertility is generally not an issue when a special needs adoption is being contemplated.

Optional adopters or preferential adopters are individuals who are fertile but prefer to adopt rather than reproduce.

Good Character and Emotional Stability

Most agencies require at least three written references of the applicants' good characters. In addition, in the case of either a public or private agency or independent adoption, there is nearly always a HOME STUDY made of the adoptive family. Part of that home study is to determine if the prospective family is of good character. In addition, police checks are run to ensure the applicant has no criminal record, and the state abuse registry is checked to verify the applicant has not been accused of child abuse. Agencies operated under religious auspices may require a reference from a member of the clergy of the applicants' faith group.

Some applicants must provide a statement from a mental health professional that the applicant is of sound mental health.

Citizenship

United States citizenship may be required by agencies or attorneys arranging the adoption of children in the United States; hence, it can be assumed that most adoptive parents are U.S. citizens. If a couple in the United States wishes to adopt a child from another country, at least one of them must be a U.S. citizen.

Number of Children in the Home

Agencies that place infants born in the United States may restrict their applications to childless couples or couples with one child. In contrast, most international adoption agencies will accept families who already have one or more children, because most countries outside the United States do not insist on families who are childless.

When agencies place children from other countries and/or children with special needs, the number of children already in the home is not usually seen as a barrier, but the ages of the children in the home may determine the age(s) of the child or children to be placed. For example, the social worker may not wish to place teenagers with a family who has preschoolers because the small children will require a great deal of the family's time. Many social workers prefer that children newly placed in the home be younger than children already living there.

Parent Preparation

The success of an adoption is directly linked to the preparedness of the parents, particularly if it is an adoption from foster care, or of children with special needs from the United States, or an international adoption. In one study of parental preparation in relation to the adoption of children with special needs based on responses of 368 adoptive parents, reported in *Child & Adolescent Social Work Journal* in 2004, parents felt insufficiently prepared particularly when the child had many foster care placements before the adoption, known sexual, emotional or physical abuse, or physical neglect in the past, difficulty in attaching to the adoptive parents, and known behavioral or emotional concerns that were noted during the placement.

Said the authors, "These factors all result in an increased level of special-need that a family system must accommodate when an adoptive child with a complicated history of social relationships is placed in a permanency focused environment. Parents may have difficulty preparing for their children's needs, especially when they lack knowledge about the child's history and lack the experience and skills necessary to address the needs, impacted by that history."

The level of support that the parents perceived receiving from the agency both before and after the adoption was also associated with how prepared the parents felt. Some parents, such as former foster parents, rated themselves as well-prepared and made such comments as "After having the girls for a year and working with the doctors, we knew what we were getting ourselves into. We have no regrets."

Some parents complained of a lack of support and information from the agency. For example, one parent said, "We were told they were children who did not have many problems. We found out that we faced attachment disorder, sexual abuse, children who had been taught to fight and shoplift. We were in no way prepared for that."

According to the authors, the more knowledge and experience the parents had on parenting children with special needs, the more prepared they felt. Said the authors, "The best way to have gained experience, as expressed in parents' qualitative responses was receiving adequate training and information, adopting previously, and having experience with other children as foster or biological parents."

Attitudes of Others

Often support or the lack of support from family and friends for an adoption is important to adoptive parents. Some experts have reported on the "stigma" some adoptive parents feel, and the impression they have that adoption is perceived as "second class." (See ATTITUDES ABOUT ADOPTION.)

Adoptive Parents Evaluating Adoption

A British study of adopted adults and their adoptive parents yielded valuable information, reported in Lois Raynor's book, *The Adopted Child Comes of Age.* Of the adoptive parents who were interviewed, 85 percent reported that their overall experience with the child had been "very satisfactory" or "reasonably satisfactory." Of the families disappointed in the adoption experience and their child, several were unhappy because of severe health problems experienced by the child. It seems unlikely that the families knew about these health problems at the time when they adopted the children because Raynor said, "Probably very few parents would have found their experience really satisfying with these four children who developed such serious handicaps, and three of these families certainly had made the best of the situation."

The other families who were unhappy said that they did not like the child's personality, and most felt they were unable to "mold" the child to their own ways.

One family was very negative about illegitimacy, considering it a "curse." Raynor believed their child ultimately disappointing them was a self-fulfilling prophecy.

According to Raynor's study, the adoptive parents' perception of similarities between themselves and the child was critically important to parental satisfaction: 97 percent who thought the child was like them in appearance, interests, intelligence, or personality were happy with the adoption, while about 62 percent were satisfied when the child was perceived as different in these areas.

The child did not necessarily actually resemble adoptive parents nor was he or she very similar to them when observed by an outsider—it was the adoptive parents' perception of the similarity that was key.

See also ADOPTION SUBSIDY; ADULT ADOPTED PERSONS; DISRUPTION/DISSOLUTION; EMPLOYMENT BENEFITS; ENTITLEMENT; LARGE FAMILIES; PARENTAL LEAVE; SIBLINGS; SPECIAL NEEDS.

Chandra, Anjani, et al. "Adoption, Adoption Seeking, and Relinquishment for Adoption in the United States," Advance Data Number 306, National Center for Health Statistics, May 11, 1999.

Egbert, Susan C., and Elizabeth LaMont. "Factors Contributing to Parents' Preparation for Special-Needs Adoption," *Child and Adolescent Social Work Journal* 21, no. 6 (December 2004): 593–609.

Nelson, Katherine A. *On the Frontier of Adoption: A Study of Special Needs Adoptive Families.* New York: Child Welfare League of America, 1985.

Office of the Assistant Secretary for Planning and Evaluation. *Understanding Adoption Subsidies: An Analysis of AFCARS Data.* U.S. Department of Health and Human Services, Washington, D.C., 2005.

Raynor, Lois. *The Adopted Child Comes of Age.* London: George Allen & Unwin, 1980.

adult adopted persons   A person over age 18 who was adopted as a child or, in some cases, (usually for reasons of inheritance) as an adult, also known as adult adoptees. Most adopted adults were adopted as infants or children.

Some adopted adults have stated they resent the label of "adopted child" that society often places on all adopted persons, regardless of age. They believe this phrase connotes an aura of immaturity and diminishes the adopted person's responsible adult status.

Psychological Adjustment of Adopted Persons

Most adults who were adopted as children appear to have successfully resolved any conflicts stemming from their adoption.

Studies of adopted adults reveal those who are the most well-adjusted and confident have known of their adoptive status for a long time; however, some who learned of their adoption later in life are able to accept this information constructively.

Katherine A. Kowal and Karen Maitland Schilling reported on adult adopted persons in the *American Journal of Orthopsychiatry.* They studied 110 adopted adults, ages 17 to 77, recruited through adoption agencies and a "search" group; 75 percent were female, and 108 were white.

The adopted adults were asked for their perceptions of their adoptions and could agree or disagree with one or more of the suggested statements. The results: 35.45 percent reported they felt "chosen or special"; 21.82 percent reported they felt "no different from anybody else"; 20.91 percent reported "feeling different, but neither better nor worse than others"; 25.45 percent were "worried or insecure about being adopted"; and 17.27 percent were "embarrassed or uncomfortable with the fact of their adoption."

When asked what information they wish adoption agencies would provide to adoptive parents, presumably to be passed on to them later, the adults reported medical information as the most desired data—75 percent of the subjects wanted information on the birthparents' medical history.

Seventy-one percent said they wanted information on personality characteristics of the birthparents. (This information was actually given to only about 4 percent of the adopted persons.)

It is unclear whether adoption agencies had provided such information to the adoptive parents, but it seems likely that a personality appraisal probably was not given. In addition, the researchers stated that other studies had revealed that adoptive parents tend to present a very positive and euphemistic view of the birthparent. They wrote,

> Many subjects had been given a reason why they were placed for adoption, yet this information still ranked high on their list of things they wanted to know. . . .

Some other information desired by adopted adults included a physical description of birthparents; the ethnic background of the birthparents; information on the adopted person's early medical history; the names of the birthparents (in most cases, unknown to the adoptive parents); interests of the birthparents; the reasons why an adoption decision was made for the adopted person; the education and occupation of the birthparents; where they resided as young children before the adoption took place (in a foster home, with a relative, etc.); and other factors.

At least one study has found adopted persons to be better adjusted than those who were not adopted. Kathlyn Marquis and Richard Detweiler reported on their findings.

Wrote the authors, "Contrary to expectations, adopted persons are significantly more confident and view others more positively than do non-adopted persons."

In addition, the attitudes of adopted adults toward their parents was compared to the attitudes of nonadopted persons toward their parents. The researchers found that "adoptive parents are experienced as significantly more nurturant, comforting, predictable, protectively concerned and helpful than nonadoptive parents." (See also ADJUSTMENT.)

Adopted adults were also found to have a stronger sense of control over their lives and demonstrated more self-assurance of their own judgement.

The authors concluded,

> The adopted may be different but, in contrast to the literature, may be different by being more positive rather than more negative than their non-adopted peers . . . If, as the earlier literature implies, there were large numbers of mentally ill adopted adults, one would expect to find some indication of this in the community population

when compared with a similar community population of nonadopted peers . . .

It is important to note the overwhelming majority of adult adopted persons studied by Marquis and Detweiler were adopted as infants: 89 percent were adopted within three months of birth, and 95 percent were adopted within one year of birth.

The social and psychological adjustment of adopted persons who were adopted at an older age could yield very different results, particularly if they had been victims of child abuse or were placed in one or more foster care settings prior to the adoption. (See DISRUPTION for further information.)

Lois Raynor studied adopted adults among adopted Britons and reported her findings in her book *The Adopted Child Comes of Age*.

Out of 104 adopted adults interviewed, 80 percent reported their adoption experience was "very satisfactory" or "reasonably satisfactory" (58 percent reported very satisfactory, and 22 percent reported reasonably satisfactory).

Reported Raynor, "Of the three who were very unhappy in their adoption, one was a young woman who had been placed in a very busy and incredibly class-conscious family, who attributed everything, good or bad, to heredity." In another case, a very intelligent boy was placed in an "unsophisticated" family, and the parents were unable to control the child.

The third very unhappy adopted person had been placed shortly after his adoptive parents had lost a beloved infant because his birthmother had reclaimed him. "Apparently the adoptive mother had not been able to work through her grief at the time, as nearly 25 years later at the research interview she wept bitterly for her lost baby. The son said he had always been compared unfavourably with the reclaimed child."

It's readily apparent this family was in no way ready to accept a child at the time they were placed with one. Most social workers today would refuse to place a child in a home where the adoptive parents were grieving such a loss.

Adopted persons were also far happier about their adoption when they perceived some common grounds with their adoptive parents in interests, appearance, or other factors. Of the adopted adults who felt "very much like" their adoptive parents, 97 percent rated their adoption experience as satisfactory. Conversely, 52 percent who perceived themselves as "unlike or uncertain" rated the experience as satisfactory.

Individual satisfaction with information provided to the adopted person about the adoption was related to the perception of the adoption experience. It was not the amount of information provided but whether or not the individual felt it was a sufficient amount that was the critical element.

Raynor noted, "Some were content with very little while others wanted much more. No apparent relationship was found between satisfaction and how *often* the adoption was discussed within the family—this seemed to be a highly individual matter—but there *was* a clear relationship with the degree of ease and comfort people felt in being able to ask their adoptive parents for further information if they wanted it."

The adopted persons were also rated by Raynor on current levels of adjustment: 70 percent were rated as "excellent" or "good," 25 percent were "marginal," and 5 percent were "poor."

Among the 5 percent who were poorly adjusted, Raynor interviewed one man who was in prison and very depressed and had been delinquent since age eight. "The adoptive mother had died before he went to school, his uninterested father somewhat later, and he was brought up by an adoptive relative who felt it was her Christian duty but who had no enthusiasm for the task," reported Raynor.

Raynor also observed that biological parents are rarely contrasted with adoptive parents, nor are biological children asked later in life if they were and are happy.

No one knows what proportion of parents are satisfied with the children born to them, or vice versa. No one can say what proportion of young adults would be considered well-adjusted by the rather stringent criteria which we used in this project . . . the cost and technical problems in finding a properly matched sample of adopted adults have defeated all researchers so far.

In a unique longitudinal study of adopted adults in the United Kingdom, researchers found positive results, particularly among adopted women, who fared better than their nonadopted cohort in some cases.

In this study, drawn from the National Child Development Study in England, the adopted children were followed at age seven, 11, and 16 years and then at age 33. Nearly all (about 92 percent) were adopted under the age of one year. Researchers compared the adopted adults to individuals who were born to nonmarried mothers but who were not adopted. The adopted adults were similar to the nonadopted group in that they were of lower than usual birth weight and were born to young mothers who received little or no prenatal care. The adopted adults were also compared to nonadopted individuals born to married couples.

Researchers obtained data from members of the original study group at age 33, including 84 adopted adults (37 women and 47 men), 137 birth comparison subjects, and 1,489 subjects in the general population.

They found that adopted females were in the best socioeconomic situation, with general population subjects second and birth comparison subjects last. They also found that adopted males fared better in housing and occupation than the birth comparison subjects. They did find that the adopted males were more likely to have been fired from a job than subjects in the other groups, although the reason for this was unclear.

In looking at relationships, men and women in the birth comparison groups were the most likely to have experienced a marital/cohabitation breakdown as compared with the adopted adults or general population adults, who experienced about the same rate of marital breakdowns.

Birth comparison women were more likely to have had unplanned pregnancies and to smoke during pregnancy than the other two groups. Interestingly, adopted women delayed childbearing the longest. The mean age for the adopted woman having her first child was 26.2 years, compared to 24.4 in the general population group and 23.1 years in the birth comparison group.

In terms of emotional disorders, the birth comparison group fared worst and the birth comparison group males had higher rates of alcoholism than the other groups.

In terms of social supports available to them, women across the board reported higher levels of support than men; however, adopted women reported experiencing the highest levels of support from friends, parents, and others, while birth comparison individuals reported the lowest.

In general, the birth comparison group fared the worst in nearly all measures. Said the authors, "Members of the birth comparison group were in less favorable social and material circumstances than the majority of cohort members." Both men and women had been vulnerable to relationship breakdowns, and women in particular reported high rates of current depressive affect and past help-seeking for emotional problems, as well as somewhat restricted social support.

"Adopted women, by contrast, showed no elevated rates of problems in any of these domains; indeed, their levels of emotional problems were rather lower than in the population comparison group, and their perceived social supports in some ways more extensive."

It was unclear why the adopted women fared better than the adopted men, although the researchers speculated that perhaps genetic differences caused more difficult adjustments in males than females.

See also ADOLESCENT ADOPTED PERSONS; ADOPTIVE PARENTS; FOSTER CARE; PSYCHIATRIC PROBLEMS OF ADOPTED PERSONS; REUNION; SEARCH; SPECIAL NEEDS; TRANSRACIAL ADOPTION.

Brinich, Paul M., and Evelin B. Brinich. "Adoption and Adaptation," *The Journal of Nervous and Mental Disease* 170, no. 8: 489–493.

Collishaw, S., et al. "Infant Adoption: Psychosocial Outcomes in Adulthood," *Social Psychiatry and Psychiatric Epidemiology* 33, no. 2 (February 1998): 57–65.

Howe, David. *Patterns of Adoption.* Oxford: Blackwell Science, 1998.

Kowal, Katherine A., and Karen Maitland Schilling. "Adoption through the Eyes of Adult Adoptees," *American Journal of Orthopsychiatry* 55 (July 1985) 354–362.

Smith, Jerome, and Franklin I. Miroff. *You're Our Child: The Adoption Experience.* Lanham, Mo.: Madison Books, 1987.

Marquis, Kathlyn S., and Richard A. Detweiler. "Does Adopted Mean Different? An Attributional Analysis," *Journal of Personality and Social Psychology* 48, no. 4 (1985): 1,054–1,066.

Raynor, Lois. *The Adopted Child Comes of Age.* London: George Allen & Unwin, 1980.

adults, adoption of   Refers to the adoption of a person who is over age 18 by another adult, usually for reasons of inheritance or to make official a long-standing informal parent-child relationship. The adopted adult voluntarily consents to the adoption, as does the adopter. In some states, notice of the adoption to birthparents may be required despite the adult status of the adopted person, and in other states, permission from the adopted person's spouse is required.

The overwhelming majority of all adoptions are of adults adopting children; however, it is legally permissible in all states for adults to adopt other adults if no fraud is intended. The laws governing the adopting of adults vary from state to state, as do restrictions. In many cases, the adopting party must be older than the person adopted.

In some cases, an adult homosexual may have attempted to adopt another adult homosexual as a way to create a legal relationship since they may not legally marry. However, some courts have denied such petitions on the grounds that such an adoption is not in the best interests of society in general; for example, in 1984 an adoption was denied in New York because of a lack of a "genuine" parent-child relationship.

Gay couples who are interested in protecting each other's right of inheritance would be better served by contacting an attorney to draw up wills. In addition, several courts have held that homosexual individuals who have been involved in long-term relationships may inherit on the principle of an implied trust.

Adult adoption does not usually involve any HOME STUDY, since presumably the adult to be adopted can manage his or her own affairs and does not need the protection of a social worker's analysis of the adopter; however, some states may require a social worker's report for all adoptions.

advertising and promotion in adoption   Methods to attract individuals interested in adopting children or attract individuals wishing to place children (usually infants) for adoption. The INTERNET is increasingly used to recruit both adoptive parents and parents considering placing their children for adoption. Paid advertising is used by some adop-

tion agencies and attorneys (such as yellow pages advertisements or advertisements in newspapers and magazines) as well as by some prospective parents who are seeking to adopt infants. Some agencies that place children from other countries advertise, seeking adoptive parents.

State or county agencies that seek to recruit adoptive parents for WAITING CHILDREN who are in foster care are usually not charged a fee by the media, since the adoption of foster children is perceived as a public good.

Promoting the Adoption of "Waiting Children"

A popular form of advertising used by state social services departments nationwide is the "WEDNESDAY'S CHILD" type of program (or Thursday, Friday, or whatever day the feature runs). Usually showing an older or minority child who needs adoptive parents, and sometimes a sibling group, the television media show a videotape of the child interacting with others and offer information on the child, such as the child's age and first name, with a number to call for further information. The goal is to interest people who are viewing the program and inspire them to investigate adoption.

Adoptive parent support groups sometimes assist state or private adoption agencies by publishing photos and descriptions of older children or children with SPECIAL NEEDS in their newsletters.

Couples Advertising for Babies

In addition to advertisements or promotions run by adoption agencies to seek prospective adoptive parents, people hoping to adopt infants sometimes use advertising to identify a pregnant woman interested in placing her child. This is a controversial type of advertising and is not lawful in some states, such as California, Connecticut, Georgia, Idaho, Kansas, Kentucky, Louisiana, Maine, and Massachusetts. In some states, prospective parents may advertise their desire to adopt in newspapers, if they have a completed home study, such as in North Carolina, Texas, Washington, and Wisconsin. In some states, such as Florida, only agencies and attorneys may place advertisements for prospective couples.

Some couples advertise their desire to adopt on a variety of Web site locations on the Internet. It is important for individuals seeking to adopt to contact a competent attorney experienced in adoption or a reputable adoption agency before advertising in the newspaper or on the Internet, to avoid common pitfalls. (See FRAUD IN ADOPTION.)

Individuals who wish to adopt and who place advertisements seeking pregnant women interested in placing their babies for adoption usually refer to a couple's infertile status and state in emotional language that they "long for" a child and will provide a good home. In many cases, these advertisements are sincere. In some cases, advertisements that appear to have been placed by people desperately seeking a baby are actually placed by an attorney or agency trying to identify pregnant women for adoptive parents. (There is no way to know the prevalence of misleading advertising, but it does exist.)

Those who oppose advertising for babies do not approve of a direct immediate contact between a pregnant woman and prospective parents, and they prefer that the initial contact be made through a social worker or attorney. They also believe that advertising demeans adoption and treats babies as commodities rather than human beings.

There are also risks involved for pregnant women responding to advertisements, including the risk of contacting an unscrupulous person who plans to sell the baby and defraud the woman. Most pregnant women considering adoption are in a crisis situation and unable to judge the sincerity or reputation of a person through a phone call. They are likely to be completely unaware of adoption laws and are highly vulnerable.

Others who support advertising believe that it enables prospective parents to reach pregnant women who may be interested in adoption but who would otherwise not make direct contact with an adoption agency or an attorney. Many, but not all, adoptions that result from contacts that are made by prospective adoptive parents with birthparents through advertising are OPEN ADOPTIONS.

Agency Outreach Ads

In recent years, some adoption agencies have begun aggressive advertising campaigns, primarily to attract pregnant women considering adoption for their babies. In addition to an ad in the telephone book's yellow pages, larger agencies often offer a toll-free hotline, and some agencies use billboards, brochures, and other marketing techniques.

When contacted by a pregnant woman, such responsive agencies act immediately rather than waiting until office hours to contact the woman, while less responsive agencies are not staffed or prepared to handle cases except during business hours. Responsive agencies may meet the woman at her home or in a designated place, such as a local fast-food chain, so she need not seek transportation to drive to the agency office so that they can obtain the needed information.

See also ADOPTION AGENCIES; ADOPTIVE PARENTS; BIRTHMOTHER; PHOTOLISTINGS.

Adamec, Christine. *The Complete Idiot's Guide to Adoption.* New York: Alpha Books, 2005.

AIDS   See HUMAN IMMUNODEFICIENCY VIRUS.

alcohol abuse and birthmothers   See FETAL ALCOHOL SYNDROME.

alcoholism and adopted persons   Alcoholism is the excessive and chronic consumption of alcohol over time, causing severe problems in the individual's life as well as the lives of immediate family members. Alcoholism is also known as alcohol dependence. Some studies indicate that children whose birthparents were alcoholic have an increased risk to develop alcoholism themselves as adults, although the risk may be decreased by positive environmental influences or increased by negative environmental influences. Some studies have shown that males, whether adopted or not, have a greater risk for developing alcoholism than females, while other studies have found no gender differences. Alcoholism is a common problem in many eastern European countries, from where many children are adopted.

According to the National Institute on Alcohol Abuse and Alcoholism (NIAAA), alcoholism is characterized by an individual with three or more of the following indicators:

• A tolerance to alcohol (more alcohol is needed to achieve intoxication than in the past)

- Withdrawal symptoms (when alcohol is not consumed, physical symptoms occur, such as nausea, sweating, and shakiness)
- Use of the substance in a larger quantity than intended
- The persistent desire to cut down or to control the use of alcohol
- A significant amount of time spent on obtaining, using, or recovering from alcohol
- Drinking that occurs to avoid the symptoms of withdrawal
- Neglect of an individual's normal social, occupational, or recreational tasks
- Continued use of alcohol despite physical and psychological problems of the user

The NIAAA reported that an estimated 3.8 percent of the population in the United States was estimated to have a problem with alcoholism in 2002, which means that about 7.9 million people were alcoholics in the United States. Worldwide, many millions of people have alcohol dependence problems.

Studies on Substance Abuse and Alcoholism

According to a 2002 article in *Alcohol Research & Health* on sex differences among alcoholics, five adoption studies of individuals showed that males whose birthparents were alcoholics had a 1.6 to 3.6 times greater risk for alcoholism compared with adopted men with no birth family history of alcoholism. Studies of adopted females had mixed results, with some studies showing an increased risk for alcoholism among women with a family history of alcoholism, while others did not. Said the authors, "These results provided some evidence of possible sex differences in heritability, but are inconclusive because of the small numbers of alcoholic female adoptees in the study."

In a large study of greater than 1,000 alcoholic subjects and their families, the Collaborative Study on the Genetics of Alcoholism (COGA), described in a 2002 issue of *Alcohol Research & Health*, the researchers evaluated the genetic, psychological, and physiological traits of the participants. They found evidence for a genetic linkage in sibling pairs on the traits of alcoholism and depression, located

on chromosome 1. They also found evidence of a possible genetic link to alcohol dependence on chromosome 4. Further studies are likely to find other genetic links.

More recently, a 2003 article in *Archives of General Psychiatry* reported on the genetic and environmental influences on substance abuse of adolescents. The subjects were 345 monozygotic twin pairs (identical twins), 337 dizygotic twin pairs (fraternal twins), 306 biological sibling pairs, and 74 adoptive sibling pairs who were recruited through the Colorado Adoption Project. The researchers also found that in males and females, genetics appeared to play a greater part in the development of substance abuse, alcoholism, or drug addiction, and the environment was less important, although it played a role.

There are numerous studies on alcoholism among adopted adults, and one might wonder why there are so many studies if adopted adults are not at higher risk for alcoholism than the nonadopted population. Perhaps British author and researcher David Howe explained it best in his book *Patterns of Adoption:*

> The choice of behaviours [that are studied] by scientists is often that which also concerns policy makers and practitioners: education, mental health and antisocial behavior. To this extent, the knowledge produced about adopted children's development appears a little imbalanced, concentrating mainly on the disturbed and the deviant. More "normal" behaviours receive less attention. Thus, a digest of behavioural genetic research that might interest adoption workers needs to be read with this distortion in mind. By association, one can have the feeling that because these scientists write a lot about schizophrenia or crime using adoption as one of their "natural experiments," then adoptions themselves are beset with these behaviours. This, of course, is not the case.

Environmental Impacts

In an article on substance abuse (including alcoholism, drug addiction, and alcohol and drug abuse), published in a 2000 issue of *Alcoholism: Clinical and Experimental Research*, the researchers studied 442 adopted adults of alcoholic and nonalcoholic adoptive parents and 1,859 adult stepchildren of alcohol and nonalcoholic stepfathers. The researchers found that being reared by an alcoholic adoptive mother was associated with an increased risk for alcohol abuse but not dependency (alcoholism) in the adopted adult. Similarly, alcoholism in the stepparents did *not* increase the risk for alcoholism in stepchildren. Thus, the environment increased the risk for an alcohol abuse problem but not for an alcohol dependency.

The researchers also found that being reared by an alcoholic adoptive father predicted the use of illegal drugs and drug addiction in the adopted adults. Being raised by an alcoholic stepfather was correlated with alcohol abuse, illegal drug use, and drug addiction in the stepchildren.

A 1998 study in *Psychiatry* was on adult twins separated as infants, one adopted and the other reared by a biological parent (drawn from the Colorado Adoption Study). The study showed few differences between the twins, and both groups were within the normal range of behavior. However, the twin reared by the biological mother had attained a lower socioeconomic status and was more likely to drink excessively than the adopted twin. The researchers speculated that the more positive socioeconomic status of the adopted adult probably mitigated against excessive use of alcohol.

It should also be noted that PRENATAL EXPOSURES to alcohol, drugs, and even stress may increase the likelihood of addiction in adolescence and adulthood, and further studies are needed to evaluate this possibility.

See also FETAL ALCOHOL SYNDROME; GENETIC PREDISPOSITIONS; PSYCHIATRIC PROBLEMS OF ADOPTED PERSONS.

Bierut, Laura Jean, M.D. "Defining Alcohol-Related Phenotypes in Humans: The Collaborative Study on the Genetics of Alcoholism," *Alcohol Research & Health* 26, no. 3 (2002): 208–213.

Bohman, M., and S. Sigvarsson. "Outcomes in Adoption: Lessons from Longitudinal Studies," in *The Psychology of Adoption*. New York; Oxford University Press, 1990.

Grant, Bridget F., et al. "The 12-month prevalence and trends in DSM-IV alcohol abuse and dependence: United States, 1991–1992 and 2001–2002," *Drug and Alcohol Dependence* 74 (2004): 223–234.

Gwinnell, Esther, M.D., and Christine Adamec. *The Encyclopedia of Addictive Behaviors and Addictions*. New York: Facts On File, 2006.

Howe, David, *Patterns of Adoption*. Oxford: Blackwell Science, 1998.

Li, Ting-Kai, M.D. "The Genetics of Alcoholism," *Alcohol Alert* 60 (July 2003): 1–4.

Newlin, David B., et al. "Environmental Transmission of DSM-IV Substance Use Disorders in Adoptive and Step Families," *Alcoholism: Clinical and Experimental Research* 24, no. 12 (December 2000): 1,785–1,794.

Prescott, Carol A. "Sex Differences in the Genetic Risk for Alcoholism," *Alcohol Research & Health* 26, no. 2 (2002): 264–273.

Rhee, Soo Hyun, et al. "Genetic and Environmental Influences on Substance Initiation, Use, and Problem Use in Adolescents," *Archives of General Psychiatry* 60 (December 2003): 1,256–1,264.

Smyer, Michael A., et al. "Childhood Adoption; Long-Term Effects in Adulthood," *Psychiatry* 61 (Fall 1998): 191–205.

almshouses   Institutions designed in the 1800s to house poor children, adults, the elderly, and the mentally ill, generally with no distinctions made between these groups in terms of services; also known as "poorhouses."

Because of reports condemning such facilities as unsafe and unclean, almshouses fell out of favor with the public by the late 1800s and no longer exist today. An alternative to almshouses at that time was "outdoor relief," which was financial aid to the poor in their own homes, usually provided by a town "overseer of the poor" and in later years by the county or state public agencies. (See "A Brief History of Adoption" in the introduction of this book.)

According to author Homer Folks in his book, *The Care of Destitute, Neglected and Delinquent Children*, published in 1902, the first American almshouses were built in the latter part of the 1700s in such large cities as Philadelphia, New York City, Baltimore, and Boston.

Almshouses were later created in other states as one means of caring for the poor. In some cases, parents actually lived with the children in the almshouse. Orphans were also housed together with the indigent elderly and the mentally ill, as well as with juvenile delinquents. The percentages of families, orphans, and elderly varied with the facility, the state, and the conditions at the time. Later reformers decided it would be far preferable to separate children in orphanages, and separate institutions were created for different groups, such as children, the mentally ill, and the indigent elderly. (*In the Shadow of the Poorhouse: A Social History of Welfare in America* provides a depiction of almshouses and institutions.)

A Michigan report in 1870 revealed there were more than 200 children under age 16 in Michigan almshouses. Subsequent to the report, the state legislature created a state public school for dependent children in 1874.

Massachusetts began separating poor children from poor adults in 1872. Then in 1879, legislation required overseers of the poor to place the children of paupers either in families or orphan asylums.

The state of New York passed legislation in 1875 requiring the removal of all healthy children over age three from almshouses and placement of them into orphanages, families, or other institutions. (The age of the children to be removed was dropped to age two in 1878 and no longer exempted children who were not healthy.)

In 1878, Wisconsin followed suit with legislation ordering the removal of all children from almshouses. A state school housing the children was built in 1885.

The trend continued among states until the early 20th century, when orphaned, abandoned, and indigent children were cared for apart from almshouses with funds for outdoor relief, orphanages, and such social experiments as the ORPHAN TRAIN.

Folks, Homer. *The Care of Destitute, Neglected and Delinquent Children*. New York: Macmillan, 1902.

Katz, Michael B. *In the Shadow of the Poorhouse: A Social History of Welfare in America*. New York: Basic Books, 1986.

ambivalence The existence of two conflicting desires. When children over age 10 are offered an opportunity to be adopted, they often experience ambivalent feelings, for example, the desire to be loved in an adoptive home versus the fear of leaving the familiar foster home or group home.

The wishes of older children are almost always taken into account when an adoptive placement is considered, and many daylong or weekend visits may occur before the child feels ready to make a change and ultimately be adopted.

When sibling groups are involved, some siblings may wish to be adopted while others do not, causing feelings of ambivalence among all the children. A sibling who wants to be adopted may feel guilty about leaving behind the child who is unready or unwilling to be adopted, and conversely, a sibling who does not wish to be adopted may believe she or he is holding back the other children.

In addition, being adopted may signify to an older child a painful renouncement of the birthparents. Even though a child may have been abused severely enough for the state to have terminated parental rights, he or she may fear the final severing of psychological ties to the birthparents.

Trained social workers understand the ambivalence felt by older children who are to be adopted and can assist both foster parents and adopting parents with suggestions to ease the transition.

anemia, iron deficiency A blood disease that results in insufficient red blood cells. It is caused by an iron deficiency in the diet, poor absorption of iron, or blood loss. Sometimes anemia is linked to lead poisoning among children. Anemia is also found among girls and women with very heavy menstrual periods. Some medications may induce anemia, such as chemotherapy medications that are given to treat cancer.

An iron deficiency can affect the attention span and learning ability of a child or adolescent and consequently cause children to perform worse in school than they would otherwise perform with normal blood levels. Before a diagnosis of attention deficit/hyperactivity disorder (ADHD) is given, iron deficiency should be ruled out with blood testing. Iron supplementation can measurably improve academic performance among children and adolescents who were deficient in iron.

Anemia in children is also linked to developmental delays and mood problems.

Some foods that are often given to children in orphanages, such as teas, inhibit iron absorption, thus increasing the risk for iron deficiency anemia.

In considering internationally adopted children, as described by Dr. Miller in *The Handbook of International Adoption Medicine: A Guide for Physicians, Parents, and Providers,* the prevalence of iron deficiency anemia varies with the child's country of origin. In newly arrived Asian children, the rates range from about 2–3 percent among Korean children to 18.5 percent in children from India and 35 percent in children from China.

Symptoms and Diagnostic Path

Patients with iron deficiency anemia may have no symptoms if the anemia is mild. They may also have the following symptoms:

- Shortness of breath
- Pallor
- Sore tongue
- Brittle fingernails
- Headache
- Lethargy
- Dizziness
- Pica (A chronic compulsion to eat nonfood items, such as ice or dirt; however, a young child eating a nonfood item once or twice usually does not indicate pica.)

When anemia is suspected, the patient is given a complete blood count (CBC) laboratory test. If the CBC indicates that anemia is present, further testing is needed to determine whether the underlying problem is iron deficiency anemia or another form of anemia such as sickle-cell anemia, thalessemia, or other hereditary type of anemia. A serum ferritin test and serum iron test will reveal if patients have iron deficiency anemia. Physicians may also wish to check for microscopic or visible blood in the stools, because gastrointestinal bleeding may indicate anemia. Some intestinal parasites found in internationally adopted children may cause anemia.

Treatment Options and Outlook

If the patient has iron deficiency anemia, usually iron supplements will resolve the problem within a few months, although physicians may wish to continue patients on supplements for an additional six to 12 months.

Adults who think that they may be anemic (or that their children may be) should not attempt to treat themselves or their children with iron supplements unless a physician specifically recommends this course of action subsequent to confirmation with blood testing. The reason for this caution is that excessive levels of iron in the blood can cause illness.

Because iron can upset the stomach, some patients also take antacids along with the iron; however, iron supplements should not be taken at the same time as antacid medications because the antacids will reduce the absorption of the iron into the bloodstream. In contrast to the effect of antacids, vitamin C *increases* the absorption of iron, although patients should check with their doctors first before taking vitamin C on a regular basis since excessive doses of vitamin C (or other vitamins or minerals) can be harmful to children and adults.

Iron is also available in an intravenous form that can be given to patients who have difficulty tolerating iron supplements, though this is rarely needed.

Children with iron deficiency anemia should not drink more than 32 ounces of milk per day, according to the National Library of Medicine, in part because excessive milk intake reduces the volume of calories of iron-rich foods that can be consumed.

Risk Factors and Preventive Measures

According to the National Center for Health Statistics, about 7 percent of children ages 1–2 years old in the United States have iron deficiency anemia. Children between the ages of nine and 24 months are at risk for iron deficiency anemia and should be screened. Adolescents may also be at risk, particularly during a growth spurt.

Among females ages 12–49 years in the United States, about 12 percent have anemia. As many as half of all pregnant women in the United States may have iron deficiency anemia. However, only about 3 percent of adult males have anemia.

Foster children in the United States face an increased risk for the development of iron deficiency anemia. Internationally adopted children are also at risk for anemia. For example, orphanages nearly always fail to provide iron-fortified formula to infants. In addition, the foods that are given to children in orphanages may lack sufficient iron.

Some children are at an increased risk for developing iron deficiency anemia, including the children who

• Had mothers with poor or no prenatal care
• Either had or now have intestinal parasites

In addition to taking iron supplements, children and adults with iron deficiency anemia should eat foods that are rich in iron, such as raisins, meat, fish, egg yolks, whole grain bread, and iron-fortified cereals.

To avoid iron deficiency anemia, others should eat a healthy diet and have regular physical examinations.

Miller, Laurie C., M.D. *The Handbook of International Adoption Medicine: A Guide for Physicians, Parents, and Providers.* New York: Oxford University Press, 2005.
Minocha, Anil, M.D., and Christine Adamec. *The Encyclopedia of the Digestive System and Digestive Disorders.* New York: Facts On File, 2004.

Asians See INDIA, ADOPTIONS FROM; INTERNATIONAL ADOPTION; SOUTH KOREA, ADOPTIONS FROM.

assisted reproductive technology (ART) As defined by the Centers for Disease Control and Prevention (CDC) in the United States, assisted reproductive technology includes all fertility treatments in which *both* eggs and sperm are handled. This generally involves the surgical removal of a woman's eggs from the ovaries, combining them with the man's sperm in the laboratory, and subsequently returning the resulting embryo to the woman's body or giving them to a female donor. (In some cases, embryos are frozen rather than implanted.) Some women undergo extensive fertility treatment including ART before they decide

they wish to adopt a child. Others who cannot create a genetic child decide to remain childless.

Treatments in which only sperm are handled, as with donor insemination, or procedures in which a woman takes medications to stimulate ovulation with no intention of having her eggs removed, do not constitute assisted reproductive technology.

According to the CDC, infants born in the United States as a result of ART represented about 1 percent of all children born in the United States. However, they represented 15.5 percent of all twins born and 43.8 percent of all triplets or higher multiple deliveries.

Fertility clinics in the United States are required to provide statistical data to the CDC, based on the Fertility Clinic Success Rate and Certification Act passed by Congress in 1992, and this is why statistical data is available on ART. Each year, the CDC publishes nationwide data as well as information on individual clinics in *National Summary and Fertility Clinic Reports.*

Fertility and the Effectiveness of ART Declines with Age

ART is most effective among younger women; pregnancy and live birthrates are low for women who are age 40 and older. For example, according to the CDC, the live birthrate for women using ART and their own (nondonor) eggs or embryos who were 40 years old was about 16 percent in 2002. By the age of 43 years, this rate had declined to 6.3 percent. For women older than age 42, the live birthrate was about 2 percent. In general women who are age 40 and older have a significantly higher success rate when they use donor eggs. The majority of women using ART who are older than age 45 (77 percent) used donor eggs in 2002.

The miscarriage rate with ART is less than 14 percent among women younger than age 34, but is 30 percent at age 40, and 45 percent at age 43.

Types of ART

Some examples of ART are

• In vitro fertilization (IVF), in which the woman's eggs are extracted, fertilized in the laboratory, and one or more embryos are then transferred to the

NUMBER OF REPORTED ASSISTED REPRODUCTIVE TECHNOLOGY (ART) PROCEDURES PERFORMED, NUMBER OF PREGNANCIES, OF LIVE-BIRTH DELIVERIES, AND NUMBER OF INFANTS BORN, BY PATIENT'S STATE/TERRITORY OF RESIDENCE AT TIME OF TREATMENT, UNITED STATES, 2002

Patient's state of residence	No. ART procedures started	No. pregnancies	No. live birth deliveries	No. infants born
Alabama	549	210	181	258
Alaska	94	32	29	41
Arizona	1,661	561	463	668
Arkansas	407	136	118	161
California	15,117	5,258	4,344	6,001
Colorado	1,624	783	681	973
Connecticut	1,656	553	460	625
Delaware	414	131	114	154
District of Columbia	488	167	138	177
Florida	4,999	1,751	1,469	2,020
Georgia	2,553	922	768	1,082
Hawaii	775	203	167	233
Idaho	371	164	140	203
Illinois	7,492	2,368	1,891	2,598
Indiana	1,871	575	470	668
Iowa	998	376	309	422
Kansas	706	252	221	317
Kentucky	868	343	306	450
Louisiana	605	206	173	231
Maine	176	68	56	84
Maryland	4,200	1,327	1,062	1,423
Massachusetts	8,631	2,807	2,318	3,086
Michigan	3,288	1,089	931	1,282
Minnesota	2,211	860	714	942
Mississippi	370	122	101	145
Missouri	1,260	508	423	608
Montana	111	44	39	55
Nebraska	675	223	190	260
Nevada	603	223	175	251
New Hampshire	512	162	137	191
New Jersey	7,744	2,805	2,266	3,106
New Mexico	223	121	99	149
New York	13,276	4,358	3,471	4,742
North Carolina	1,947	691	612	896
North Dakota	207	66	61	85
Ohio	3,411	1,193	1,033	1,457
Oklahoma	535	238	203	280
Oregon	815	353	300	425
Pennsylvania	4,329	1,264	1,045	1,449
Puerto Rico	318	110	83	119
Rhode Island	759	257	216	285
South Carolina	772	324	265	362
South Dakota	146	47	45	59
Tennessee	787	302	249	366
Texas	5,716	2,159	1,828	2,559
Utah	574	207	183	258

(continues)

(Table continued)

Patient's state of residence	No. ART procedures started	No. pregnancies	No. live birth deliveries	No. infants born
Vermont	175	75	65	95
Virginia	3,364	1,227	994	1,324
Washington	2,101	803	677	931
West Virginia	172	61	54	75
Wisconsin	1,231	397	337	478
Wyoming	68	39	33	48
Non-U.S. resident	1,414	520	429	589
Total	115,392	40,046	33,141	45,751

Source: Clay Wright, Victoria, et al. "Assisted Reproductive Technology Surveillance, United States, 2002," *Morbidity & Mortality Weekly Report Surveillance Summaries* 54, SS02 (June 3, 2005): 1–24.

woman's uterus. In some IVF procedures, a specialized procedure using a single sperm, known as intracytoplasmic sperm injection (ICSI) is used to inject the sperm directly into the egg.

- Gamete intrafallopian transfer (GIFT). With this procedure, a laparoscope is used to guide the transfer of unfertilized eggs and sperm (gametes) into the woman's fallopian tubes.

- Zygote intrafallopian transfer (ZIFT). In this procedure, the woman's eggs are fertilized in the laboratory, and then a laparoscope is used to guide the fertilized eggs (zygotes) into the fallopian tubes.

In most cases, the woman uses her own eggs, but in other cases, donor eggs are used. In some cases the transferred embryos are fresh while in other cases they were previously frozen and have been thawed. In a few cases, an embryo previously produced by another couple and then frozen is donated to an infertile woman because the couple has decided they do not wish to have any more children. Complicating matters further, the infertile woman who wants the child (and who is also the intended parent) may be the gestational mother (the woman who carries the child), or alternatively, she may rely upon a surrogate to be the gestational mother.

Statistical Data on ART

In 2002, there were 391 fertility clinics operating in the United States. These clinics reported 33,141 deliveries in 2002, including 45,751 babies. (Some births were multiple births.)

As can be seen from the table, the greatest number of infants born using ART were in California (6,001), followed by New York (4,742) and New Jersey (3,106).

See also INFERTILITY.

Centers for Disease Control and Prevention. *2002 Assisted Reproductive Technology Success Rates: National Summary and Fertility Clinic Reports.* U.S. Department of Health and Human Services, December 2004.

Clay Wright, Victoria, et al. "Assisted Reproductive Technology Surveillance, United States, 2002," *Morbidity & Mortality Weekly Report Surveillance Summaries* 54, SS02 (June 3, 2005): 1–24; Also available online. URL: http://www.cdc.gov/mmwr/preview/mmwrhtml/ss5402a1.htm. Accessed on July 12, 2005.

at-risk placement   Also known as legal risk placement or fost-adopt placement. It refers to the placement of a child into an adoptive family when the birthparents' rights have not yet been legally severed by a court or when birthparents have not yet signed a voluntary relinquishment of their parental rights.

Such placements are made only when the social worker is reasonably confident that a termination of the biological parents' rights is imminent.

attachment disorder   A psychological disorder present in some infants and older children who have difficulty relating to or accepting a parental figure as the primary caregiver. This problem more commonly occurs in children who experience difficult circumstances in early life; most children with attachment disorders have been previously neglected and/or abused, and many have had multiple caregivers and placements. Attachment disorder is not limited to adopted children.

Attachment disorder is not common in children adopted as infants, although it may occur. It is also a problem among some children adopted from other countries, particularly among children who have spent considerable time living in orphanages under conditions of severe emotional deprivation or those who were emotionally neglected while living with their birth families prior to institutional placement.

Even in well-staffed orphanages, children may develop attachment disorders. Some children may have 10 or more caregivers in the first year of life, due to staff schedules, turnover, and orphanage protocols that mandate the transfer of children to a new room (and a different set of caregivers) as they grow. As a result, children may never know who will feed, bathe, diaper, and comfort them. Because of the inconsistent responses to their needs, some children develop outgoing personalities with a somewhat superficial charm. Others have more severe attachment disorders.

Babies form attachments to their primary caregivers through such behaviors as crying and reaching for their mothers. They learn to differentiate their parents from others, and by the time they crawl, they cry when the parent or other caregiver is gone. They also develop a fear of strangers. These are all normal behaviors. However, children who do not receive loving care in response to their needs develop maladaptive behavioral patterns which may progress to attachment disorder. The impact on children who receive abusive or neglectful care as infants can be profound.

In *Attachment & Human Development,* David Howe discussed adopted children who exhibited attachment disorders, based on abuse or neglect that occurred prior to the adoption. He wrote, "Distinctively, any adopted children with histories of maltreatment not only fail to experience safety and regulation in relationship with their new attachment figure, *the actual provision of safe and sensitive caregiving itself seems to generate feelings of considerable anxiety and fear, culminating in aggressive/controlling behaviors.*"

Howe says that institutionalized children may have failed to form selective attachments, but in contrast, abused and neglected children did form attachments but they are maladaptive. "In the first sense, there is a disorder because an attachment has not formed. In the second, there is a disorder because the attachment relationship itself activates negative arousal, the very thing it is supposed to help regulate."

Howe says that the internal mental state of children with attachment disorders may be seen in their drawings and in their play, in which monsters frequently appear, to be vanquished by the child. "Children typically represent themselves as both powerful and dangerous as well as frightened and confused. Having survived extreme abuse and neglect, some children also see themselves as invulnerable and immune to danger. They have experienced starvation and beating and survived. There is little that the world can throw at them that could be worse than that which they have already endured."

Minde, however, challenges that parental pathology is a prerequisite for the development of an attachment disorder, and says, "In my personal clinical experience with some 150 biologically and cognitively fragile small premature infants I have observed at least three children who had bewildered yet 'good enough' parents but nevertheless showed the signs of 'disordered attachment,' i.e., they displayed significant and pervasive role reversal and/or excessive clinging at age 4."

Types of Attachment Disorders

One form of attachment disorder, reactive attachment disorder of infancy or early childhood, is recognized and described in the *Diagnostic and Statistical Manual of Mental Disorders* (*DSM*) used by psychiatrists. According to this source, the child's disturbed and inappropriate behavior begins before the age of five years and is associated with having received pathological care. With the Inhibited Type of reactive attachment disorder, the child is hypervigilant and excessively inhibited, as well as resistant to comfort. With the Disinhibited Type, the child is indiscriminately sociable or does not seem to care who takes care of him or her.

Said Dr. Fahlberg, "It is difficult for foster or adoptive parents to feel close to a child who is acting close to everyone else. In addition, children who are willing to go with strangers pose real supervision problems for their parents."

Gregory Keck and Regina Kupecky describe reactive attachment disorder in their book, *Parenting the Hurt Child: Helping Adoptive Parents Heal and Grow.* The authors say,

The types of problems that adoptive parents see in their children are most likely the result of breaks in attachment that occur within the first three years. They are problems that impair, and even cripple, a child's ability to trust and bond—or attach to other human beings.

These issues with attachment are the ones that cause the greatest problems in adopting a child with special needs. As adoptive parents attempt to attach to a child whose attachment ability is impaired by developmental delays, the attachment will either be nonexistent, distorted, or focused around negative behaviors.

The authors further say that "Therapy with hurt children needs to include high energy and intense focus, close physical proximity, frequent touch, confrontation, movement, much nurturing and love, almost constant eye contact, and fast-moving verbal exchanges."

In the realm of attachment disorders, some children form insecure attachments to caregivers, while others form disorganized attachments. Only the reactive attachment disorder is recognized by the American Psychiatric Association, but many therapists also refer to disorganized attachment. According to Van Ijzendoorn and Bakermans-Kranenburg, disorganized attachment "can be described as the breakdown of an otherwise consistent and organized strategy of emotion regulation." These authors say that children with disorganized attachment may be stressed in infancy and aggressive in kindergarten.

While some children never develop an attachment, others may have suffered an interrupted attachment or experienced unresolved separation issues.

Some therapists have their own definitions of attachment disorders. In her book, *Attaching in Adoption: Practical Tools for Today's Parents,* clinical social worker Deborah Gray describes attachments as either secure (normal attachment) or insecure. She subdivides insecure attachments into subtypes, including avoidant attachment; insecure, ambivalent attachment with anxious, clingy presentation; insecure, ambivalent attachment; and insecure, disorganized attachment.

With avoidant attachments, children feel a connection with caregivers but they are unsure how caregivers will react to them. Says Gray, "Children who have an avoidant attachment style do not know whether they will be hugged or hurt when they express needs." Avoidant attachments are also seen in families that are not abusive but are insensitive to the child's needs.

She describes children with insecure, ambivalent attachment with clingy presentation: "They convey that they have finally found someone whom they can trust, within limits. The limit comes at the time that they are expected to believe that their parents can be trusted to return. Their love for and trust in a parent are always in the moment. They seem to believe that the parent will disappear once out of sight. Children tend to show this anxious style after neglect, or after sudden and shocking moves in the first several months of life."

With the other form of insecure, ambivalent attachment, the child alternately clings to the parents or pushes them away. The child may ask for help and then tell the parent she is not helping in the way that is needed. The child may ask the parent for a hug and then complain that it was too tight. Says Gray, "The parent is enticed to continue to try to find ways to satisfy this child, but he ends up feeling sabotaged much of the time." Gray says some children adopted from eastern European orphanages present with this form of attachment disorder.

Children with insecure, disorganized attachment are those who have difficulty relating to their caregivers and do not exhibit consistent ways to show what they need. Says Gray, "Children become fearful, frozen, or disoriented in the midst of signaling some need to their parent. The children show levels of extreme rage. They seem to be either unable to play, or only able to play out violent themes that involve separation." She says that often the original caregivers have "set the child up for overwhelming situations and then responded in a rejecting, frightening, or abandoning manner. Children with disorganized attachments tend to have a sense of helplessness about their relationship with parents."

Symptoms and Diagnostic Path

Dr. Fahlberg has said that the most apparent trait of a child with an attachment disorder is the psychological and physical distancing from adults. In addition, the child may see himself or herself as an unworthy person. In most cases, the child is either overly dependent or greatly independent. Learning problems are common.

Some indicators of attachment disorders include

- Cruelty to animals
- Self-destructive behavior
- Sleep disorders
- Stealing from parents
- Obvious lying
- Preoccupation with fire or weapons
- Intense rages, particularly toward female care-givers
- Inappropriate emotional responses, such as laughing at another's pain
- Showing little or no eye contact
- No remorse when harm is caused by the child
- Above or below average tolerance to pain
- Poor personal hygiene

Treatment Options and Outlook

Attachment can be encouraged; for example, a child's temper tantrums could be used to encourage attachment. After a tantrum, a child is usually exhausted, and she is relaxed and is more open to bonding with the parent.

Support groups are often extremely useful to parents trying to help children with attachment disorders, as are respite care providers. Gray and Keck offer many suggestions for adoptive parents in their books.

It should be noted that there are no specific treatments known to be effective with children with attachment disorders. Say O'Connor and Zeanah, "Despite more than 20 years since the establishment of 'disorders of attachment' in the DSM-III in 1980, there is still no consensual definition or assessment strategy; nor are there established clinical guidelines for treatment or management. Perhaps more alarming is the fact that there is little evidence that the diagnostic definitions currently in favor (DSM-IV and ICD-10) drive current clinical research."

However, parents can receive assistance and therapy. Lieberman studied parental interactions of adoptive parents with attachment-disordered children and says she found four major findings based on her review of 83 clinical charts of foster children who were adopted between the ages of 10 months and 43 months. In general, the request for the referral for mental health services occurred about six months after placement.

Lieberman found four recurrent themes. First, the adoptive parents were distressed by the child's behavior and often internalized their guilt or were angry at the child for failing to respond to them. They were also ambivalent and some expressed regret about adopting the child.

Second, she found that sometimes parents completely missed subtle signs of attachment. For example, a 15-month-old girl looked momentarily worried when the father left the room, and then she smiled almost imperceptibly upon his return. He remarked: "she did not notice I was gone, did she?"—completely missing the subtle behavior of the child. Lieberman says that parents misinterpreted temper tantrums or defiance as indications that the child did not like them rather than seeing them as age-appropriate indicators of fear of loss or anxiety.

The third finding she made was that parents failed to respond in the best way to the child, often due to a lack of knowledge or education about what the child needed. "Specifically, they often responded with disciplinary measures when they perceived the child's behavior as inappropriate, instead of responding with firm but comforting behavior that would have reassured the child about the parent's ongoing ability." Lieberman says that the use of "time-outs," a common method of discipline used with many children, reinforces the child's fear of being unwanted and consequently should be avoided.

The fourth finding that Lieberman made was that adoption agencies had failed to adequately prepare the adoptive parents. "Even parents who were reasonably knowledgeable about child development were not sufficiently aware of the special needs of children who had been deprived of a primary attachment figure."

She also advised that parents need to accentuate their own responses to the muted signs of the child's need, indicating extreme sadness if the parent and child must be separated and showing great joy when they are reunited.

Some therapies have been proven to be dangerous to children, such as "holding therapy," in which the child is held tightly against his or her will in an attempt to force bonding to occur. This is in contrast to therapeutic holding, in which the child is held back from aggressive or violent behavior or from holding to which the child consents. (Some therapists still believe that holding therapy can be effective.)

Even more dangerous was a therapy called "rebirthing therapy," in which a child was compelled to force his or her way through blankets in order to simulate childbirth. This form of therapy is actually illegal in Colorado, because of the death of a 10-year-old girl who suffocated during the so-called therapy.

Risk Factors and Preventive Measures

As mentioned, early deprivation and/or abuse or neglect are risk factors for the development of an attachment disorder. It is unknown if PRENATAL EXPOSURES, including prenatal exposure to maternal stress, may also contribute to attachment disorders, and further research is needed.

The best preventive measure against attachment disorder is for children needing families to be placed with loving adoptive families at as young an age as is possible. If that is not possible, children should be placed with foster families with whom it is likely they may stay. If an institutional setting is needed, then it should be staffed with sufficient and consistent caregivers such that infants and small children can be given individual attention.

See also BONDING AND ATTACHMENT; PSYCHIATRIC PROBLEMS OF ADOPTED PERSONS.

American Psychiatric Association. *Diagnostic and Statistical Manual of Mental Disorders.* Fourth Edition Text Revision. (DSM-IV-TR). Washington, D.C.: American Psychiatric Association, 2000.

Boris, Neil W. "Attachment, Aggression and Holding: A Cautionary Tale," *Attachment & Human Development* 5, no. 3 (September 2003): 245–247.

Fahlberg, Vera, M.D. *Attachment and Separation: Putting the Pieces Together.* Chelsea, Mich.: National Resource Center for Special Needs Adoption, 1979.

Fahlberg, Vera, M.D. *Residential Treatment: A Tapestry of Many Therapies.* Indianapolis, Ind.: Perspectives Press, 1990.

Gray, Deborah D. *Attaching in Adoption: Practical Tools for Today's Parents.* Indianapolis, Ind.: Perspectives Press, 2002.

Howe, David. "Attachment Disorders: Disinhibited Attachment Behaviours and Secure Base Distortions with Special Reference to Adopted Children," *Attachment & Human Development* 5, no. 3 (September 2003): 265–270.

Howe, David, and Sheila Fearnley. "Disorders of Attachment in Adopted and Fostered Children: Recognition and Treatment," *Clinical Child Psychology and Psychiatry* 8, no. 3 (2003): 369–387.

Hughes, Daniel. *Facilitating Developmental Attachment: The Road to Emotional Recovery and Behavioral Change in Foster and Adopted Children.* New York: Jason Aronson, 2000.

Hughes, Daniel A. "Psychological Interventions for the Spectrum of Attachment Disorders and Intrafamilial Trauma," *Attachment & Human Development* 5, no. 3 (September 2003): 271–277.

Keck, Gregory C., and Regina M. Kupecky. *Parenting the Hurt Child: Helping Adoptive Parents Heal and Grow.* Colorado Springs, Colo.: Pinon Press, 2002.

Lieberman, Alicia F. "The Treatment of Attachment Disorder in Infancy and Early Childhood: Reflections from Clinical Intervention with Later-Adopted Foster Care Children," *Attachment & Human Development* 5, no. 3 (September 2003): 279–282.

Miller, Laurie C., M.D. *The Handbook of International Adoption Medicine: A Guide for Physicians, Parents, and Providers.* New York: Oxford University Press, 2005.

Minde, Klaus. "Attachment Problems as a Spectrum Disorder: Implications for Diagnosis and Treatment," *Attachment & Human Development* 5, no. 3 (September 2003): 289–296.

Minnis, Helen, and Gregory Keck. "A Clinical/Research Dialogue on Reactive Attachment Disorder," *Attachment & Human Development* 5, no. 3 (September 2003): 297–303.

O'Connor, Thomas G., and Charles H. Zeanah. "Attachment Disorders: Assessment Strategies and Treatment Approaches," *Attachment & Human Development* 5, no. 3 (September 2003): 223–244.

O'Connor, Thomas G., and Charles H. Zeanah. "Current Perspectives on Attachment Disorders: Rejoinder and Synthesis," *Attachment & Human Development* 5, no. 3 (September 2003): 321–326.

Robinson, Jane R. "Attachment Problems and Disorders in Infants and Young Children: Identification, Assessment, and Intervention," *Infants and Young Children* 14, no. 4 (2002): 6–18.

Steele, Howard. "Holding Therapy Is Not Attachment

Therapy: Editor's Introduction to This Invited Special Issue," *Attachment & Human Development* 5, no. 3 (September 2003): 219.

Van Ijzendoorn, Marinus H., and Marian J. Bakermans-Kranenburg. "Attachment Disorders and Disorganized Attachment: Similar and Different," *Attachment & Human Development* 5, no. 3 (September 2003): 313–320.

attitudes about adoption   An attitude is an overall outlook and may encompass positive, negative, or neutral views. Some people have a generally positive attitude toward adoption while others see adoption as a problematic institution, and others are neutral in their attitude. A belief is a premise that is accepted or rejected, such as a generalized belief that adopted children are more likely to have mental health problems than are nonadopted children. In fact, many adopted children exhibit no psychiatric problems, while some have serious problems. (See also PSYCHIATRIC PROBLEMS OF ADOPTED PERSONS.)

Some beliefs are stereotypical, such as the common belief that Asian-born children are inevitably adept at math and science. This belief, although seemingly positive, can present a problem, such as when Asian-born children have difficulty with math or science.

Even when a belief is not supported by evidence or is actively refuted by research, sometimes it is nonetheless accepted by many people. Such beliefs may have an impact on individuals who are directly affected by adoption, particularly adopted children. For example, if teachers hold the belief that (non-Asian) adopted children usually struggle in school, they may act on this underlying belief by lowering their expectations for adopted children and failing to challenge children who are bright or gifted.

If members of the ADOPTION TRIAD are given the impression that adoption is not considered acceptable by society, consequences may result; for example, a pregnant woman considering adoption for her child may feel discouraged away from this choice, even though she may feel unwilling or unready to become a parent and she may decide against an abortion. An adopted person may feel "second-best" when societal attitudes seem to support the view that adoption is not an acceptable choice. The adoptive parent, particularly the infer-tile adoptive parent, may perceive adoptive parenthood as inferior to biological parenthood because of a societal emphasis on the overwhelming importance of "blood ties."

Societal attitudes about adoption appear to be changing in a positive and more realistic direction, although it is also true that adoption TERMINOLOGY has not kept pace with this change; for example, when a birthmother decides adoption is the right answer for herself and her child, she is often said to "give up" or even "give away" her baby, indicating both a lack of control and a negative act, rather than the more neutral terms of "to plan" or "to choose" or "decide on" adoption for her child. However, despite the use of negative adoption language, some positive inroads have occurred in public attitudes toward adoption, based on studies of attitudes toward adoption.

Studies on Attitudes toward Adoption

In 2002, the National Adoption Attitudes Survey was published. This study, sponsored by the Dave Thomas Foundation for Adoption and the Evan B. Donaldson Adoption Institute and performed by polling company Harris Interactive, provided important information on the prevailing attitudes about adoption among the general public. The pollsters surveyed 1,416 Americans aged 18 and older in 2002, including whites, African-Americans, and Hispanics.

Some areas of concern were identified; for example, the study revealed that many respondents believed that adopted children were at greater risk for experiencing problems with drugs and difficulties in school. Said the study authors, "Although adopted children undergo an adjustment period, the reality is that the majority of adopted children have similar long-term outcomes as biological children."

Another very common concern, expressed by 82 percent of the respondents, was that birthmothers would reclaim the child after the adoption was finalized—although this situation rarely happens. (Most birthmothers who "change their minds" about adoption do so before the child is placed with the family.)

This belief of the lurking birthmother largely stems from a few sensationalized stories in the media in which birthparents have tried (and occasionally succeeded) in overturning an adoption. These stories are somewhat similar to extensive media coverage about catastrophic train wrecks, airplane or car crashes, although in those cases, most people realize that trains, airplanes, and cars usually do not crash, and they continue to travel. However, because of a lack of unbiased (or any) information about adoption among the general public, often when people hear or read about something that is very negative (or positive) they may generalize the situation to all adopted children.

One consequence of the generally accepted and erroneous belief that birthmothers will inevitably come to reclaim their children is that some people who would otherwise consider adopting infants and older children, including children in foster care, decide it is too risky for them. In addition, some people who fear adopting a child in the United States will adopt a child from another country, believing that the birthparents in other countries present no risk.

On the positive side, the research revealed that 75 percent of the respondents believed that adoptive parents loved their children as much as parents whose children are born to them. In the past, many adoptive parents have complained that others viewed them as inauthentic or not "as good as" parents of children who were born to them. The research also revealed that the prevailing perception about adoptive parents was that they were compassionate and caring people.

The National Adoption Attitudes Survey poll takers reported that almost two-thirds (63 percent) of Americans have positive feelings about adoption. This is an increase from 56 percent who reported positive feelings in a 1997 survey on adoption attitudes by the same pollster.

Attitudes were mitigated by a personal experience with adoption and having a family member or a friend who has adopted a child, was an adopted person, or who had placed a child for adoption. Those with a personal connection to adoption had a greater percentage of having a very favorable opinion about adoption (69 percent) compared with those with no connections to adoption (51 percent).

Attitudes were also affected by age and other factors, and although the majority favored adop-

tion, those groups who were the *least* supportive included individuals aged 18–24 years old and those aged 65 and older, those with less education and also African-Americans.

In another study on adoption attitudes, performed in Canada, preliminary results indicate that Canadians have positive attitudes about adoption. In this survey, performed in 2000, researchers Charlene E. Miall and Karen March interviewed 82 families in their homes and later randomly interviewed 706 adults by telephone.

The researchers found that about 75 percent of Canadians were strongly supportive of adoption and about 75 percent also believed that mothers feel the same way about their adopted children as they do about children born to them. In addition, about one-third strongly approved of birthmothers who made a plan to place their children for adoption and one-third somewhat approved. The majority (more than two-thirds) believed that birthparents were responsible and unselfish by making an adoption plan for their children.

This finding is very significant because in past decades, relinquishing birthparents in North America were perceived very negatively, as lazy or uncaring people. In fact, in the mid-twentieth century, unmarried birthmothers were given the mixed message that they should place their babies for adoption, yet at the same time, they were stigmatized for doing so.

Harris Interactive Market Research. *National Adoption Attitudes Survey Research Report.* Sponsored by Dave Thomas Foundation for Adoption in cooperation with the Evan B. Donaldson Adoption Institute. June 2002. Available online. URL: http://www.adoptioninstitute. org/survey/Adoption_Attitudes_Survey.pdf, downloaded February 14, 2005.

Miall, Charlene E., and Karen March. "Social Support for Adoption in Canada: Preliminary Findings of a Canada-Wide Survey," press release, 2002. Available online. URL: http://www.carleton.ca/socanth/Faculty/News% 20Release%20Adoption%20Survey.pdf, downloaded March 3, 2004.

attorneys Lawyers are almost invariably involved in adoptions, although the extent of typical legal involvement varies from state to state.

Lawyers may be involved in an agency adoption by preparing and filing the appropriate court papers to finalize an adoption. Attorneys may also be heavily involved in an adoption by overseeing all phases of an INDEPENDENT ADOPTION—from offering advice to prospective parents or birthparents to preparing finalization papers.

In the case of an independent adoption, in those states that do not allow attorneys to advertise their adoption services or to seek out pregnant women considering adoption for their babies, attorneys may advise prospective adoptive parents on how they might search for a birthmother and what legal and practical matters they should consider, for example, what expenses of the birthmother may be paid by the adoptive parents and what risks are involved in an independent adoption. In addition, the attorney will also advise the prospective adoptive parents of their options if the birthfather refuses to consent to the adoption or if there are other concerns or problems.

In some cases, the attorney will also represent the birthparents while in others the attorney will represent only the birthparents or the adopting parents. If the lawyer works with the birthparents, legal advice will be provided, and information, such as medical and ethnic background, will be collected on the birthparents.

In the case of an INTERSTATE ADOPTION, attorneys from each state work with interstate compact offices to ensure that state laws are complied with.

Attorneys may also be appointed when state or county social workers attempt to terminate parental rights so a child can be placed for adoption. In some cases, there may be an attorney assigned for the parents, another attorney for the child, and a third attorney for the social services agency as well.

The primary role of the attorney in a SPECIAL NEEDS ADOPTION is to finalize the adoption in court. Lawyers may also represent the state, when social workers are attempting to terminate the parental rights of abusive or neglectful parents. In addition, some states require that minor children be represented by counsel in court hearings on adoption.

Lawyers may also be involved in lawsuits. An example is WRONGFUL ADOPTION suits in which the adoptive parents allege that they were not provided with sufficient information about a child when they were considering whether or not to adopt. Lawyers are also providing services to those interested in adopting internationally.

Attorneys involved in adoption may belong to the American Academy of Adoption Attorneys, the American Bar Association, or be attorney members of the National Council for Adoption.

autobiography   Often requested by adoption agencies, the autobiography is a written history of the adoptive parent, including educational background, career, and a variety of other information; also called a profile or a RÉSUMÉ.

Often guided by the agency on the type of information to include, the prospective adoptive parent prepares the autobiography for review by agency staff.

The agency staff may use the autobiography to help them evaluate the family in the HOME STUDY or family study process. Some agencies also provide nonidentifying autobiographies to pregnant women or birthmothers considering adoption and ask them to select which adoptive parents they would like to consider for their child. Some agencies will then arrange a meeting between the pregnant woman and the prospective adoptive parents.

baby selling   Refers to the selling of an infant to adoptive parents or other persons by the birthparent and/or an intermediary. Baby selling is unlawful in every state in the United States; however, desperate couples and unscrupulous individuals apparently continue to risk the legal penalties.

It is extremely risky for a couple to try to buy a baby because of the distinct possibility of that adoption being overturned at a later date. In addition, the fear that state or federal authorities may eventually "catch up" with them can generate intense anxiety in the adopting parents or persons who buy the infants; however, unscrupulous individuals involved in baby selling will continue to operate as long as there is a profit to be made.

Some individuals may try to buy a baby to avoid a HOME STUDY investigation of the family because they believe they would not be approved after such a study. This is a morally reprehensible reason for buying a child and failing to protect a child's legal rights.

It is unclear how many babies are actually "sold" in the United States, although it is clear from people who are identified in baby selling rings that such practices do occur.

Periodically, there are rumors of baby selling among INTERNATIONAL ADOPTION agencies. It is often extremely difficult to determine where the truth lies and how many of these reports are generated by groups opposed to Americans adopting children from abroad.

Some mistakenly equate INDEPENDENT ADOPTION with baby selling. Independent adoption is lawful in most states, and if the adoptive parents and their attorneys comply with state laws, then no baby selling has occurred.

Every state has its own laws on adoption and the lawful expenses related to adoption. Payments that would be considered excessive and perhaps baby selling in some states are acceptable in others; however, in no state is a birthmother allowed to accept a direct payment solely in exchange for her baby.

States that allow pregnant women to receive any sums of money consider the money to be for her support and maintenance during the latter part of her pregnancy and directly thereafter. Some states ban any payments of money at all to the pregnant woman.

In some cases, it is clear when a mother or father attempts to sell their baby, for example, if they request enough money for a worldwide cruise, car, or other significant expenditure unrelated to the maintenance during pregnancy, or if they request other similar payments.

In other cases, it is less clear where to draw the line between legitimate support payments and unreasonably excessive payments. It is always best to identify and rely on a reputable adoption agency or attorney's judgment on what constitutes an acceptable sum of support.

It is usually through independent adoption that attorneys or other intermediaries provide support money to indigent pregnant women planning to place their babies for adoption; however, increasing numbers of adoption agencies will also provide a limited amount of support to pregnant women needing financial assistance.

Some attorneys and social workers require an exact accounting of how the money will be spent before they will approve any payment to a pregnant women making an adoption plan for her child.

They may insist on making vendor payments directly, for example, paying the woman's landlord for her rent, the phone company and electric company for her utilities, and the doctor for the obstetric bill. Other attorneys will give the woman a lump sum or a weekly payment, and she will take responsibility for paying her own bills. Many state laws require an accounting of how support money was spent, which is given to the court before FINALIZATION.

Although attorneys are blamed for most of the baby selling that occurs in the United States, it is also true some agencies and facilitators charge unusually high fees for their adoptions. They claim these fees are necessary to cover advertising costs and salary expenses.

baby shortage   Refers to few healthy babies that are available for adoption in the United States and/or Canada. Because the number of people who are interested in adopting healthy infants from the United States and Canada exceeds the number of infants who are in need of adoption, some experts have called this problem a "baby shortage." However, others actively dispute how severe the baby shortage really is.

In the past, some reports said that a million people wished to adopt infants, yet this statistic was based on individuals actively seeking to create a pregnancy. It was unknown how many of these individuals were interested in adopting infants. The most modest estimates are that 50,000 to 100,000 people in the United States wish to adopt babies.

One factor that is known is that some infertile couples will only be satisfied with a biological child, and if they cannot have a biological child, then they will remain childless. They feel that they would perceive an adopted child as somehow "second-best." With such an attitude, it is preferable for such families to avoid adopting children, who need the unconditional love of a parent.

Because of the perceived baby shortage and/or because families are not interested in participating in an OPEN ADOPTION (an adoption in which the identities of the birthparents and the adoptive parents are known to each other), many families seek to adopt children from other countries. There is no baby shortage in orphanages throughout the world, and many children urgently need families.

background information   Data provided to prospective adoptive parents on the child they are considering adopting and also on the child's biological family if available. Background information on the birthparents may be unavailable if children are adopted from orphanages. Also known as the referral.

In the case of an infant adoption, background information generally includes such nonidentifying information as the pregnant woman or birthmother's age, a physical description, her racial and ethnic background, religion, education, and medical and family history. Information on the birthfather is usually gathered by caseworkers as well, and caseworkers may also obtain data on birth grandparents.

Some workers also include information on personality or hobbies, for example, the birthmother's good sense of humor or the birthfather's musical talent.

If the adoption is an OPEN ADOPTION, then the adopting parents and birthmother (and birthfather, if possible) usually meet and may exchange extensive identifying information beyond that provided by the social worker.

Particular attention is paid to recent illnesses the pregnant woman or birthfather may have suffered, and social workers attempt to determine if there has been any drug or alcohol abuse before or during the pregnancy. Whether or not the birthmother has obtained any prenatal care is also determined. (See PRENATAL EXPOSURES.)

In the case of an older child's adoption, workers will try to obtain the same information on biological parents as they do in an infant adoption as well as data on the child since birth. (Most older children have been in foster care for several years, and the information should be included in their case files or should be accessible by social workers with some effort on their part.)

Background information on an older child will include a medical history, immunization records, previous foster and/or adoptive placements, information on behavioral problems, the existence of any siblings, and other information that could be valuable to the child in the future or to his or her adoptive parents.

If the child has been abused and the social worker knows this, that information should be shared with adopting parents. This knowledge will help the adopting parents with their own adjustment to the child; for example, if a child shrinks from her adoptive father's hugs, it helps to know that she is fearful of men because of attacks she suffered from her biological father or her biological mother's boyfriend.

Sometimes the adopting parents will meet foster parents in advance of the adoption and discuss the child's likes and dislikes and information that could aid the parents in helping the child with the adjustment. However, in many cases of adoption of older children, the foster parents become the adoptive parents.

Studies have revealed that parents who are well informed are far less likely to disrupt an adoption, and workers should make every effort to ensure that the adopting parents feel they have as much information as caseworkers can give them.

biographical information   Usually refers to information on prospective adoptive parents, including age, interests, reasons why they wish to adopt, hobbies, and other information needed by the caseworker and/or the birthparents.

Some agencies ask prospective adoptive parents to write a special RÉSUMÉ or profile that will be seen by birthparents considering adoption. Such a résumé will usually include nonidentifying information, such as the individual's profession (if this information is nonidentifying), hobbies, and so forth.

See also AUTOBIOGRAPHY; BACKGROUND INFORMATION.

biological parents   Also known as genetic parents, birthparents, or natural parents, the man and woman who conceive a child.

See also BIRTHFATHER; BIRTHMOTHER.

biracial   A child of mixed race; usually refers to a child born to a black parent and a white parent.

Some agencies place biracial children with white families, while others are opposed to such placements believing biracial children should be placed with black families. The presumption is that society identifies biracial children as black.

See also TRANSRACIAL ADOPTION.

birth certificate   See SEALED RECORDS; OPEN RECORDS.

birthday   An adopted child's birthday is important and should be celebrated with cake, presents, and the usual birthday accoutrements. A child who is adopted as an older child may be unfamiliar with birthday celebrations, and if he or she appears bewildered, parents should explain what will happen and what the child should do.

Some adoptive parents celebrate both "adoption day"—the day the child arrived in the home—and the child's birthday as well. Experts have mixed views on celebrating two holidays each year. Therapist and adoptive parent Stephanie Siegel, author of *Parenting Your Adopted Child,* advises against celebrating both days and instead urges concentrating on the child's birthday.

She says that "adoption is a memorable occasion and should be treated as such. A birthday, however, is the day to be celebrated each year. Do not confuse your children by celebrating their adoption day as well."

A birthday may also be a time when questions about birthparents arise, particularly as the child reaches adolescence and adulthood.

Siegel, Stephanie E. *Parenting Your Adopted Child.* New York: Prentice Hall, 1989.

birthfather   Term applied to the biological father of an adopted child. In most adoptions that occur in the United States, the birthfather agrees to the adoption or he does not challenge it. In international adoptions, however, the birthfather may not be aware that he conceived a child with the birthmother, who may abandon or relinquish the child without his permission or knowledge. In such cases, the birthmother is usually unmarried, and it would bring great shame to herself and her family to parent a child out of wedlock. As a result, most of this essay concentrates on birthfathers in the United States.

In the latter part of the 20th century, the issue of unmarried birthfathers and their rights in adoption came to the forefront in many parts of the United States. It was argued that if a biological mother does not wish to parent a child, then the child should be placed with the biological father, unless he specifically states that he does not wish to parent the child. Also, because a mother's fitness to parent a newborn baby is rarely challenged, fathers argued that neither should their fitness have to be proven; it should be assumed, absent compelling evidence otherwise. This is the position taken by Toni L. Craig in her article for the *Florida State University Law Review* in 1998. In her opinion, "When an unwed father contests the at-birth adoption of his child, the federal Constitution requires application of the biological rights doctrine."

Some also argue that birthfathers should not be given veto rights over an adoption because they may use their parental rights as a psychological weapon to maintain contact with the birthmother.

Some states have taken the position that notice of a planned adoption must be given to a birthfather. Others have taken the position that "notice" occurs at the point of sexual intercourse, when a man should know that he may have conceived a child with a woman. Some states rely upon whether or not a birthfather has registered with a state putative father registry (see BIRTHFATHER REGISTRY) to determine if his parental rights may be exercised. Some states consider whether the birthfather provided financial support to the birthmother during her pregnancy. If he did not, it is assumed he is not sufficiently interested in the child.

If notice is required and the birthmother does not know who or where the birthfather is (or says that she does not know), some states require that legal notices or advertisements be taken out to protect the birthfather's interests. If he does not come forward, it is then assumed he is not interested in the child and the adoption can go forth.

Problems have arisen when birthmothers have lied about who the birthfather is, and some states have yet to resolve complex issues, such as how long a biological father has to come forward and claim his parental rights, assuming that he was denied knowledge of the child. If the child was born in one state but adopted by individuals in another state and the birthfather resides in a state where he is entitled to notice, these circumstances may leave the adoption open to legal challenge by the birthfather. It should be noted that such situations occur infrequently and by no means are as prevalent as many adopting couples fear.

Of course, not all birthfathers are opposed to adoption, and many willingly sign consent to the adoption or sign a document or statement (some-times called a waiver) that disclaims any personal interest in the adoption. Some states allow birthfathers to sign consent to an adoption before the child is born. This is known as PREBIRTH CONSENT TO AN ADOPTION.

Whenever possible, social workers and/or attorneys obtain information about and from the birthfather, not only to protect his legal rights but also to ensure that important medical and genetic background information is provided to adoptive parents.

If birthparents are married, the birthfather must usually consent to an adoption along with the birthmother. In almost all cases, the married man is presumed to be the biological father and is also the LEGAL FATHER.

Highly Publicized Legal Battles

The birthfather rights issue came to the forefront most dramatically in 1993, when an Iowa birthfather successfully challenged an adoption by a Michigan couple after a battle of several years (*In re Claussen*). The case became publicized throughout the United States as the adoptive parents openly struggled with the birthfather over custody of the child the adopters had named "Jessica DeBoer."

In this case, the birthmother had named one man as the father of her child and he had signed consent to the adoption. After the child was placed, the birthmother stated that the biological father was really another man, and she sought the return of the child. The actual birthfather sought custody, and he won his court struggle when the child was about three years old. She was placed with him and the birthmother, whom he had married.

Another case, known popularly as "the Baby Richard case" in Illinois, also received national notice, primarily because of stories written by Chicago columnist Bob Greene and nationally prominent author Dennis Prager. In this case, a birthmother placed a child for adoption and told the birthfather that the baby had died. She later admitted to him that an adoption had occurred, and the birthfather actively sought custody. He prevailed when the child was about three years old. The birthparents later divorced and the child purportedly was then reared by his birthmother.

Because these two cases received an unusually high level of media attention, nearly all state legislatures subsequently reviewed their laws on birth-fathers, and many new laws were enacted. Some states created putative father registries, while other states created laws allowing prebirth consent from birthfathers. Some states required the birthfather to appear in court within a certain time frame or to submit documents to a particular court or organization in order for paternity to be established.

History of Birthfathers' Rights

Prior to 1972, unwed birthfathers were rarely involved in adoption proceedings, and a birth-mother could decide to place her child for adoption or parent the child as she chose. It was generally presumed that unwed fathers had no interest in parenting their children born out of wedlock or, if they did, that they would make unfit parents.

Married men whose wives desired to place their children for adoption are in a different category. They must consent to an adoption of their child unless their parental rights are lawfully terminated or special circumstances are met.

U.S. Supreme Court decisions about unmarried fathers indicate that the court is clearly interested in whether or not the birthfather has or had a parental relationship with the child and the nature of that relationship.

Important U.S. Supreme Court Cases

In 1972, the landmark case of *Stanley v. Illinois* was heard by the U.S. Supreme Court. Stanley was an unwed father who had lived with the birthmother periodically for 18 years and had a parental relationship to their three children.

When the birthmother died, the state sought to remove the children from Stanley's custody and denied him a hearing based on his nonmarital relationship with the deceased and the out-of-wedlock status of the children.

Stanley ultimately won his case and custody of the children because the court believed he had been denied due process. The court was sympathetic to Stanley's case because he had maintained a relationship with his children and had acted in a paternal manner. In this case, the court apparently strove to maintain an already existing family unit.

The next landmark birthfather case was *Quillon v. Walcott,* which the Supreme Court heard in 1978.

Quillon was an unmarried father; the mother of his child later married another man. The child lived with her mother and stepfather as a family unit, and Mrs. Walcott's husband sought to adopt her.

Quillon attempted to block the adoption of the 11-year-old child, but he had never taken responsibility for the child, nor did he seek custody. He lost his case.

The next major case was *Caban v. Mohammed* in 1979. The unmarried couple had lived together for five years and parented two children. Ms. Mohammed later moved away and married, and her husband petitioned to adopt the children. New York law held that a birthmother, but not a birthfather, could block an adoption, so there was no bar to this stepparent adoption.

The Supreme Court rejected the distinction between birthmothers and birthfathers; however, very important to the court was the fact that the children were older and were known to and by the father. In addition, Caban had established "a substantial relationship" with his children and he had admitted paternity. (He was also listed on the birth certificates as the father.) As a result, Caban was successful in blocking the adoption of his children.

The case of *Lehr v. Robertson* was another case of birthfather's rights and was heard by the U.S. Supreme Court in 1982. Mr. Lehr had never provided financial support to Ms. Robertson or the baby, nor did they live together after the child's birth. His name was not listed on the birth certificate, and he never registered with New York's Putative Father Registry.

Robertson later married and her husband sought to adopt the child. Lehr tried to block the adoption and asked for visitation rights. The court rejected Lehr's claims and held that "the mere existence of a biological link" does not guarantee due process unless the unwed father "demonstrates a full commitment to the responsibilities of parenthood" and is involved in the rearing of his child.

These cases were all interesting to birthfather rights advocates, but not until 1988 was an adoption case involving unrelated adoptive parents scheduled. Edward McNamara was a birthfather whose child was conceived as the result of a casual affair. When he learned the birthmother had placed the child for adoption in 1981 through a

San Diego, California, county agency he began his fight to stop the adoption. (*In re Baby Girl M.*)

While he began his legal battle, the agency placed the baby with Robert and Pamela Moses, an adoptive family selected by the birthmother.

When his case was heard initially the court decided it would be in the "best interests" of the child for the child to remain with the adoptive parents. McNamara continued to fight until his case was heard in 1988, seven years after the child's birth. He sought to have himself declared the legal father and to obtain visitation rights with the child. A California court denied his claim, contending that his parental rights could be terminated in the best interests of a child.

The U.S. Supreme Court dismissed the case and said that no federal question had been raised.

The most recent Supreme Court case involving birthfathers as of this writing was *Michael H., and Victoria D., Appellants v. Gerald D.* (June 13, 1989), wherein an alleged birthfather and the child's legal father were in conflict.

The mother had had a relationship with an unmarried man, and together they had a child. Because she was married, the legal father was presumed to be her husband. The alleged birthfather had a relationship with the child; however, the mother elected to return to her husband. The alleged birthfather sued for visitation rights.

The Supreme Court found the presumption of the legal father's paternity in this case was irrefutable and was upheld, and consequently the birthfather's requests for visitation and a continuing relationship were denied. (However, in many states the contention of paternity based on marriage to the child's mother may be rebutted and may also require proof, such as genetic testing.) The court also stated that had the husband or wife wished to challenge the law, then the request would have been considered; however, the unmarried man who alleged paternity had no standing.

See also BIRTHMOTHER; MARRIED BIRTHPARENTS.

Boccaccini, Marcus T., and Eleanor Willemson. "Contested Adoption and the Liberty Interest of the Child," *St. Thomas Law Review* 10 (Winter 1998).

"Michael H. and Victoria D., Appellants v. Gerald D.," *United States Law Week*, June 13, 1989, 4,691–4,705.

birthfather registry   A legal device in the United States whereby biological fathers who are not married to the BIRTHMOTHER may register their paternity, usually to block an adoption before it may occur. Birthfather registries are also known as putative father registries. The birthfather may wish to obtain legal custody of the child or he may wish to block an adoption so that his mother or another relative can rear the child. In some cases, a birthfather wishes to block the adoption in an attempt to compel a birthmother to rear the child, knowing or suspecting that she would not wish him to obtain custody of the child and that, if the child could not be adopted, she would rather raise the child herself.

Many states have birthfather registries, according to the "Summary of U.S. State Adoption Laws" in the second edition of *The Complete Idiot's Guide to Adoption*, including as follows: Alabama, Arkansas, Arizona, Florida, Georgia, Idaho, Illinois, Indiana, Iowa, Louisiana, Massachusetts, Michigan, Minnesota, Missouri, Nebraska, New Mexico, New York, Ohio, Oklahoma, Pennsylvania, Tennessee, Texas, Utah, Vermont, and Wyoming.

Birthfather registries may be managed by the state social services department or the courts. Each state has its own laws and system set up on how and when birthfathers should register their paternity in order to prevent an adoption from going forth. Whether failing to register paternity is sufficient to block an adoption depends on the state law. Some states also require notice in the form of newspaper advertisements or other means to attempt to identify and contact birthfathers before an adoption may occur.

Supporters of birthfather registries say that the registry gives a birthfather an opportunity to prevent an adoption and to assert his paternal rights. It also provides protection to biological fathers in cases where the birthmother has failed to notify the birthfather that she has had a child and that she has decided to place the child for adoption.

Dissenters to the birthfather registry concept say that a man may not know that he has fathered a child because the birthmother failed to tell him that she has borne a child and that she plans an adoption for the child. They argue that a man should not be required to register with a birthfather registry every time he has unprotected sex with a woman that may lead to the conception of a child. Instead, dissenters believe that the birthfather should receive some form of legal notice about an impending adoption. Note that if the mother is *not* planning an adoption for her child, she is under no obligation to tell the biological father about the child's existence, although some would argue that in most cases, she has a moral obligation to do so.

In some cases, such as when the birthmother was raped, it may be possible for an adoption to go forth, even if a birthfather who was convicted of the rape that resulted in the child registers on a birthfather registry that he wishes to block the adoption.

See also BIRTHFATHER; PREBIRTH CONSENT TO AN ADOPTION.

Adamec, Christine. *The Complete Idiot's Guide to Adoption.* 2nd ed. New York: Alpha Books, 2005.

birth grandparent   The biological or genetic grandparent of an adopted child. It would be clearer to use the phrase "the birthmother's parents" or the "birthfather's parents."

Studies have revealed the tremendous impact of the birth grandparent, particularly a birth grandmother, on a birthmother's decision to parent a child or place it for adoption.

Author Leroy H. Pelton found the attitude of birth grandparents to be very critical in the adoption decision of birthmothers. The birth grandparents' unwillingness to accept the child into the family was the strongest factor that helped a birthmother decide to choose adoption rather than parenting.

Birth grandparents also face tremendous societal pressure. Those who encourage their daughter or son to choose adoption for the child rather than to parent often incur societal disapproval from friends, relatives, and others, who cannot understand how they can "give up their own flesh and blood."

If the birthmother is a teenager, her parents will often end up parenting the child themselves if the birthmother decides against adoption, particularly if the birthmother is a young teenager living at home. Sometimes the birth grandparent wants to rear the child herself, which is one reason why birthfathers who have expressed little or no interest in parenting may sometimes, just before or just after the baby's birth, decide to demand custody of the child. (See BIRTHFATHER.)

Some birth grandparents-to-be do not wish to raise another child or do not feel they can provide an adequate environment for an infant and consequently encourage adoption as the better solution, while others may still believe the proper solution is for the birthmother to parent the baby herself.

It is often difficult for birth grandparents-to-be to understand that they cannot forbid their child to choose either parenthood or adoption, although they can exert tremendous moral and economic influence. Individuals whose daughters or sons are expecting a child should take care that they are well aware of all the options available to them so regret and resentment will not overwhelm them in later years.

Jeanne Warren Lindsay addressed the emotional issues of helping your daughter make an adoption plan in her book *Parents, Pregnant Teens and the Adoption Option: Help for Families.*

Lindsay reports that birth grandparents are unlikely to receive or seek out support from their peers and may not want to discuss their daughter's pregnancy at all. "Their friends may not know how to approach them for fear of offending them," Lindsay writes. "Many birth grandparents feel terribly alone during this time."

Grandparents

Virtually every adoption agency is eager to involve birth grandparents in the counseling process, particularly the parents of the birthmother, in order to help them work through the issues of grief and loss and to know the peace of mind of having their grandchild in the family that is best for the child, all things considered.

See also BIRTHMOTHER; GRANDPARENT ADOPTIONS.

birth kin   The biological relatives of an adopted person, including birthparents, birth grandparents, siblings by birth, aunts and uncles by birth, and so forth.

See also KINSHIP CARE.

birthmother or birth mother   The biological/genetic mother of a child placed for adoption. In some cases, the woman makes the decision to place the child for adoption while she is pregnant or soon after the delivery of the child, and she seeks out the assistance of an adoption agency or attorney. In other cases, a woman abandons her child, such as to an orphanage in another country or to a firehouse in the United States. (See ABANDONMENT.)

Sometimes a child is taken from the birthmother by a state agency because of abuse, neglect, or abandonment and placed in foster care (or, in other countries, in an orphanage). In some cases, the woman's parental rights are involuntarily terminated. In all of these cases, the biological mother of the child is known as a birthmother, whether she willingly chose adoption for her child or the choice was imposed by others.

The term *birthmother* is sometimes also used to refer to all biological mothers, whether their parental rights are transferred to adoptive parents or they choose to parent their children, but in most cases, the word is used *solely* to denote a woman whose biological child was adopted, whether by design or not. If the child remains in the home, the biological mother is simply referred to as the "mother."

There is a surprising dearth of research on birthmothers, and most research about adoption has been performed on adopted children. There is also one common problem with most research on birthmothers, which is that nearly all researchers concentrate on studying pregnant adolescents or teenagers whose children were adopted, and these results are subsequently generalized to all birthmothers. It may be that pregnant teenagers are studied because teenage pregnancy is perceived as a serious social problem, whereas if a single

woman in her late teens or twenties is pregnant, it is not considered a problem to society. It may also be that it is easier to identify adolescents to study and to obtain their cooperation.

Yet experts agree that most females who voluntarily choose adoption in the United States are over age 18, as are most birthmothers who involuntarily lose custody of their children who are later adopted.

Many authors and researchers believe that females older than 17 and 18 in the United States are more likely to choose adoption today than younger birthmothers under age 17, primarily because younger women have difficulty separating their needs from the needs of the child and also because of magical thinking, in which the adolescent female assumes that everything will work out for the best, despite the enormity of her problems.

Author Leroy Pelton has stated that in past years birthmothers tended to be younger women living at home, but he hypothesized that this pattern began to reverse itself in the 1970s when older mothers became more likely to choose adoption than younger women. In addition, the women choosing adoption for their infants were more likely to be living independently, less likely to report that the baby's father was supportive during pregnancy, and less likely to receive help during the pregnancy from their family and friends than the mother who chose to parent her baby.

Parenting v. Placing

Michael Resnick studied 93 adolescents, including 67 who chose parenting, 24 who chose adoption, one who had an abortion, and one whose child was in foster care. Resnick stated that 85 percent of the "placers" (those who chose adoption for their infants) and 94 percent of those who chose parenting were satisfied with their decision.

When asked for the most crucial factor in their decision making, 80 percent of those who chose parenting stated that they were ready to assume this responsibility. Other reasons were that they felt they could not carry a child for nine months and then make an adoption plan or that the birthfather wanted them to parent the baby.

Of the placers, 75 percent said they were unable to parent a child and to offer the type of environment they believed was important. Other reasons cited for choosing adoption were that they believed

AMONG CHILDREN BORN TO NEVER-MARRIED WOMEN UNDER 45 YEARS OF AGE, PERCENT WHO WERE RELINQUISHED FOR ADOPTION, BY RACE, ACCORDING TO YEAR OF BIRTH

Race	Before 1973	1973–1981	1982–1988	1989–1995
All women	8.7	4.1	2	0.9
Black	1.5	0.2	1.1	—
White	19.3	7.5	3.2	1.7

Source: National Center for Health Statistics

adoption was in the child's best interest. Some cited their plans to continue their education.

In a later article by Resnick (1992), he stated that the pregnancy decision of an adolescent was most influenced by the teenager's mother, the birthfather of the baby, and the adolescent's peers.

In a study that compared unmarried adolescent parents to "placers," Debra Kalmuss et al. in *Family Planning Perspectives* looked at the short-term consequences of young women who made this choice. Researchers studied 311 women who chose parenting and 216 who chose adoption. The sample was heavily skewed toward young women living in maternity homes, while others were recruited from prenatal clinics, teenage pregnancy programs, and adoption agencies. The mean age of the women was 17.5 years.

The researchers found significant differences between the two groups and said, "Placers were considerably more likely to have lived in a maternity residence during pregnancy, they were somewhat older and were more likely to have graduated from high school. Moreover, they were more likely to be white and to have come from intact families, and less likely to have grown up in a family which received public assistance, or to have been receiving public assistance themselves at the time that they became pregnant."

In contrast, the researchers also found that 60 percent of those who chose parenting were receiving public assistance at the post-birth interviews, versus 4 percent of the placers. These findings support earlier research.

In looking at the psychological area, researchers found that parents and placers were about equal in stability, although placers were happier with their lives and their relationships with their own mothers. Placers had a more positive outlook on the future achievements they expected to make by the age of 30. They were also more likely to return to high school after the birth than were parents.

Both groups were generally satisfied with their choices, and 56 percent said they had few or no regrets about their adoption decision. About 80 percent of the placers said they would have made the same decision again. Although both groups expressed high comfort levels with their decision, the parents were more likely to say they would make the same choice again. Researchers were unclear if this was the result of the birthmothers still dealing with feelings of loss or if the parents felt inhibited about saying they were unhappy to be parents.

In a study reported in 1993, researchers studied 162 unmarried pregnant teenagers. Fifty-seven percent initially planned adoption for their babies, but about half ultimately changed their mind and decided to parent the babies. The teenager's perception of what her mother preferred affected her initial decision. However, the researchers found that the birthfather's preference was the driving force in the final decision.

Said the researchers, "A perception that the birth father would prefer that the infant be placed for adoption more than tripled the odds that the teen mother would remain consistent in her choice to place." Interestingly, adoption knowledge and attending adoption seminars did not affect the decision significantly. Socioeconomic status and race did not have statistically significant impacts in this study.

Birth Order

According to a report by Christine Bachrach for the National Center for Health Statistics, a birthmother in the United States who chooses adoption is usually placing her first child for adoption. An estimated 75 percent of all infant adoptions are firstborns, 12 percent are second children, and 13 percent are later children.

Race

Many birthmothers are white, and infants born to white single mothers are more likely to be placed for adoption with nonrelatives than are the newborns of African-American mothers, according to studies by the National Center for Health Statistics.

This does not mean, however, that African-American and other nonwhite birthmothers are uninterested in learning about adoption. In addition, some African Americans utilize informal adoptions, in which no legal transfer is made but others care for the child, such as a relative.

A study by Margaret Klein Misak in 1981 of 387 women of all races (217 white, 111 black, 50 Latina, and 9 racially designated as "other") revealed that as many as 51 percent of the African-American clients were considering adoption, compared with 53 percent of white women in crisis pregnancies.

An apparent factor affecting the number of African-American women choosing adoption for their babies was the insufficient number of families interested in adopting African-American infants. It is unknown if researchers today would have similar findings. However, both public and private agencies continue to find it difficult to recruit enough adoptive families for minority infants and children. Public agencies, of course, may not discriminate, because of the MULTIETHNIC PLACEMENT ACT.

Attitudes Affecting the Choice of Adoption

It has been hypothesized by some that birthmothers who plan for their babies' adoptions have a lower self-esteem than those who choose to parent. Dr. Steven McLaughlin of the Battelle Human Affairs Research Centers in Seattle, Washington, compared adolescent "relinquishers" (adolescents who chose adoption) to adolescents who chose parenting in his 1987 study, "The Consequences of the Adoption Decision," and found both groups had about the same levels of self-esteem.

Some have speculated that women who elected adoption for their babies may quickly become pregnant again to replace the child they lost, but McLaughlin found this was not the case. Instead, the teenagers who chose parenting were more likely to become pregnant again shortly after the first child's birth, and many of these pregnancies ended in abortion.

A small study of 21 pregnant adolescents revealed that societal pressure was strongly perceived as a factor in choosing parenting over placing for adoption among adolescents. According to researcher Marcia Custer, in her article in a 1993 issue of *Adolescence,* teenagers believed there were no social sanctions against them parenting their children but there were strong societal sanctions against the adoption choice. Teenagers believed that parenting was the responsible and socially acceptable choice.

Custer also found that most of the teenagers as well as professional counselors had very little knowledge about adoption. Only two of the adolescents had received any information about adoption. She stated, "This low level of adoption knowledge nurtures the stereotypical beliefs held by society in general, including pregnant teenagers and the professionals who interact with them."

Marital Status

Although most birthmothers in the United States are single (or divorced), some birthmothers are married. The National Center for Health Statistics estimates at least 5 to 6 percent of all infants placed for adoption in the United States were born to married couples. The couple may be in the process of divorcing or may be poor and financially unable to support an additional child.

In some cases, the child may be the result of an extramarital affair, and although the husband would be the legal father if he opted to raise the child, he and his wife choose to place the baby for adoption.

Married couples who elect adoption for their children may also face mental or physical problems, drug addiction, alcoholism, or a wide variety of social problems. They decide placing the child with a stable two-parent couple is in the best interests of the child.

See MARRIED BIRTHPARENTS.

Socioeconomic Status

Researcher Carmelo Cocozzelli found a correlation between socioeconomic status and the decision to rear or place the baby. Women receiving welfare are more likely to decide to parent the baby than women who are not on public assistance. (This finding has been reported in study after study—women who choose adoption are usually of a higher socioeconomic level than women who choose parenting.)

Some studies indicate that women whose fathers are employed or whose fathers are professionals are more likely to make an adoption plan. The socioeconomic finding was backed up by a study in 1987 by Jane Bose and Michael Resnick, who found a higher socioeconomic status among adolescents who chose adoption than among adolescents who chose parenting for their children. Similar findings were also reported by researchers Debra Kalmuss and associates in a 1991 issue of *Family Planning Perspectives.*

Other Factors

In a study by Jane Bose and Michael Resnick on placers and adolescents who chose parenting, they found that placers tended to come from suburban areas rather than rural or urban areas. In addition, the placers were more religious than were teenagers who chose to parent.

The researchers also found that both placers and parents came from a "high proportion" of families who had already faced a teenage pregnancy. In addition, placers were more likely than parents to have a family member who was adopted or to have been adopted themselves. If a placer's sister became pregnant, the sister was more likely to choose adoption than the sisters of birthmothers who chose parenting. Apparently the past experience of other family members had a direct impact on the decision of what to do about an unplanned pregnancy.

Birthmothers of Past Years

Many birthmothers who are 45–50 years old and older today and who placed their infants 25 or more years ago found a cultural climate of the time that was vastly different from today.

Adoption was the expected action, and was not really a choice, when one was a young unwed mother before the early 1970s. Pressure was common from parents to place the baby for adoption, and women really did not have much of a choice at that time. If single women were in their 20s or older and became pregnant, they were often pressured into marriage to "give the baby a name," while some obtained abortions, often illegal and dangerous procedures at that time. Others chose adoption.

In 1961, a parent frequently said to a pregnant teenage girl, "You're pregnant, and you're not ready to be a parent. Either have the baby adopted or get out of the house."

In 2006, the message is very different, and a parent frequently says, "You're pregnant, and you're not ready to be a parent. Either have an abortion or get out of the house." Often adoption is not considered as an option. Conversely, some parents with pregnant teenager daughters urge them to parent their babies, and their message is, "Don't come home from the hospital without the baby."

Thousands of young women before the 1970s went or were sent to maternity homes, but many more were quietly kept at home or taken to relatives, where they received no counseling or emotional support and little or no information about pregnancy and childbearing.

Before 1970, very few agencies provided résumés of prospective adoptive parents to choose from, and the women retained little or no control. Some women report that they were not even

informed on what labor and delivery would be like. Alone and terrified in a strange hospital, they experienced childbirth.

The women were urged to then go home and forget. Yet even though she had been told she had done the "right thing," people who knew about the baby often looked down on the birthmother as a bad person. In essence, she was in a no-win situation. She would have been condemned if she had tried to raise the child as a single parent, but she was also condemned when she made the adoption plan that others insisted was the one right choice.

Some birthmothers who suffered such conditions are intensely bitter today. These birthmothers who have suffered should be treated, belatedly, with the compassion they were denied in their time of need. Their desire for confidentiality, or a chance to speak their minds, should be equally honored.

Birthmothers and Trends in Adoption

Over time, more agencies began to question the practice of prohibiting birthmothers from having input in the adoption process. Today nearly all agencies and increasing numbers of adoption attorneys provide extensive nonidentifying background information about the adopting couple to pregnant women in the United States, for example, their age, religion, why they want to adopt a child, and many other factors. (This type of information is not usually shared with birthmothers in other countries.)

Many adoption agencies in the United States also offer OPEN ADOPTION to pregnant women considering adoption, which may mean they meet the prospective adoptive parents and may have continuing contact between birthparents and adoptive parents subsequent to the adoption.

Short-term and Long-term Impact of the Adoption Decision on Birthmothers

Adoption counselors report that many birthmothers, no matter how committed they were to the adoptive placement and how certain they were that they had made the right choice, usually suffer a grieving period. Said O'Leary Wiley and Baden in their 2005 article for *The Counseling Psychologist*, "During the early postrelinquishment period (defined broadly as the first two years following relinquishment), the reported effect of relinquishment on birth parents, but especially birth mothers, varies greatly depending on their coping skills, support system, and degree of involvement in planning the adoption—that is, to what degree the birth mother is involved in choosing the adoptive parents and meeting them."

The authors also pointed out that if the adoption is a "closed" adoption rather than an open one, the birthmother may worry about the child. However, there are also issues involved with open adoptions, particularly just after the child is placed with the adoptive family. They say, "Birth mothers in more open arrangements may become childlike in their dependence on the adopting parents only to feel discarded and betrayed by them once the baby is born." Some adoptive parents have reported anecdotally that they almost felt like the birthmother wished she could be adopted too, along with her child. If the birthmother is an adolescent, they may be right about this speculation.

Over the long term, birthmothers may continue to suffer from the adoption decision. Say O'Leary Wiley and Baden, "Clinicians report that the birth mothers they see in therapy alternate between denial of the relinquishment of their child and feelings of continuing shame, depression, and negative self-image. They feel they carry a serious secret and that they are unacceptable and unlovable. They report difficulty attaching to romantic partners and, sometimes, their subsequent children. If the birth mother has had an open support system, one that she can honestly communicate within, then these intense emotional sequelae seem to be reduced."

Note, however, that the authors are talking about a clinical population, and it is not known if these feelings can be generalized to birthmothers who have not felt a need to seek out therapists.

Birthmothers in Intercountry Adoptions

Although researchers have done very little research on birthmothers in countries outside the United States, primarily because of cultural and financial restraints, most agencies and attorneys who handle INTERNATIONAL ADOPTIONS believe that many of these birthmothers are young and/or poor. However, it is known that some are married, such as in China, where because of governmental population control concerns, the number of chil-

dren per family is limited. In addition, the stigma of unwed parenthood is still very powerful in many countries of the world.

Children from other countries who are adopted by Americans usually live in orphanages prior to adoption (although, in some cases, the child may reside in a private foster home), and the child must be legally considered as an "orphan" or officially "abandoned" to be adopted. As a result, few American adoptive parents have the opportunity to gain much, if any, information on the birthmother. However, whether information on the birthparents is available depends on the policies of the country.

Many birthmothers in South Korea reside in maternity homes prior to delivery; social and family medical histories are often available to adopting parents. Individuals seeking to adopt should always ask the agency for any available information on the birthparents, because this information (whether medical, social, or another type of information) could be useful to the child as he or she grows and even in later adulthood.

See also ADOPTIVE PARENTS; BIRTHFATHER; SEARCH.

Adamec, Christine. *Complete Idiot's Guide to Adoption.* New York: Alpha Books, 2005.

Bachrach, Christine A. "Adoption Plans, Adopted Children, and Adoptive Mothers," *Journal of Marriage and the Family* 48 (May 1986): 243–253.

Bose, Jane, Michael D. Resnick, and Martha Smith. *Final Report: Adoption and Parenting Decisionmaking among Adolescent Females.* University of Minnesota, July 1987.

Chandra, Anjani, et al. "Adoption, Adoption Demand, and Relinquishment for Adoption," Washington, D.C.: National Center for Health Statistics, May 11, 1999.

Cocozzelli, Carmelo. "Predicting the Decision of Biological Mothers to Retain or Relinquish Their Babies for Adoption," *Child Welfare* 63 (January–February 1989): 33–44.

Custer, Marcia. "Adoption as an Option for Unmarried Pregnant Teens," *Adolescence* 28 (Winter 1993): 891–902.

Kalmuss, Debra, Pearila Brickner Namerow, and Linda F. Cushman. "Adoption versus Parenting among Young Pregnant Women," *Family Planning Perspectives* 23 (January–February 1991): 17–23.

Klein Misak, Margaret. *Experience of Multiple Unwed Pregnancies: A Report from Selected Catholic Agencies.* Chicago: Catholic Charities of Chicago, 1982.

McLaughlin, Steven I., et al. "To Parent or Relinquish: Consequences for Adolescent Mothers," *Social Work* 33 (July–August 1988): 320–324.

O'Leary Wiley, Mary, and Amanda L. Baden. "Birth Parents in Adoption: Research, Practice, and Counseling Psychology," *Counseling Psychologist* 33, no. 1 (January 2005): 13–50.

Pelton, Leroy H. "The Institution of Adoption: Its Sources and Perpetuation," in *Infertility and Adoption: A Guide for Social Work Practice*. New York: Haworth, 1988.

Resnick, Michael D. "Adolescent Pregnancy Options," *Journal of School Health* 62, no. 7 (September 1992): 298–303.

———. "Studying Adolescent Mothers' Decision Making about Adoption and Parenting," *Social Work* 29 (January–February 1984): 5–10.

birth order/family order Refers to the child's ordinal position among children in the family. According to psychologists, whether a child is the class clown or a serious striving person is strongly related to whether the child is the oldest or youngest in the family or somewhere in the middle.

Because adoptive families may be composed of both biological and adopted children, perhaps *family order* is a more appropriate term when considering their relative age.

Most social workers seriously consider the ages of children already in the family when they are considering a placement; for example, they may not wish to place a child who is older than the oldest child already in the home.

Often the oldest child already in the home occupies a position with some privileges, and this role is very important to the child. To bring a new child in who is older and probably worthy of even greater privileges could be disturbing to the formerly oldest child.

The much-cherished baby of the family may find her or his nose out of joint when a newly adopted baby or younger child receives a great deal of attention and seemingly everything done by the new child is perceived as amazing by the adoptive parents. Being bumped from the privileged status of the baby of the family to the role of the middle child requires a considerable adjustment, whether the new baby is born to the family or is adopted into the family.

Of course, bringing any child into the family will change the family order. A new child will become either the baby, be in the middle, or be the oldest. Anyone who formerly occupied those positions—with the possible exception of the middle child—may evince resentment until adjustments have been made.

Author, therapist, and adoptive parent Claudia Jewett disputes the common practice of placing only children younger than the children already in the home and says many families can successfully adopt a child who is older than children already in the home. Jewett says the practice of placing only younger children is unfair to older children who may need to behave younger than their chronological age would permit.

Jewett, Claudia L. *Adopting the Older Child.* Boston: Harvard Common Press, 1978.

birthparent Biological or genetic mother or father of a child; usually refers to a biological parent who places the child for adoption.

See also BIRTHFATHER; BIRTHMOTHER; MARRIED BIRTHPARENTS.

black/African-American adoptive parent recruitment programs Programs designed to encourage African-American couples and singles to adopt children of all ages, from infancy through adolescence. Although black adoptive parents adopt at about the same rate or greater than white adoptive parents, there are more African-American children in need of families, largely because there are greater numbers of African-American children in the foster care system.

Some social workers believe that the social work system is dominated by whites who do not provide sufficient assistance to blacks interested in adoption. Some experts believe that blacks face numerous obstacles in their attempts to adopt and, as a result, may begin the adoption process, become exasperated, and forget the idea.

Some adoption agencies concentrate on the recruitment of black parents. Yet despite often outstanding efforts on the part of many black social workers, there are still large numbers of black children of all ages waiting to be adopted. Even though there are numerous black children awaiting adoption, and despite the MULTIETHNIC PLACEMENT ACT prohibiting racial and ethnic discrimination in adoption, there are some black social workers (and social workers of other races) who are adamantly opposed to the placement of African-American children with white adoptive parents. (See TRANSRACIAL ADOPTION). Others believe that a loving adoptive home is the priority for children without families, and that racial matching is secondary to the need for the timely placement of young children.

black families Because at least half of all the "WAITING CHILDREN" available through public welfare agencies are black, black children of all ages are often considered children with SPECIAL NEEDS.

Census studies indicate that blacks adopt at about the same rate as whites, but to successfully place all the black children available for adoption, experts estimate blacks would need to adopt children at three times the rate of white families.

A cultural/racial bias against adoption is blamed as one reason why black birthmothers often choose not to place babies for adoption and other blacks choose not to adopt, but the reasons are much more complex than this. For example, some blacks have alleged that adoption agencies are dominated by whites who impose similar criteria on black families as they do on white prospective parents.

Whites have also adopted some of the available black children, and TRANSRACIAL ADOPTION has been one of the most hotly debated topics of the past 30 years. Those who disapprove of whites adopting blacks, notably the National Association of Black Social Workers, believe that whites cannot truly understand blacks, that children will be deprived of their heritage, and that their development will be harmed. They also worry that black children will feel inferior, particularly if raised in a predominantly white neighborhood.

Supporters of transracial adoption when suitable black adoptive families cannot be identified, cite longitudinal studies, especially by researchers Rita Simon and Howard Altstein, that indicate black children raised by whites are generally well-adjusted. In addition, they state that permanence is the real issue and that loving, appropriate white parents are better than continuous foster care or other less suitable arrangements.

Research has revealed that black adoptive parents adopt for essentially the same reasons stated by Caucasian adoptive families.

A study by Gwendolyn Prater and Lula T. King discussed the motivations of black adoptive parents. According to their article, the primary reasons given for adopting by the 12 families who participated in the study were "unable to have children biologically," the desire to "share their love with a child" and a desire to "give a child without a home, a home and a family." Three couples wanted to adopt a girl because they already had boys.

The researchers concluded that black adoptive parents would make a valuable resource in recruiting other black adoptive parents. They warned, however, that families were reticent about discussing adoption with strangers, and thus adoption workers should be sure to maintain confidentiality unless the parents indicated their willingness to talk about adoption with prospective parents.

See also BLACK/AFRICAN-AMERICAN ADOPTIVE PARENT RECRUITMENT PROGRAMS.

Prater, Gwendolyn, and Lula T. King, "Experiences of Black Families as Adoptive Parents," *Social Work* 33 (November–December 1988): 543–545.
Illinois Department of Children and Family Services. *Mostly I Can Do More Things than I Can't.* Chelsea, Mich.: National Resource Center for Special Needs Adoption, 1987.

blended families Families with both biological and adopted children and/or families with children of different races. The term *blended family* is more commonly used to refer to stepparenting relationships resulting from remarriage when the parents already have children from a previous marriage or relationship.

blood ties See ATTITUDES ABOUT ADOPTION.

bonding and attachment Refers to the mutual affectionate connection that is cemented between a child and a parent, whether the child is a birth child or an adopted child. The process of establishing this connection includes a growing feeling of ENTITLEMENT to family life, love, responsibility, and a variety of other emotions normally experienced by a parent and child. "Bonding" is the process and "attachment" is the result.

Some people extend the "bonding and attachment" concept to apply to any two individuals who fit certain parameters. For example, psychologist Tiffany Field defines attachment as "a relationship between two beings which integrates their physiological and behavioral systems."

In his book *Parenting Your Adopted Child,* Dr. Andrew Adesman cites some key bonding concepts. Says Adesman, "Decades of research on bonding and attachment have produced some key observations:

- Children and parents usually form strong attachments with each other.

- Attachments can often be observed in the behavior of the child and the parent.

- If children don't form attachments in early life, it can be harder (or in rare cases, impossible) for them to attach to others.

- Strong attachments in early life enable children to form other attachments to people later, such as parents, friends, spouses, and others.

- Adoptive parents can and do love their children as much as biological parents. "Love doesn't require a genetic link."

Past Studies on Bonding

Psychoanalyst John Bowlby first wrote about bonding and attachment in 1951, based on his research with institutionalized children. Bowlby believed that if children did not form a close attachment to a parent by the age of about two and a half, then the child's future character was in jeopardy. Although researchers and physicians have since challenged this conclusion, it is important to note that, before Bowlby's work, the potential impact of institutional life on a child was largely unexplored.

In another commonly cited study on bonding, published in 1972 by Dr. John Kennell and Marshall Klaus in the *New England Journal of Medicine,* the doctors studied the impact of early contact between newborns and their mothers. They believed that their findings proved that early-contact mothers had a better chance at having a positive relationship with their children, based on a study of 28 new mothers. In one group, the mothers had extended contact with their newborns, and in the other group, mothers were allowed to hold their newborns for five minutes and then were separated from them for up to 12 hours. Other experts challenged these findings based on the tiny sample; however, the doctors' work did result in changed policies in hospitals, which began to offer much more extended contact with newborns with their mothers.

Bonding and Attachment: Misunderstood Concepts

Some experts believe the terms *bonding* and *attachment* are far too loosely used. Said Jean Nelson-Erichsen, codirector of adoption at Los Ninos International Adoption Center in The Woodlands, Texas, in *Is Adoption For You? The Information You Need to Make the Right Choice* (John Wiley & Sons, 1998), "this overused word 'bonding' sometimes drives me wild. You don't usually just fall in love with people and become all warm and cuddly in days! And a lot of people whose babies are born to them don't immediately love their babies. The way you bond with children is to hold them and play with them and read to them. All the holding and caring things are important." Likewise, parents who report "instant bonding" are usually misinterpreting the child's anxious response to the trauma of the recent transition.

Concern about Bonding and Attachment in Relation to the Child's Age

Most adoptive parents and adoption experts are concerned about the timing of bonding in relation to the age of the child who is adopted, whether the child is six months old or six years old. In general, children adopted as infants or young children have a more rapid rate of attachment than older children. Or, as social worker Deborah Gray stated in her book *Attaching in Adoption,* "Children adopted as infants have been shown to enjoy higher-than-average rates of secure attachment with their parents."

Psychiatrist Michael Rutter provides further information on this point. Rutter found the idea that there are "sensitive periods" when environmental factors are critical is an issue that has some validity, although the upper age limits of the sensitive periods may be at an older age than originally postulated by some scientists. His study showed that children who were adopted before the age of four bonded well with their parents while children who were over age four experienced many of the same problems as children who had remained in an institution. Yet Rutter supported the idea that even children adopted after the age of four years could bond with adoptive parents. He concluded that the "sensitive period" was either wrong or that the timing occurred at a later age than was previously thought.

The First Meeting

The first meeting with the child is a very dramatic moment for most parents, be they biological parents or adoptive parents. If they are adopting an older child, the parents usually will have seen photographs or a VIDEOTAPE of the child and will have received information about the child as well.

Many adoptive parents have reported that they felt they bonded to the child based on his or her picture alone, before the first meeting with the child occurred. This is especially true in the case of an international adoption, when the decision to adopt was based solely on the photo, a sketchy description, a videotape, or an Internet Web site introduction. In fact, when such an adoption has fallen through for some reason, adoptive parents experience a grieving process, even though they have never actually met the child. In their minds, the child was theirs.

If the child to be adopted is an infant, the adoptive parents will have virtually no idea what the child will look like until they first see her or him, although they will know his or her racial and ethnic background and have general information about the birthparents' appearance and may have met the birthparents, as in an open adoption.

The time when they first view their baby or older child is very important and unforgettable to most adoptive parents, as if it were imprinted in their brains along with other important scenes of their lives. Both adopting parents should be present at the first meeting along with older children and, if possible, the rest of the nuclear family (the members who reside together in the same home). In general, however, it is best for extended family members, such as grandparents, aunts, and uncles,

to meet the child later on, to avoid overwhelming the child.

The Bonding Process

Part of bonding is physical touch, and because infants require much touching in the course of their care, most adoptive parents bond more rapidly to infants than to older children. Some research indicates that when parents are adopting siblings, they appear to bond more rapidly with the younger child, probably because of the greater amount of care that is needed by that child.

Parents bond to older children by teaching them how to cook, taking them shopping, and performing other similar activities with them as a parent and a child.

Some older children do not respond to affection at first and, if they have been abused, they may shrink from hugs and kisses. Adopting parents learn to "go slow" until the child is ready to accept love.

Studies indicate that parents seem to bond the most quickly and with the most lasting bond when they perceive that the adopted child is similar to them in physical appearance, intelligence, temperament, or some other aspect. As a result, adoptive parents will see "Uncle Bob's nose" and "Mom's smile" in an infant, even though they realize the child is genetically or even ethnically unrelated to them.

Sometimes strangers may point out apparent similarities between the parent and child, and the adoptive parent may respond with embarrassment, confusion, pride, or a mix of all of these emotions. New parents sometimes feel compelled to tell these friendly strangers that they adopted the child, and there is no genetic link. This is unnecessary, because passing strangers were merely making pleasant conversation and do not need details about the adoption.

It is important to note that bonding is not always instantaneous, even when the child is a newborn baby (nor is bonding always instantaneous between a biological mother and her child), and it rarely occurs immediately when a child is an older child.

Often the bonding process is a slow evolution of a myriad of tiny events in the course of days, weeks, or months, for example, the older child's first visit, the time when he or she first comes to stay, is registered for school, taken to the doctor, and so forth.

Many parents of older adopted children report that the first time they really *knew* they were parents was when they felt someone had threatened their child by speaking harshly to him or pushing him. The rush of parental anger and protectiveness is a clear-cut sign that this parent has bonded to this child.

The support of the extended family is very important to the bonding process and helps legitimize the feeling of closeness the adoptive parents are developing with their child. Unfortunately, sometimes extended families are distant or negative about the adoption, which causes considerable anxiety and may affect the bonding process. Adoptive parent support group members can help such families with their need for a feeling of importance and belonging.

Societal attitudes about the urgency of early bonding can sometimes make adoptive parents feel inferior. However, the inability to parent a child in the first days of infancy (because the child is in the hospital, a foster home, or someplace other than where the adoptive parents are) should not make adoptive parents feel that they are somehow less valid parents. Certainly professionals do not claim that early contact at birth is essential to successful attachment.

In a study of infant bonding that compared adoptive mothers to nonadoptive mothers, researchers Leslie M. Singer, David M. Brodzinsky, Douglas Ramsay, Mary Steir, and Everett Waters studied infants ages 13 to 18 months. Some of the parents had adopted children of another race.

The researchers found no differences in mother-infant attachment between nonadopted and same-race or transracially adopted children. They did, however, find a greater incidence of "insecure attachment" in the transracial mother-infant groups compared to the nonadoptive groups. In addition, they reported that mothers who had adopted transracially were less willing to allow other people to care for their children.

The researchers also said they found no relationship between "quality of mother-infant attachment and either perceived social support, infant development quotient, infant temperament, number of foster homes experienced by the infant, or infant's age at the time of placement."

Researchers Leon J. Yarrow and Robert P. Klein studied the effect of moving an infant from a foster home to an adoptive home. They reported that ". . . change *per se* in the environment is less important than change associated with less adequate care. Infants who experience a marked deterioration in quality of the environment following adoptive placement show disturbances in adaptation, whereas infants who are moved to an environment where there is a significant improvement in maternal care are less likely to show significant disturbances following the move."

One aspect that can seriously impair the bonding process is if the adopted child is very different from the type of child that the parent had dreamed of, for example, if the child's behavioral problems far exceed what the parent is ready to cope with or the child's physical or emotional problems are more severe than what the parent had said she or he could handle.

Consequently, it is very important for social workers to share as much nonidentifying information as possible about a child with prospective parents before a placement occurs.

Attachment Problems

Sometimes children experience difficulty attaching to adoptive parents or others, because of early deprivation, institutional living, past abuse, or other reasons. They may develop an ATTACHMENT DISORDER.

Adamec, Christine. *Is Adoption for You? The Information You Need to Make the Right Choice.* New York: John Wiley & Sons, 1998.

Adesman, Andrew, M.D. *Parenting Your Adopted Child: A Positive Approach to Building a Strong Family.* New York: McGraw-Hill, 2004.

Bowlby, John. *Maternal Care and Mental Health.* Geneva, Switzerland: World Health Organization, 1951.

Field, Tiffany. "Attachment and Separation in Young Children," *Annual Review of Psychology* 47 (1996): 541–561.

Gray, Deborah D. *Attaching in Adoption: Practical Tools for Today's Parents.* Indianapolis, Ind.: Perspectives Press, Inc., 2002.

Klaus, M., et al. "Maternal Attachment: Importance of the First Postpartum Days," *New England Journal of Medicine* 286, no. 9 (1972): 460–463.

Rutter, Michael. "Family and School Influences on Behavioural Development," *Journal of Child Psychology and Psychiatry* 26, no. 3 (1985): 349–368.

Singer, Leslie M., and David M. Brodzinsky, Douglas Ramsay, Mary Steir, and Everett Waters. "Mother-Infant Attachment in Adoptive Families," *Child Development* 56 (1985): 1,543–1,551.

Yarrow, Leon J., and Robert P. Klein. "Environmental Discontinuity Associated with Transition from Foster to Adoptive Homes," *International Journal of Behavioral Development* 3 (1980): 311–322.

breast-feeding an adopted infant Providing nutrition to an infant through the breast. A small number of adoptive mothers choose to nurse their infants, and it is sometimes possible to induce lactation in a woman who has never borne children, never been pregnant, or who has not recently been pregnant. Even if an adoptive mother produces a tiny amount of milk or no milk at all, the tactile closeness to her infant is a very positive experience.

The baby's suckling at the breast will further stimulate the production of milk. In some cases, the adoptive mother may have breast-fed biological or adopted children previously. She will need to "relactate" for her new baby.

If the adopting mother knows weeks or months ahead of time that the baby will be arriving, she may opt to use a breast pump to begin stimulating the breasts to induce a milk supply. Because it is unlikely that sufficient breast milk will be produced, the breast milk must be supplemented by bottle feeding or by special devices that are designed for adoptive mothers who are nursing. If the bottle is used, mothers may use larger than usual nipple holes on the bottle, because the baby will quickly receive what she or he needs yet will still have a natural desire to suck and can then be breast-fed.

Devices that stimulate nursing are commercially available. Such devices include an external bag of formula that is placed atop the mother's nipple while the child nurses. The baby can simultaneously nurse at the breast and the supplemental device or the device may be slipped into the infant's mouth after nursing has begun.

Experts say newborn infants are the best candidates for nursing; however, adoptive mothers may also nurse older infants as well, and adoptive mothers have been successful with infants as old as six to nine months.

It is important for the adoptive mother who nurses to obtain moral support from others. Relatives and friends may not understand the value of the experience to the adoptive mother and may try to discourage her from nursing or find her efforts humorous or bizarre.

As a result, finding other adoptive parents who have successfully nursed can be a major boon to a new mother. The La Leche League may be able to recommend local adoptive mothers or provide advice.

Peterson, Debra. *Breastfeeding the Adopted Baby.* San Antonio, Tex.: Corona Publishing, 1999.

Canada and adoption   Canadian adoption rules are determined by the province in which prospective adoptive parents live, and Canadians interested in adoption should call their provincial social services office for further information. In addition, there are adoptive parent groups throughout Canada that can provide assistance and advice. The Adoption Council of Canada, the national adoption organization, also offers helpful information to adoptive parents throughout the country. (The address of the organization is: Adoption Council of Canada, Bronson Centre, 211 Bronson Avenue, Suite 210, Ottawa, Ontario, Canada, K1R 6H5.) One useful publication for Canadians interested in adoption is *Family Helper,* produced by content specialist Robin Hilborn.

According to the Adoption Council of Canada, there are an estimated 66,000 children in Canada who are in the custody of child welfare organizations (the counterpart to the U.S. foster care system). Of these children, in 22,000 cases, the parental rights have been terminated by the courts and the children are available for adoption. About 1,700 of children in the custody of child welfare organizations are adopted by Canadians in a year, and most are between ages one and six years, according to *Waiting Kids in Canada: All About Domestic Adoption.* More information is available at the site for Canada's Waiting Children, at http://www.canadaswaitingchildren.ca. In addition, some provinces have photo listings of waiting children.

Some Canadians adopt children (usually babies) privately, although the number of private adoptions is unknown. A home study is required.

Many Canadians adopt children from other countries through adoption agencies, and in 2004, 1,955 children were adopted internationally by Canadians. Of these children, about half (1,001) were from China, according to the *Canadian Guide to Intercountry Adoption.* Canadians also adopted children from Haiti (159), Russia (106), South Korea (97), the United States (79), the Philippines (62), Thailand (40), India (37), and other countries. The largest number of adoptions occurred in Quebec (783), followed by Ontario (673), and British Columbia (227). Of adoptions from China, Quebec led with 423 adoptions, followed by Ontario at 358 adoptions.

Note that after the implementation of the HAGUE CONVENTION ON INTERCOUNTRY ADOPTION by the United States, which is expected to occur in 2007, it is likely that it will become more difficult for Canadians to adopt children from the United States.

Attitudes about Adoption in Canada

Canadians are generally supportive of adoption, based on a Canada-wide telephone survey that was conducted by the Institute for Social Research at York University in 2000. Based on this survey, more than 75 percent of Canadians strongly approved of adoption. When asked how they felt about adoption, and if they strongly approved, somewhat approved, somewhat disapproved, or strongly disapproved of adoption, 77 percent said they strongly approved and 21 percent said they somewhat approved. Only 2 percent somewhat disapproved, and none strongly disapproved of adoption.

In addition, the majority (77 percent) of the respondents said that mothers feel the same way about their adopted or biological children, while 70 percent said that fathers felt the same way about their adopted or biological children. Most Canadians (about two-thirds) said that birthmothers and birthfathers were unselfish, caring, and responsible to make an adoption plan. In addition, more than two-thirds of the surveyed Canadians said that adopted children were no more likely to be a problem than nonadopted children.

Tax Benefits

In 2005, the federal government in Canada passed a law allowing for a tax benefit of up to $1,600 for adoptive families. This is considerably less than the tax credit of about $10,000 available to citizens in the United States, but it is a long-awaited benefit nonetheless.

See also EASTERN EUROPEAN ADOPTIONS; INTERNATIONAL ADOPTION; ROMANIA, ADOPTIONS FROM; RUSSIA, ADOPTIONS FROM.

Hilborn, Robin. "Adoption Tax Credit of up to $1,600," Adoption Council of Canada, http://www.adoption.ca/news/050223.tax.htm, downloaded on May 20, 2005.
———. *Canadian Guide to Intercountry Adoption.* 4th ed. Ontario, Canada: Family Helper Publishing, 2004.
———. "China Leads Adoption Statistics for 2004." Available online. URL: http://www.adoption.ca/news/050527stats04.htm, downloaded on June 27, 2005.
———. *Waiting Kids in Canada: All about Domestic Adoption.* Ontario, Canada: Family Helper Publishing, 2004.
Miall, Charlene E., and Karen March. *Social Support for Adoption in Canada: Preliminary Findings of a Canada-Wide Survey.* Available online. URL: http://www.carleton.ca/socanth/Faculty/News%20Release%20Adoption%20Survey.PDF, downloaded on June 5, 2005.

case records The file maintained by the adoption agency on the child to be adopted, the biological parents, or the prospective adoptive parents. In some cases, records may be very voluminous, particularly if the child has been in foster care for several years or more.

Case records include confidential and personal information about individuals and families that is generally not shared outside the agency, for example, information obtained during professional counseling, allegations of child abuse, and results of investigations.

Prospective adoptive parents of children with SPECIAL NEEDS should request as much nonidentifying information as possible about the child they are planning to adopt, including permission to review appropriate portions of the case records when legally permissible.

See also OPEN RECORDS; SEALED RECORDS; SEARCH.

case study HOME STUDY or family study of prospective ADOPTIVE PARENTS, also involving counseling and the preparation for adoption.

child abuse See ABUSE.

Child Citizenship Act of 2000 A law passed in 2000 in the United States that took effect in 2001, which automatically confers U.S. citizenship on children adopted from other countries. (Some forms must be filled out by the adoptive parents and some fees paid for the citizenship to proceed.) The law was an amendment of Section 320 of the Immigration and Nationality Act.

The Act has the following requirements:

- At least one parent of the child must be a U.S. citizen by birth or by naturalization.
- The child must be under age 18.
- The child must reside in the United States with the adoptive parents.
- The adoption must be finalized (including finalization in the foreign country).

Before the passage of the Child Citizenship Act, it was cumbersome for adoptive parents to obtain citizenship for their children, and the process often took at least 18 to 24 months. The new law streamlines the process, and children who are adopted under the IR-3 entrant program will automatically become citizens and their parents will receive certificates of citizenship within several months. The IR-3 entrant program encompasses children who are adopted abroad and who are seen in the foreign country by both their adoptive parents. Otherwise, the child is granted an IR-4 visa.

Adoptive parents should be sure to check with their adoption agencies to determine if there are any actions they need to take to facilitate the citizenship process. For further information on the Child Citizenship Act on the Internet, individuals may go to the U.S. Citizenship and Immigration Services Web site at http://uscis.gov.

In past years and before the passage of the Child Citizenship Act, some parents failed to obtain citizenship for their adopted children, either assuming that citizenship was automatically granted, forgetting to apply for citizenship for the child, and/or not realizing its importance. As a result, some children who reached adulthood faced serious legal and immigration challenges, even deportation, since they were not lawful citizens of the United States. For example, John Gaul was adopted from Thailand by a Florida family in 1979 when he was four years old, and his parents subsequently obtained a U.S. birth certificate. They did not realize that he was not a U.S. citizen until they sought a passport for him at age 17. They immediately applied for citizenship, but delays resulted in John Gaul reaching his 18th birthday without having attained U.S. citizenship.

Gaul subsequently got into trouble with the law and was incarcerated. Upon his release, and to his shock, immigration officials immediately took him to a detention center in preparation for deportation. There were many appeals and many delays, but ultimately, Gaul was deported to Thailand at the age of 25, despite not speaking Thai and having no familial contacts or memories of Thailand. He may not return to the United States.

Similar cases have been reported for other adopted adults prior to the passage of the law. It is believed by many people that the Child Citizenship Act should rectify these problems.

See also INTERNATIONAL ADOPTION.

children, adopted   See ADOLESCENT ADOPTED PERSONS; INFANT ADOPTION; SPECIAL NEEDS ADOPTION.

Children's Aid Society of New York   The oldest formal child-placing agency in the United States, founded in 1853 by the Reverend Charles Brace; still in existence today in New York City.

Brace formed the organization to help the thousands of homeless children who roamed the streets of New York. He initiated the ORPHAN TRAIN program, which sent an estimated 150,000 children to families in the West, Midwest, and other areas outside New York.

Wheeler, Leslie. "The Orphan Trains," *American History Illustrated* 18 (December 1983).

children's rights   Although children do not have many of the civil rights of adults, they do have limited rights that were not afforded them in the earlier part of this century. At that time, children were considered "chattel" or possessions and were expected to work and earn their keep.

Today children are protected from exploitation by labor laws. They are also entitled to a free public education and in fact are required by law to attend school until reaching an age determined by the state (usually age 16), at which time they may choose to drop out.

Children are also protected by law from abuse, even when that abuse occurs at the hands of their parents. State social service workers are empowered with the authority to remove children from abusive homes and place them in foster homes or institutional shelters until a court decides what disposition to make of the children and whether or not abuse did occur.

Children are not automatically entitled to a permanent home and may wait in a series of foster homes for several years to be adopted.

See also ADOPTION AND SAFE FAMILIES ACT; TERMINATION OF PARENTAL RIGHTS.

China, adoptions from   Although virtually no adoptions of children from mainland China occurred prior to 1994, 787 children were adopted from mainland China by United States citizens in 1994. The number of adoptions further surged to 2,193 in 1995. The numbers of children adopted from China continued to increase to 7,906 children adopted by citizens of the United States in fiscal year 2005, representing about a third of all international adoptions. The numbers of children adopted from China are likely to continue to increase for the foreseeable future, as of this writing.

International adoption is increasingly popular in Canada, and Canadian citizens adopted 1,001 children from China in 2004. (See CANADA AND ADOPTION.)

The government manages adoption in China and oversees the institutions in which the children live. The Chinese government works with many international adoption agencies to place the children with adoptive families.

Reasons for Adoptive Placements

There are many reasons why so many Chinese children are in orphanages and need families, but the most important relates to the governmental concern about China's burgeoning population, which led to the "one child per family" policy. A second cultural issue reflects that male children are valued more highly than female children, because it is usually assumed in China that males will support the parents in their declining years, while girls will live with their husband's family. This has made male babies more highly valued, and female babies are often a second choice.

As a result of the one child per family policy (which had and still has some exceptions), many families who had girls abandoned them to orphanages so the parents could "try again" for a male child. Many of the abandoned girls are the second girl born to the family.

Since many adoptive parents in the U.S. and other countries are eager to adopt baby girls, the easy availability of female infants was and continues to be greatly appealing to American adopters.

Chinese Attitudes toward International Adoption

In a unique study reported in *Adoption Quarterly* in 2004, the researchers interviewed 25 government officials, 15 administrators of institutions that housed children, and 180 individuals from the general public in China. This study showed a positive attitude toward adoption. The researchers said that the government officials seemed genuinely positive about international adoption, seeing it as a good way to protect orphans as well as an opportunity to create a bridge to the West.

Among the general participants, the overwhelming majority (94 percent) viewed international adoption positively. Among the 6 percent who viewed international adoption negatively, the two primary concerns were that they were ashamed that the children would become foreign citizens and also that they were worried about the children losing their Chinese roots and culture.

Among the institution directors, there were three key themes to their views about international adoption. First, they saw adoption as an opportunity for a child to have a family. Said the authors, "They believed the prognosis for healthy development is greater through international adoption than if children remain in the welfare institutions [orphanages]. The directors emphasized that the institution's role should be that of a temporary or transitional home, and that the care from the welfare institution cannot substitute the love from birth or adoptive parents."

Next, the directors were worried about the lack of funding that they had for the children in their care, and international adoption eased their financial burden. Said the authors, "One director reported that there were so many children in care that they really could not afford to take care of more prior to beginning international adoption. Consequently the directors viewed international adoption as a win-win proposition: providing families for parentless children while also strengthening the welfare institutions' abilities to care for more children in need." Last, the institution directors emphasized that the postplacement reporting of the children was very important. American agencies are generally very diligent about providing follow-up reports to Chinese officials.

Stereotypes about Chinese Children

Many Westerners generally perceive Chinese and other Asian children in positive but stereotypical terms; for example, assuming that they are clean, bright, obedient, and so forth.

Another stereotype about Chinese children and other children adopted from Asia is that they are invariably adept in math and science; however, this is not so.

CHILDREN ADOPTED FROM CHINA IN THE UNITED STATES, FISCAL YEARS 1994–2005											
	1994	1995	1996	1997	1998	1999	2000	2001	2002	2003	2004	2005
Number of children adopted from China	856	2,193	3,388	3,637	4,206	4,101	5,053	4,681	5,053	6,859	7,044	7,906

Source: United States Department of State

Adoptive parents need to be aware of these stereotypical attitudes that they and their children will face.

Health of Chinese children   Chinese infants are often perceived by adopting parents as far healthier than orphaned children from orphanages in eastern Europe or Latin America and, because of social controls, less likely to experience FETAL ALCOHOL SYNDROME or suffer from the DRUG ABUSE ADDICTION of the biological mother. (In the majority of cases, that perception about the lower rate of fetal alcohol syndrome is correct.)

It should not be assumed, however, that Chinese children are inevitably healthy. Children from China have a high rate of lead poisoning. In addition, about a third of the children adopted from China suffer from iron deficiency ANEMIA. Rarely, children adopted from China have unrecognized, untreated congenital SYPHILIS. In addition, the longer the period that children remain in the orphanages, the higher the probability of physical and emotional health risks.

Other health risks for children adopted from China include the following:

- HEPATITIS B and C
- Thyroid disease
- TUBERCULOSIS
- Rickets
- Malnutrition
- DEVELOPMENTAL DISABILITIES

Language Delays

As with all young children who have been institutionalized, LANGUAGE DELAYS are common in newly arrived Chinese children.

Some anecdotal reports indicate that school and learning difficulties may be more common among Chinese adopted children than previously thought. For example, a Massachusetts support group published an article in their newsletter on such problems and subsequently received more than 8,000 requests for reprints of the article.

See also INTERNATIONAL ADOPTION; MEDICAL PROBLEMS OF INTERNATIONALLY ADOPTED CHILDREN; PRENATAL EXPOSURES.

Chen, Lin H., M.D., Elizabeth D. Barnett, and Mary E. Wilson, M.D. "Preventing Infectious Diseases during and after International Adoption," *Annals of Internal Medicine* 139 (2003): 371–378.

Luo, Nili, and Kathleen Ja Sook Bergquist. "Born in China: Birth Country Perspectives on International Adoption, *Adoption Quarterly* 8, no. 1 (2004): 21–39.

Miller, Laurie, C., M.D. *The Handbook of International Adoption Medicine: A Guide for Physicians, Parents, and Providers.* New York: Oxford University Press, 2005.

Miller, Laurie C., M.D., and Nancy W. Hendrie, M.D. "Health of Children Adopted from China," *Pediatrics* 105, no. 6 (June 2000). Available online. URL: http://www.pediatrics.org/cgi/content/full/105/6/e76.

Nicholson, Laura A. "Adoption Medicine and the Internationally Adopted Child," *American Journal of Law and Medicine* 28 (2002): 473–490.

Sullivan, Sharon, M.D. "Cultural and Socio-Emotional Issues of Internationally Adopted Children," *International Pediatrics* 19, no. 4 (2004): 208–216.

"chosen child"   A concept that social workers in past years encouraged among adoptive parents to convey to their adopted children and that told how the child had been "chosen" by them. This story was urged because it was believed the child would feel special and unique, and this feeling would overcome any anxiety or negativism about being adopted.

A problem with the "chosen child" story is that it was not always accurate in the past and is less likely to be so now, except in some international adoptions.

Very few adoptive parents now actually select the child they wish to adopt. Instead, a social worker, agency team, attorney, or other individual decides a particular couple or single person would be most likely to meet the needs of a particular infant.

As a result, when an older child starts asking for details on *how* or *why* she was chosen, the whole "chosen child" story falls apart.

Parents can instead explain that they chose to adopt as a way of building their family and that, once the child was placed, they chose to follow through and legally finalize the adoption in a court of law.

Today it is more often birthmothers who do the choosing—in such cases, adoptive parents are selected by a pregnant woman from a number of nonidentifying résumés or profiles written by prospective adoptive parents who were selected by professional staff as all being appropriate parents for a particular child. In many cases, the pregnant woman meets the prospective adoptive parents.

Another problem with the "chosen child" story is that sometimes adoptive parents have biological children, either before or after they adopt a child. Given current technology, biological children are not handpicked and come out however nature decrees. The parents are not "stuck with" the biological child, although the "chosen child" story does imply that they are when a child is born into a family.

The "chosen child" story also has an underlying implication that the child should feel grateful he was chosen when, in fact, most adoptive parents feel very grateful themselves that they have had an opportunity to adopt this child.

Most social workers and adoption experts urge adoptive parents to tell the child about adoption in a positive yet honest way, such as that they wanted a child to love and that the birthparents who were not ready or able to be parents themselves wanted the child to be placed in a loving home.

See also EXPLAINING ADOPTION.

classes for adoptive parents   See EDUCATION OF ADOPTIVE PARENTS.

confidentiality   In adoption, the practice of preserving privacy or anonymity and refraining from providing information on the identities of birthparents and adoptive parents, either to each other or to the adopted children or adult adopted persons.

An adoption agency social worker, attorney, or other intermediary is aware of the identities of all concerned and retains this information in confidence. Original birth certificates become SEALED RECORDS upon FINALIZATION of the adoption, and a new amended birth certificate is issued with the names of the adopting parents as parents.

Confidentiality in U.S. Adoptions

Confidentiality in adoptions has been the standard in the United States since infant adoptions became widespread in the 1930s. A particular focus on

confidentiality arose during and after World War II, according to historian E. Wayne Carp.

Today confidentiality is under attack by a variety of groups and individuals who seek to open all records and insist that OPEN ADOPTION is in the best interests of all concerned. They are greatly opposed to any confidentiality in adoptions.

Critics of confidentiality believe "secrecy" in adoption is wrong and also argue that, should the adopted person need to contact his birthparents for whatever reason, NO SEARCH would be necessary—the adopted person would know who his birthparents are and probably could learn exactly where they are. These critics believe it is wrong to deprive a birthparent or an adopted child of identifying information.

Advocates of continued confidentiality assert that all parties in an adoption, including the adopted person, birthparents, and adoptive parents, are protected by confidentiality. They believe these groups could be negatively affected if identities were revealed. They also insist that some birthparents might choose abortion over adoption if confidentiality and privacy were banned in all cases.

In addition, advocates state that the child benefits when only NONIDENTIFYING INFORMATION is provided and the child can be raised by parents who have a stronger sense of ENTITLEMENT.

Confidentiality in International Adoptions

Information that is available to families adopting internationally varies from country to country and may depend on what facts are available as much as the confidentiality policies of the country. In China, virtually all children who are adopted are foundlings, so no information is available. In contrast, in South Korea detailed but nonidentifying demographic information about the birthparents is supplied. In Russia the names and addresses of the birthparents are often supplied to the adoptive families, although sometimes this information has been falsified, as when the birthmother has provided incorrect information to the maternity hospital. In Ethiopia, adoptive parents may sometimes visit the child's birth family.

consent (to an adoption)   Voluntary agreement of those with PARENTAL RIGHTS to make an adoption plan. Who may give legal consent for an adoption varies from state to state.

If the birthmother was married at the time of the conception or birth of the child, both she and her husband must consent to any adoption, even if the husband is not the biological father. If the mother is unmarried, her consent is necessary. In most states, consent of the PUTATIVE FATHER is also necessary if he fulfills certain statutory criteria. Often these criteria are modeled after the *Stanley v. Illinois* case. (See BIRTHFATHER.)

An adoption agency that was asked to help arrange the adoption may also consent to the adoption by writing a report to the court.

Consent is waived if the state has terminated parental rights of the person whose consent would otherwise be required. In most states, parental rights may be terminated only on "fault" grounds (such as abuse, neglect, abandonment) or for serious incapacity (such as severe mental retardation or serious and incurable mental illness).

See also PREBIRTH CONSENT TO AN ADOPTION; TERMINATION OF PARENTAL RIGHTS.

corporate benefits   See EMPLOYEE BENEFITS FOR ADOPTION.

costs to adopt   Expenses associated with adopting a child. There are always costs involved in adoptions, but because of ADOPTION SUBSIDIES and taxpayer underwriting for some adoptions, the term usually applies to the fees for adoptions that are paid by the adoptive families, including adoption agency and/or attorney fees as well as other expenses related to the adoption. For example, many states in the United States allow (and may require) adoptive parents to pay for counseling for a pregnant woman who is considering adoption.

Payment of the birthmother's prenatal and delivery medical fees is allowed in some states, while reasonable living expenses in the latter part of pregnancy are also allowed in some states. Some states permit payment of the pregnant woman's medical expenses while they prohibit payment for living expenses. If living expenses are allowed, they must be documented, and many states require the disclosure of these expenses to the court.

Other additional expenses incurred by adopting parents include physical examinations for themselves and sometimes for children already in the home, phone calls to out-of-state agencies, and photographs (sometimes required by the agency). Parents adopting children overseas must also pay for special immunizations (if not covered by health insurance), visas, and passports. Some adoption agencies encourage adopting parents to donate to the orphanage where their child has been residing in another country, and to provide gifts to the orphanage director, other staff, and to foreign officials. Some of these gifts are in the form of cash.

Fees paid by adopting parent(s) vary greatly, depending on whether the child is an infant or older child, whether it is an agency or nonagency adoption, a state/public agency or private agency adoption, an international or U.S. adoption, and many other factors. For example, in an international adoption, the fees vary depending on the country from where the child will be adopted. Travel fees vary as well, since some countries require two trips to the foreign country, while others require only one trip.

There are no fees charged to birthparents: all fees are charged to the adopting parents, whether the adoption is primarily managed through an agency or through an attorney.

Children Adopted through State Foster Care

Parents who adopt their children through the state public social services adoption system usually incur few or no expenses. In addition, many children with SPECIAL NEEDS are also eligible for continuing MEDICAID coverage after FINALIZATION of the adoption, as well as adoption subsidies. INCOME TAX LAW BENEFITS may apply to the adoption, even when there are few or no expenses, in the case of the adoption of children with special needs. The reason for this was that the Congress wished to encourage the adoption of foster children from the public system.

Different Types of Fees in Agency Adoptions

In the adoption process, the first cost usually incurred by prospective adoptive parents working with a private (nongovernment) adoption agency is the agency application fee, which may start at $50 or more. Application fees in excess of $1,000 should be questioned. Note that public (government) agencies do not charge an application fee.

When the agency accepts the adoptive parents for a HOME STUDY (the thorough assessment of the family, prior to their approval to adopt), many agencies then charge a home study fee, which may be several thousand dollars. Other fees may be payable to the agency at a later date, with the remainder of the payment usually due when the child is placed with the family. These fees are usually the largest part of expenses.

Prospective adoptive parents should fully understand an agency's fees prior to deciding to work with a particular agency.

Some agencies will allow a family to make payments for the adoption on a regular basis or will even finance the fee for the parents, rather than requiring that the entire fee be paid initially or by the time of placement. The willingness to make such an arrangement is probably more likely when the family is adopting a child with special needs, whether domestically or internationally.

Some agencies charge SLIDING SCALE FEES. In this case, the fee is dependent on the income of the adopting parents, with a floor (minimum) fee and a ceiling (maximum) fee. The maximum fee is paid by more affluent individuals.

Fees for adoption attorneys   In general, the attorney's fees are reflected by how much work is required. State laws vary greatly on how much assistance attorneys may provide in an adoption. In some states, they may advise on an adoption only after the prospective parents themselves find a pregnant woman interested in adoption. In other states, attorneys may arrange the match between the pregnant woman and the adoptive parent(s), and attorneys are actively involved in all stages of the adoption. Prospective adoptive parents should ask attorneys for an estimate on their fees for adoption before agreeing to work with an attorney.

Attorneys usually require some initial payment, often referred to as a retainer, and probably expect at least $200 for a one-hour consultation fee. If prospective adoptive parents and a pregnant woman wish to make an adoption plan, the adopting parents generally give the attorney money for expenses, and that money is usually placed in a special restricted bank account.

If an adopting parent is unsure where the money is going, he or she should ask the attorney for an accounting. Most ethical attorneys will be willing to provide such information within a reasonable time.

Interstate adoption fees   If the child is adopted from another state, there will usually be additional fees and costs associated with complying with the INTERSTATE COMPACT ON THE PLACEMENT OF CHILDREN. This is an agreement between the states that governs interstate adoption, and it is administered by the public agency in each state. If the adopting parents are adopting a child from another state, they will pay an agency in their own state to study them, and they will pay the agency or attorney in the other state to oversee the paperwork involved with that state.

Affording Adoption

Many prospective adoptive parents save the money needed for an adoption, and some parents work two jobs to earn the required amount. However, some individuals are able to obtain several thousand dollars or more from their employer in adoption reimbursement expenses. (See EMPLOYMENT BENEFITS FOR ADOPTION.) In addition, the $10,000 income tax benefit is helpful to many adoptive parents in the United States. Some states also offer state income tax deductions or credits for adoption.

In Canada in 2005, the federal government passed a law allowing for a tax benefit of up to $1,600 for adoptive families.

Some families take a second mortgage on their homes or borrow money from relatives to pay the adoption fees. Others borrow on their 401(k) plan with their employer. Some employees request low-interest loans through their credit union. Some parents borrow on their insurance policies.

The image of adoptive parents as all affluent people is inaccurate. It is true, however, that few parents adopting healthy infants are living in poverty.

See also ADOPTION AGENCIES.

Adamec, Christine. *The Complete Idiot's Guide to Adoption.* 2nd ed. New York: Penguin, 2004.

counseling   Advice and discussion provided to adopting parents, birthparents, or adopted persons.

One of the primary advantages of an adoption arranged by a good, ethical agency is the counseling services offered. Caseworkers assist both birth-parents and prospective adoptive parents in working through a variety of issues, for example, the grief and pain associated with infertility and felt by most adopting parents. The grief associated with placing a child for adoption is another issue that the birthparents and particularly the birthmother must face.

Although nonagency adoptions traditionally did not include any form of counseling, and adoptive parents and birthparents were often not ready or able to cope with the myriad of feelings associated with an adoption, counseling of some sort is being increasingly provided.

See also PREGNANCY COUNSELING.

crisis pregnancy An unplanned pregnancy or a planned pregnancy that becomes a serious problem to the pregnant woman because of the desertion by the birthfather, the lack of support from her own parents, financial problems, or other factors.

A woman in a crisis pregnancy may need shelter and certainly also needs PREGNANCY COUNSELING. Many women in crisis pregnancies choose to abort, while others carry their pregnancies to term and either parent the child or place it for adoption.

MATERNITY HOMES provide shelter to pregnant women, usually young and unmarried but not necessarily indigent. Adoption agencies can advise women with crisis pregnancies who need a home.

cultural differences See CULTURE SHOCK; INTERNATIONAL ADOPTION.

culture camps Summer camps, either day camps or weeklong camps, for Indian, Korean, Latin American, or other groups of adopted children. Some camps are extremely well run and any adoptive family could feel comfortable enrolling their child. Other camps are lacking in substance or are thinly veiled programs to promote SEARCH. Parents can best check out camps by reading camp literature and talking to other adoptive parents whose children attended camp.

The goal of the culture camp is to promote the adopted child's awareness of and pride in his native origins and also enable him or her to meet other children of the same racial and ethnic background.

Culture camps cover history, music, dance, and other aspects of the child's native culture, and campers often eat foods prepared as they are in the country where the campers were born. Extracurricular activities such as arts and crafts and recreation are usually also provided.

Korean culture camps were initially the most prominent, because until 1990, the largest population of foreign-born adopted children came from Korea.

culture shock A feeling of disorientation and confusion experienced by a person visiting or relocating to a culture different from his or her own.

Adults

Adoptive families who adopt children internationally often must travel to the country and stay for days or several weeks until legal procedures are completed and they may leave with their children and return home.

Many families report a feeling of dismay at being strangers who do not speak the common language. Adoptive parents of children born abroad report that it is very helpful, whether they travel to the child's birth country or not, to learn some basics of the child's native language. Even if the child is an infant, he or she is used to the sounds of the language. And if the child is older than an infant, it is really considered a must by adoption experts for parents to learn some basics: "I love you." "Do you need to use the toilet?" "Come here." "What do you want?" "I am your mother (father)." Learning simple words and phrases can help both parents and child with problems of culture shock. The parents will feel more comfortable if they can communicate with the child at a basic level while in the foreign country. The child will feel more comfortable with the parents in her new country if the parents can use some familiar words.

If parents have already traveled abroad, they will probably understand that attitudes and the overall atmosphere of another country may be very different from what the adopting parents consider "normal"; for example, the host country's prevailing attitude may be flexible when it comes to time, whereas Americans like punctuality.

To alleviate culture shock, preparation well ahead of time is the best defense. Prior to traveling to a foreign land, it is advisable to read about the country and talk to other North Americans who have traveled there recently. Often an adoptive parents support group can advise how to find a fellow traveler or one who could provide good advance information.

Another aspect of culture shock can be fear. One American reported a sick feeling in his stomach as he viewed armed soldiers on every street corner of a Latin American city: the local residents appeared not to notice.

Concentrating on the objective of legally adopting the child and relaxing as much as possible by taking deep breaths and reassuring oneself aloud and silently are several helpful steps. It can be helpful to travel with fellow Americans and stay in the same hotel as well.

Children

If adults who are well aware of their goals in traveling abroad to adopt a child experience culture shock, how much greater a shock must be felt by a small child who is adopted from overseas. Children placed in intercountry adoptions usually contend with a complete language change as well as new parents and a totally different lifestyle.

Videocassette recorders, microwave ovens, fast foods, television, and computers are all unknown in an overseas orphanage. The way Americans dress, think, behave, even how they beckon people or wave to them is different from the behavior and gestures of people from other countries.

As a result, the culture shock to an adopted child who is not an infant can be profound, and new parents should take this into account. Experts advise limiting parties and visits for at least a few days after the child's arrival to give the child an opportunity to begin the cultural assimilation process.

Even children adopted from within the United States can sometimes face a form of culture shock, although there are usually a shared language and many commonalities. For example, one adoptive parent was amazed when her child asked what an ocean was and drove the child to the ocean to see for herself.

Children raised in small towns or big cities need time to adapt to a radically different environment.

Social workers generally try to place older children with families in environments similar to what they are accustomed, such as placing a child from a rural area with a family living in the country, but sometimes this is not possible.

Whether children are adopted from abroad or within the United States, most children are flexible and will, given the chance, adapt to their new families and their new homes.

See also INTERNATIONAL ADOPTION.

custody Legal control of a child, usually of a child who resides with the custodial parent. FOSTER PARENTS do not have legal rights over the child, and they are not considered to have legal custody: state social services departments retain control over major decisions to be made about a child. Adoptive parents obtain complete and permanent custody of a child upon FINALIZATION of an adoption in a court of law.

Custody battles abound in the courtrooms, and most suits are between divorcing parents, although single parents as well as gay partners have also argued over the custody of a child. In addition, relatives have argued for custody, including grandparents versus birthparents, aunts versus stepparents, and many other variations. The court usually considers such factors as the "best interests of the child" as well as blood relationships, where the child has resided in the past, and other issues, depending on state laws.

It is important for attorneys and judges to avoid making judgments involving psychological issues when psychologists, social workers, and psychiatrists are trained to provide such information. Conversely, mental health workers should avoid making legal decisions and should instead rely on legal counsel. For example, according to the authors of *The Best Interests of the Child*, in one case in which a judge stated reasons why he decided to award custody to a mother, he said that he found the father to be a "demeaning person" and made other psychological judgments about the father. This action was inappropriate because he was, in effect, acting as a psychologist but not one who could be cross-examined.

In recent years, unmarried birthfathers have begun to attempt to gain custody of their children.

In some cases, they have prevailed, while in others they have not. (See BIRTHFATHER; BIRTHMOTHER.)

There have also been custody battles between adoptive parents seeking to retain custody of an infant or toddler and birthparents who wished to revoke their consent to an adoption. Judges must decide the custody issue based on state law, legal precedents, the "best interests of the child," and a variety of factors.

Often the custody battles and appeals take years and cause serious emotional anguish to both sides—with the worst potential damage to the child.

See also CONSENT TO AN ADOPTION; PREBIRTH CONSENT TO AN ADOPTION; TERMINATION OF PARENTAL RIGHTS.

Goldstein, Joseph, et al. *The Best Interests of the Child: The Least Detrimental Alternative*. New York: Free Press, 1996.

demographics   See BIRTHMOTHERS; SOCIOECO-
NOMIC STATUS; STATISTICS ON ADOPTED CHILDREN.

developmental disabilities   Chronic severe disabilities such as mental retardation, cerebral palsy,
FETAL ALCOHOL SYNDROME (FAS), autism, and other
potentially long-term handicapping conditions.
Some children with severe attention-deficit/hyper-
activity disorder (ADHD) may be identified as having a developmental disability, while others with
ADHD may perform adequately or well in mainstream classes.

A developmental disability that occurs before the
age of 22 years can be attributed to a physical
and/or mental impairment, and is likely to continue. In addition, the individual experiences limits
in three or more of the following areas: self-care,
language, learning, mobility, self-direction, potential for independent living, and the potential for
economic self-sufficiency as an adult.

Within the many different categories of developmental disabilities, children may face a range
from mild to severe problems. Some children may
have a disability such as blindness, epilepsy, or
spina bifida, and yet they are not classified as
"developmentally disabled" if they are able to
function acceptably with medical or technological
support.

Developmental disabilities are not always
detectable in infancy, and they may not show up
until the child enters school and must compete
with other children of the same age.

A number of legal issues affect developmentally
delayed children. Some of these issues are the right
to a free public education (a right that was denied
to many disabled children in the recent past), the
right to live in a community, and the right to have
appropriate modifications made at school.

In some cases, children with developmental disabilities who are adopted may show considerable
improvements, especially when the disability was
exacerbated by a negative early environment, such
as orphanage living.

It should not be assumed that adoptive parents, no matter how loving, can overcome a
developmental disability. For example, a child
with FAS will continue to have the medical and
other problems associated with this developmental delay, despite a loving home. However, studies
have shown that once adopted, children with FAS
are less likely to engage in problem behaviors,
such as those that may cause suspensions from
school.

In another example, a child with Down syndrome may flourish in an adoptive family but will
never achieve above-normal intelligence. There
appears to be a basic ceiling of behaviors and
achievements for each child, although for many
children, the extent of their maximum abilities
may be difficult to predict.

Developmental delays may be caused by genetic
defects, malnutrition, metabolic diseases, toxic
exposures (such as lead poisoning), and birth
defects. As mentioned, they may also be caused or
exacerbated by an adverse environment, such as
early abuse or orphanage life.

Delays Caused by Institutional Living

Children who reside in institutions such as orphanages in foreign countries are more likely to have
developmental delays than children reared with
families. Says Dr. Laurie C. Miller in her book on
international adoption medicine, "Orphanage routines do not promote the expression of opinions or
preferences by the children, and leave little room
for discussion or response to novelty." Russian

researchers found that among three-year-old children residing in Moscow region orphanages, only 14 percent of children used two-word phrases." (See LANGUAGE DELAY.)

Some researchers have found that children with developmental delays likely caused by the deficits they experienced from orphanage life may experience remarkable "catch up" improvements in growth and development and even in INTELLIGENCE. This means that in some children developmental delay is largely environmental. These children may improve to the extent that they are either equivalent to or at about the same level of typically developing children of their own age in their new country.

Children with developmental delays related to their environment who are then adopted may sometimes show dramatic improvements. However, adoptive parents should not assume that a loving and supportive family can overcome all developmental delays. Some studies of children adopted internationally have shown that the children needed long-term modified educational programs in school.

Individuals who are considering adopting a developmentally delayed child should obtain as much information as possible on the particular challenges of the child and should also have appropriate specialists carefully review the medical records of the child before assuming parental responsibility.

Dr. Miller says the duration and the extent of the environmental deprivation, balanced by the biological potential of the child and the post-adoption support the child receives, are the key factors that determine children's cognitive (thinking) improvements after adoption. Thus, less severely deprived children are generally more likely to improve in their cognitive abilities. In most cases, improvements occur within about two years of arrival into the adoptive family.

Children should be screened for developmental disabilities with an age-appropriate test, for example, the Bayley or Mullen scales. Children should not be tested immediately after their adoption, when they are still becoming adjusted to the family, but screening should occur within the first month or so after arrival into the new family.

Dr. Miller says in her book on international adoption medicine that the following preadoption risk factors for serious developmental disorders are important (and these indicators may also be useful to consider in children born in the United States, Canada, or other Western countries):

- Prenatal alcohol exposure (which may be determined by the maternal history of alcohol abuse and/or the facial appearance of the child)
- Premature birth (less than 35 weeks gestation)
- Low birth weight (less than 2.5 kg, which may reflect either prematurity or intrauterine growth retardation)
- Microencephaly (small head size, reflecting poor brain growth, especially if severe or prolonged)
- Malnutrition (reflected in growth measurements)
- Social neglect (which may occur in the birth family, foster care, or orphanage)
- Physical neglect
- Physical abuse (which is based on the child's history, although in international adoption this information is usually not available)

Past Discrimination against the Developmentally Delayed

In much of the 20th century, many physically and mentally delayed individuals were placed in institutions as children and they remained there for life, usually in state hospitals. They were not taught necessary skills and behaviors, and then, because they did not exhibit the "normal" behaviors that they were never taught, many people believed that this *proved* that disabled individuals could neither learn nor function in society. This belief has been discarded by most people, who instead believe that developmentally disabled children can learn far more than was past believed. However, many developmentally delayed children and adults still have difficulty functioning in the community without help.

Laws Protecting the Developmentally Delayed

In 1975, Congress enacted the Education for All Handicapped Children Act, comparing the case of disabled children to that of minority children who were denied schooling prior to the ruling of *Brown v. Board of Education* in 1954. In 1990, the act was retitled the Individuals with Disabilities Education Act (IDEA), which was reauthorized in 1997.

IDEA covers many different disabilities, including learning disabilities as well as severe mental disorders, mental developmental disabilities, and other disabilities. This law states that a free public education is an entitlement of disabled children as well as nondisabled children.

In 2004, the law was reauthorized again, and the law took effect in 2005. The federal government in the United States authorized $10.6 billion in grants to the states for the education of children with disabilities, the largest annual amount of educational funding ever allocated. The law encompasses children enrolled in private schools and charter schools.

One new requirement of the law was the requirement that states develop policies and procedures to prevent an over identification of nonwhite children. This provision was included because numerous reports indicated that a disproportionate number of nonwhite children were placed in special education programs.

Another new requirement was that teachers or administrators could not compel parents to place their children on psychiatric medications, such as Ritalin, before they were allowed to attend classes and/or receive an evaluation for a disability. Teachers could still share information on the child's academic performance and behavior and, if they wished, parents could consult with physicians who could determine if medication was indicated.

When Developmentally Delayed Children Are Adopted

Adoptive parents of developmentally delayed children should be flexible people with realistic goals who can be positive about small improvements and changes in a child. In addition, it is very helpful if a support group of other adoptive parents or parents of disabled children is available to them. Support groups can also assist adoptive parents in learning about community resources for their children.

The outcome for families who have adopted children with developmental disabilities has been surprisingly positive. For example, a study of 52 families who had adopted 114 children with devel-

opmental disabilities, reported in *Children and Youth Services Review* in 1996, found that the majority of parents (79 percent) were "highly satisfied" that they had adopted their child. In fact, 60 percent had adopted other children with disabilities.

The study revealed that the parents found that an ADOPTION SUBSIDY and MEDICAID were very important and said that they could not have afforded to adopt without these supports in place. When asked which services were most important to the families, parents indicated: special education (88.5 percent of the families cited as important), dental care (63.5 percent), counseling (59.6 percent), and respite care (7.7 percent). The parents were most likely to receive counseling services; however, less than 25 percent found it adequate. They were least likely to receive respite services (time off while someone else cared for the child).

Said the researchers, "Families often challenge themselves to do what the lay person, and even the professional, may see as the 'impossible.' However, as noted earlier, the demands of caring for an adopted child with chronic illness or disabilities has much less of a negative impact on family life than might be expected. Quite the contrary, most of the families spoke often of the joy and meaning their children had brought to their lives. However, when they did need help, they did not want their reaching out to be seen as failure." Researchers also found that the parents wanted to be taken seriously by professionals and to work *with* them rather than to be dictated to by an agency staff person.

See also ATTACHMENT DISORDER; EARLY INTERVENTION; FOSTER CARE; MEDICAL PROBLEMS OF INTERNATIONALLY ADOPTED CHILDREN; ROMANIA, ADOPTIONS FROM; RUSSIA, ADOPTIONS FROM.

Babb, L. Anne, and Rita Laws. *Adopting and Advocating for the Special Needs Child.* Westport, Conn,: Bergin & Garvey, 1997.

Boehner, John, and Mike Castle. *Individuals with Disabilities Education Act (IDEA): Guide to "Frequently Asked Questions,"* February 17, 2005. Available online. URL: http://www.house.gov/ed_workforce/issues/109th/education/idea/ideafaq.pdf, downloaded on April 3, 2005.

Brown, Eva. "Recruiting Adoptive Parents for Children with Developmental Disabilities," *Child Welfare* 67 (March–April 1988): 123–135.

Hannon, Robert Captermon. "Returning to the True Goal of the Individuals with Disabilities Education Act: Self-Sufficiency," *Vanderbilt Law Review* 50, no. 3 (April 1997): 715.

Lightburn, Anita, and Barbara A. Pine. "Supporting and Enhancing the Adoption of Children with Developmental Disabilities," *Children and Youth Services Review* 18, nos. 1–2 (1996): 139–162.

Miller, Laurie C., M.D. *The Handbook of International Adoption Medicine: A Guide for Physicians, Parents, and Providers.* New York: Oxford University Press, 2005.

disabilities, developmental   See DEVELOPMENTAL DISABILITIES.

disruption   A disruption is an adoption that fails. Sometimes the child is removed from the home and returned to foster care or to the placing agency. The child may be placed with relatives of the adoptive family in some cases. In a few cases, the child is placed for adoption again by the adoptive parents. Disruptions are not common, but they do occur. Statistics about disruptions center on children adopted from within the United States (usually from foster care); however, international adoptions sometimes disrupt.

Adoptive parents should strive to educate themselves as thoroughly as possible about adoption in general and the child they plan to adopt in particular before making the serious commitment of adoption, particularly when they plan to adopt an older child or a child who has experienced severe deprivation.

Considering Disruptions

Prior to the 1970s, most adoptions were of infants, and very few disrupted. Even today infant adoption disruptions probably occur at about a 1 percent level at most. Disruptions of older children are more common, and estimates of older child adoptions that have disrupted have ranged from as low as 5 percent to as high as 10 to 25 percent. (The disruption rates vary according to the child's age and other factors.) The highest disruption rates occur among children adopted as teenagers, generally because adolescents usually present the most difficult and challenging problems to parents.

Some factors increase the likelihood of an adoption disruption. These may include the following:

- Children who have been in many foster care placements
- Children who have been sexually abused in the past
- Children with severe emotional and/or behavioral problems
- Children who were adopted previously and that adoption had failed

An early study by Trudy Festinger on disrupted adoptions among 1,500 adoptive placements in New York City yielded valuable information that is still useful today. Festinger reported her findings in 1986 in *Necessary Risk: A Study of Adoptions and Disrupted Adoptive Placements.* (Festinger also studied dissolutions in 2002, discussed later in this entry.)

The children studied were all over six years old, and the average age was 10.2 years. Her research revealed that the disruption rate over the course of two years was about 8 percent for the adopted children ages six to 10, whereas the disruption rate for children 11 and up was 16 percent over the same period of time.

The Festinger study revealed a significant success rate when children were placed with their own siblings. She found a 5.6 percent disruption rate for children placed with siblings contrasted to a 10.7 percent disruption rate with children placed alone. Children who were placed alone and who had siblings living elsewhere disrupted at a very high rate: 20.6 percent.

The separation may have been the source of the problem, or the reason for the separation itself may have caused problems; for example, siblings are separated when one child is sexually or physically abusive to the other child.

Some studies have indicated a relationship between the adoptive parent's education and the disruption rate. Adoptive mothers with higher educations were more prone to disrupt than adoptive mothers who were less educated, particularly when the children involved were between the ages of three and nine. Interestingly enough, educated mothers did not disrupt at a greater rate when they adopted teenagers unless the teenagers were emotionally disturbed.

Educated mothers are also less likely to have been foster parents, because foster parenting is often perceived by them as a blue-collar, working-class activity. Since foster parent adopters were more successful, this could be a factor in the comparisons to disruption rate of educated mothers.

Adoptive parents who had very high expectations of their children were often disappointed and sometimes did disrupt, which may relate to the better-educated mothers.

Stages of Disruption There appear to be several basic stages leading to a disruption, and caseworkers should be particularly sensitive to these stages in order to save an adoption, if at all possible, that looks like it may disrupt. These stages were described by a University of Southern Maine research study in 1986, which is still relevant today.

The first stage of a disruption is the stage of "diminishing pleasures," when the parent starts to see the hardships of raising the child as overtaking the joys of parenthood. Many adoptive parents have moments when they wonder "why in the world" they ever adopted this child, but when that attitude becomes foremost and prominent, it has become a major problem.

A second stage occurs when the child is perceived as a major problem—one the adoptive parents are not sure how to manage. The parents want the child to change his behavior, but the child cannot or will not change.

The next stage occurs when adoptive parents begin to complain freely to other people about problems they face with this child. Invariably they will receive some feedback from people who urge them to give up. An adoptive parent support group can possibly provide the positive reinforcement needed by parents in this stage to stop them from proceeding to a more advanced stage of disruption.

The fourth stage is a turning point: a critical event occurs that leads the adoptive parents to believe that they can no longer accept the child's behavior. The child may be extremely cruel to other family members, and this behavior could frighten the parents. Or he may run away yet again, despite having received numerous warnings, counseling, and other attempts to help him

resolve this behavior. The adoptive parents begin to envision life without the child, and they no longer actively strive to assimilate him into their everyday life.

The fifth stage is a deadline stage. Either the child is given a direct ultimatum or the parents decide between themselves that if the negative behavior occurs just one more time, they will return the child to the agency.

The final stage occurs when the adoptive parents give up and decide they will return the child to the agency. They feel that they have done everything they can, and can no longer cope with this child any further.

This stage is extremely painful for the child and for the parents, and it is also difficult for the caseworker. The stricken child may promise to "be good." It is easy for the worker to blame the parents at this point or for the parents to blame the agency, even when blame cannot reasonably be conferred.

The child's self-image is especially fragile at this point. Even if the child realized that his behavior was disturbing the parents but deliberately continued the distressing actions, the child will experience a profound feeling of rejection and failure with a disruption. The child may not have believed the parents would give up, despite what they said, and is genuinely shocked by the disruption.

Considering Dissolutions

The few studies that exist on adoption dissolutions indicate that only about 1–3 percent of finalized adoptions are dissolved.

For example, in Festinger's 2002 study of 497 children adopted in New York in 1996 from foster care, she found few children (3.3 percent) who had gone back into foster care again sometime after they were adopted, indicating a dissolution. The median age of the children when placed for adoption was about three years old.

Said Festinger, ". . . such a small number can be taken as a clear signal that families are loath to dissolve a relationship established by legal adoption." She noted, however, that some of the families seemed close to burning out, and they most frequently cited two barriers, including a lack of knowledge about where to turn when they needed help and the cost of services.

Factors associated with dissolutions In general, some factors associated with adoption dissolutions include as follows:

- The child was older at the time of adoption.
- The child was male.
- The adoptive family faced barriers in obtaining services that were needed by the child.
- The child had severe emotional or psychiatric problems.

See also ACTING OUT; FOSTER CARE; OLDER CHILD; SEXUAL ABUSE, CHILDHOOD.

Barth, Richard P., and Marianne Berry. *Adoption and Disruption: Rates, Risks, and Responses.* New York: Aldine De Gruyter, 1998.
Festinger, Trudy. "After Adoption: Dissolution or Permanence?" *Child Welfare* LXXXI, 3 (May/June 2002): 515–533.
———. *Necessary Risk: A Study of Adoptions and Disrupted Adoptive Placements.* Washington, D.C.: Child Welfare League of America, 1986.
Partridge, Susan, Helaine Hornby, and Thomas McDonald. *Learning from Adoption Disruption: Insights for Practice.* Portland, Maine: Human Services Development Institute, 1986.

divorce of adoptive parents It is unknown how many adoptive parents ultimately divorce their spouses or how many single divorced parents adopt children, but with the high divorce rate nationwide, it is virtually certain that some number of adopted persons' parents will divorce.

Divorce is a traumatic event and process for any child, biological or adopted. In some cases, divorce may be even more painful for an adopted child, especially when that child was adopted at an older age. In addition, even children adopted as infants may feel acutely rejected, both because of loss and separation issues related to adoption and because of the normal losses all children suffer. (The child's age at the time of the divorce is significant in how the child copes with this radical change.)

Researchers Dorothy Le Pere and Carolyne B. Rodriguez explored and wrote about how divorce affects adopted children at various stages of life. According to the two experts, the impact on the child depends in part on the age of the child when the parents divorce. For example, during infancy, the loss of an adoptive parent could be a serious "first loss." During toddlerhood, a child whose parents have just divorced may become unduly clingy and have difficulty striving for autonomy, an important aspect of this stage of life.

Preschoolers may blame themselves for the divorce, presuming some action or inaction on their part was the cause. The egocentrism of this stage of development causes such reasoning on the part of the child. The child may reason that because he had angry thoughts about his father, the father is now leaving, a form of "magical thinking" common to preschoolers.

School-age children may tend to see divorce as a personal rejection of themselves rather than of the other parent.

Adolescence is the rockiest point for many children. A severe reaction to divorce could be abuse of drugs or alcohol or promiscuous sexual behavior. The adolescent may also become concerned or confused by his or her own relationships.

In addition, adopted children may have more emotional baggage with which to struggle if they were adopted at an older age. They need to understand that their place in the family is still secure. Most adopted children, however, can resolve difficulties with the help of the parents and, as needed, professional assistance.

Le Pere, Dorothy, and Carolyne B. Rodriguez. "Adoption and Divorce: The Double Life Crisis," in *Adoption Resources for Mental Health Professionals.* Butler, Pa.: Mental Health/Adoption Therapy, September 1986, 270–281.
Seidman, Matthew Sanford. "Effects of Separation for Divorce of Adoptive Parents on the Adopted Child." Ph.D. diss., University of Southern California, 1989.

doctors See PHYSICIANS.

Down syndrome A chromosomal defect that results in physical and developmental abnormalities. (Also known as Down's syndrome). The syndrome is named after British physician Langdon Down, who initially identified many features of this syndrome.

Down syndrome is caused by an additional chromosome, known as trisomy 21, which means that there are three instead of two 21st chromosomes present. The syndrome results in a complex pattern of birth defects, including some degree of mental retardation. However, the retardation may not be severe, and most children and adults with Down syndrome are mildly or moderately retarded. A child with Down syndrome is developmentally disabled and considered a child with SPECIAL NEEDS.

Some parents choose to place their children with Down syndrome for adoption. It is probably not the appearance of the child that causes biological parents to choose adoption as much as their concern about current or future developmental delays and health risks, particularly if they fear that the child will need lifelong care.

According to the National Institute of Child Health & Human Development, Down syndrome occurs in about one of every 800 live births. It occurs within all races and socioeconomic classes.

Prenatal Testing

It is possible to obtain a prenatal diagnosis of Down syndrome. What expectant parents do with this information depends on the individual. According to one study of mothers whose fetuses had a prenatal diagnosis of Down syndrome, reported in the *American Journal of Obstetrics and Gynecology* in 2005, about half the mothers reported that they felt that their physicians had pressured or rushed them into the decision about whether to continue their pregnancies. Some mothers said the physician tried to change their minds about continuing the pregnancy. The study indicated that most mothers who continued their pregnancies did so for personal or religious reasons.

Prenatal testing can detect Down syndrome in the fetus as early as the first trimester of pregnancy with screening blood tests. Several methods are used. For example, the mother's blood may be checked for markers for Down syndrome. Screening tests are usually done in conjunction with an ultrasound. These tests have about at least a 60 percent accuracy, and there are some false positive readings (meaning that the test incorrectly identifies that the fetus has Down syndrome) and some

false negatives (meaning the test does not correctly identify a fetus with Down syndrome).

These tests cannot definitively confirm Down syndrome, and therefore other tests are needed. For example, an amniocentesis, a test in which a small sample of fetal cells is withdrawn from the amniotic fluid no earlier than the 14th to 18th week of pregnancy, can provide confirming evidence. Chorionic villus sampling is another test for Down syndrome. This test can be performed as early as the ninth to the 12th week of pregnancy.

Another test, percutaneous umbilical blood sampling, can also be used to detect Down syndrome in the fetus, and it is the most accurate test; however, it cannot be performed until the 18th to the 22nd week of pregnancy, and it carries a higher risk of miscarriage than earlier tests.

Symptoms and Diagnostic Path

Down syndrome can be detected at birth, if it has not been detected prenatally. A child with Down syndrome usually has somewhat slanted eyes, with epicanthal (extra) folds at the inner corners, and small hands, feet, ears, and nose. The tongue may be enlarged. About 50 percent of children with Down syndrome have heart defects, and about 10 percent of children with Down syndrome have defects in their gastrointestinal systems. Many of these birth defects are correctable by surgery.

A majority of children with Down syndrome have hearing loss, which may be correctable. Seizure disorders may be present and affect 5–13 percent of individuals with Down syndrome according to the National Institute of Child Health & Human Development. Vision disorders may also be a problem. An estimated 3 percent of children with Down syndrome develop cataracts. Children with Down syndrome have an increased risk (10 to 15 times greater than other children) of developing leukemia. They may be treated with chemotherapy or other cancer treatment options.

Children with Down syndrome are more susceptible to infectious diseases because of their abnormal immune systems. As a result, they have a greater likelihood than other children of developing chronic respiratory infections or pneumonia.

Treatment Options and Outlook

The average life expectancy of children with Down syndrome is at least 50 years (compared to only nine years in 1929), according to the National Institute of Child Health & Human Development.

Adults with Down syndrome may hold jobs and some marry. However, males with Down syndrome can only rarely father children because of low sperm counts. Females with Down syndrome generally have normal fertility; however, they have a high risk of bearing a child with Down syndrome.

In the past, many parents were urged to institutionalize their affected children. Today parents of a child with Down syndrome may choose other courses, such as parenting the child or placing the child for adoption. It is also important to note that children with Down syndrome are eligible for EARLY INTERVENTION programs through the school system.

Risk factors and Preventive Measures

Older mothers have an increased risk for having a child with Down syndrome, and the probability of a woman under age 30 of having a child with Down syndrome is less than one in 1,000. The probability increases to one in 400 among women who become pregnant at age 35. The odds increase further to one in 60 for a 42-year-old woman and one in 12 for a 49-year-old woman. However, experts report that maternal age alone is insufficient to detect most cases of Down syndrome. In addition, most women who have babies are younger women, and thus, only about 25 percent of the babies born with Down syndrome are born to women ages 35 and older.

There are no preventive measures against Down syndrome other than avoiding pregnancy altogether.

For further information on Down syndrome, contact the National Down Syndrome Society at their toll-free number of (800) 221-4602 or their Web site at http://www.ndss.org

See also DEVELOPMENTAL DISABILITIES.

National Institute of Child Health & Human Development, "Facts about Down Syndrome." Available online. URL: http://www.nichd.nih.gov/publications/pubs/downsyndrome/down.htm, accessed on June 6, 2005.

Skotko, Brian G. "Prenatally Diagnosed Down Syndrome: Mothers Who Continued Their Pregnancies Evaluate Their Health Care Providers," *American Journal of Obstetrics and Gynecology* 192 (2005): 670–677.

drug abuse/addiction Excessive use or dependence on illegal drugs or prescription drugs. When pregnant women abuse drugs, it is possible that the infant will suffer serious birth defects or later neurodevelopmental problems. (See PRENATAL EXPOSURES.) Drugs such as cocaine, "crack" cocaine (cocaine that is smoked), heroin, and other drugs such as prescribed pain medications and psychiatric drugs, as well as drugs that are not normally dangerous, can be perilous for the developing fetus and may cause problems to the child after birth.

Alcohol abuse is also a problem to the fetus, and children born to alcoholic mothers may suffer FETAL ALCOHOL SYNDROME and other effects. If the drug or alcohol abuse of the birthmother is known, it should be reported to prospective adoptive parents prior to the adoption. Often the abuse is not known, however, particularly in the case of infants and children who are abandoned to orphanages in other countries.

Abusive or Neglectful Parents

If addictive parents abuse or neglect their children, the state will usually remove the children from the home and place them in foster care. If the parent is able to recover from the drug abuse or addiction, then she or he may be able to parent children effectively; however, there is also a high recidivism rate of individuals who return to drug abuse and addiction. As a result, in many cases the parental rights are terminated. Such TERMINATION OF PARENTAL RIGHTS is more common as a result of the ADOPTION AND SAFE FAMILIES ACT.

Children remaining in their biological homes with drug-abusing parents generally have very unfavorable environments, and some aspects of their learning difficulties could theoretically be attributed to environment, while some aspects could be a result of actual neurological damage. The longer the children remain with drug-addicted parents who do not receive treatment, the higher the probability that they will suffer harm.

Finding Foster and Adoptive Homes

It is difficult to identify enough foster homes or adoptive homes for infants born addicted to drugs as well as children who were exposed to drugs during pregnancy. Social workers struggle to deal with babies and children returned by foster parents who cannot cope with the extra care and attention the children need.

Yet it should be noted that children are affected in different ways by drugs, and by such factors as when and how much of the drug was ingested. For example, some children who test positive for cocaine in their urine at birth appear normal and behave normally. It is unknown what long-term effects may occur, but some adoptive parents believe the risk is well worth their efforts.

Individuals who are considering adopting drug-exposed infants from the United States should request copies of the child's medical records. An in-office review of the records is inadequate, and the couple (or single person) should be able to take the copy of the medical record to their own physician for review, whether the child is still an infant or is an older child who was exposed to cocaine in utero. (The agency will almost always delete the identities of the birthparents for purposes of confidentiality.)

If the family or single person is adopting a child in the United States from foster care but are not the child's foster parents, they should also ask to speak to the child's foster parents to learn as much as possible about the child. The prospective parents should also ask the agency for names of local physicians and psychiatrists or psychologists who are knowledgeable in the area of treating children who were exposed to drugs in utero.

If the child is being adopted from another country, the prospective parents may wish to consult with a physician who is expert in international ADOPTION MEDICINE and who can provide a professional opinion about the child's medical status.

See also FOSTER CARE; MEDICAL PROBLEMS OF INTERNATIONALLY ADOPTED CHILDREN.

early intervention Educational programs offered in the United States to children from birth to age three who have or are deemed at risk for DEVELOPMENTAL DISABILITIES, under the Individuals with Disabilities Education Act (IDEA). (In some states, eligibility extends to age five.) The reauthorization to this act was signed by President George W. Bush in 2004. IDEA was first enacted by Congress in 1975, and it has been reauthorized numerous times. As of this writing, new regulations are being written to support the 2004 reauthorized law.

Any children who fit the program criteria are eligible for services. It is unknown how many adopted children are receiving early intervention program assistance.

Early intervention programs are provided at no cost to families with supporting federal funds. Infants and toddlers with delays in physical, adaptive, or cognitive development, as well as children with communication difficulties or social or emotional developmental delays are eligible for these programs. If a foster parent or adoptive parent thinks a child might be eligible, he or she may ask for an evaluation for developmental delay. The child's pediatrician should be able to refer the parent to the intervention services in the community. Alternatively, a parent may directly request an evaluation through the local department of public health (usually listed in the blue pages in the front of the telephone book.)

According to the National Center for Health Statistics, in 2001–02 about 10.7 children per 1,000 children under age five had speech problems, 6.8 per 1,000 had mental retardation or other developmental delays, 3.0 per 1,000 had other mental, emotional, or behavioral problems, and 2.6 per 1,000 had learning disabilities.

Some services that may be provided to the child in an early intervention program include

- Speech therapy
- Physical therapy
- Occupational therapy
- Psychological services
- Assistive technology devices
- Feeding team and nutritional advice
- Supervised play groups

Therapists come to the home or to the child's day care or preschool to provide needed services.

National Center for Health Statistics. *Health, United States, 2004 with Chartbook on Trends in the Health of Americans.* Hyattsville, Md., 2004, page 85.

early puberty/precocious puberty Development of signs of sexual maturity that occur well before age eight in girls and age nine in boys. Some children have shown pubertal changes as young as age three or four years. This uncommon hormonal problem can reflect abnormalities of the pituitary, hypothalamus or adrenal glands, or gonads. Chromosomal or genetic disorders can also trigger early puberty. In other cases, it is idiopathic, which means there is no obvious cause for the early puberty.

Early puberty has been reported among children adopted from other countries, especially among those who have shown dramatic catch-up growth after adoption. It is primarily seen among girls although rarely, precocious puberty may be seen in boys adopted from other countries.

Sometimes a seemingly early puberty is not "precocious," but it is actually appropriate for the child's age. For example, the age of the onset of puberty varies among ethnic groups. Unfortunately, little information is available about the normal onset of puberty in many of the ethnic groups represented by children adopted from other countries. Furthermore, a child's age may have been unknown and then underestimated (because of deprivation or small size) when he or she entered institutional care; thus, the child was inappropriately assigned a younger age. Bone age X-rays may aid in determining a child's actual age; however, results are affected by many different factors.

In one study reported in *Archives of Disease in Childhood* in 1998, Italian researchers studied 19 girls adopted by families in Sweden from developing countries (15 children were from India) and who were referred to a specialist for the onset of early puberty.

The researchers reported that the children showed signs of "chronic undernutrition" at the point of adoption. They divided the girls into those adopted before and after the age of four. The age at adoption had little association with the age at the onset of puberty (six and one-half to seven years), but the girls adopted younger were somewhat taller. Hormonal treatment to suppress the precocious puberty was not very successful, in part because many girls were referred when the puberty was too advanced.

The theory suggested by some researchers for an early puberty in some children adopted from other countries is that the abrupt change from deprivation and malnutrition to relative affluence, adequate diets, and psychological security may trigger the body into launching into an early puberty. Thus, the altered diet of the girls in the study could have exacerbated puberty.

Said the researchers, "Before adoption these girls were mostly on a low protein, low energy vegetarian diet, which changed to a balanced enriched diet after adoption. . . . Improved nutritional conditions increase insulin-like growth factor 1, which would stimulate both the maturation of ovarian follicles and their oestrogen production, and also the hypothalamic secretion of gonadatrophin releasing hormone, favouring sexual maturation."

Some researchers believe that the age of the child when adopted is a factor, and that children adopted as infants have a lower risk of an early puberty. However, in some studies, the adopted children who developed early puberty were only a median age of four and one-half months when they arrived in the family, so adoption at a young age is not necessarily protective.

Symptoms and Diagnostic Path

Early puberty is characterized by physical body changes in a child that are typical of children undergoing adolescence, such as the development of breast tissue in females, the appearance of underarm and pubic hair in both males and females, and enlarged testicles in males. Females may begin to menstruate. Children with even subtle signs of early puberty such as acne or body odor should be evaluated by an experienced pediatric endocrinologist to check for serious illnesses that need treatment.

Physicians should rule out diseases and disorders that may cause precocious puberty, such as McCune-Albright syndrome. Girls should be screened for ovarian tumors or follicular cysts and boys for testicular tumors. Boys and girls should be screened for adrenal and brain tumors.

In one study reported in *Pediatrics* in 2003, researchers found that 12 percent of the patients with early puberty had endocrine diseases or disorders, such as McCune-Albright syndrome, a rare condition that is often accompanied by early puberty and short stature. Other patients had growth hormone deficiency, neurofibromatosis, or pituitary adenomas (tumors of the pituitary gland that are often benign).

Physicians may order a gonadotropin-releasing (GnRH) stimulation test, which will help to diagnose the presence of precocious puberty. In girls, a pelvic ultrasound may be ordered to rule out an ovarian tumor. Boys who may have precocious puberty should have their androgen levels tested. Elevated androgen levels may indicate a tumor of the adrenal glands or congenital adrenal hyperplasia, a genetic disorder that causes the adrenal glands to increase in size.

In both girls and boys with signs and symptoms of early puberty, thyroid blood levels should be checked. If the child is hypothyroid (below normal in thyroid production), treatment with thyroid hormone may cause a remission or halt the progression of early puberty, if it has not already advanced too far.

Treatment Options and Outlook

When children have precocious puberty, the cause is sought and, if found, the decision is made as to whether it can or should be treated. Sometimes hormones to suppress puberty are used, especially if the child is younger than five or six years old. If the treatment works, the puberty may be delayed until it would normally occur. If it does not work, the child will often have a short final stature that is significantly lower than their peers.

Researchers reported on their findings in 2001 in the *Journal of Clinical Endocrinology & Metabolism* on the treatment of 98 children with early puberty. They found that treatment with deslorelin, a medication to suppress puberty, given in boys before age nine and in girls before age eight, was effective in improving the final height that the children achieved. The children were treated with the drug for more than two years. However, they were still of smaller stature than their peers, although taller than they would have been without treatment. According to the researchers, even girls whose bone age was 13 years old at the onset of treatment showed improvement in growth.

Risk Factors and Preventive Measures

Some illnesses, as mentioned, may predispose children to an early puberty. Adopted young girls who show a dramatic growth spurt within two years of adoption are more likely to experience an early puberty. Most of the reported girls with this condition have been adopted from South Asia, especially from India.

Consequences of Precocious Puberty

Early puberty can be difficult for a child and family to deal with. The child may be more sexually mature than her classmates or older siblings, causing teasing and resentment. Parents may have their own difficulties coping with puberty that occurs early. The child may be expected to behave more maturely than his or her chronological age. Many children adopted from a background of abuse or neglect may be emotionally very immature, exacerbating the problems of dealing with puberty. However, some research indicates that families and children take early puberty in stride.

See also GROWTH DELAYS; MEDICAL PROBLEMS OF INTERNATIONALLY ADOPTED CHILDREN.

Mason, Patrick, M.D., and Christine Narad. "Growth and Pubertal Development in Internationally Adopted Children," *Current Opinion in Endocrinology & Diabetes* 9 (2002): 26–31.

Midyett, L. Kurt, M.D., Wayne V. Moore, M.D., and Jill D. Jacobson, M.D. "Are Pubertal Changes in Girls Before Age 8 Benign?" *Pediatrics* 111, no. 1, (2003): 47–51.

Miller, Laurie, C., M.D. *The Handbook of International Adoption Medicine: A Guide for Physicians, Parents, and Providers.* New York: Oxford University Press, 2005.

Oerter Klein, Karen, et al. "Increased Final Height in Precocious Puberty after Long-Term Treatment with LHRD Agonists: The National Institutes of Health Experience," *Journal of Clinical Endocrinology & Metabolism* 86, no. 10 (2001): 4,711–4,716.

Petit, William A., Jr., M.D., and Christine Adamec. *The Encyclopedia of Endocrine Diseases and Disorders.* New York: Facts On File, 2005.

Virdis, Raffaele, et al. "Precocious Puberty in Girls Adopted from Developing Countries," *Archives of Disease in Childhood* 78 (1998): 152–154.

eastern European adoptions Children adopted from such countries as Russia, Kazakhstan, Ukraine, and Poland. In fiscal year 2005, there were 6,288 children adopted from eastern European countries by Americans, including 4,639 children adopted from Russia, 755 from Kazakhstan, 821 from Ukraine, and 73 from Poland. The total number of eastern European adoptions represented 27 percent of all international adoptions by U.S. citizens. In contrast, 7,906 children were adopted from China in 2005.

Historical Background

With the exception of some children from eastern Europe who were adopted during a brief period after World War II, before 1989 nearly all intercountry adoptions were of children from Latin American or Asian countries, and Korea was the principal country from which children were adopted by Westerners. With the downfall of despot Ceauşescu in Romania came the revelation that many thousands of children languished in Romanian orphanages, often under horrific conditions. The plight of these children motivated many Americans to rush to adopt them. More than 2,590 Romanian children were adopted by American parents in 1991 alone.

It was subsequently realized that many children lived in orphanages throughout eastern Europe, needing adoptive families. In the 1990s and to the present, countries of the former Soviet Union, such as Russia, Ukraine, and Kazakhstan, have accounted for many adoptions by families in the United States. Meanwhile, the number of Romanian adoptions declined dramatically as adoption abuses were uncovered, and Romanian officials struggled to put appropriate controls in place. In fiscal year 2003, only 200 children were adopted from Romania, and in 2004, the number fell further to 57 children. A moratorium was placed on the adoption of Romanian children in 2004, and this moratorium is still in effect as of 2006.

Reasons for These Adoptions

Experts have postulated a variety of reasons for why so many Americans have chosen to adopt children from eastern Europe. One reason is that many of the children are Caucasian, and white parents from the United States and other countries believe that it can be difficult to adopt white children from within their countries or that it would be difficult to parent an ethnically different child adopted from the United States or another country. However, some children adopted from eastern Europe are of a mixed racial heritage.

Another reason is that many prospective adoptive parents do not wish to engage in the OPEN ADOPTION that is the standard practice among most domestic adoption agencies placing infants in the United States. Some prospective adoptive parents fear that a birthmother in a domestic adoption may change her mind, putting the placement at risk. Others believe (rightly or wrongly) that their personal characteristics (age, sexual orientation, marital history, and so forth) may disqualify them from domestic adoption. However, many choose international adoption out of their generous spirits, feelings of sympathy and love for the children abandoned to orphanages, and an altruistic desire to share their home and family with those needy children.

Who Adopted

In contrast to most adoptive American parents who adopt children domestically from the United States, some adoptive parents of eastern European children already have biological children, and many could have had more children if they chose

to do so. In contrast, most people who adopt from adoption agencies that place infants born in the United States are infertile and childless. This difference lies largely in the fact that many domestic adoption agencies placing infants seek childless couples, while for international adoption agencies, it is acceptable if there are already children in the home.

Much Success and Some Problems

The vast majority of parents who have adopted children from eastern Europe have expressed satisfaction with their children. Children who came to them with serious problems usually showed dramatic catch-up growth and improvements that have amazed pediatricians and researchers. However, to the dismay of some parents, some of the DEVELOPMENTAL DISABILITIES caused by orphanage living and other problems were not as easily surmountable as they initially believed.

Some of the children adopted from eastern European countries have been found to have FETAL ALCOHOL SYNDROME (FAS) or fetal alcohol spectrum disorders (FASD), conditions which may not be clearly detectable by experts, but which may cause significant learning and behavioral problems. (See ADOPTION MEDICINE; PRENATAL EXPOSURES.) Many individuals in Russia and other eastern European countries have a serious problem with ALCOHOLISM, and women may fail to give up drinking during pregnancy, as there is little awareness of the adverse effects of prenatal alcohol consumption on the developing child.

Some children adopted from eastern Europe have problems with ATTACHMENT DISORDER or with specific disorders, such as SENSORY INTEGRATION DISORDER.

As with foster children adopted within the United States, research has revealed in many cases that the older or more complex the background of the child at the time of placement, the higher the probability that the child may have more long-lasting and severe developmental, behavioral, and emotional problems. A considerable number of children in eastern Europe are placed in orphanages after parental rights are terminated due to abuse or neglect. Such difficult early life experiences may have enduring effects on the emotional stability of the child.

As the large cohort of eastern European children adopted in the 1990s enters their late teens and early adult years, increasing numbers of severe problems are being identified. Current research efforts as of this writing are attempts to track the number of eastern European adoptees—now young adults—who are homeless or institutionalized (incarcerated in psychiatric facilities or jails) in the United States.

To complicate matters, according to Dr. Miller, medical records available from eastern European countries are often confusing, although generally prepared in good faith. Says Dr. Miller in her book, *The Handbook of International Adoption Medicine,* "Concerns about possible maternal drug or alcohol use or smoking are seldom addressed, even if the infant is low birth weight." Moreover, much of the medical terminology used is obscure, archaic, or alarming to those unfamiliar with eastern European usage. For example, terms such as "perinatal encephalopathy," "hypertensive-hydrocephalic disorder," or "vegetal-visceral syndrome" appear frequently yet have little clinical importance.

The Future

As with all intercountry adoptions, it is difficult to impossible to predict what will happen even six to 12 months in the future. The only certainty is that countries will continue to "close" and "open" their doors to adoption. The adoption of children in eastern Europe, especially from Russia and Kazakhstan, may continue for years to come or it may cease altogether, and quite abruptly. Should that happen, it is likely that the plethora of intercountry adoption agencies will turn their sights to other eastern European countries that may agree to the adoption of their institutionalized children.

See also HAGUE CONVENTION ON INTERCOUNTRY ADOPTION; INTERNATIONAL ADOPTION; MEDICAL PROBLEMS OF INTERNATIONALLY ADOPTED CHILDREN; ROMANIA, ADOPTIONS FROM; RUSSIA, ADOPTIONS FROM.

Miller, Laurie C., M.D. *The Handbook of International Adoption Medicine: A Guide for Physicians, Parents, and Providers.* New York: Oxford University Press, 2005.

eating disorders in adopted children   Abnormal eating patterns, including excessive eating or an unusual lack of interest in food, despite the presence of malnutrition in the child. The eating disorders of adopted children often stem from their past deprivation, particularly among some children newly adopted from other countries, who may eat ravenously because they have never had enough food in the past. They may also engage in food hoarding, hiding food under the bed or in their closet.

In such cases, according to Dr. Miller, "Parents should be encouraged to offer food freely; usually the voracity diminishes within a few days or weeks when the child becomes confident that the food supply is reliable."

Some children adopted from other countries may be very resistant to trying new foods, possibly because they are used to the extremely bland tastes and textures of orphanage food. In such a case, it is best to introduce new foods slowly and not press the child to try many different types of foods at once. Some children may never find eating an enjoyable activity, but as long as they consume sufficient nutrition to maintain normal health, this should be considered acceptable.

In some cases, young children who have been fed only liquids for a prolonged period may resist textured foods and also have difficulty accepting food on a spoon due to overactive tongue thrust. Many children have been exclusively bottle-fed with an enlarged opening in the nipple and have not developed good sucking and swallowing muscles or coordination. Some children "store" food in their cheeks, as they may have difficulty sensing that their mouths are full and they need to swallow. These problems often resolve within weeks, but sometimes parents need help from the physician or feeding specialists.

Some children may engage in eating nonfood items, which is a condition known as pica. This behavior may be indicative of ANEMIA, and the child should be evaluated by a physician if the behavior is seen frequently.

Treatment Options and Outlook

Children with eating disorders of any type should be evaluated by a physician. If there are no illnesses that are noted by the doctor, a feeding specialist (often through an EARLY INTERVENTION program) may provide useful advice.

Risk Factors and Preventive Measures

Children most at risk for unusual eating behaviors are those who

- Lived previously in an orphanage
- Were or are malnourished
- Had a past life of deprivation, in which food was scarce
- Missed feeding milestones in early life, such as the delayed introduction of solids and textures

See also MEDICAL PROBLEMS OF INTERNATIONALLY ADOPTED CHILDREN.

Miller, Laurie C., M.D. *The Handbook of International Adoption Medicine: A Guide for Physicians, Parents, and Providers.* New York: Oxford University Press, 2005.

economics of adoption See COSTS TO ADOPT.

education of adoptive parents Numerous adoption agencies nationwide hold adoption classes for prospective adoptive parents as part of the family assessment process (HOME STUDY) and preparation process.

Policies of the agency are fully explained during the course of the classes.

Adoption issues are usually covered, such as when and how to talk to a child about adoption, how to deal with relatives and acquaintances, and problems the child may have if the child does not resemble the parents' racial or ethnic background.

Parents adopting children with SPECIAL NEEDS will usually learn about physical and sexual abuse along with suggestions on how to handle problems that may occur as a result of previous abuse. Social workers usually encourage parents to ask for help and not fear that they will be unable to finalize their adoption if they let the social worker know about a problem.

The classes are held primarily to help prospective parents prepare for parenthood and to educate them as much as possible about adoption. Classes are usually small groups of up to 20 couples, and the couples often develop a strong camaraderie that may last for years after they have adopted their children.

In some cases, social workers bring in birth-mothers, adult adopted persons, and adoptive parents as speakers, either singly or on a panel. Social workers encourage prospective parents to ask many questions.

Specifics of Child Care

Because of the anxiety associated with the adoption process, even when adoption agencies offer classes, the prospective parents may not fully listen and take advantage of the information offered. In addition, they usually concentrate on adoption issues rather than basic child care, such as how to change a baby, give it a bath, and so forth.

As a result, some educators offer child care classes to prospective parents or individuals who have recently become adoptive parents, combining information about adoption with basic child care information. Some experts believe that there are some issues that should be covered by educators, including issues rarely covered by agency classes; for example, some adoptive parents may actually feel a postpartum depression after their infant arrives home.

Confused by this feeling and fearful about such feelings, they can be tremendously relieved to learn other adoptive parents often feel an initial overwhelming tiredness, especially during the first six weeks after adoption.

emotional problems See ACADEMIC PROGRESS; ACTING OUT; BONDING AND ATTACHMENT; CULTURE SHOCK; OLDER CHILD; PSYCHIATRIC PROBLEMS OF ADOPTED PERSONS; SPECIAL NEEDS.

employee benefits for adoption Paid or unpaid benefits given to adoptive parents. Companies vary widely on adoption benefits provided to employees. Some companies offer financial assistance in the form of reimbursement for adoption expenses to their employees. According to the National Adoption Information Clearinghouse in Washington, D.C., the average maximum corporate reimbursement for adoption expenses was $3,879 in 2004.

In most cases, the benefit is paid after FINALIZATION of the adoption, although some companies will reimburse the employee when the expenses are incurred or after the child is placed with the family. Some employers exclude benefits from stepparent adoptions.

Leave/Vacation Benefits

Leave policies for adoptive parents vary widely as well. Some companies provide adopting parents with the same parental leave that would be given to new biological parents.

Of course, since the passage of the Family and Medical Leave Act, adoptive families are entitled to the same unpaid leave time (up to 12 weeks) to care for a newly adopted child (or a child who is sick) as are other employees. It must be stressed, however, than FMLA leave is unpaid and thus many workers will only use a few weeks of unpaid time. However, some employers offer paid time off to new adoptive parents.

Prospective adoptive parents who would like to discover more about what adoption benefits their company may offer should check with the human resources or benefits office of their companies to learn what is covered in the areas of reimbursement, parental leave, and insurance coverage. Note that not all human resources personnel are knowledgeable about adoption benefits provided by the company. It is not an everyday occurrence for people to apply for such benefits, which is why a clerk may not be aware of these benefits.

For information on corporations that provide employee benefits for adoption, the following Web site may be helpful: http://www.adoptionfriendly workplace.org/employers.asp.

See also ADOPTION SUBSIDY; COSTS TO ADOPT; INCOME TAX LAW BENEFITS FOR ADOPTIVE PARENTS.

entitlement   The term is usually used to describe the feeling of the adoptive parents that they deserve their adopted child and can truly bond to him or her. This term can also be used to describe such feelings of anyone in the adoptive family.

Authors Jerome Smith and Franklin Miroff write in their book, *You're Our Child,*

> The sense of entitlement of the parents to child, of child to parents, and siblings to each other is a task unique to adoption. This is a relatively easy procedure in having a biological child and usually occurs at an unconscious level. For adoptive parents, however, there is this extra psychological step involved.

Author Patricia Johnston maintains that entitlement is not always an immediate feeling. "Developing a sense of entitlement is an ongoing process of growth rather than a single task identifiably completable, and the success of an adoption is related to the degree to which this sense of entitlement has been acquired by each family member rather than to its being seen as achieved or not achieved."

Some adoption experts believe infertile couples continually struggle over feelings of entitlement to their adopted child. Other researchers believe societal attitudes inhibit or enhance the feeling of entitlement. Charlene Miall studied how adoptive parents perceived community attitudes and found those she interviewed were dismayed by the attitudes and behavior of people they knew.

Miall observed that the absence of entitlement in some infertile adoptive parents was probably caused more by a knowledge of the attitudes of the surrounding society than by a failure to adequately deal with the infertility. She said the focus on blood ties in much social work literature relegates adoption to a second-rate position. (See also ATTITUDES ABOUT ADOPTION.)

Critics of OPEN ADOPTION state that when an adoptive family and the birthfamily know each other's identity and periodically exchange information, it may be difficult for the adoptive family to feel an entitlement to the child. (And visits with the child are becoming increasingly more common in open adoptions.) As a result, they will feel the child is really the birthfamily's child and not their own.

Proponents of open adoption as well as proponents of meetings between birthfamilies and adopting families hypothesize that when adoptive families believe they were actually selected by the birthfamily, they feel more of an entitlement than when they were simply selected from an adoption agency waiting list.

Johnston, Patricia Irwin. *An Adoptor's Advocate.* Indianapolis, Ind.: Perspectives Press, 1984.

Miall, Charlene E. "The Stigma of Adoptive Parent Status: Perceptions of Community Attitudes toward Adoption and the Experience of Informal Social Sanctioning," *Family Relations* 36 (January 1987): 34–39.

Smith, Jerome, and Franklin I. Miroff. *You're Our Child: The Adoption Experience.* Lanham, Md.: Madison Books, 1987.

environment Scientists have argued the "nature-nurture" controversy for years and will probably continue to disagree on whether heredity or environment is more important; however, most experts agree that both the child's genetic heritage and the environment are critical factors to a child's personality and development.

There are some indications that INTELLIGENCE levels can be positively affected by adoption. There are also indications that both heredity and environment play a role in an adopted person's contracting cancer.

etiquette In adoption, refers to the polite way to discuss or mention adoption-related issues or to refrain from mentioning them.

Most adoptive parents, adopted children and adults, and birthparents would probably appreciate some generally accepted basic rules of etiquette regarding adoption. The following list is a set of several rules the authors have drawn up, based on their knowledge of adoption, for the friends and relatives of individuals whose lives are somehow affected by adoption:

1. If a woman says she is considering placing her child for adoption, it is impolite to react with extreme horror and exclaim, "How could you give up your own flesh and blood? I could never do that!" A woman who is thinking about adoption would prefer to hear empathetic comments, such as, "That must be a hard decision to make."

2. If a couple is considering adopting a child, it is impolite to say, "You mean you can't have kids of your own? How sad!" It is also not polite to tell about your cousin who waited nine years on a waiting list or ask how much money the adoption will cost. Instead, it is preferable to say something like, "That sounds very exciting."

3. If a family member or friend discovers someone has just adopted, it is inappropriate to ask if the "real mother" is known, what she looks like, how old she is, and whether or not she is married. It is even less acceptable for the mail-

man or supermarket checkout clerk to ask these questions. It is appropriate to say, "Congratulations! How wonderful!"

4. If a family has adopted an infant from another country, it is inappropriate—and silly—to say, "How wonderful! She will be bilingual!" (Yes, people do say such things.)

5. In the case of an intercountry adoption, it is impolite to ask if the child was abandoned or had many unusual diseases or if the mother was starving to death.

6. It is always impolite to refer to a child's adoption in front of the child over age two as if she or he did not exist.

7. If a family has a biological child after adopting, it is unacceptable to tell them it is too bad they did not wait a little longer before adopting.

8. When a family adopts an older child, it is impolite to ask them if the child had been abused.

9. It is impolite to ask an adopted adult if he plans to "search" for his birthparents. Adults who do not wish to search will feel embarrassed and may think they have to explain why they do not wish to search. Adopted adults who wish to discuss a planned or past search will talk about it if they wish.

10. It is equally impolite to ask a birthmother if she plans to search for her birth child or if she is worried he or she will someday search for her.

These are basic rules of etiquette for individuals who have not adopted. Hopefully, individuals who have adopted, placed, or were adopted will also follow them.

expenses to adopt See COSTS TO ADOPT.

explaining adoption Discussions with children, usually between children and their adoptive parents, about the reasons why adoption exists for children in general and why they in particular were adopted. Whether children were adopted as newborn infants or as older children well aware of their adoption, it is important for adoptive parents to explain adoption and clarify what adoption is and is not. If no explanations are provided, children may develop erroneous and negative ideas. Adoptive parents also need to explain adoption issues to curious family members, friends, and other individuals.

Parents should keep in mind that they need not share all the personal information that they know about a child's background and/or birthparents with many different people. For example, some parents have later regretted sharing some information, such as that a birthmother was not sure which of two men fathered her child, or that the birthmother used drugs during her pregnancy, or that a child was abandoned outside an orphanage in another country.

Such information is often remembered for years by family members and friends, who may judge the child negatively because of it and may make cruel and/or unthinking comments to the child or within earshot. One rule of thumb is that if the information could be hurtful to the child, it generally should not be shared with others. (One exception is the child's physician, who may need to know about medical problems of the birthparents.)

Another way to consider the issue is whether the parent would wish the information to appear on the front page of the *New York Times* or the *Wall Street Journal*. If the answer is "no," then it is sufficiently personal to withhold from others, including comments, letters, or public postings on the Internet.

Mistaken Assumptions Adoptive Parents Sometimes Make

Many parents who adopt children presume that if a child is curious about adoption, then he or she will ask a question. However, adoption experts and researchers have learned that children are often afraid to bring up the subject of adoption because they fear their parents will become angry, offended, or hurt. Even adopted adults are often inhibited about asking questions about their adoption. Some adopted adults who wish to search for their birthparents are so fearful that the search will upset their adoptive parents that they take no action to search until the adoptive parents are very old or have died.

As a result, although adoptive parents should not continually or obsessively talk about adoption,

it is a subject that should be brought up occasionally to show the child that the parents are willing to discuss it and to offer information as needed and available. The child will then learn and remember that parents are comfortable with being asked questions and will retain this information for the future when he or she may have more questions.

Another common mistake is to misinterpret the child's question. If the child asks where she came from, she may mean what state or what country, and if so, could become confused or upset by a detailed discussion of how babies are made and/or why children are adopted. Asking one or two questions can determine what the child is asking about, for example, "Do you mean what state you were born in? It was Kansas." If the child wants more information, she will say so.

Yet another mistake is to assume that it is sufficient to talk about adoption a few times and that the information will somehow "stick." Parents should realize that adoption is not a subject that can be explained once and then forgotten, with an attitude on the parent of "I'm glad that's over now!" In addition, it should not be assumed that the child remembered or understood what was said about adoption, even if it was last week and the child is an adolescent. The parent may wish to say something like, "You may remember that we talked about how you were adopted as a baby from China, and you had lots of hair that stuck straight up in the air!" After capturing the child's attention, some information sharing and discussion can ensue. However, parents should not compel children to talk about adoption. Sometimes they are not interested.

Sharing Information about Adoption Is Important

In the past, some parents were advised against sharing the very fact of adoption with the child. They were urged to treat and raise the child in every way as if born to the family. One problem with this advice was that adopted persons usually found out that they were adopted anyway, often at a difficult time in life or in awkward circumstances, such as when a relative blurted out the fact. One man reported that he had a major argument with his father when he was 19 years old, and at the height of his anger, the father told the son he was adopted. The father apologized immediately for blurting such important and long-withheld information, but the two men were estranged for years and both suffered from this mutual loss until a later reconciliation occurred.

When parents withhold the fact that the child was adopted, the trust level in the ongoing parent-child relationships may suffer seriously because of the strain of keeping the secret. It can be stressful for the parents, who may constantly worry about someone else telling the child about the adoption, such as another family member.

Also, this approach of withholding the fact of the adoption deprives adopted individuals of any available appropriate health and genetic information that may be important, not only to the adopted adult's own health but to the health of their children that are later born to them.

When to Explain

Although most experts agree that it is important for a child to know that he or she was adopted, they disagree on when and how often to explain and discuss adoption.

Some adoption authors insist that the child should hear the word *adoption* from infancy onward, repeating such phrases as "my beautiful adopted baby," whereas most say a child cannot possibly begin to understand such a complex subject as adoption until at least age five or six.

A study of 200 adopted and nonadopted children by David Brodzinsky, Leslie Singer, and Anne Braff revealed that children under age six did not have a very good understanding of adoption, and few of them "differentiated between adoption and birth as alternative paths to parenthood or understood anything about the adoption process, or the motives underlying adoption."

The researchers found that children from about age six to eight understood that there is a difference between adoption and birth but were apparently unaware of the reasons for adoption. Between the ages of eight and 11, the children's understanding increased. Preadolescent and adolescent children had the best understanding of their adoption.

Despite this research, many adoption experts think that the child should know about the fact of the adoption prior to entering kindergarten or first grade. One very practical reason is that children constantly tease each other about a variety of real or imagined traits—wearing glasses, chubbiness, and so forth—and if the adoption has been disclosed to others who may tell the child, or it is obvious because of ethnic differences between the child and the parent, the child should have long since been given a basic explanation of adoption.

The chosen child explanation Until recently, many social workers encouraged parents to tell a version of the "CHOSEN CHILD" story, wherein it was maintained that the adopted child was "special" because he or she was specifically chosen by the parents. However, the problem with this advice is that it may make the child feel undue pressure to be worthy of having been chosen. In addition, in many cases, the child was *not* personally selected by the adoptive parents, and the first time they met the child was after the adoption was already arranged. Thus, the chosen child story is untrue in such cases. However, some experts continue to believe that telling a small child that he or she was chosen to be adopted may be acceptable, as long as the realities of adoption are explained when the child is older.

Adoption Explanations Should Be Tailored to the Child's Age and Level of Understanding

Small children will enjoy hearing their own adoption story, of positive comments about how excited the parents were to see and hug the child for the first time. Simple stories are all most small children need. A child of 11 or 12 will usually have a more sophisticated understanding of adoption, and an adolescent will have more questions and a greater understanding. However, adolescents are undergoing challenges related to their bodies and personal identities and may react negatively to discussions about adoption. The parent may offer to table the discussion until later, if resistance is met. (See also ADOLESCENT ADOPTED PERSONS.)

It is also advisable for adoptive parents to use positive adoption terminology when explaining any aspect of adoption. Even when said by the most loving parent, such phrases as "given away," "surrendered," and "real parents" almost invariably evoke a very negative image of both the birthparents and adoption itself. Far more preferable are such phrases as "made an adoption plan" or "chose adoption"—if the adoption was in fact a voluntary choice of the birthparent. "Transferred parental rights" could be used in the case of involuntary or voluntary termination of parental rights. Birthparent, birthmother, and birthfather are preferable to "real parents."

At the same time, parents should not become unduly upset if their children do use negative words and phrases, since they are so common in society. Instead of angrily correcting a child who asks about his real parent, it is best for the adoptive parent to use the words "birthmother," "birthfather," and "birthparents" in the explanation to the child. Some parents also use humor, such as saying, "Look at me! I'm real and I'm your parent!" The child may then state that the parent *knows* what is meant, and the parent can say that birthparent is a better phrase for the person who the child was born to, even if many people do not know this.

Parents should also realize that the MEDIA often presents distorted and negative views of adoption, and stereotypical or unfair depictions should be challenged aloud by parents, whether the child asks a question or not.

In addition, parents should note that the word *adopt* is sometimes used in an unusual context; for example, pet shelters may solicit new pet owners by advertising that they want people to "adopt" a pet or a highway. Some adoption professionals, adoptive parents, and adopted children are very upset by this usage, while others are not.

Avoiding Explanations That Can Be Distorted in a Child's Mind

The one best explanation about adoption is that the birthparents were unable to parent the child. However, there are a variety of pervasive simplistic explanations about adoption that parents have used and some continue to use. Some of these have proven to be problematic. The explanations were well-meant, but they involved sophistication not present in small children or preadolescents. For example, in past years, many adoptive parents were counseled to tell their child that he or she was placed for adoption because "his mother loved him so much." Another potentially problematic explanation was that the birthparents were too poor to raise him.

One problem with the explanation that the child's mother loved him or her, therefore she chose adoption, according to child psychiatrist and author Denis Donovan, is that true as it usually was, a child could logically conclude that if his adoptive parents also love him very much, then they may ultimately decide the child should be adopted by others, for example, if the adoptive parents decide to divorce.

In addition, the adoptive family may not *know* how the birthparents felt about the child. They may presume it was a difficult decision but can only guess about the birthparents' emotions about the adoption, sometimes even when the adoption is an open adoption. This is true whether the child was adopted in the United States or from another country.

One approach is for the adoptive parents to explain to the child that though the birthmother (or birthparents) loved the child, this love was not the main reason for the adoption. Instead, she (or they) cared about the child's happiness and wanted the child to be with a family who could care for him or her, which they could not do.

Note that some children have been removed from their parents because of abuse or neglect, while others have been abandoned. This does not necessarily mean that their parents did not love them (although they may not have), but it does mean that their parenting was inappropriate and dangerous. The decision for adoption was also not theirs to make: an involuntary termination of their parental rights was made.

The poverty explanation of adoption, which is commonly used by adoptive parents to explain why an adoption occurred, can create unanticipated fears and concerns. For example, if the birthparents chose adoption because they were poor, a child may worry if his adoptive parents start complaining about money. She may wonder if she will be adopted by another family, since this family also has financial problems. Although it is true, especially in countries overseas, that birthparents may have chosen adoption for their child because of poverty, the issue is more complicated and may involve such factors as nonacceptance of single motherhood or, if the child is of mixed race, potential discrimination against the child if he or she remained with the birthparent. Older children may be able to understand these issues but they will usually be too difficult to grasp for younger children.

Preadolescents and even many adolescents think in either-or terms, such as, if a birthmother was poor, someone should have helped her, or that his or her adoptive parents should have helped her (even though they did not know her). Many children also know other children born to single mothers who are struggling financially but who have not chosen adoption for their children. As a result, the one best explanation for most children is to tell them that their birthparents were not able to be parents, because of their own problems, and that the adoptive parents could not resolve the situation.

Types of Questions Children May Ask

Children can come up with a wide variety of questions but there are several common questions that many children ask their parents, such as questions that were covered by Dr. Adesman in *Parenting the Adopted Child: A Basic Approach to Building a Strong Family.*

Some common questions that children may ask about adoption include the following:

- Why was I adopted?
- Why did *you* adopt me?
- What happened to my birthparents?
- Was it my fault?

Explaining Why Adoption Occurs: Birthparents Were Unable to Parent the Child

Dr. Adesman explains that often it is best to explain adoption in general and then move to discuss the specific reasons why a particular child was adopted. In addition, whether referring to all adopted children or to one child, it is important to explain that the biological parents were unable to parent the child. This explanation fits a variety of cases, whether the birthparent was a young adult who decided that she could not handle parenthood or was a single woman in another country whose child would have been shunned in the society. In addition, the explanation incorporates birthparents who were abusive and/or neglectful and whose parental rights were terminated.

Says Dr. Adesman, "This reason—that some parents are unable to manage parenthood—encompasses the gamut of reasons why children are placed for adoption, including a birth parent's desire for a child to have a stable family, as well as possible struggles with drug abuse or mental illness, physical abuse, and poverty."

Once the general reasons for adoption are provided, the parent can move into specifics on what is known about the child's particular adoption, such as the age of the birthparents (if known), where the child was born, and the reasons (if known) for the adoption. If very little (or no) information is known, the parents may wish to concentrate on when they first heard about or met the child and how excited they were. If the child persists with questions, the parents should answer honestly that they do not know. This may be difficult for younger children to believe, since their parents loom so large in their lives, but parents may say that although parents know a lot, they do not know everything. They wish they could answer all questions but they cannot.

Explaining Why Adoptive Parents Adopt Their Children

Eventually the child will wish to know why the adoptive parent adopted him or her. Some adoptive parents are infertile while others could have borne children but preferred to adopt them, sometimes called "preferential adopters." If the reason is infertility, it is best to avoid providing clinical details that might frighten or confuse children. Simply stating that the parents could not have children should suffice.

If the adoptive parents were not infertile, then the explanation may be that they wished for a family (or a larger family) and wanted a child who was already born, rather than adding to the population.

Explaining What Happened to the Birthparents

In discussing adoption, some children worry about their birthparents coming back to take them while others may wish to go meet them, immediately. (It is also true that the same child may have opposing reactions, at different times.) If the adoption is an open one, then the child knows about and often has had contact with at least one birthparent. Yet explanations are still in order for why the child was adopted, even when there is a continuing relationship between the birthparents and the child.

If the adoption is not an open one or the birthparent is unavailable, or if the adoptive parents say no to a meeting (because the child is too young, they do not know who or where the birthparents are, or they are opposed to a meeting), then the child may feel angry and upset. These are normal emotions. The parents may wish to tell the child they realize the child is not happy with their decision but parents must make decisions for children, including some decisions that children do not like.

Adoptive parents are very mixed in their feelings about meetings with birthparents. Some are open to meetings that occur before the child reaches the age of 18 while others are opposed. They may believe that only adults have the maturity to manage an adoption REUNION with birthparents.

See also OPEN ADOPTION; OPEN RECORDS.

Explaining That the Adoption Was Not the Child's Fault

Many children have magical thinking and assume that if something important happened, such as their adoption, then it was because they were not attractive or there was some other flaw in them. They need to be told that the adoption was planned before their birth, if this was the case. If the adoption was planned after birth or the child was older, they need to be told that the adoption plan was made because the birthparents were unable to parent them, and this was not the child's fault, in any way.

Even if the child has a serious medical problem, and this may be one reason why the birthparent chose adoption, it is important to emphasize that the birthparents were unable to manage parenting, and as a result, another family was found.

It is important to avoid demonizing the birthparents in the explanation, even in the event that the birthparents exhibited problematic behavior, such as drug or alcohol abuse or physical or sexual abuse of the child. The explanation that the birthparent was unable to parent the child removes any guilt feelings from the child, while at the same time it avoids casting blame on the birthparents. The reason why it is important to avoid criticizing the birthparents is that when they *are* blamed, the child may later start to wonder if he or she is bad,

like his birthparents, who were alcoholic, drug-addicted, physically abusive, or may have exhibited other problem behaviors.

Explaining Adoption to Family Members and Friends

Often relatives, grandparents, and friends may have a very limited knowledge or no knowledge of adoption. (See also ATTITUDES ABOUT ADOPTION.)

Dr. Adesman suggests that the following basic points be made to others about adoption: that adoption is permanent, that it is legal and involves a court proceeding, that it is another good way to form a family, that some information about the adoption should be kept private, and that most adopted children grow up to be normal adults.

Many people confuse adoption with foster care and do not realize that adoption is a permanent change, nor do they realize that adoption is a legal process that transfers the parental rights to the adoptive parents, giving them all the rights and obligations of a family whose child was born to them.

A positive attitude about adoption as another good way to create a family is also an important point for parents to convey to extended family members, friends, and others.

Although some adopted children have psychiatric and behavioral problems, most lead normal lives as adults, and this is another important point to convey to others in explanations about adoption. Because some people have watched made-for-TV movies in which the adopted child was the criminal or the emotionally disturbed person, they may mistakenly generalize this stereotype to all adopted children.

If the child is of another ethnicity or race from the adoptive parents, it is more likely the parents will be asked questions about the child by their extended family as well as friends and even total strangers. (See also ETIQUETTE.) Families adopting internationally or transracially should be prepared to deal with the intense curiosity of the general public, and negative comments should be politely deflected.

See also INTERNATIONAL ADOPTION; TRANSRACIAL ADOPTION.

Explaining at the Child's Level of Understanding

Some experts have compared explaining adoption to explaining sex. What a parent tells a five-year-old is very different from what is told to a 15-year-old child.

However, sometimes children's understanding of adoption and their insights are more comprehensive and accepting than parents realize. For example, an adoptive mother who was open in discussing adoption with her child said her daughter was only six years old when she and her mother were discussing adoption and the child suddenly said (of her birthmother and mother), "She gave me starting life. You gave me growing life."

Adesman, Andrew, M.D., with Christine Adamec. *Parenting the Adopted Child: A Basic Approach to Building a Strong Family.* New York: McGraw-Hill, 2004.

Bothun, Linda. *Dialogues about Adoption: Conversations between Parents and Their Children.* Chevy Chase, Md.: Swan Publications, 1994.

Brodzinsky, David M., Leslie M. Singer, and Anne M. Braff. "Children's Understanding of Adoption," *Child Development* 55 (1984): 869–878.

Donovan, Denis M., and Deborah McIntyre. *Healing the Hurt Child.* New York: W. W. Norton Company, 1990.

failed adoptions   See DISRUPTION.

family preservation   A phrase used to describe efforts made by state and county social workers to enable children to stay with a family despite severe problems that prevented good parenting, such as DRUG ABUSE/ADDICTION, alcoholism, mental illness, and/or criminal behavior. The problem or combination of problems led to child maltreatment, in the form of ABANDONMENT, ABUSE, or NEGLECT, and the child was removed from the home and placed in FOSTER CARE.

The ADOPTION ASSISTANCE AND CHILD WELFARE ACT OF 1980 included strong provisions for holding families together through various means: counseling, parenting classes, contracts between the parent and the social services department, and other attempts to "preserve" the family.

In some cases, these efforts were successful and the child and family were reunited. In others, the process was one of the child being returned to the family, abuse or neglect recurring, and the child being returned to a foster home. Some children flip-flopped between their biological family and a series of foster families for years and sometimes for their entire childhoods until they "aged-out" at age 18 and were no longer eligible for foster care assistance.

In more dire cases, the child was returned to a very abusive family and was severely abused or even murdered. Such incidents enrage the public for a short period, and then the incident is forgotten. Then a similar incident would happen to another child.

For years, adoption advocates said it was wrong to warehouse children in foster care, and also made a statement quite heretical to most social workers: "Some families cannot be saved." Many social workers continued to believe that with

enough time, money, and hard work, virtually every family could be "fixed."

Other social workers said that there were three basic elements that had to be present in order to salvage an extremely dysfunctional family: means, ability, and motivation. They said that the social service system could provide "means," or the resources necessary to help a family. For example, social workers might be able to help the family find an affordable apartment that was much better than where they were living. They might be able to improve the client's living situation in many other ways with "means," by using money and professional skills.

What the social workers could not provide were the other two essential elements: ability and motivation. The family had to have the capacity to change, whether it was the intellectual or cognitive capacity (or some other capacity). Then, even if they had help from excellent social workers *and* the ability to implement changes, they needed the final piece of the puzzle—motivation. No matter how bright the family was and how enormous their capabilities, the fact remained that if they did not want to change and did not acknowledge the need to change, the dysfunction would continue. This would apply whether the dysfunction was caused by alcohol or drugs or emotional disorders or some other problem.

After years of lobbying, the ADOPTION AND SAFE FAMILIES ACT (ASFA) was passed in 1997. This did not wipe out attempts to preserve families, but rather it was a law that took into account the child's needs as paramount. It was an attempt to prevent children from spending their lives in foster care. Instead, the child either was returned to their families when possible or, in some cases, the parental rights of their parents would be ended so that the children could be adopted, often by their foster parents who had cared for them for years.

The idea of family preservation was a very positive and optimistic one. The problem was that public social service departments interpreted the concept in an extremely rigid way, often assuming that children *had* to be sent back to abusive homes and families, even when they were likely to be reabused. A major part of the problem was also the judiciary. State social workers and their attorneys often presented what they thought was a "perfect" case for leaving a child in foster care, if not terminating parental rights altogether. And then a judge would inexplicably send the child back to abusive parents.

Because the Adoption Assistance and Child Welfare Act was so misinterpreted in its application, Congress passed ASFA to rectify this error.

family tree A genealogical chart denoting parents, grandparents, and other relatives in the family as far back in history as information allows. The chart has many branches and consequently resembles a tree in appearance.

Family trees are routinely assigned as a project to schoolchildren. The assignment can be used to advantage in helping adopted children straighten out identity issues over belonging to their adoptive families, if well-informed guidance is provided to the child.

The child will not be as likely to be disturbed by the exercise if adults explain why he belongs on the family tree, namely via the legal and socially approved action of adoption. Each family member's genetic ancestry tree is another reality that should merit discussion; for example, the genetic ancestry of the mother and her parents and relatives is completely different from the genetic ancestry of the father and his parents and extended family. When they married, they formed a new legal entity and together they create their own family tree with their children.

Older children will need caring clarification, pointing out that with adoption, there was a transfer of family membership from one family to another family system. Their birth families still comprise their genetic ancestry trees.

If a family-tree exercise is assigned as a means of teaching genetic inheritance, e.g., eye color, hair color, etc., some experts say that such an exercise could be problematic for the adopted child while others say that the simplest solution is for the adoptive family to be used in the child's "tree." Some experts recommend that the "family tree" assignment should be discarded from school curricula.

See also SCHOOL.

father, legal See LEGAL FATHER.

federal government Although states set their own adoption laws, the federal government also plays a role in adoption, particularly in the area of SPECIAL NEEDS in FOSTER CARE. In order for states to receive federal funds, they must comply with federal regulations on the length of time children may spend in foster care before returning to their parents or being placed for adoption. The federal government also provides funds for ADOPTION SUBSIDIES, MEDICAID, and numerous other entitlements. The federal government also oversees INTERNATIONAL ADOPTIONS, and it prohibits racial discrimination in adoption, as with the MULTIETHNIC PLACEMENT ACT.

See also INCOME TAX LAW BENEFITS FOR ADOPTIVE PARENTS.

fertile adoptive parents Also known as OPTIONAL ADOPTERS and preferential adopters; individuals who could conceive a child if they wished, but for a variety of reasons choose to adopt instead in order to introduce or expand the number of children in their family. They may believe in ZERO POPULATION GROWTH and believe it is better to care for already WAITING CHILDREN or children with SPECIAL NEEDS rather than to bring another child into the world.

fetal alcohol syndrome (FAS) Fetal alcohol syndrome (FAS), or more commonly, fetal alcohol spectrum disorder (FASD), encompasses a range of developmental disabilities and birth defects in a child whose mother abused alcohol during pregnancy. The mother may have been an alcoholic and/or have engaged in binge drinking (defined as consuming five or more drinks on at least one occasion in the past two weeks).

Physicians from ancient Greece through the present day have recognized that alcohol abuse by a pregnant woman was harmful to children born to her, yet it was not until 1968 that French researcher P. Lemoine and colleagues identified the characteristics of fetal alcohol syndrome among 127 children born to alcoholic mothers. Little attention was given to this discovery. Then in 1973, Kenneth Jones and David Smith at the University of Washington in Seattle independently identified the same problem in children born to alcoholic mothers. They provided the name "fetal alcohol syndrome," and their article in *Lancet* received a great deal of attention.

Some families adopt children with FAS or another form of fetal alcohol spectrum disorder. If the family is aware of the problem in advance, they can prepare to help the child with the challenges that lie ahead. If they are not prepared, they may face great disappointment and challenges. Children born to mothers in the United States and other countries, including eastern Europe, may suffer from FAS.

Symptoms and Diagnostic Path

FAS can be difficult to diagnose, except by experienced physicians. However, there are some indicators that should be evaluated. For example, children with FAS are often premature and underweight, with small heads, and they are likely to remain unusually small and thin.

Many children with FAS are developmentally delayed (mentally retarded). Children with FAS may also experience seizures and a host of other medical and psychological problems that are not outgrown as the child ages. Hyperactivity and poor attention span are common problems.

A low intelligence level is not inevitable, however, although it is more likely among children with FAS. Dr. Ira Chasnoff, a noted expert on FAS, treated twin girls who clearly had FAS, including such symptoms as small head circumference, abnormal facial features, low developmental scores, and slow growth. The mother's parental rights were terminated and the girls were adopted into a family that provided opportunities for the children to develop at their own level. At the age of two and one-half, they showed considerable improvement. By the age of 17, they both were enrolled at a public school in

a program for gifted students. Of course, it should not be interpreted from this encouraging story that FAS children are exceptionally gifted intellectually. To the contrary, most are either below average or of average intelligence.

According to the Task Force on Fetal Alcohol Syndrome and Fetal Alcohol Effect in their 2004 booklet, *Fetal Alcohol Syndrome: Guidelines for Referral and Diagnosis,* a diagnosis of FAS requires all three of the following:

1. Documentation of all three facial abnormalities, including a smooth philtrum (the area of the face between the nose and the upper lip. The normal ridges separated by a groove are underdeveloped and flattened in children with prenatal alcohol exposure), a thin upper lip with poorly defined cupid's bow, and small palpebral fissures

2. Documentation of growth deficits

3. Documentation of central nervous system abnormalities, such as structural, neurological, functional, or a combination of abnormalities. Central nervous system dysfunctions may lead to impulsivity, memory problems, and learning disorders.

Identifiable facial features of children with fetal alcohol syndrome may also include folds in the inner aspect of the eyelids (epicanthal folds), short upturned noses, small chins, and a "flattened" midface. An estimated 30 percent of children with FAS suffer from heart defects and one-quarter to one-half of the children have heart murmurs. Another characteristic of children with FAS is poor muscle coordination. Other problems sometimes seen are cleft lip and palate, skeletal anomalies, and kidney malformations.

Fetal Alcohol Spectrum Disorders

The term *fetal alcohol spectrum disorders* is used to connote the full range of developmental disorders caused by the mother's alcohol abuse during pregnancy. These include FAS, which is the most serious form of fetal alcohol spectrum disorder, and alcohol-related neurodevelopmental disorder (ARND), which leads to defects in the central nervous system, behavioral problems such as hyperactivity, and cognitive delays such as LANGUAGE DELAY. In addition, alcohol-related birth defects (ARBD) are part of the fetal alcohol spectrum disorders, and these defects may affect various organs of the body.

Learning disabilities Children with FAS may experience serious shortfalls in learning, partly in arithmetic and, as adults, in managing money. Some studies have indicated that the children of women who were binge drinkers during pregnancy are subsequently more likely to experience difficulty in math and reading and other areas of learning. As a result, the school setting can be a very frustrating environment for the child with FAS, and parents should work to obtain as much academic assistance for the child as possible.

Children who have been diagnosed with FAS are eligible for EARLY INTERVENTION programs, and their adoptive parents or other caregivers should ensure the child receives this opportunity.

Risk for social problems Some studies have revealed that children with FAS are more likely to become alcoholic adults, experience unplanned pregnancies, and become involved in car accidents. These problems could be a function of poor judgment, poor impulse control, and lower intelligence, alcohol abuse, or other issues.

A study reported in a 1998 issue of *Alcoholism: Clinical and Experimental Research* on adopted adults ranging from 18 to 45 years included children exposed to alcohol before birth and children who were not. The study concluded that fetal alcohol exposure was a risk factor for adult use of nicotine, alcohol, and drug dependence.

Late diagnosis Most children with FAS are not diagnosed until after age six. In one study of 400 children and adults with FAS, only 11 percent had been diagnosed before age six. The average age of diagnosis is age 10 or 11. Part of the reason for this late diagnosis is there is no laboratory test or X-ray that will definitely prove that a person has FAS, although the CDC has developed diagnostic guidelines for physicians. The diagnosis for this syndrome is based on physical appearance, medical problems, behavioral problems, and other issues.

Risk Factors and Preventive Measures

Alcohol consumption during pregnancy is the cause of FAS. The only certain way to avoid the risk of FAS or any other form of fetal alcohol spec-

trum disorder is for pregnant women to abstain from all drinking during their entire pregnancies.

According to the Centers for Disease Control and Prevention, some doctors mistakenly believe that only alcoholics have babies with these illnesses. However, binge drinking may also lead to FAS in a child. In addition, fetal damage may be caused by as little as 0.5 drinks per day, and thus physicians recommend that pregnant women avoid alcohol altogether during pregnancy. The extent of the damage to the child varies greatly and may be mild to severe. Alcohol exposure during pregnancy is the number-one cause of preventable mental retardation.

Alcoholic women who are pregnant and plan to continue their pregnancies should definitely seek prenatal care and treatment so they can recover from alcoholism and avoid the possibility of birth defects in their children. Indeed, any pregnant woman who normally drinks alcohol in any quantity whatsoever, including as little as one drink per day, should stop drinking immediately, to avoid continuing potential harm to the child. They should also consult their physicians to obtain information and advice about alcohol consumption during pregnancy.

FAS Prevalence in the United States

As can be seen from the table, in 2002 many women continue drinking during their pregnancies. About 10 percent of pregnant women in the United States drink during pregnancy. Of these, 1.9 percent were binge drinkers, and an additional 1.9 percent were frequent drinkers. Among those who might become pregnant, the percentages were higher, and nearly 55 percent used alcohol, including about 12 percent binge drinkers and 13 percent frequent drinkers.

According to the CDC, an estimated 1,000 to 6,000 infants of the approximately four million babies born each year in the United States have FAS. This is a rate of about 0.5 to 2.0 cases per 1,000 live births. Some groups, such as Native Americans, have FAS rates that are much higher: three to five cases per 1,000 children. Studies by Dr. Sokol and his colleagues indicate that African-American children have a five times greater risk of having FAS than white children, and American Indian/Alaskan Native children have a 16 times greater risk than white children.

PREVALENCE OF ALCOHOL CONSUMPTION AMONG CHILDBEARING-AGED WOMEN (18–44 YEARS) BY DRINKING PATTERN AND PREGNANCY STATUS, UNITED STATES, 2002

Pregnancy Status	Drinking Pattern	Percentage
Pregnant	Binge*	1.9
	Frequent use	1.9
	Any use	10.1
Might become pregnant	Binge	12.4
	Frequent use**	13.1
	Any use	54.9
All respondents	Binge	12.4
	Frequent use	13.2
	Any use	52.6

*Five or more drinks on one occasion
**Seven or more drinks per week or binge drinking
Source: Centers for Disease Control and Prevention, "Alcohol Consumption among Women Who Are Pregnant or Who Might Become Pregnant—United States, 2002," *Morbidity and Mortality Weekly Review* 53, 50 (December 24, 2004): 1,178–1,181.

As a result of the higher rate of FAS among some racial and ethnic minority groups, some physicians mistakenly conclude that it is primarily or solely minority women who have children with FAS, which is untrue. A white woman who binge drinks or drinks heavily during her pregnancy is at risk for bearing a child with FAS. The primary risk factor for FAS is the alcohol consumption by the mother, rather than her ethnicity.

FAS Prevalence in Other Countries

Statistics are difficult to locate but experts estimate that between one in 1,000 and one in 300 infants worldwide experience a prenatal exposure to alcohol. Some experts estimate that the prevalence of FAS in children in Russian orphanages is as high as 14 percent. FAS is most common among children adopted from countries such as Russia, Ukraine, and other former countries that comprised the Soviet Union. FAS is much less commonly seen among children adopted from China, Guatemala, and South Korea.

Studies on FAS

In 2004, Ann P. Streissguth and her colleagues described their research in the *Journal of Develop-*

mental and Behavioral Pediatrics, based on interviews with caregivers and other informants about the life span experiences of 415 child, adolescent, and adult patients with either FAS or fetal alcohol effect (FAE), which they defined as a less severe form of FAS. The subjects included 236 males and 179 females. The patients had a median intelligence quotient (IQ) of 86. (An IQ of 100 is average.) The children included 60 percent white patients, 25 percent Native Americans, 7 percent blacks, and 6 percent Hispanics.

Most of the children were not reared by their biological mothers, and most (80 percent) were raised by adoptive and foster families. The patients were diagnosed in the 1970s, 1980s, and the 1990s and were enrolled in the Fetal Alcohol Follow-up Study of the University of Washington's Fetal Alcohol and Drug Unit. The study respondents were the children's adoptive mothers (33 percent), foster mothers, biological fathers or stepmothers (25 percent inclusive), biological mothers (17 percent), other relatives or current or former caretakers (20 percent), and others. Most of the respondents (80 percent) had known the children with FAS for half or more of the patients' lives.

The researchers considered the presence of problem behaviors in the subjects with FAS or FAE and found that promiscuity (26 percent) and inappropriate sexual advances (18 percent) were the most frequently mentioned inappropriate sexual behaviors.

Many of the adolescents and adults with FAS had a disrupted school experience. Fifty-three percent of the FAS/FAE adolescents had been suspended from school, 29 percent had been expelled, and 25 percent had dropped out of school. Learning problems were common, especially attention problems (70 percent) and difficulty completing schoolwork (58 percent).

The researchers found that many of the adolescents and adults had been in trouble with the law, including 14 percent of the children and 60 percent of the adolescents and adults with FAS. Thirty-five percent of the adults had been incarcerated for a crime.

In Streissguth's study, some of the study individuals with FAS or FAE had a two- to fourfold improvement in their odds of escaping the adverse life experiences that are typically predicted by FAS and FAE, such as confinement for criminal violations, inappropriate sexual behavior, and problems with drugs and alcohol. The researchers found two key protective factors—an early diagnosis of FAS/FAE and living in a stable and nurturing environment—that were conducive to an improved outcome.

Said the researchers, "In summary, this study documents the adverse postnatal environments and the corresponding risk of adverse life outcomes among many patients diagnosed FAS or FAE. These include major disruptions in schooling, trouble with the law, inappropriate sexual behaviors, extensive confinements, and alcohol and drug problems. Adverse life outcomes are not restricted to those with or without the classic facial features of FAS or to those with or without mental retardation. We find that good stable families, with enduring relationships with their children with FAS/FAE, appear to be a critical protective factor for helping children avoid adverse life outcomes.

"We also observed a significant reduction in the risk of adverse life outcomes with an earlier diagnosis."

Families Who Adopt Children with FAS

In many cases, an adoptive family will adopt their FAS child through the state social services system, although they may also adopt through a private adoption agency placing children from the United States or other countries. Families who adopt children with FAS should obtain as much information and assistance as possible from social workers, physicians, and parent groups. They must understand that tender, loving care, although extremely important, cannot entirely alleviate the damage that occurred in utero to the child. Families should also learn about adoption subsidies and the child's eligibility for MEDICAID.

Families adopting internationally who suspect that the child may have FAS, based on the birthmother's history, the country of origin, and concerns raised by an international adoption medicine expert, should press the agency for more information. However, definitive information is usually unavailable.

In some cases, families unknowingly adopt children with FAS, which can be traumatic for everyone concerned. (See DISRUPTION.) Most studies indicate that the adoptive parents who regard themselves as happiest are also the ones who felt they were aware and prepared for the child, whether any disabilities were present or not.

According to Dr. Miller in *The Handbook of International Adoption Medicine,* the following problems are parenting concerns for families who adopt children with FAS:

- Sleep disorders (insomnia, frequent wakening)
- Poor appetite
- Developmental delays
- Language and speech delays
- Frequent infections
- Dental problems
- Hyperactivity
- Inappropriate social behaviors, such as poor judgment and below-normal responsiveness to social cues
- Difficulty with making and keeping friends
- Overall parenting stress

Dr. Miller also points out that some children with FAS have positive features as well. These may include the following:

- Cheerful nature
- Trusting and loving attitude
- Curious
- Energetic
- Artistic or musical

Treatment Options and Outlook

FAS is not curable, but when it is identified in infants and small children, intervention and treatment can begin so that the children's abilities can be optimized. Streissguth's approach is to minimize "secondary disabilities" to improve outcome. Children may benefit from EARLY INTERVENTION programs provided within the public school systems. Treatment of medical problems associated with FAS, such as cardiac or kidney problems, should be provided. Psychological and emotional problems should be treated by a professional experienced in treating children and/or adolescents with FAS, and support should be provided to parents.

See also DEVELOPMENTAL DISABILITIES; FOSTER CARE.

Miller, Laurie C., M.D. *The Handbook of International Adoption Medicine: A Guide for Physicians, Parents, and Providers.* New York: Oxford University Press, 2005.

National Task Force on Fetal Alcohol Syndrome and Fetal Alcohol Effect. *Fetal Alcohol Syndrome: Guidelines for Referral and Diagnosis.* Centers for Disease Control and Prevention, Atlanta, Ga., July 2004.

Minugh, P., et al. "Drinking of Alcoholic Beverages—Health Aspects, Health Behavior—Surveys," *American Journal of Drug and Alcohol Abuse* 24, no. 3 (August 1998): 483–498.

Sokol, Robert J., M.D., Virginia Delaney-Black, M.D., and Beth Nordstrom. "Fetal Alcohol Spectrum Disorder," *Journal of the American Medical Association* 290, no. 22 (December 10, 2003): 2,996–2,999.

Streissguth, Ann P., et al. "Risk Factors for Adverse Life Outcomes in Fetal Alcohol Syndrome and Fetal Alcohol Effects," *Journal of Developmental and Behavioral Pediatrics* 25, no. 4 (2004): 228–238.

Warren, Kenneth R., and Laurie L. Foudin. "Alcohol-Related Birth Defects—The Past, Present, and Future," *Alcohol Research & Health* 25, no. 3 (2001): 153–158.

Weinburg, Naimah Z. "The Adverse Effects That Parental Alcohol Use May Have on Children Are Numerous, Pervasive, Costly and Often Enduring," *Journal of the American Academy of Child & Adolescent Psychiatry* 36, no. 9 (September 1997): 1,177–1,187.

Yates, William R., et al. "Effect of Fetal Alcohol Exposure on Adult Symptoms of Nicotine, Alcohol, and Drug Dependence," *Alcoholism: Clinical and Experimental Research* 22, no. 4 (1998): 914–920.

finalization   The process in a court of law by which an adoption is decreed to be permanent and binding by a judge. After this point, it is extremely difficult to overturn an adoption unless fraud, duress, baby-selling, or other allegations can be proven. In many cases of INTERNATIONAL ADOPTION, the finalization occurs in the court of the native country of the child. Sometimes parents perform a RE-ADOPTION once they return to the United States, so they can obtain a U.S. birth certificate for the child.

States have varying amounts of time before which children born in the United States may be adopted; however, the average time is about six months from when the child was placed with a family.

The day of finalization is an exciting day for the adoptive parents and for the adopted child as well (if the adopted child is old enough to understand what is going on).

The JUDGE reviews appropriate papers, health reports, recommendations from the social worker, and other documents and approves the adoption in writing.

Subsequent to the court hearing, most states require the original birth certificate to become sealed and a new amended birth certificate will be issued with the adoptive parents' names as the parents.

foreign adoption   See INTERNATIONAL ADOPTION.

forever family   Term used by adoptive parents to describe themselves and their tie with their children and to emphasize the permanency aspect; often used by families who adopt children from countries outside the United States although also used by families who adopt older children and children with SPECIAL NEEDS.

foster care   Refers to the system set up in the United States to protect children who have been abused, neglected, or abandoned. The parents or primary caretakers of these children are unable to fulfill their parenting obligations because of ALCOHOLISM and/or DRUG ABUSE/ADDICTION, serious physical illness, emotional problems, incarceration in jail or prison, or a host of other reasons. Often there are multiple causes of the placement, such as a combination of abuse, alcohol dependence, and emotional problems in the parents or other primary caregivers. In some few cases, the placement of their children into foster care by their parents is voluntary, but most placements into foster care are mandated by a court and without the desire or consent of the parents or the custodial caretakers.

It is also true that in some countries that allow international adoption, particularly South Korea and Guatemala, infants usually spend a few months in foster homes while awaiting adoptive placement. The remainder of this essay refers solely to foster children in state care in the United States.

Foster care (as well as the reasons that led to placement into foster care) has a profound and life-long effect on children who enter this system, and the longer the time that they remain in foster care, the greater the potential impact on children.

Children in Foster Care

According to the Adoption and Foster Care Analysis and Reporting System (AFCARS), there were 523,000 children in foster care in the United States as of September 30, 2003, the most recent information as of this writing. The average age of the children in care was 10.2 years and slightly more than half (53 percent) were males. The ages of the children were widely distributed, with 14 percent under age one, 26 percent aged one to five years old, 20 percent aged six to 10 years old, 29 percent aged 11 to 15 years old, and 11 percent aged 16 to 18 years old.

A third of the children had been in foster care for 30 months or longer. Of these third, 16 percent had been in foster care for five years or more. About half of all the children (46 percent) were living in a nonrelative family foster home, while 23 percent were living with a relative yet under the control of the state. Of the others, 10 percent were living in an institution, 9 percent lived in a group home, 5 percent were in a pre-adoptive home, 4 percent were on a trial home visit, 2 percent had run away, and 1 percent were on supervised independent living (for older children).

The goal set by caseworkers for nearly half of all the foster children (48 percent) was to be reunified with a parent or another principal caretaker. For 20 percent, the goal was adoption. For the rest of the children, the goals were as follows: case plan goal not yet established (10 percent), long-term foster care (8 percent), emancipation (6 percent), live with other relatives (5 percent), and guardianship (3 percent).

There is also some slightly older information on foster care that is instructive and that can be seen from the table. For example, in 2001, many children in foster care were WAITING CHILDREN, which means that their parental rights had been terminated and they needed adoptive families.

Of these children, there were a disproportionate percent of African-American children. As shown in the table, African-American children represented only 14.9 percent of all children in the United States in 2001; however, they represented 39.1 percent of children in foster care and nearly half (46.8 percent) of children waiting to be adopted.

In contrast, about 61 percent of all children were white non-Hispanics, but these children represented more than a third (about 39 percent) of children in foster care, and about 36 percent of children in foster care were white children waiting to be adopted. In 2003, based on the AFCARS data, white children still represented 39 percent of the entire population. They represented 37 percent of the children waiting to be adopted.

PERCENTAGE OF CHILDREN IN THE GENERAL POPULATION, IN FOSTER CARE, WAITING TO BE ADOPTED AND CHILDREN WHO WERE ADOPTED, BY RACE/ETHNICITY, 2001

Race/Ethnicity	General Population of Children	Children in Foster Care	Waiting Children	Adopted Children
White, non-Hispanic	60.7	38.7	35.6	38.4
African-American, non-Hispanic	14.9	39.1	46.8	34.8
Hispanic	17.6	17.1	12.7	16.3
Other	6.9	5.1	4.9	5.3

Notes:

1. The general population and adopted children data only include children less than 18 years of age; whereas children in foster care and waiting children include those 18 and older.

2. Foster care and waiting children data include all children in foster care, regardless of age, and exclude cases where the race/ethnicity was unknown or unable to be determined. Waiting children excluded children who have a goal of adoption and/or had parental rights terminated, excluding those aged 16 and older with a goal of emancipation.

3. "Other" category includes American Indians, Asians, Native Hawaiians, and children with more than one race designation.

Source: Adapted from Office of the Assistant Secretary for Planning and Evaluation, *Understanding Adoption Subsidies: An Analysis of AFCARS Data.* U.S. Department of Health and Human Services, Washington, D.C.: 2005, page 3-3.

In 2001, about 18 percent of all children in the United States were Hispanic and about 17 percent of the foster care population were Hispanic. In addition, Hispanics represented about 13 percent of children in foster care waiting to be adopted. Based on AFCARS data for 2003, Hispanics still were 17 percent of the foster care children, and they were 14 percent of the children waiting to be adopted.

Of the children who left foster care in 2003, these children had the following outcomes:

- Reunification with parent(s) or primary caretaker(s): 55 percent
- Living with other relatives: 11 percent
- Adoption: 18 percent by relatives or nonrelatives
- Emancipation: 8 percent
- Guardianship: 4 percent
- Transfer to another agency: 2 percent
- Runaways: 2 percent

Requirements for Foster Parents

Foster care providers must be licensed by the state or county, and a limit is set on the number of children that may be placed in a home. However, practicality often rules, and sometimes foster parents are given more children than they are specifically licensed for because of the shortage of foster parents. (See FOSTER PARENT.) Before they may receive foster children, however, the family undergoes at least a cursory background check, such as a state official making a check with a state abuse registry to verify that they have not been accused of child abuse, and a police check to verify that they have not committed crimes. Most states also require foster parents to take classes so that they will be better prepared to understand the problems that the children may have experienced and be better able to help them. Relatives who become foster parents may be exempted from some of the requirements, such as classes.

The Process of Entering Foster Care

In most cases, a child enters the foster care system after removal from the parents or permanent caretaker on an emergency basis after abuse, neglect, or abandonment has been alleged, and/or the child is perceived as at risk for being abused. (The process may be different when a parent voluntarily requests that the child be placed in foster care, depending on state laws.)

The child is then placed with a foster family or in a group home while the case is adjudicated. The social worker will then request a court date, at which time the court will decide the conditions under which the child should either return home or continue to stay in foster care. Rules on foster care vary from state to state, but federal regulations also apply; for example, the federal government requires that "reasonable efforts" be made to prevent a removal from the home; however, if the caseworker believes a child is in danger, the primary goal is to protect the child, which usually necessitates the child's removal from the home.

If the neglect or abuse is substantial, a judge will order that the child should remain in foster care, and the state usually must create a plan to help the parents overcome their problems that led to the child's removal, whether they are drug and/or alcohol problems, mental health issues, or other problems. In some cases, the state may terminate the parent's rights rapidly, as when the child has been egregiously abused or another child or the child's other parent was murdered by the parent. If the child is an abandoned infant, the state may also terminate parental rights quickly. However, in most cases, the social service system seeks ways to help the child and parents reunite.

Parents are given goals to meet, such as obtaining a job, going to a rehabilitation facility if the problem is alcoholism or drug dependence, taking parenting classes and/or anger management classes, and so on. If the parents fulfill all the goals they are given within the time allotted, then the state usually returns the children to them; however, parents often are still subject to some overview by social workers because of the past abuse and neglect.

If the parents fail to meet the goals that they have been given within about two years or less (depending on state law), the state may seek to terminate their parental rights involuntarily in court. (See TERMINATION OF PARENTAL RIGHTS and Appendix V.) In general, if children have been in foster care for 15 of the past 22 months, then parental rights may be terminated. There are some exceptions to this rule, such as that the child is living with relatives or the state has failed to provide needed services to the parents. These provisions are federal rules within the ADOPTION AND SAFE FAMILIES ACT (ASFA), and some states have stricter rules than ASFA.

Expenses of Caring for Foster Children

Foster parents usually receive a monthly stipend to cover the child's expenses, and this amount varies from state to state. However, many foster parents consider this amount highly inadequate to cover all the child's expenses and as a result, they often spend their own money to cover basic expenses for food and clothes. Foster children also usually receive MEDICAID benefits to cover the medical expenses and prescriptions that may be needed. If the foster parents adopt the child, the Medicaid coverage usually continues. Often the adoptive parents may receive an ADOPTION SUBSIDY as well. If the foster parents are relatives of the child, whether they may receive a monthly subsidy for the child depends on state law.

In many cases, the child may arrive in a foster home with the clothes on his or her back and nothing else because of the hurried nature of the move. Foster parents often are not provided with the child's family medical/genetic history. This can be a serious problem, and some physicians urge that adequate medical records, including immunizations, be maintained because good records are essential, especially in medical emergency situations. Some experts recommend that two sets of medical records be kept: one by the foster parents and one by the social worker. The foster parents may wish to keep their own set of records because often records are misplaced by bureaucrats and they may never be recovered.

Children's Behavioral and Development Problems in Foster Care

Often ungrateful about being "saved" from their parents, and resentful of the social worker, older foster children sometimes act out. Their ACADEMIC PROGRESS may plummet. They may overeat or undereat (see EATING DISORDERS), and they may behave aggressively. Conversely, some children withdraw from contact.

If possible, siblings are placed together in the same foster home in order to reduce the stress of the move as much as possible. If there are many children in the family, however, the probability that they will stay together in the same foster home is low.

Visitations with parents are usually arranged by social workers. The child's social worker will attempt to arrange visits between the child and parents on a weekly basis or as frequently as is feasible. The child may act out in the foster home after parental visits because he or she is upset and may wish to return to the parent, but social workers generally believe that visits with parents are in the child's best interests.

Visits may be supervised in the social services office or may occur at the foster home, depending on the individual case.

Foster-Care Disruptions

Some children in foster care are transferred from family to family, which can be very traumatic for the child, who must often change schools as well. These moves may have nothing to do with the child, and instead, usually may be caused by such factors as the foster family deciding to retire, moving to another state, becoming ill, and so forth. One researcher, Sigrid James, studied foster children movements, reporting on her findings in a 2004 issue of *Social Service Review*. She studied 580 children from birth to 16 years old who entered foster care between 1990 and 1991. Most of the children were female (55 percent) and most had been neglected (74 percent) rather than physically abused (27 percent).

James found that about 70 percent of the children were transferred from one foster care placement to another because of system or policy changes, such as a move that was made in order to place a child with a family member or to move a child to a less restrictive setting.

However, in about 20 percent of the disruptions, the child's behavior was cited as the reason for the change. About half the children who were removed for behavior-related reasons experienced one change, while 22 percent experienced two changes, and 8.5 percent experienced three changes. The rest of the children, about 20 percent, had four to 14 behavior-related placement changes over the course of 18 months.

According to James, the risk of a behavior-related change increased by 48 percent if the child had entered foster care because of emotional abuse. Children exhibiting externalizing behaviors (acting out) had a 243 percent increased risk of having a foster care placement change related to behavior. In contrast, living with a relative reduced the risk of a placement disruption, and according to the study, "A child's hazard of experiencing a behavior-related placement change is reduced by 1 percent with each day spent in kinship care."

Factors that were *not* found relevant to foster care disruptions were the child's gender, age, ethnicity, the presence of internalizing behavior problems, or any specific type of maltreatment.

Concluded the researcher, "The majority of children who experienced behavior-related moves in this cohort did so shortly after entering out-of-home care. This suggests that a percentage of children might enter care with attributes or conditions (older age, evidence of externalizing problems) that demand immediate intervention if the risk of experiencing behavior-related placement change is to be reduced."

Foster Children Grown Up

One study looked at former foster children, now adults, to determine the possible long-term effects of foster care. This study is instructive because it may be predictive for other foster children in the United States. However, it is impossible for researchers to isolate the effects on the child of the reasons for placement into foster care (such as abuse and/or neglect) from the effects of foster care itself. Despite this, the study findings are of merit because they reveal important information on the outcome of foster children as adults.

In the Northwest Foster Care Alumni Study, researchers studied the outcomes for 659 adults, aged 20 to 33 years old, who had been in foster care as children between 1988 and 1998 in Washington and Oregon. In this sample, about 61 percent of the subjects were female and 54 percent were nonwhite. The researchers reviewed 659 case records, and 479 of the subjects were interviewed between September 2000 and January 2002. Many of the adults had experienced frequent foster care moves and about a third had experienced eight or more different placements. However, most of the adults (82 percent) reported that they felt loved by their foster parents.

When they were placed in foster care, the most prominent problems of their parents were substance abuse (65 percent of mothers and 45 percent of fathers) and criminal justice problems (35 percent of mothers and 37 percent of fathers).

Of these former foster children, 20 percent were doing well as adults. The large majority, however, were experiencing problems in major areas of their lives, such as education, finances, mental health, and employment.

With regard to mental health, the majority (54 percent) of the former foster children experienced one or more mental health problems, such as depression, post-traumatic stress syndrome, drug addiction, and other mental health problems. For example, the rate of major depression was 20 percent for the former foster children, compared to 10 percent among the general population in the United States. The researchers also found that 25 percent of the adults had post-traumatic stress disorder, a rate that was about twice as high as that experienced by military veterans of Vietnam (15 percent) or Iraq (12 to 13 percent).

The prevalence of other psychiatric problems was much higher in the former foster children than among the general population, such as 15 percent with panic syndrome in the "alumni," compared to 3.5 percent in the general population; 11.5 percent of the alumni with generalized anxiety disorder, compared to 3 percent of the general population; 8 percent of the alumni with drug dependence (addiction), compared to less than 1 percent of the general population; and about 4 percent of the alumni with bulimia, compared to less than 1 percent of the general population. About 20 percent had three or more mental health problems. About 22 percent had experienced homelessness at some point after leaving foster care. Clearly, the former foster children experienced profound impacts on their mental health.

Most of the alumni (85 percent) had completed high school or obtained a general education development (GED) credential. However, few had gone on to higher education, and about 16 percent had received a vocational degree. The rate of college graduation was significantly lower than their age group peers, or 2 percent compared to 24 percent among peers.

Many of the former foster children were employed (80 percent). However, this percentage of employed individuals was lower than the average for their age peers, or 95 percent. About a third of the former foster children were living at or below the poverty level and a third had no health insurance. About 17 percent of the alumni were receiving cash public assistance, compared to 3 percent of the general public.

Children Adopted from Foster Care

The numbers of children adopted from foster care each year have more than doubled since the passage of the Adoption and Safe Families Act in 1997, and many children are adopted by their foster parents. (See FOSTER PARENT ADOPTION.) In 2003, 50,000 children were adopted from foster care. Of the adopted children, the majority (88 percent) received an ADOPTION SUBSIDY, which is a monthly payment given to the adoptive parents on the child's behalf to defray expenses.

Most of the children who were adopted from foster care in 2003 were adopted by married couples (67 percent), followed by single females (28 percent), single males (3 percent), and unmarried couples (2 percent). In most of the cases (62 percent), the children were adopted by their foster parents. Twenty-three percent were adopted by relatives, and 15 percent were adopted by nonrelatives.

If parental rights are legally terminated, the child may then be adopted. (See TERMINATION OF PARENTAL RIGHTS.) However, some older children who probably could be placed with adoptive families may decide against adoption for themselves. If a child is over a certain age, for example, 12 years in some states, often he or she has the option of declining adoption. In such a case, a legal guardianship and/or extended foster case may be feasible. In other cases, the state may seek a legal emancipation of the child before he or she reaches the age of majority at 18 years.

In some cases, foster children are adopted by their foster parents or they are placed in a "legal risk situation" with a family that is interested in adopting the child, and thus, if the child is adopted, there is no need to relocate him or her to another home, another school, new parents, or new friends. The legal risk is not to the child but to the family because there is a chance that they will not be able to adopt the children, since the parental rights have not been terminated upon placement with the foster family.

Recruitment for adoptive parents is achieved through MEDIA advertising, PHOTOLISTING books and listings on state and national computer data banks. In addition, the caseworker may already know about a family who appears a good match for the child. Some public and private agencies recruit adoptive parents through Web sites on the INTERNET.

Increasingly, older children and children with SPECIAL NEEDS are successfully placed with adoptive parents who may be older parents, single parents, or parents with children in the home already.

See also DISRUPTION; FOSTER PARENT; FOSTER PARENT ADOPTION; OLDER CHILD; SIBLINGS.

Studies on Foster Children Who Were Adopted

Richard P. Barth and his associates studied foster children who were adopted, and they found some key factors related to a child's likelihood to be adopted. The researchers evaluated data from 1,268 families who had adopted 1,396 children. From this sample, they based their findings on about 500 children who had been in foster care and subsequently were adopted.

Said the researchers, "The items found to be negatively related to timely adoption were exposure to sexual abuse, physical abuse, and neglect; history of multiple foster care placements; severe behavioral problems; greater age at entry into foster care; and the fact that the social worker and foster family did not plan that the child would be adopted by the family at initial placement."

In another study, published in a 1998 issue of *Children and Youth Services Review*, researchers studied factors that mitigated for or against adoption. The study included 150 children in foster care. The average age was 11 years.

They found three variables that were significant. First was age, and this had the strongest correlation of the variables. Next was the number of siblings placed together, and last was a genetic or family history of a problem. They found that an adolescent in foster care was 33 times more likely to remain in foster care than a preschool child.

Children *not* placed with siblings were more likely to stay in foster care, contrary to what most people might think. (Although it is not clear if this was because of social workers' desire to keep families together or because of other reasons.)

Another intriguing finding was that children with a genetic or family history indicating possible problems were *more* likely to be placed, which seems to fly in the face of what one would expect. The researchers said it was "surprising that what may be considered a deficiency would sway the permanency plan towards adoption. Perhaps when considered with other factors such as age, the presence of a risk which has not yet blossomed does not emerge as a prohibiting factor in the workers' or adoptive parents' estimations of adoptability."

One factor that was found significant was race, with nonwhite children more likely to remain in foster care. This remains a problem in 2006. Another factor was the presence of DEVELOPMENTAL DISABILITIES, with disabled children being more likely to remain in foster care than nondisabled children.

How Children Feel about Foster Care

In the book *The Heart Knows Something Different: Teenage Voices from the Foster Care System,* a poignant work that shares first-person stories from foster children, one can gain a feeling for how foster care feels from the inside. This revealing book, which is still meaningful in the 21st century, only deepens the sense of urgency to help so many children who are lost in a complex system.

Wrote a 17-year-old girl,

My biological mother used to beat me for no reason, just because she was angry. She told me to keep the bruises on my body a secret from everyone, but if she was in a good mood she'd be very nice to me and say, "I'll be there for you."

My foster mother doesn't know about my past. She doesn't know that everything I once owned has been taken away from me.

My brother has been adopted and I haven't seen him in years. Perhaps he wouldn't have been adopted if I could have shown him I loved him.

My mother abused me and I take some of the blame. I just wish I could have been a better child.

See also ABUSE; FOSTER PARENT; FOSTER PARENT ADOPTION; GRANDPARENT ADOPTIONS; KINSHIP CARE; PSYCHIATRIC PROBLEMS OF ADOPTED PERSONS; RESILIENCE; SEXUAL ABUSE, CHILDHOOD; SPECIAL NEEDS ADOPTION.

Adoption and Foster Care Analysis and Reporting System (AFCARS), "The AFCARS Report: Preliminary FY 2003 Estimates as of April 2005," U.S. Department of Health and Human Services, Administration for Children and Families, Administration on Children, Youth and Families, Children's Bureau. Available online. URL: http://www.acf.hhs.gov/programs/cb/publications/afcars/report10.pdf, downloaded on July 17, 2005.

Austin, Lisette. "Mental Health Needs of Youth in Foster Care: Challenges and Strategies," *Connection* 20, no. 4 (Winter 2004): 6–13.

Barth, Richard P., et al. "Timing Is Everything: An Analysis of the Time to Adoption and Legalization," *Social Work Research* 18, no. 3 (September 1994): 139–148.

Desetta, Al, ed. *The Heart Knows Something Different: Teenage Voices from the Foster Care System.* New York: Persea Books, 1996.

James, Sigrid. "Why Do Foster Care Placements Disrupt? An Investigation of Reasons for Placement Changes in Foster Care," *Social Service Review* 78, no. 4 (December 2004): 601–627.

Lieberman, Florence, Thomas K. Kenemore, and Diane Yost. *The Foster Care Dilemma.* New York: Human Sciences Press, 1987.

McDonald, Thomas P., et al. *Assessing the Long-Term Effects of Foster Care: A Research Synthesis.* Washington, D.C.: CWLA Press, 1996.

Office of the Assistant Secretary for Planning and Evaluation. *Understanding Adoption Subsidies: An Analysis of AFCARS Data.* U.S. Department of Health and Human Services, Washington, D.C., 2005.

Pecora, Peter J., et al. *Improving Family Foster Care: Findings from the Northwest Foster Care Alumni Study.* Seattle, Wash.: Casey Family Services, revised March 14, 2005.

Schmidt-Tieszen, Ada, and Thomas P. McDonald. "Children Who Wait: Long-Term Foster Care or Adoption?" *Children and Youth Services Review* 20, nos. 1–2 (February 1998): 13–28.

foster parent   An individual who cares for children on a temporary basis, which may mean days, weeks, or months, and who has been previously screened and approved by a government or private agency. In some cases in the United States, the child remains in the home for years, and sometimes the foster parents adopt the child subsequent to termination of parental rights. In other cases, such as with teenagers, legal guardianship may be used rather than adoption if the foster parents do not wish to adopt the child for reasons considered acceptable by the child's social worker. Children adopted from other countries sometimes reside with foster parents prior to the adoption, most commonly in GUATEMALA or SOUTH KOREA, and occasionally in other countries.

Most foster parents in the United States are under the jurisdiction of the state or county public social services department; however, some private adoption agencies that arrange infant adoptions place babies in temporary foster care until the birthparents are certain adoption is the best plan for them and the child. This type of foster care generally lasts only a few weeks at most and has largely fallen out of favor with the practice of OPEN ADOPTION.

Foster parents who provide care for children in state custody have undergone a licensing and/or certification process, and they have also attended classes prior to receiving their first foster child. Their homes are also inspected for cleanliness and safety. At least a basic background check will be done on the prospective foster parents, to ensure that they have not been accused of child abuse in the past and they have not committed any crimes.

Foster parents have an ongoing relationship with the state or county social worker with regard to the child's progress, future plans for the child, and so forth. Conversely, some foster parents complain that they receive inadequate support from social workers, and the constant turnover of social workers makes it difficult to create a relationship with one social worker.

Foster parents for the county or state receive a monthly payment for the foster child and the child's medical care is covered by MEDICAID. Most foster parents reportedly do not believe that the monthly check adequately covers all the expenses that are involved in caring for a child.

See also FOSTER CARE; FOSTER PARENT ADOPTION.

foster parent adoption   The adoption of a child by his or her foster parent. In many cases, the children have been living with the foster parents for years, and the foster parents are also the PSYCHOLOGICAL PARENTS. Most children adopted from the foster care system are adopted by their foster parents.

Studies have also revealed that adoption DISRUPTION is less likely to occur in foster parent adoptions than in "new" parent adoptions. As a result, foster parents are far more frequently considered as possible adoptive parent candidates than in past years. However, there are insufficient numbers of foster parents interested in adoption to accommodate all the children who need adoptive families. Some foster parents regard themselves as too old to adopt or have other reasons for not adopting their foster children. This means that states need to actively recruit adoptive parents with little or no foster parent experience.

Some states mandate that public agencies give foster parents first consideration should the child become free for adoption.

See also ADOPTION AND SAFE FAMILIES ACT; FOSTER CARE.

fraud in adoption   Active and purposeful deception of individuals, usually prospective adoptive parents and sometimes pregnant women considering adoption, and which are nearly always for the purpose of obtaining money. There are many different types of frauds. The best defense against fraud is to deal with a reputable adoption agency or adoption attorney. Some countries have had scandals related to baby selling, which led to a requirement in GUATEMALA for DNA testing of the relinquishing mother to verify her parenthood of the child.

In domestic adoptions, prospective adoptive parents should advise the social worker or attorney if any requests for money are received from the pregnant woman or anyone else interested in the adoption, so that these requests can be reviewed and a determination made as to their legality.

It is best to avoid giving any money directly to the pregnant woman and, instead, to allow the agency or attorney to disburse funds. If the prospective parents give the pregnant woman money directly, this may constitute "baby selling" and could invalidate the adoption in many states, particularly when the amounts total thousands of dollars. Some states have limits on how much money a pregnant woman may receive in living expenses.

Some states require an accounting of such expenses to the court at the time of FINALIZATION. (See also COSTS TO ADOPT.)

In some cases, it may be acceptable to provide rent money by paying the landlord directly; however, it is best to consult with an attorney or social worker before doing so. The pregnant woman may be innocent of any intent to defraud and may be truly indigent; however, it is best for a person experienced in adoption to make this determination.

In the United States, some individuals pretend to be pregnant so that they can obtain money for their living expenses from individuals seeking to adopt. They may weave elaborately sad stories that take advantage of prospective adoptive parents. Rather than seeking advice from an adoption agency or an adoption attorney, the person seeking to adopt may send money directly to the person faking the pregnancy. Multiple families may be scammed at the same time by the same woman using this strategy.

Sometimes the woman truly is pregnant but has no intention of placing her child for adoption, and she (and often a male partner) will simultaneously seek out funds from many couples. The people committing the fraud may tell themselves that the couples are wealthy and that they will never miss the money. However, the individuals seeking to adopt may become so traumatized by the experience that they decide against adoption altogether. In addition, many couples seeking to adopt save up their money for years, and they may not be able to afford to adopt after being defrauded.

In other countries, individuals may contact citizens in the United States or Canada, proclaiming that they wish to place their child for adoption once it is born. They may find prospective adoptive parents who advertise their desire to adopt on the INTERNET. The Internet has made it possible to expand the reach of those seeking to defraud families wishing to adopt children.

In some countries, fraud in adoption became so rampant that the country shut down adoptions altogether. This situation occurred in ROMANIA in 2004.

Sometimes an actual placement of a child does occur, and later the adoption proves to be invalid, because the adoptive family unknowingly has failed to follow the laws of their state and/or the federal government. This is yet another reason why it is important to engage the services of an experienced adoption agency or attorney before actively seeking to locate a pregnant woman who may wish to place her child for adoption.

Families seeking to adopt should be particularly wary of any organization or individual that uses one or more of the following tactics:

- The family is told about a baby or child and it is said that they must decide by *today* if they want the child, otherwise the child will be given to someone else. Pressure tactics should always be questioned.

- The family is told they must pay an extra fee that was not discussed earlier and that sounds suspicious. This does not include such fees as increased medical expenses because the mother needed a cesarean section instead of a vaginal delivery.

- The family is told that a baby may die/not be adopted/needs surgery or some other urgent request. This request is also tied to an increased demand for money.

- The family is told the child is one race when it is known that the child is actually of another race or ethnicity. This does not include unborn children, in which case the pregnant woman may have not reported (or not known) that she was having a child of another race or ethnicity.

- The family is told there is no information on the birthparents of a child born in the United States. There is nearly always some information available on the birthparents of U.S.-born children. However, such information is often unavailable on children born in other countries.

- The same child is promised to two or more families. They may discover this fact later. The only protection against this scam is to deal with reputable adoption agencies and/or attorneys.

- Individuals advertise a fee of a relatively small amount of money in exchange for assisting individuals with locating agencies or midwives so they can adopt a baby. The prospective parents pay the fee and never hear from the individual or organization again. In one case, hundreds of couples nationwide paid $200 each before one woman's online fraud was discovered.

- Rarely, children from other countries are stolen from their parents for adoption. In 2005, a Seattle, Washington, woman was convicted for placing children illegally from Cambodia.

Note that most ADOPTION AGENCIES and adoption attorneys behave in a reputable manner, and it is only a few individuals that actively seek to defraud individuals who are seeking to adopt or to place their child for adoption.

See also WRONGFUL ADOPTION.

gays and lesbians adopting children Homosexuals who adopt children, whether as single parents or as a couple. The laws of the state where the individual lives determine whether gays and lesbians may adopt, as well as the policies of the agency or attorney and other factors. In open adoptions, the sexual orientation of the adoptive parent(s) may be a concern for the birthparent or may not.

Adoptions by gays and lesbians are considered controversial by many people, while others have no problem with this policy. Some individuals believe that only a married heterosexual couple or a single heterosexual person should adopt a child, while others believe that whether adoption should be allowed should be decided on a case-by-case basis, and that the sexual orientation of the prospective parent should not be considered as relevant.

Some individuals believe that if gays and lesbians adopt children, they then will be preventing heterosexuals from adopting; however, many gays and lesbians adopt children from foster care or from other countries, and it is difficult to find enough families for these populations of children.

Some states have had specific bans in the past against the adoption of children by gays and lesbians. New Hampshire rescinded its ban on homosexual adoption in 1999. Florida law continues to ban adoption by homosexuals, as not in "the best interests of the child." The Florida law was upheld by the U.S. Supreme Court, which refused to hear a challenge to the law. Other states do not address the issue directly. Some countries, such as China, specifically ban homosexuals from adopting children. Some adoption agencies assist gays and lesbians to adopt.

When the partner of a homosexual person wishes to adopt a biological child of one of them or they both wish together to adopt an unrelated child, they may encounter difficulties in many states. For example, some states require a biological mother to relinquish her parental rights before another woman may adopt her child; however, a lesbian mother would not wish to lose her parental rights, and she would instead prefer to share the legal parenting with her partner.

In some cases, the biological parent has retained parental rights while at the same time an unrelated person was allowed to adopt the child. As a result, a child can have two parents.

In a 1985 Alaska case, *Adoption of a Minor Child,* a minor child's GUARDIAN AD LITEM recommended that a lesbian couple be allowed to adopt a child they had both parented since birth. The adoption was allowed because the court determined the mother's lesbian relationship was not a factor in whether she would be a good parent. Same-sex couples have also been allowed to adopt in California, Connecticut, and Vermont. In addition, the courts have also recognized second parent adoptions in Illinois, New Jersey, New York, Pennsylvania, and the District of Columbia. Courts in other states have approved joint adoptions by unrelated same-sex couples.

Increasingly, both gay and lesbian parents may become adoptive parents, although in the vast majority of cases, it is one of the partners who adopts rather than both. It is unclear what the effect of gay marriages, as in Massachusetts, will have on the adoption of children.

gender preference International and domestic adoption agencies report a very strong preference of adopting parents in the United States to adopt girls, whether they are childless couples or individuals or whether they already have children. This sex preference is seen in adopting parents of all races, socioeconomic status, and all ages.

Many domestic adoption agencies, however, refuse to allow adoptive parents to make a sex preference on their first child. If the parents wish to adopt again at a later date, the agency may sometimes allow the parents to express a sex preference then. If a family already has three boys or three girls and the agency allows them to adopt again, the agency will usually be far more amenable to the family adopting a child of the opposite sex than they now parent. Thus, the manifestation of this preference can be most clearly charted in INTERNATIONAL ADOPTION.

The reverse is generally true when people have biological children: Most want a boy to be their first child. According to an article by Cosette Dahlstrom, Dr. Nancy Williamson of the Population Council reviewed preferences of biological parents in 1976 and concluded:

1. For an only child, 90 percent of men and 67 percent of women would choose a boy.

2. Eighty percent of both parents prefer to have a boy as their firstborn child.

3. For a three-child family, most prefer two boys and one girl.

There are many theories on why adoptive parents tend to prefer to adopt girls. One theory is that girls are perceived as easier to raise than boys, and adoptive parents prefer that things go smoothly. They may have an unrealistic image of a cute little girl in a frilly dress, beaming at them and obeying every command.

Males, however, are perceived as more aggressive, getting into fights as boys, and are viewed as far less passive and submissive. Apparently, these are positive traits in a biological child but less positive to those who prefer to adopt a female child.

Female children may also appeal to the protective and altruistic side of people, and it is possible that adoptive parents have a higher level of such feelings than the average person, particularly in the case of international adoption. Male children do not fulfill this protective instinct as effectively as female children, at least in the abstract perception of many people planning to adopt.

Carrying on the family name is an important reason for many biological families wishing to bear male children; however, sometimes the family is opposed to adoption and opposed to an adopted male child with no genetic connection to the family carrying on the family name.

Other reasons include the expectation that a girl will stay closer to the family even after marriage and the fact that society permits a more open show of affection toward female children.

Extended family support may be much stronger when the family adopts a girl for many of the reasons described here, and the adopting family may realize, consciously or unconsciously, that an adopted female would be more accepted than an adopted male.

The gender preference of adoptive parents in international adoption may also derive from the expectation of parents who believe females from other parts of the world can blend in with American society easier than a male.

Adoptive parents may think that boys adopted from abroad tend to be shorter and thinner than American boys and would be teased about their appearance by other schoolchildren, especially other boys. Petite and dainty girls, however, are seen in a positive light.

This sexist preference, when it exists, presents a particular problem to international adoption agencies and children abroad. In some countries, people have an even more pronounced protective and positive preference for females than for male children.

Based on this view, females are to be protected, while males are expected to fend for themselves. Females are economically more valuable: They can ultimately serve as maids and perform other menial tasks, whereas boys are often seen as a burden on their societies. As a result, at many international agencies male infants and older children are more readily available for adoption, and prospective adoptive parents who want to adopt females face a longer waiting period. However, in some countries (such as China and India), there is a strong preference for male children. Girl fetuses are more likely to be aborted and girl children to be abandoned.

In the case of an independent or an open adoption, a particular family is usually matched to a particular pregnant woman, so it is very seldom that a family is offered a sex preference. However, many obstetricians routinely perform ultrasound examinations, which often detect the sex of a child.

Adamec, Christine. "Adopt a Boy," *OURS* (July/August 1988): 30–31.

genetic parents The individuals who together conceive a child; this term is generally used to refer to the genetic parents of an adopted child. More popularly used descriptive terms are *birthparents* or *biological parents* of a child. Sometimes the term *genetic parents* is contrasted to the term *psychological parents*. The psychological parents are the individuals the child mentally and emotionally identifies as parents although there is no genetic link.

See also BIRTHPARENT; PSYCHOLOGICAL PARENT.

genetic predispositions The propensity to inherit traits from biological parents. Children inherit many traits from their birthparents, including their eye color, natural hair color, potential physical build, potential talents, and others. In addition, children may also inherit propensities to certain diseases, such as diabetes or obesity. Some studies indicate that adopted children born to alcoholic parents have an increased risk for developing ALCOHOLISM themselves. Some studies have found genetic predispositions to the development of attention-deficit/hyperactivity disorder, depression, and other psychiatric disorders. For example, a news release from the National Institute of Mental Health in 2005 revealed that a suspect gene might increase an individual's susceptibility to developing depressive or anxiety disorders.

Sometimes the combination of a genetic predisposition combined with extreme stress may lead to the development of psychiatric problems. According to Dr. Miller, individuals "with a short form of the serotonin transporter gene (5-HT T) are more likely to experience depression after emotional stress than those with the long form of this gene. Similarly, a functional polymorphism in the gene encoding the neurotransmitter-metabolizing enzyme monoamine oxidase A (MAOA) influences the response to maltreatment in early childhood. Individuals with lower activity of the MAO gene are more likely to develop behavioral and mental disorders after stressful experiences in early childhood."

However, a genetic predisposition means that a person may exhibit a trait but may not necessarily do so. Many characteristics are thought to stem from the confluence of heredity and environment. Neither should be denied its importance.

Children may also inherit predispositions to talents or abilities. For example, if a birthmother has musical talent, then her child, now adopted, might have a genetic predisposition to musical ability. On the other hand, it is also true that this genetic predisposition may never appear, especially if the child is never exposed to music.

Individually considered, genetic predispositions may seem "good" or "bad" to the prospective adoptive parent or other individual who is considering the trait. However, genetic characteristics are often expressed in negative terms when it comes to adopted children and adults. When scientists study populations of adopted children and adults, they often look at social problems such as alcoholism, drug abuse, and so forth. This research bias may make it seem as if these characteristics are the only or the most important aspects of adoption.

Rarely, if ever, do researchers analyze whether the "good" traits that are inherited from biological parents are later evidenced in their children who were adopted. This is a reality of how research is performed. (See RESEARCH, PROBLEMS WITH.)

Studies of twins separated at birth and studies of adopted children and their birth and adoptive families have revealed a wide variety of possible inherited predispositions, such as intelligence levels, temperaments, a propensity to suffering from allergies, and many more.

Intelligence

Researchers have identified a strong heritability of general mental ability and intelligence. (See also INTELLIGENCE.) Studies which provide information that compares adopted children's intelligence levels to those of their birthparents are usually not performed on children adopted from other countries, where such information is not available. Instead, they are derived from studies performed in the United States. Many studies are also performed in Scandinavia, based on data from Scandinavian children adopted by Scandinavian parents.

The Colorado Adoption Project is a longitudinal study of 245 adopted children, their adoptive parents and birthparents. The children were studied at ages one, two, three, four, and seven years of age with age-appropriate tests of intelligence.

The researchers reported on their findings in *Nature,* stating that there were strong indicators of a relationship between the child's intelligence and that of the birthparents. This relationship increased as the child grew older. Apparently adoptive parents have a strong impact on a child's intellectual level in the early years, and genetics may "kick in" at a later date.

Researchers on the Texas Adoption Project, a study of children measured twice at 10-year intervals, also found an increased heritability of intelligence, a relationship that strengthened until adolescence or even into adulthood.

In a longitudinal study of 100 identical twins raised apart, the Minnesota Study, the researchers found a strong correlation for intelligence and other traits; however, they do not denigrate the value of environment and good parenting in promoting intellectual ability.

There have also been studies comparing the IQ levels of children who have been adopted to those of their half-siblings who were raised by birthparents. A study by M. Schiff and R. C. Lewontin in 1986 compared the IQ levels of adopted children whose birthmothers were "socially disadvantaged" with the IQ levels of half-siblings raised by the birthmother. They found that the adopted children scored as much as 16 points higher in IQ levels than did the siblings who remained with the birthmother. This finding indicates that the impact of the environment was a positive one.

Temperament

There are both genetic and environmental components in temperaments, or the overall mood and outlook of a child, including whether the child is active or passive, fearful or calm, and many other traits. Said David Howe in his book *Patterns of Adoption,* "For many temperaments, adopted children are more like their biological than their adopted parents. However, some traits appear to be more heritable than others."

Allergies

Many other correlations have been found, including some surprising ones. For example, in a 1998

issue of the *Annals of Allergy, Asthma & Immunology,* researchers studied 367 adoptive parents from Iowa with and without asthma and their young adult children.

They found that if an adoptive mother had asthma and allergic rhinitis, the adopted child's risk for asthma increased. Even if the adoptive mother had only asthma or only allergic rhinitis, that too increased the risk of asthma in the adopted child. If the adoptive father had asthma or allergic rhinitis there was a trend, although a lower probability than with the mother, toward increased asthma in the adopted person.

The researchers speculated that there could be an environmentally triggered propensity to some allergies, and it seems that the results suggest they were mostly environmentally mediated and not genetic, but that they might be triggered by an environmental agent, such as a virus. Allergens could also be the cause. That could explain the increased existence of asthma in the adopted adults with mothers who had allergic rhinitis and/or asthma. The researchers did not have information on the birthparents, but it seems apparent that it is very unlikely that the children were matched with their adoptive parents on the basis of whether or not their biological parents had allergic rhinitis or asthma.

Attempts to Elicit Genetic Data

Most scientists agree that both heredity and environment are important to a child's development. However, genetic markers cannot always be identified nor can the interaction of heredity and environment be clearly delineated.

Because some genetic predispositions can be very important to a child's future, many states require that child-placing agencies and adoption attorneys placing children born in the United States provide extensive nonidentifying medical and social information to the adoptive parents.

It should also be noted that adopted adults in numerous studies have stated their desire for medical information, hobbies, and interests of birthparents, so obviously the information would be valuable to them, when available. (One country outside the United Stages in which such information often is gathered is SOUTH KOREA.) Whether the adoption is a confidential adoption or an open adoption, such information should be obtained from the birthparents, when possible.

It is important, however, to remember that many children who were adopted in the past, as now, did not come with this genetic and other information as part of their "passports." Orphaned children and foundlings such as the thousands of children adopted from other countries indicate that many adopted children can make excellent adjustments despite the lack of this information.

Also, most qualified medical practitioners realize that careful testing and physical examination may offset the absence of detailed medical background information in their patients.

Preadoption Genetic Testing

Because of interest and concern about genetic predispositions, some adoptive families have indicated a strong interest in genetic testing. As our knowledge of genetics grows, so should our ability to obtain such data. However, one serious problem with preadoption genetic testing is that it may unfairly screen out children to be adopted. A "predisposition" is just that: a possibility, a propensity. It is not a certainty. However, if genetic testing could show, for example, that the child carried a gene for a serious health problem, it is likely that child would be regarded as a child with SPECIAL NEEDS and might not be adopted at all.

In addition, even if a child with an identified particular genetic predisposition was adopted, that child might experience a variety of subtle or overt discrimination, in the family, at school, or in the workplace. The child's self-esteem could also be affected quite profoundly, leading to low expectations and poor achievement, as well as in other ways. For example, diagnosis of a genetic potential may lead to an unintended outcome, such as that of adult women who, when they learned that they had a genetic predisposition to breast cancer, have insisted on a mastectomy even though there was no cancer present in the breast.

Another problem with genetic testing is the "self-fulfilling prophecy." For example, if a child and his parents believe that the child is likely to develop an emotional disorder, then the disorder may present as a result of the expectation, rather than as a result of genetics. Psychiatrists Andre Derdeyn and Charles L. Graves expressed their concern over parents who may overlay their negative expectations on adopted children based on the biological parents' attributes. Said the doctors:

"Parents' over-concern about their adopted children may contribute significantly to the family's problems. A source of this concern relates to the parents' fantasies of the behavior and personalities of the people whose union produced the child and whose imagined weakness, immorality, or instability led to the child's adoption. These ideas can lead to the construction of a defective mental portrait of the child."

And when this scrutiny occurs, say the doctors, "Parents' over-concern about problematic behavior has had its paradoxic effect, whereby the child has started to identify with the parents' expressed expectations and has started to act accordingly. Insufficient working through of the loss of the biologic child and the acceptance of the adopted child may make the parents feel underentitled to the child, undermining their confidence and their ability to set limits. Parental frustration leads to increasing hostility, which triggers the child's separation anxiety. The child typically deals with the separation anxiety in a counter-phobic manner in terms of provocative behavior." In other words, the child acts out in the feared (but apparently expected) manner.

Although the doctors did not address the issue of preadoption genetic testing, it seems likely that if adoptive parents were able to obtain information about genetic predispositions for problem behaviors, they would be even more likely to watch out for such behaviors in their children.

It is also not clear that the "best interests of the child" are represented by requiring genetic testing.

See also ALCOHOLISM AND ADOPTED PERSONS; PSYCHIATRIC PROBLEMS OF ADOPTED PERSONS.

National Institute of Mental Health, "Depression Gene May Weaken Mood-Regulating Circuit," press release, National Institutes of Health, May 2, 2005.

Derdeyn, Andre P., M.D., and Charles L. Graves, M.D. "Clinical Vicissitudes of Adoption," *Child and Adolescent Psychiatric Clinics of North America* 7, no. 2 (April 1998): 373–388.

Freundlich, Madelyn D. "The Case against Preadoption Genetic Testing," *Child Welfare* 77, no. 6 (November 1, 1998): 663.

Howe, David. *Patterns of Adoption: Nature, Nurture and Psychosocial Development.* Oxford: Blackwell Science, 1998.

Rutter, Michael, et al. "Genetic Factors in Child Psychiatric Disorders—I. A Review of Research Strategies," *The Journal of Child Psychology and Psychiatry and Allied Disciplines* 31 (January 1990): 39–83.

Smith, Jeanne M., M.D., et al. "Asthma and Allergic Rhinitis in Adoptees and Their Adoptive Parents," *Annals of Allergy, Asthma & Immunology* 81 (1998): 135–139.

girls, adoptive parents' preference for   See GENDER PREFERENCE.

grandparent adoptions   It is not known how many grandparents have adopted their biological grandchildren, but laws in many states ease the way for RELATIVE ADOPTIONS. Most states waive the requirements for a HOME STUDY and also waive age criteria and other requirements used for non-relative adoptions.

Grandparents may adopt for a variety of reasons. The birthmother may be a teenager and unready or unwilling to parent her child, while the grandparent is young enough to handle the task. Some grandparents who adopt their grandchildren are probably about the same age as adoptive parents who adopt nonrelatives—in their late thirties or early forties.

The birthmother may have abandoned a child or children to the custody of grandparents, and such situations are increasingly more common with the rise of cocaine and crack cocaine abuse. (See DRUG ABUSE/ADDICTION.)

If the birthmother remains in the home with the grandparents and adopted child, the situation may be difficult or awkward. In the past, some grandparents who raised an adopted child as their own biological child did not tell the child he or she was adopted, and the child grew up thinking his birthmother was his sister. The actor Jack Nicholson has talked about such a situation in his own case.

Experts today urge candor with adopted persons and believe it is better for a adopted man or woman to know as much as possible about his or her heritage (especially that he or she was adopted) rather than learning the information from a third party outside the family.

Because single parenthood is far more socially acceptable now than it was 20 or 30 years ago, many a young woman who becomes pregnant chooses to raise the child herself or place the child for adoption rather than pretend the child is actually her parents' child.

The difficulties of a relative adoption exist when a grandparent adopts a child. Most of the family is aware of the adoption and many approve or disapprove very actively.

grandparent caregivers   According to a 2003 U.S. Census Bureau report, about 2.4 million adults were grandparent caregivers in 2000 to their grandchildren under age 18 years who lived with them and for whom they had primary responsibility. More than a third (39 percent) of all grandparent caregivers provided care for their grandchildren for five or more years. In considering different races and ethnicities, American Indian or Alaska Native grandparents are most likely (56.1 percent) to be grandparent caregivers, followed by African-American grandparents (51.7 percent) and white grandparents (41.6 percent). Asian grandparents, however, have a low rate of being the caregiver to their grandchildren (20 percent). (See table.) Most grandparent caregivers are females.

Other grandparents have a more traditional role, and they have a range of contacts with their children's children, whether adopted or not.

Grandparents Raising Grandchildren

Life spans have increased and a grandmother could be as young as 30 or as old as 80 years or older. Their adult children may have problems with drugs or alcohol and thus be unable to care for their child, and so the grandparent provides that care. Grandparents may also provide care because of an adult child's incarceration. Over half of the children of incarcerated mothers live with their grandparents. Sometimes grandparents adopt their grandchildren, while in other cases they act as foster parents or as informal parents.

With the passage of the Adoption and Safe Families Act (ASFA) of 1997, it is likely that many more grandparents will adopt their grandchildren, particularly if they are allowed to continue receiving MEDICAID and an ADOPTION SUBSIDY for the child.

See also FOSTER CARE; KINSHIP CARE.

GRANDPARENTS LIVING WITH GRANDCHILDREN, RESPONSIBLE FOR CORESIDENT GRANDCHILDREN, AND DURATION OF RESPONSIBILITY BY RACE AND PERCENT: 2000

Characteristic	Total	White	African American	American Indian and Alaska Native	Asian	Native Hawaiian and Other Pacific Islander	Some Other Race	Two or More Races	Hispanic or Latino
Responsible for grandchildren	2,426,730	1,340,809	702,595	50,765	71,791	6,587	191,107	63,076	424,304
Percent of coresident grandparents	42.0	41.6	51.7	56.1	20.0	38.7	33.7	39.7	34.7
By duration of care (percent)									
Total	100.0	100.0	100.0	100.0	100.0	100.0	100.0	100.0	100.0
Less than 6 months	12.1	12.6	9.8	13.0	13.6	12.7	15.6	13.5	14.6
6 to 11 months	10.8	11.6	9.3	10.5	11.0	8.4	11.4	11.2	11.2
1 to 2 years	23.2	23.8	21.2	22.5	25.2	23.8	26.1	23.4	25.1
3 to 4 years	15.4	15.8	14.6	13.9	17.6	11.7	15.7	16.0	15.8
5 years or more	38.5	36.3	45.2	40.0	32.7	43.3	31.1	35.9	33.3

Source: U.S. Census Bureau, "Grandparents Living with Grandchildren: 2000," C2KBR-31, U.S. Department of Commerce, Economics and Statistics Administration, October 2003, page 3.

U.S. Census Bureau. "Grandparents Living with Grandchildren: 2000," C2KBR-31, U.S. Department of Commerce, Economics and Statistics Administration, October 2003.

grief   See LOSS.

group homes   Residential facilities for children. Group homes may receive funding from state or federal sources, or they may be privately funded by religious organizations or other groups. Some group homes receive a mixture of federal, state, and private funding. The children may be in state custody but unable to live in a foster home, or they may be children who have been placed in the group home voluntarily by the parents.

Group homes usually house children over age five and provide temporary shelter for emergency situations or long-term shelter for hard-to-place children, such as teenagers or large sibling groups. Some children may have experienced adoption disruptions and need a group environment rather than a foster home environment because of their difficult behavior problems.

Once a popular solution for all orphaned or abandoned children, or those removed from their parents, group homes have been largely displaced by individual foster homes. However, the entry of increasing numbers of children into the foster care system has made social worker experts and some politicians reconsider the group home as an appropriate venue for housing children. (See also FOSTER CARE.)

Children who have been severely physically or sexually abused may not be able to fit into the family environment of a foster home and may instead need the facilities and structure of a group home, where it is hoped they can receive readily available psychiatric counseling.

growth delays   A delay or deficiency in the growth of the child, referring to height, weight, and/or head circumference. Ongoing growth delays are sometimes termed as "failure to thrive."

Many children adopted from other countries have growth delays. Growth delays are most commonly due to ORPHANAGE living. It may be surprising, but children need love and affection in order to grow adequately.

Said Dr. Miller in her article for *Pediatric Annals,* "Growth delays result from a variety of causes, including insufficient food, improper feeding techniques such as bottle propping, lack of nurturing physical contact, depression leading to poor appetite or poor absorption and use of calories, or almost any concurrent medical problem."

Of course, medical problems can interfere with growth as well. These may be relatively minor problems, such as recurrent diarrhea (sometimes caused by INTESTINAL PARASITIC INFECTIONS) or respiratory infections—both common in children residing in group care—or by more serious medical problems, such as hypothyroidism, kidney disease, gastrointestinal disease, or chronic serious infections (such as TUBERCULOSIS). Some medications may also cause or contribute to growth delays. Children who have been chronically and severely deprived of food, a situation which may occur in the United States and other countries, will show growth delays. (This is a form of neglect.)

Dr. Miller notes that many adopted children with initial growth delays will recover and said, "Nearly all children show rapid improvements in weight, height, and head circumference within 6 months of arrival. Younger children have more potential for recovery than older children, especially for linear growth. Because rapid catch-up is so frequent in this population, children who do not display this must be carefully assessed for medical reasons for poor growth."

Note that ethnic differences should not be used to account for poor growth. Well-nourished, healthy children have similar growth patterns and growth velocity regardless of their racial or ethnic origins. The standard growth charts available in pediatric offices (and at www.cdc.gov/nchs) can be used to monitor the growth of any child. Poor growth patterns should be carefully evaluated by a pediatrician or family physician, as many treatable causes of poor growth are often found.

See also ADOPTION MEDICINE; INTERNATIONAL ADOPTION; MEDICAL PROBLEMS OF INTERNATIONALLY ADOPTED CHILDREN.

Mason, Patrick, M.D., and Christine Narad. "Growth and Pubertal Development in Internationally Adopted Children," *Current Opinion in Endocrinology & Diabetes* 9 (2002): 26–31.

Miller, Laurie C., M.D. "Initial Assessment of Growth Development, and the Effects of Institutionalization in Internationally Adopted Children," *Pediatric Annals* 29, no. 4 (April 2000): 224–232.

guardian ad litem An individual, usually an attorney, appointed by the court to represent a child's best interests, often in relation to CUSTODY. Social workers will present the state's view of who should be given custody, and parents may also retain attorneys to represent their rights.

The guardian ad litem may also be a lay person who is dedicated to helping children. The guardian ad litem is given information from social workers and other authorities and may perform additional investigations as needed before making a recommendation to the court.

The guardian ad litem should contact attorneys to gather additional information from them and determine the status of the case and what problems exist. In addition, the guardian ad litem should also ask for copies of affidavits and pleadings related to the case.

The guardian ad litem should meet with the parents, making it clear that he or she is not their attorney and information they provide will not be held in confidence. Other actions the guardian ad litem should take are to determine and discuss parental views on custody and to gather background information on the child's education, activities, religion, and other relevant factors.

The guardian ad litem should also investigate any possible problems that could harm the child, such as drug or alcohol abuse or the battering of a spouse, if the child were placed with the family.

See also FOSTER CARE; FOSTER PARENT.

Guatemala, adoptions from Adoptions that occur from Guatemala, a Central American country. In fiscal year 2005, 3,783 children were adopted from Guatemala by Americans, and adoptions from Guatemala represented the third greatest number of international adoptions. (The greatest number of adoptions occurred from China, followed by Russia.) Guatemala has consistently been in the top five countries from which Americans have adopted children internationally since 1992.

According to Dr. Miller, Guatemala is the only country that provides DNA test results that prove the relationship of the mother and child, along with a signed consent document from the birthmother. The reason for the DNA test results are that some women in the past had falsely claimed to be the birthmother of a child placed for adoption, defrauding the adoptive parents and violating the laws of Guatemala and the United States.

Most Guatemalan infants adopted by Americans live in foster care before the adoption, rather than in an ORPHANAGE. Often the child placed for adoption is the third or fourth child in the family and the older children remain with the birthparent(s).

Health Issues

Most children adopted from Guatemala are healthy, although some have ANEMIA, parasitic infections, or TUBERCULOSIS.

Travel

Most adoptive parents travel to Guatemala to receive their child. This will provide an opportunity to meet the foster parents and obtain useful and practical information about the child. However, some adoptive parents arrange for their children to be escorted to the United States.

Adoptive parents Mary McKay and Richard Stollberg with Bea Evans offer a free guide replete with helpful information for new adoptive parents: *Guatemala Travel and Etiquette: A Guide for Adoptive Parents.* The guide has many good suggestions for new parents, such as terms of endearment that may be familiar to the baby, including *niña bonita* (beautiful little girl) or *niño guapo* (handsome little boy), or *mi bebé* (my baby). The second edition of this guide, published in 2005, may be downloaded online.

See also INTERNATIONAL ADOPTION; LATIN AMERICAN ADOPTIONS; MEDICAL PROBLEMS OF INTERNATIONALLY ADOPTED CHILDREN.

McKay, Mary, Richard Stolley, and Bea Evans. *Guatemala Travel and Etiquette: A Guide for Adoptive Parents.* 2nd ed., June 2005. Available online. URL: http://www.guatadopt.com/documents/travelguide.pdf, downloaded on July 2, 2005.

Miller, Laurie, C., M.D. *The Handbook of International Adoption Medicine: A Guide for Physicians, Parents, and Providers.* New York: Oxford University Press, 2005.

Hague Convention on Intercountry Adoption
An international agreement that set forth the norms and procedures to safeguard children involved in INTERNATIONAL ADOPTION, and to protect the interests of birth and adoptive parents in the participating countries in the world. These safeguards are designed to discourage trafficking in children and to ensure that international adoptions are made in the best interests of the children involved.

The United States signed the agreement in 1994, and in 2000, the Intercountry Adoption Act, which enacted the Hague provisions, was passed in the United States. The U.S. State Department is the regulating arm of the Hague Convention in the United States. As of this writing, state agencies and other nonprofit entities are seeking to become accrediting organizations that can approve adoption agencies which will manage international adoptions. It is expected that the full provisions of the law in the United States will take effect by 2007.

handicapped children See DEVELOPMENTAL DIS-ABILITIES.

hard-to-place children This phrase, now out of favor with most adoption professionals, has been replaced by "children who have SPECIAL NEEDS." Depending on the definition—and the definition varies from state to state and adoption program to adoption program—the category may include black and biracial children of all ages, sibling groups, healthy and intellectually normal children over age eight, and physically or mentally handicapped children of all ages.

Many families are eager to adopt children with a variety of special needs, and children who were once considered UNADOPTABLE are now being placed in good families.

See also DEVELOPMENTAL DISABILITIES.

health insurance See INSURANCE.

Helicobacter pylori (H. pylori) A chronic and common bacteria that is present worldwide and that may cause gastrointestinal symptoms, although many patients have no symptoms. If untreated, chronic infection with *H. pylori* can lead to the development of ulcers of the stomach and/or the small intestine, as well as stomach cancer. In the past, it was believed that most stomach ulcers were caused by severe stress; however, physicians now know that most ulcers are caused by either *H. pylori* or by the chronic use of medications, particularly prescribed and over-the-counter non-steroidal drugs (NSAIDs) used for pain. Of course, stress may exacerbate an existing ulcer.

Children who have been living in crowded institutional care (such as orphanages) have a greater risk of harboring *H. pylori* bacteria, although *H. pylori* can be found in every country. According to *The Encyclopedia of the Digestive System and Digestive Disorders,* the incidence of *H. pylori* infection ranges from about 20 to 50 percent in developed countries and is greater than 80 percent among individuals living in poor countries. In general, children are infected before they are one or two years old.

One study evaluated the presence of *H. pylori* antibodies in the blood of 226 children ranging in age from newborns to children older than three years, and who were adopted from 18 countries, including Cambodia, China, Colombia, Ecuador, Eritrea, Guatemala, India, Kazakhstan, South Korea, Latvia, Lithuania, Nigeria, Paraguay, Philippines, Romania, Russia, Ukraine, and Vietnam. The children were evaluated by the International Adoption Clinic at the New England Medical Center in Boston, and the results were described in a 2003 issue of *Helicobacter*. Although antibodies are not considered diagnostic of infection, the researchers found that 31 percent of the children had antibodies to *H. pylori* in their blood. This was significantly higher than is found among pediatric populations in the United States or Canada.

In considering individual countries, the highest incidence of *H. pylori* was found in children adopted from Russia (49 percent), Romania (20 percent), and China (16 percent).

Symptoms and Diagnostic Path

Chronic diarrhea and gastritis may indicate an infection with *H. pylori*. Other signs and symptoms may include chronic indigestion or acid reflux. However, as mentioned, many patients have no symptoms.

When *H. pylori* infection is suspected, whether because of symptoms or because the patient has other possible indicators, such as former residency in an area of high prevalence, physicians can check the stools or blood for the evidence of the bacteria. However, sometimes the patient's blood may test positive for antibodies to the bacteria, but the *H. pylori* is no longer present, which means that the patient no longer harbors any active *H. pylori* bacteria and treatment is not indicated. In contrast, the stool test can be used to check for an active and current infection with *H. pylori*, for which treatment is needed.

A urea breath test is also sometimes used to detect *H. pylori*, although it is not reliable in children under age six and most physicians do not use this test for young children. If an endoscopy procedure is performed, in which a special tube is inserted down the throat and into the digestive tract, a biopsy of the stomach can be taken at that time to test for *H. pylori*.

Treatment Options and Outlook

H. pylori is treated with a combination of two or more antibiotics for two weeks or longer. The bacteria can be eradicated; however, it is also possible for patients to become reinfected at a later date. As of this writing, such antibiotics as

metronidazole (Flagyl) and/or clarithromycin (Biaxin) are often used in combination with other medications to treat *H. pylori*. Some medication regimens come in special packages (dosepaks) that include two or more medications that should be taken, to make the regimen simpler and increase patient compliance.

Patients with gastric symptoms may also be prescribed a proton pump inhibitor medication.

Risk Factors and Preventive Measures

Some children have a greater risk for harboring *H. pylori* than others. In the study discussed in *Helicobacter*, several key risk factors for the presence of *H. pylori* and/or its antibodies among children adopted from countries outside North America included the following:

- Residence in an orphanage (versus living in foster care in the same country or living in a combination of family care and institutional care)
- Older age at the time of the adoption (children who tested positive for *H. pylori* were an average age of 43 months, compared to children without the bacteria, who were an average age of 17 months)
- Simultaneous infection with intestinal parasites (44 percent of the children with intestinal parasites also had *H. pylori*, compared to 19 percent of the children who did not have parasites but did have *H. pylori*)

Factors that were found *not* related to infection with *H. pylori* were the presence of diarrhea or ANEMIA. In addition, infection with *H. pylori* did not appear to directly affect the height or weight of the children, although there may be indirect effects, and it is possible that the bacteria may cause growth delays in some children. Further research is needed on this issue.

The authors of the *Helicobacter* article concluded, "International adoptees rapidly recover from many of the effects of institutionalization after placement in their adoptive homes. However [about] 1/3 may harbor *H. pylori* infection. Physicians caring for these children should be aware of [the] possibility of early acquisition of *H. pylori*, and the risks of long-term problems associated with chronic infection."

See also INFECTIOUS DISEASES, SERIOUS; INTESTINAL PARASITIC INFECTIONS; MEDICAL PROBLEMS OF INTERNATIONALLY ADOPTED CHILDREN; ORPHANAGE.

Miller, Laurie C., et al. "Serologic Prevalence of Antibodies to *Helicobacter pylori* in Internationally Adopted Children," *Helicobacter* 8, no. 3 (2003): 173–178.

Minocha, Anil, M.D., and Christine Adamec. *The Encyclopedia of the Digestive System and Digestive Disorders.* New York: Facts On File, 2004.

hepatitis   Inflammation of the liver, commonly used to refer to infections of the liver caused by viruses. Hepatitis A and B are the most commonly known viruses, but hepatitis C also affects the liver.

Children in the United States are routinely immunized against hepatitis B in the first year of life. Unvaccinated children may acquire hepatitis B through sexual contact, blood transfusions, or at birth to a mother infected with the virus. However, ordinary household contact may sometimes transmit the virus between household members. Few people are vaccinated against hepatitis A, although many people have had unrecognized infections and have developed immunity. There is no immunization for hepatitis C as of this writing.

General Information on Hepatitis A, B, and C

Hepatitis A   Hepatitis A is very common worldwide, and is usually transmitted through contaminated food or water. It is rarely if ever contracted through blood transfusion. It is also not contracted through sexual acts.

In the United States, the rate of infection with hepatitis A has declined dramatically from 12.64 cases per 100,000 people in 1990 to 3.77 cases per 100,000 people in 2001, the most recent information available as of this writing from the Centers for Disease Control and Prevention (CDC). There were 31,441 cases of hepatitis A in 1990 in the United States, and by 2001 that number had declined to 10,609.

Hepatitis B   Hepatitis B is usually transmitted by exposure to blood from an infected person (or to medical equipment, such as needles contaminated with this blood) or by sexual contact with an infected person. Hepatitis B can be spread from an infected mother to her infant at the time of delivery.

Since 1991 in the United States, the American Academy of Pediatrics has recommended that all infants be immunized at birth against hepatitis B. Thus, routine preadoption screening of children adopted in the United States is not recommended unless there are medical risk factors (for example, the mother is a known hepatitis B carrier, has a history of intravenous drug use, there is known or suspected sexual abuse of the child, or the immunization record is incomplete).

Immunization against hepatitis B is not routine in other countries; therefore internationally adopted children should be tested upon arrival in the United States or Canada, even though most have had testing done in their birth countries prior to adoptive placement. Preadoptive testing in the native country is not always reliable.

As with hepatitis A, the rate and number of cases of hepatitis B has declined greatly over past years in the United States. For example, in 1990 the rate was 8.48 per 100,000 people in the United States. By 2001, this rate had declined to 2.79 people per 100,000. There were 21,102 cases of hepatitis B identified in 1990. In 2001, the number had plummeted to 7,843 individuals. Most of these individuals were born in other countries.

Worldwide, an estimated 300 million people are infected with hepatitis B, and most of them reside in Asia.

Hepatitis C   The prevalence of hepatitis C varies from country to country. In some countries, such as China, Russia, Guatemala, Vietnam, and Kazakhstan, about 2.5 percent of the population is infected.

Mothers who are infected with hepatitis C may pass on the virus to their newborn children, and according to the CDC an estimated five of every 100 infants who are born to women infected with hepatitis C will become infected, or a rate of 5 percent. Infants infected at birth generally show no symptoms and are well during childhood. According to the CDC, children born to hepatitis C-infected mothers may harbor maternal antibodies until the child is about 18 months of age, somewhat complicating the determination of the child's infectious status.

Some high-risk behaviors, such as intravenous use of illegal drugs, body piercing, or tattooing, can lead to infection with hepatitis C (or hepatitis B). Having received a blood transfusion in the United States prior to 1992 (when screening of blood for hepatitis was instituted) is another risk factor for infection. However, most children to be adopted do not fall into these risk categories, although some are born to mothers who do fit them.

According to the CDC, the number of new infections of hepatitis C identified each year has declined from about 240,000 in the 1980s to about 25,000 in 2001. In addition, most of these infections are contracted through illegal injected drug use. About 3.9 million Americans are infected with hepatitis C, and of these, 2.7 million have a chronic form of the infection.

Symptoms and Diagnostic Path

Hepatitis A is often asymptomatic. When symptoms occur, they may include fatigue, headache, light-colored stools, dark urine, jaundice, and abdominal pain. Routine liver enzyme tests such as for serum alanine aminotransferase (ALT) will show an elevated level in patients with hepatitis A.

With hepatitis B and C, patients also may have no symptoms. If symptoms occur, they may include jaundice, fatigue, darkened urine, abdominal pain, a loss of appetite, and nausea. Routine liver enzyme tests are elevated. Special blood tests must be used to detect the virus; occasionally (especially with hepatitis C), there are false-negative results, which means that although they test negative for the virus, the patients really are infected.

Treatment Options and Outlook

There is no cure for any form of hepatitis at present, although some patients, especially those infected with hepatitis A, usually recover completely without specific therapy. However, there are treatments and/or recommendations for patients with hepatitis. With hepatitis A, the only common recommendation is for the patient to avoid alcohol, which could, along with the hepatitis A infection, injure the liver. (Patients with any form of hepatitis should avoid alcohol.)

With hepatitis B, treatment may include the injection of interferon and other antiviral medications. Patients should be vaccinated against hepatitis A to avoid further liver damage. With hepatitis C, ribavirin may be given along with interferon. In addition, patients diagnosed with hepatitis C should be vaccinated against hepatitis A and hepatitis B, to avoid any further damage to the liver.

The liver enzyme levels of patients diagnosed with hepatitis B or C should be checked periodically. Patients with hepatitis B and C also have an increased risk for developing liver cancer (hepatocellular carcinoma). Hepatitis B and C may also progress to cirrhosis, which, if severe, may necessitate a liver transplant. With hepatitis C, about 70 percent of infected individuals eventually develop chronic liver disease, according to the CDC, although this usually takes many years.

Risk Factors and Preventive Measures

Individuals at risk for contracting hepatitis A may live with a person who either has the disease or work in a facility such as a day care center or eat in a restaurant staffed by an infected worker. Children who are sexually abused or who are born to infected mothers are at risk for hepatitis B or C infection. Children living in ORPHANAGES also face an increase risk of infection for hepatitis B, which is highly contagious. Children living in other countries may contract hepatitis B or C infection via exposure to contaminated blood or medical equipment.

Those individuals most at risk for developing liver cancer as a result of long-term hepatitis C are Asians, Hispanics, Native Americans, and Pacific Islanders. In most cases, the younger the child was at time of the initial infection with hepatitis B or C, the more likely he or she is to be an asymptomatic carrier.

In terms of preventive measures, all children should be vaccinated against hepatitis B. Hepatitis A vaccines are generally reserved for those planning to travel to endemic areas.

Other preventive measures against hepatitis B and C include avoidance of shared needles, such as is common with illegal intravenous drug use, not having body piercing or tattoos or ensuring that the equipment used is sterile, and wearing surgical gloves if the blood of another person must be touched.

See also IMMUNIZATIONS; INFECTIOUS DISEASES, SERIOUS; MEDICAL PROBLEMS OF INTERNATIONALLY ADOPTED CHILDREN.

Miller, Laurie, C., M.D. *The Handbook of International Adoption Medicine: A Guide for Physicians, Parents, and Providers.* New York: Oxford University Press, 2005.

———. "International Adoption: Infectious Diseases Issues," *Clinical Infectious Diseases* 40 (January 15, 2005): 286–293.

Minocha, Anil, M.D., and Christine Adamec. *The Encyclopedia of the Digestive System and Digestive Disorders.* New York: Facts On File, 2004.

heredity   See GENETIC PREDISPOSITIONS.

high-risk placements   Adoptive placements that have a high probability of DISRUPTION; almost exclusively refers to the placement of children with SPECIAL NEEDS who are older or who suffer medical or mental disabilities; not to be confused with AT RISK PLACEMENT.

The age at which a child is considered a high risk placement varies from state to state, but most states consider the placement of a teenager to have a high level of risk.

However, studies have revealed that children who are older when adopted can often successfully adjust to their new families, despite a troubled past that might include abuse and neglect. Also, there is a positive relationship between large family size and the success of the placement.

home study   The assessment and preparation process a prospective adoptive family undergoes to determine, among other things, whether they should adopt and what type of child would best fit the family. Some agencies refer to this process as the "family study" or "preadoptive counseling" or other phrases that are considered more accurate and descriptive.

The home study includes the entire process of evaluation and instruction about adoptive parenting and is not limited to visits to the residence of the family. (See EDUCATION OF ADOPTIVE PARENTS.)

Prospective parents initially fill out application forms for agency adoption, and agency criteria are applied to determine whether the parents fit the primary criteria, for example, age, length of marriage, number of children in home, religious affiliation (if it is a sectarian agency), infertility, and other factors.

Many adoption agencies accept applications to adopt healthy infants only from couples who have been married at least three years, are childless or have only one child, are medically infertile, and are under 45 years of age.

The criteria and application process vary from agency to agency. Some agencies may accept applications from couples who are in their mid-forties or older or who have been previously divorced. In addition, single applications may also be accepted, although married couples are much preferred by most agencies.

The criteria to adopt a child with SPECIAL NEEDS are usually different from those for a healthy infant, and often agencies will accept applications from prospective adoptive parents who are well over age 40, already have children, are still fertile, and so forth. This does *not* necessarily mean the home study will be easier.

Because children with special needs themselves need adoptive parents who can cope with whatever their special needs are, the social worker will carefully evaluate the family to ensure it is within their realm of coping to raise a child with special needs.

After initial screening, the couple or single person's name may be placed on a WAITING LIST until the agency decides it is ready to begin the home study process with the individual(s).

If the prospective parents are adopting a child through INDEPENDENT ADOPTION, the home study may be performed by a state or county social worker or by a licensed adoption agency or private social worker, depending on the laws of the state where the adopting parents reside.

The home study process often includes one or more group orientation classes in which prospective parents learn about the agency and its policies. These classes may occur prior to the application process to provide general information or after initial acceptance of the applicants by the agency as a beginning step to the home study process.

Agencies may rely on individual conferences with prospective parents, or they may offer classes or a combination of the two in the assessment process.

If classes are offered, the subjects covered will depend on whether the prospective parents are interested in INFANT ADOPTION or special needs adoption.

For those seeking to adopt healty infants, many agencies will discuss subjects such as coming to terms with infertility, birthmothers and their feelings and reasons for placing the child for adoption, when and how to tell the child he or she was adopted, and a variety of other topics that will improve the parent's ability to successfully rear the child.

The social worker may bring in a panel of adoptive parents, adopted persons, or birthmothers to share their feelings with the group. An interchange of questions and an ongoing dialogue between the adopting parents and the social worker is usually encouraged.

Parents who plan to adopt children with special needs will often learn about physical and sexual abuse and neglect, developmental delays, problems that may be exhibited by newly adopted children, and other topics.

Whether the group or individual home study approach is used, the adopting parents are always interviewed privately to obtain certain personal information from them.

The social worker will ask them together and individually why they want to adopt, what their expectations are in adopting, the type of child they hope to adopt, how their extended family feels about the adoption, whether both parents intend to work outside the home after the placement of a child, and many other questions, including sensitive questions about their marital relationship, drug and alcohol use, and philosophies about discipline for a child.

These questions are asked not only to help the social worker with the assessment of the family but also to help the family explore issues they may not have fully examined or understood.

If the prospective adoptive family already has children in the home, the children may be interviewed on their feelings about the introduction of a new sibling to ensure they are emotionally prepared for such a change.

A background investigation is also conducted to determine if the prospective adoptive parent has a criminal record or has ever been charged with child abuse or neglect. References are almost invariably requested by the social worker, and these may be written or verbal, depending on the agency, although most are written.

The agency will discuss management of the family finances, including a verification of the applicants' wages and income, to confirm that there will be sufficient income in the family to support the child. The social worker may also request copies of the previous year's income tax returns and request banks or other financial institutions to provide written verification of current balances.

A home study for an INTERNATIONAL ADOPTION will also include the requirement for the applicant to be fingerprinted, often by local police. Additional paperwork is usually required in an international adoption, and the international adoption agency or adoption lawyer should be able to assist the applicants if they have difficulty completing forms.

International adopters will need visas to travel abroad. They should obtain their visas well ahead of the time they need to travel to the country where their child awaits them.

A social worker's visit to the home of the prospective parents is also an essential aspect of any home study. Despite the fears of nearly every adopting parent, the social worker is rarely seeking to perform a "white gloves" study of the home, despite the term "home study." The house simply should be normally clean.

The home may be the site for many personal questions asked of the adopting parents regarding how they plan to discipline the child, their religious beliefs, and so forth. The social worker will usually want a tour of the home and will ask to see where the child would sleep.

The adopting family should have a plan for how they will accommodate the child. They need not have the nursery or room completely set up and decorated, but they should have a room or a plan to create a room or plan to have the child share a room with another child.

Safety is another issue the caseworker will be checking: Is the area free of safety hazards? Do the adopting parents seem sensitized to the needs of the type of children they wish to adopt? (For example, if they have a swimming pool, do they have a plan to protect a young child from wandering into that area?)

The interaction between a married couple is also observed, and the social worker will attempt to determine if both parties are committed to adopting or if the adoption is primarily the idea of one person with the other reluctantly agreeing. Although often one person is the instigator of the idea to adopt, both parties should be enthusiastic about adopting a child.

After completion of the home visit and gathering information from references, the police check, and so on, the caseworker will write up preliminary findings about the couple. The social worker will then write a formal evaluation of the couple with a recommendation to approve or disapprove the couple for adoption.

In some cases, especially cases of an INDEPENDENT ADOPTION in which a lawyer, doctor, or other nonagency person is involved in facilitating the placement of the child, the child may actually already reside in the home before the home study commences.

Ideally, however, the home study is completed prior to placement of the child so the family will be prepared for the adoption and any problems can be determined well in advance of the child's entry into the home. Such a step would markedly reduce the probability of a child being in the custody of inappropriate people.

At least one or two other visits to the home (or with the parents and child elsewhere) will ordinarily occur after placement to ensure the child and adoptive parents are happy and adjusting to each other.

After a waiting period ranging from weeks to months to as long as a year (six months on average), depending in which state the adopting parents live, the adoption will be finalized in a court. A new amended birth certificate will be issued to the adopting parents, with their names on the birth certificate as parents. The original birth certificate is "sealed" in most states, which means it cannot be reviewed by anyone without a court order.

Reasons for rejecting couples or singles who are studied vary. Although most people who pass the initial criteria set by agencies will ultimately be approved in the home study process, a small number of people will be disapproved.

The couple or single may be disapproved for adopting an infant if it is apparent they have not at all come to terms with their infertility, and it is very unlikely they could accept an adopted child as "their own." (This does not mean that infertility must be completely accepted or never cause the adoptive parents pain again. See INFERTILITY.)

If their marriage appears to be in jeopardy, this marital discord would be another reason to deny a couple the opportunity to adopt a child of any age.

The couple may be disapproved for adoption if the home study reveals the couple has provided the caseworker with false or misleading information, for example, if the investigation reveals a felony was committed in the past, perhaps a drug abuse or alcohol conviction.

Most home studies take at least 30 days to complete and may take several months before all steps can be accomplished. Frequently prospective adoptive parents are placed on a waiting list to obtain a home study. Some adoptive parents call this "a waiting list to get on a waiting list."

After a couple or single has had an approved home study, their names may be placed on a WAITING LIST until they are matched with a child. A couple may receive a child the day after their home study is approved or may not receive a child for several years.

If the parents feel able to adopt a child with special needs, this may also shorten the wait; for example, if white adopting parents are interested in adopting a biracial baby or child, they may receive their child more rapidly than if they stipulate they will only adopt a racially matching child.

Although the home study process may be perceived as nerve-racking to prospective adoptive parents, studies have revealed that individuals who are being evaluated or who have completed their home studies are significantly less anxious than couples who have not yet begun their home study. This is probably so because those who have begun or completed the process believe they will ultimately succeed in adopting a child.

homosexual adoption See GAYS AND LESBIANS ADOPTING CHILDREN.

hospitals' treatment of birthmothers Hospitals play a critical role in dealing with birthmothers who are considering an adoption plan, far beyond assisting the birthmother with the delivery of her child and providing immediate postpartum care. The attitude of hospital staff, particularly nurses, may mean the difference between a woman deciding to parent her baby or to proceed with her previous plan of adoption. Despite receiving counseling beforehand by experienced social workers, the birthmother's decision may change in the vulnerable moments after giving birth.

In addition, although she may follow through with her original plan, whether it was adoption or parenthood, the reactions and behavior of the hospital staff can affect the birthmother's own self-image, both during her stay and after she leaves. For example, if she felt the hospital staff were understanding and positive, she could begin the process of reorienting herself to her own individual goals. Conversely, if she perceived the hospital staff as very negative, the birthmother could have many lingering doubts about her decision.

Most hospitals have an adoption policy, and some hospitals even have separate policies for agency adoptions, independent adoptions, and special needs adoptions. Because of turnover in nursing staff, it is possible new staff members may not have received in-service training on adoption policies. One way to avert potential errors is to involve the hospital social worker from the time of the birthmother's admission until her discharge.

Some hospitals also offer birthmothers the opportunity to visit the hospital before the delivery, meet with the hospital social worker, and be introduced to the head nurses of labor, delivery, obstetrics, and the nursery. This advance visit can alleviate much of the anxiety of the pregnant woman, including both the fear of a first-time mother as well as a dread about later telling hospital staff about her adoption plan. Ideally, the agency social worker or attorney assisting the pregnant woman with her adoption plan formally notifies the hospital social work department about the upcoming delivery and the woman's wishes. This should be done as far in advance as possible in order to allow the hospital social worker to notify key people in labor and delivery, the nursery, and, of course, the obstetrician.

The role of the hospital social worker will vary, depending on whether the pregnant woman has an established relationship with another counselor (usually a social worker) and whether that worker is on the staff of an adoption agency or retained through private adoption intermediaries.

The hospital social worker's role should not interfere with any other counseling relationship the pregnant woman has established prior to admission, such as with a professional who specializes in working with pregnant women considering adoption. Upon admission of a pregnant woman who is considering adoption but does not have a counselor, however, the hospital social worker begins the evaluation and support process. The social worker interacts with medical personnel, the patient's family, agency social workers, attorneys, and adoptive couples.

Although the pregnant woman should have already received counseling about her options, the hospital social worker is another checkpoint to ensure adoption really is what the birthmother wants for herself and her child. The hospital social worker can discuss what plans the birthmother has made for after her recovery, for example, if she will return to work or school and what her long-term goals are.

Many issues are involved during a hospital stay; for example, the birthmother may wish to see her baby after its birth or may even opt for "rooming in" (wherein the baby stays in the room with the mother throughout her hospital stay). Policy decisions regarding birthmothers should be carefully considered by hospital staff.

The choice to have the child "room in" may not always be advisable for women considering an adoption plan. It is the view of Jerome Smith and Franklin Miroff, authors of *You're Our Child*, that at some point in such a process, the bond between the birthmother and child becomes so strong that to continue with the adoption plan could cause emotional trauma, including clinical depression over the experienced loss.

In addition, Smith advised against the birthmother nursing her child unless she plans to parent the baby. His general advice for the birthmother planning an adoption is to see the infant and hold it if she wishes but not to have constant close contact with the baby while in the hospital.

Smith also recommends that the birthmother be allowed to grieve her loss and be counseled about the feelings she will probably experience after she leaves the hospital.

Most hospital staffs know a birthmother has the right to see her child unless and until she signs consent papers for adoption (or even after signing consent, depending on state law and circumstances). Birthmothers may sometimes not realize this entitlement and wrongfully believe they have no rights.

Nurses and other well-meaning people sometimes mistakenly believe a woman "giving up" her child could not possibly want to see or hold it. They may also think it would be easier for a mother to follow through with an adoption decision if she does not risk bonding to the infant, a logical conclusion supported by some research.

Nonetheless, most social workers and other adoption practitioners today believe it is important for the birthmother to see for herself that the child is physically well and to observe the appearance of the child. (The birthmother should not, however, be overly pressured to see the child if she does not wish to.)

Some birthmothers wish to say good-bye to the child before signing the agreement to adoption. Although, as far as we know, the farewell will be meaningless to the newborn infant, the saying of good-byes may be profoundly important to the birthmother as she explains to the child (and herself) why she has made this adoption decision and what she hopes the future will hold for the child. If the birthmother is deprived of the opportunity to say good-bye, such a deprivation could make the resolution of her loss even more difficult.

Jeanne Lindsay and Catherine Monserrat wrote in *Adoption Awareness: A Guide for Teachers, Counselors, Nurses and Caring Others:*

> Hospital staff need to be reminded how vulnerable a woman is during labor and delivery and immediately afterward. She is likely to take seriously everything said by the doctor and nurses. "I don't known how you could do this" or "Adoption must be really hard. I could never do that . . ."

The authors believe such comments, combined with the guilt and emotional pain the mother may be feeling, could lead her to decide impulsively that she should parent the baby.

One author was concerned about an apparent lack of confidentiality when nurses were aware of new mothers considering adoption. She stated that one nurse examined a baby who was not supposed to be shown to the public because the nurse was considering adopting a child herself. Nurse Susan Malestic has stated that sometimes nurses providing prenatal care tell friends about single pregnant women in an attempt to arrange an adoption. She cautioned that it is better to remain neutral about adoption and to refer the woman to adoption agencies where she can obtain counseling and assistance.

Hospital social workers may wish to bring adoption up if the birthmother has not made any plans for her child and seems unsure of the immediate future.

Many birthmothers are afraid to broach such a subject, thinking they will be judged as unfeeling, but if a nurse mentions it, they may be interested. (Again, the nurse should not promote adoption or parenting at this very vulnerable time; however, the patient may be afraid to verbalize her unspoken need for assistance.) In such a case, the hospital social worker should be contacted and can then follow up the case and provide referrals and counseling as needed.

Older single mothers are also sometimes interested in adoption for their babies. The average person can understand why a teenager would want to place her child for adoption (although most teenagers choose to parent) but might wrongfully presume that a 35-year-old single woman would invariably choose to parent.

Despite her age, the older single mother should also be advised of the option of adoption, to consider or reject according to her own desires.

In addition, married birthparents sometimes opt to place their baby for adoption. The family may be divorcing or may already have several children and feel unwilling or unable to parent an additional child. Although it may be difficult to withhold judgment in such a case, it is imperative to understand adoption or parenting is their decision to make. If the birthparents felt unwilling to abort and yet believed adoption would be a positive answer for the child, they should be supported in this decision.

Sometimes when nurses and other staff members are unsure of how they should treat a new mother planning to place her baby for adoption, they may avoid the woman altogether, not wishing to make a mistake and not really knowing what to say. As a result, they may leave her alone, bringing in trays and medication and keeping the door shut otherwise.

Experts such as Lindsay and Monserrat say just listening to a birthmother can help her considerably. Rather than conveying his or her own views for or against adoption, the nurse can listen to the birthmother in a compassionate manner. If the birthmother feels the staff is trying to avoid her, she may believe she is an object of shame and what she is doing is wrong and bad. If staff members are willing to talk with her, her psychological pain can be eased, although not erased.

It may be difficult for a nurse to merely listen to the birthmother when a nurse's role is generally to offer exact advice on actions a patient should take; however, listening is often what the birthmother needs as much or more than the physical care the nurse can provide. Most hospitals are short-staffed, but even five minutes could help the birthmother.

Where the birthmother stays in the hospital is also important. Most women planning to place their child for adoption do not wish to be in the same area with other women who are joyous about the child they will bring home and are nursing or feeding their infants, nor do they wish to discuss their decision with other women who, particularly at this point in their lives, would have tremendous difficulty understanding why a woman would choose not to parent.

As a result, whenever possible, birthmothers are placed in rooms by themselves or in a surgical ward.

Hospital staff may understandably be confused by the array of options offered to birthmothers today. Although most adoptions are confidential, some birthmothers know the identity of the adoptive parents. Nurses who try to keep adoptive parents and the birthmother apart are looked at askance by both parties in an OPEN ADOPTION.

Yet if the adoption is confidential, the parties involved do wish to remain apart. If an attorney has arranged for a couple to see the baby, there is risk that they may encounter the birthmother, and hospital staff should be alerted so that an accidental meeting of the couple and the birthmother in the hallway is averted.

Even when an open adoption is planned, the birthmother may wish to be alone and not want to see the adoptive parents. The hospital social worker and her own social worker should ensure that the birthmother's desires for privacy are met.

Increasing numbers of hospitals are now offering seminars to their staffs on adoption and are enhancing staff awareness of why women choose adoption for their babies.

Seminars may include panels of adoptive parents, birthmothers, and adopted persons as well as talks by trained social workers. Seminars also provide the opportunity to bring issues and problems out in the open and help nurses and other staff members offer the compassionate care they strive to give *all* patients. Nurses and other hospital personnel may also benefit from training on adoption.

See also PHYSICIANS.

Malestic, Susan L. "Don't These Patients Have a Right to Privacy? (Pregnant Women Planning to Give Baby up for Adoption)," *RN*, March 1989, p. 21.

Lindsay, Jeanne, and Catherine Monserrat. *Adoption Awareness: A Guide for Teachers, Counselors, Nurses and Caring Others*. Buena Park, Calif.: Morning Glory Press, 1989.

Smith, Jerome, Ph.D., and Franklin I. Miroff. *You're Our Child: The Adoption Experience*. Lanham, Md.: Madison Books, 1987.

hotlines   Toll-free telephone numbers oriented to a particular group; for example, adoption agency hotlines are oriented to pregnant women considering adoption for their children, while hotlines for adoptive parents concentrate on placing special needs children.

Hotlines are sometimes staffed 24 hours per day, or they may be operated during office hours with an answering machine available to take urgent calls. Hotlines are also available to take abuse allegations, and social workers may be given a certain amount of time by state law to respond to an allegation of child abuse.

human immunodeficiency virus/acquired immunodeficiency syndrome   The human immunodeficiency virus (HIV) is a disease that is transmitted by blood or sexual contact with an infected individual. Most children with HIV contract the virus during childbirth or breast-feeding, although there are medications that HIV-infected women can take which will decrease the likelihood that their infants will contract the virus during pregnancy and childbirth. HIV infection may progress to the development of acquired immunodeficiency syndrome (AIDS), a disease for which there is no cure at present.

HIV/AIDS has a major impact on children worldwide. Globally, millions of children are orphaned by parents who have died of AIDS. The children may or may not be HIV-positive themselves. In the United States, children orphaned by mothers or other relatives who have died of AIDS are often placed in foster care. Even when the children are disease-free, it may be difficult to find adoptive families for them. Complicating the problem, many children orphaned by parents with AIDS are minority members, thus making it more difficult to find adoptive families for them.

Every year, infected children die of pediatric AIDS. In the United States, 5,406 children under the age of 13 years have died of AIDS through 2003, according to the Centers for Disease Control and Prevention (CDC). Among adolescents and adults, 500,395 have died of AIDS so far through 2003 in the United States.

Worldwide, according to the World Health Organization, 700,000 children were newly infected with HIV in 2003 alone, primarily through mother-to-child transmission during pregnancy or childbirth. Of these children, an estimated 90 percent lived in sub-Saharan Africa.

According to the World Health Organization in their 2004 guide to antiretroviral drugs, "AIDS is wiping out families, destroying communities and threatening the social, economic and political gains of recent decades."

However, with treatment, there is hope, especially for infants and children born to HIV-positive mothers. For example, there are many fewer cases of AIDS diagnosed in the United States. According to the CDC, in 1992 there were 952 children newly diagnosed with AIDS. This number began to fall in 1994 and continued to plummet until only 59 children were diagnosed with AIDS in 2003 in the United States.

Death rates from AIDS among children have also fallen in the United States. According to the CDC, in 1999, 97 children died of AIDS. By 2003, that number had fallen to 29.

In considering all children in the United States with HIV in 2003, there were 1,683 children under the age of 13 years with HIV infection (not AIDS) and 1,942 children with the disease (AIDS). (See table.)

Psychological Effect on Children

Children may not contract HIV themselves but they are still profoundly affected by it when their parents contract the virus or it develops further into AIDS. In a study by Pelton and Forehand in the *Journal of the American Academy of Child & Adolescent Psychiatry* in 2005, the researchers reported on their study of 105 African-American children from New Orleans and their HIV-infected mothers. The children and their mothers were followed for four years. During the course of the study, 35 of the mothers died, and their children were evaluated.

The researchers found a high level of borderline or clinical psychiatric problems in the children whose mothers had died (from 52 percent to 73 percent in different assessments). The researchers noted the importance of providing intervention to children before their mothers died, as well as after the deaths.

In a significant number of cases, problem behaviors emerged within two years after the death of the mothers. Some people might think that any serious behavioral problems would occur immediately after the death, and if they do not materialize then, they would not appear at all. Yet this was not the case. The researchers explained the delayed behavior problem in this manner:

"First, children may be traumatized in the first 6 months after the mother's death, and, as a consequence, problem behaviors do not emerge at a clinical level until later. Second, children are adjusting to new caregivers and residences in the first 6 months after maternal death and, as a consequence, may be less certain of the consequences of displaying externalizing and internalizing symptoms. As a result, these behaviors may be inhibited. Third, the new caregiver may not have sufficient information or may be hesitant to evaluate a

ESTIMATED NUMBERS OF CHILDREN YOUNGER THAN 13 YEARS LIVING WITH HIV INFECTION (NOT AIDS) OR WITH AIDS AT THE END OF 2003, BY STATE, UNITED STATES

State of Residence	Living with HIV Infection (Not AIDS)	Living with AIDS
Alabama	33	15
Alaska	0	2
Arizona	41	5
Arkansas	13	10
California	Unknown	138
Colorado	14	3
Connecticut	Unknown	30
Delaware	Unknown	12
District of Columbia	Unknown	63
Florida	253	361
Georgia	Unknown	60
Hawaii	Unknown	4
Idaho	1	0
Illinois	Unknown	80
Indiana	29	18
Iowa	4	3
Kansas	9	3
Kentucky	Unknown	10
Louisiana	98	43
Maine	Unknown	3
Maryland	Unknown	81
Massachusetts	Unknown	35
Michigan	Unknown	22
Minnesota	72	22
Mississippi	34	19
Missouri	39	14
Montana	Unknown	0
Nebraska	6	4
Nevada	15	6
New Hampshire	Unknown	3
New Jersey	294	119
New Mexico	0	4
New York	Unknown	349
North Carolina	86	25
North Dakota	1	1
Ohio	66	35
Oklahoma	18	4
Oregon	Unknown	6
Pennsylvania	Unknown	123
Rhode Island	Unknown	10
South Carolina	64	29
South Dakota	2	1

State of Residence	Living with HIV Infection (Not AIDS)	Living with AIDS
Tennessee	66	11
Texas	305	85
Utah	9	0
Vermont	Unknown	3
Virginia	60	53
Washington	Unknown	6
West Virginia	5	5
Wisconsin	19	11
Wyoming	1	1
Total	1,683	1,942

Source: Adapted from Centers for Disease Control and Prevention. *HIV/AIDS Surveillance Report,* 2003, page 15. Atlanta: U.S. Department of Health and Human Services, 2004.

child's behavior as problematic in the 6 months after the death of her or his mother."

Internationally Adopted Children and HIV

Children who enter the United States for adoption are not required to undergo HIV testing; however, such testing should be requested and performed on all children after arrival in the United States.

HIV is a particular problem in Africa, eastern Europe, and Central Asia. The prevalence of HIV is also especially high in Romania and Ukraine. In Central America, HIV prevalence is high in Guatemala.

Few children adopted from other countries are HIV-positive (possibly because the very sickest children die before they are adopted), although it is expected that this number will increase. Although children are usually tested in their birth countries prior to adoptive placement, the accuracy of these tests may be questionable, and children could conceivably be exposed after testing is completed.

Symptoms and Diagnostic Path

Children with HIV may have no symptoms in the early stages, although they may test positive for the virus. If children have symptoms, they may include the following:

- Opportunistic infections (infections which are unusual in those with normally functioning immune systems)

- Failure to thrive
- Developmental delays

Testing for HIV includes the use of the enzyme-linked immunosorbent assay (ELISA). However, infants who have a positive ELISA may be reflecting maternal antibodies, and consequently, they may not be infected with the virus. Thus, the test may need to be repeated later. There are also more sophisticated tests, such as DNA polymerase chain reaction tests, which may not be available or reliable in many countries.

Treatment Options and Outlook

HIV cannot be cured, but it can be controlled for years, and hopefully a cure will soon be developed for the children and adults who have contracted the virus. However, when AIDS was first identified, there were no treatments, and most people with the virus died quickly. Antiretroviral drugs were subsequently developed, such as zidovudine (ZDV) and later, lamivudine (3TC) and nevirapine (NVP).

According to the World Health Organization, in preventing the transmission of HIV/AIDS from mother to child, a combination of ZDV plus single-dose maternal and infant NVP works better than single drug regimens. If there is no medication intervention, from 15 to 30 percent of HIV-positive mothers will transmit the virus to their infants either during pregnancy or delivery.

Risk Factors and Preventive Measures

Some groups are at greater risk than others for contracting HIV and developing AIDS. For example, black children are disproportionately affected. About 16 percent of all children in the United States are black, but of all the children who have AIDS, 62 percent are black.

Other children at risk for being HIV positive include children whose parents are or were illegal drug users, especially intravenous drug use. If their parents were sex workers, the children are also at risk. Children who have been sexually abused are also at risk for HIV infection. Other children at risk are those who have been abandoned or are in state custody or foster care.

In the United States, patients in three states represented more than half (55 percent) of the 33,301 cases of infection, including Florida, New York, and Texas. In considering patients of all ages with AIDS, patients in California, Florida, and New York represented 38 percent of cases reported in 2003 to the CDC.

The survival rate was lowest among patients who were intravenous drug users and highest among children who acquired the infection from their mothers during pregnancy and childbirth.

See also FOSTER CARE; MEDICAL PROBLEMS OF INTERNATIONALLY ADOPTED CHILDREN; SEXUALLY TRANSMITTED DISEASES; SYPHILIS.

Centers for Disease Control and Prevention. *HIV/AIDS Surveillance Report,* 2003, p. 15. Atlanta, Ga.: U.S. Department of Health and Human Services, 2004.

Miller, Laurie, C., M.D. *The Handbook of International Adoption Medicine: A Guide for Physicians, Parents, and Providers.* New York: Oxford University Press, 2005.

Pelton, Jennifer, and Rex Forehand. "Orphans of the AIDS Epidemic: An Examination of Clinical Level Problems of Children," *Journal of the American Academy of Child & Adolescent Psychiatry* 44, no. 6 (June 2005): 585–591.

World Health Organization. *Antiretroviral Drugs for Treating Pregnant Women and Preventing HIV Infection in Infants: Guidelines on Care, Treatment and Support for Women Living with HIV/AIDS and Their Children in Resource-Constrained Settings.* Geneva, Switzerland: World Health Organization, 2004.

identity Developing a clear sense of one's individuality, including one's distinct personality, talents, abilities, and flaws, is difficult for the average person. Many people seriously question their values, beliefs, and identity during adolescence.

For 25 years, researchers Janet Hoopes and Leslie Stein studied families that had adopted young children. The authors in their 1985 report concluded: "Evidence suggesting that the adoptee has greater or more sustained difficulty with the tasks of adolescence was not found, indicating that adoptive status in and of itself, is not predictive of heightened stress among adolescents . . . as a group, the adolescent adoptees were doing quite well."

This finding was backed up by a large study of adopted adolescents done by the Search Institute. In this four-year study of 881 adopted adolescents, released in 1994, researchers found that the majority of adolescents were strongly attached to their adoptive parents and were emotionally healthy. In a few cases, the adopted adolescents scored higher than their nonadopted counterparts: for example, in "optimism" and the expectation that they would be happy in 10 years and "connectedness," or having three or more friends. They also placed a higher value on helping other people.

Most children with SPECIAL NEEDS who were adopted were separated from their parents because of abuse, neglect, or abandonment and may have internalized a negative sense of self. In addition, as foster children, they have experienced at least one foster home and probably several more.

Each move requires an adjustment to a new family, new school, and different values and requirements. The child may never have realized what his or her innate talents and strengths are, and consequently the adopting parents' task is to

help the child identify his or her best points and build self-esteem and self-knowledge.

The parent of the same sex as the child serves as a role model. Single parents who parent an opposite-sex child need to find appropriate role models among their families or friends. The child may also identify with a much loved teacher, neighbor, or other person in his or her life.

In a study of 49 adopted and 49 nonadopted college students, reported in 1998, researcher Margaret Kelly found that "adjustment and identity formation" were very similar, and she said, "the results of this study support a generally encouraging view of adoptees who are at the point of being launched from their adoptive families and seeking to establish their autonomy as adults. On all measures of developmental tasks, the adoptees' functioning was indistinguishable from that of the nonadopted controls. In addition, on most discrete aspects of identity formation . . . adoptees were comparable to nonadoptees."

She did find that on two scales of identity measures, moral self-approval and self-control, many of the adopted young adults judged themselves more harshly than the nonadopted adults. The exceptions to this finding were the adopted individuals from very organized and structured, yet open and expressive, families. These young people had more positive self-perceptions than the other adopted adults in the sample. They found that adopted adults whose parents had taken the lead in decision making had higher levels of self-approval and self-control. The speculation was that some adoptive parents tend to be child-dominated rather than adult-led, which could be problematic for some adopted children and adults. However, the overall findings were very positive.

Of course, studies that concentrate on children adopted as infants by two-parent married couples working through licensed agencies, as the Search Institute's was, may have different findings from studies that concentrate on children who were adopted under different circumstances; for example, older children with special needs. However, in any case, it is a good idea to compare the adopted children with similar children who have remained in the biological family. In that case, the adopted children nearly always have higher levels of functioning than their nonadopted peers.

See also TRANSRACIAL ADOPTION.

Benson, Peter L., Anu R. Sharma, and Eugene C. Roehikepartain. *Growing up Adopted: A Portrait of Adolescents and Their Families.* Minneapolis, Minn.: The Search Institute, 1994.

Kelly, Mary Margaret, et al. "Adjustment and Identity Formation in Adopted and Nonadopted Young Adults: Contributions of Family Environment," *American Journal of Orthopsychiatry* 68, no. 3 (July 1998): 497–500.

Stein, Leslie M., and Janet L. Hoopes. *Identity Formation in the Adopted Adolescent: The Delaware Family Study.* Washington, D.C.: Child Welfare League of America, 1985.

illegitimacy The legal status of a child born to unwed parents, now more properly described as "out of wedlock" or "nonmarital."

In the United States, illegitimacy, or "bastardy," was formerly a great stigma on a person, and people born out of wedlock were presumed to be "bad." Until recent years, BIRTH CERTIFICATES of those born out of wedlock were often a different color from those born legitimately and were separated and locked in special vaults.

With the increase in the divorce rate and the resulting trend toward acceptability of single parenthood, the negative connotations associated with out-of-wedlock births have radically declined; however, there are still many people who harbor negative views toward persons born out of wedlock.

There are cases today, even in our "enlightened" age, of parents casting out their unmarried daughters who are pregnant. Although out-of-wedlock births are far more common today than 10 or 20 years ago, pregnant girls are sometimes tainted with the image of being "fast" or "cheap," and their child (or children) is also looked down upon.

immigration and naturalization In adoption, refers to the entry of children from other countries for the purpose of being adopted by U.S. citizens. Also refers to citizens of other countries (immigration) and their subsequent acquisition of citizenship (naturalization). Citizenship for children adopted from other countries by Americans was expedited by the passage of the CHILD CITIZENSHIP ACT OF 2000, which took effect in 2001. This law automatically confers U.S. citizenship on children adopted from other countries and was an amendment of Section 320 of the United States Immigration and Nationality Act. Thus, internationally adopted children no longer need to be naturalized.

See also CHINA, ADOPTIONS FROM; GUATEMALA, ADOPTIONS FROM; INDIA, ADOPTIONS FROM; INTERNATIONAL ADOPTION; LATIN AMERICAN ADOPTIONS; SOUTH KOREA, ADOPTIONS FROM.

immunizations Vaccines that are given to prevent infectious diseases in a child or adult. Immunizations protect infants and children from crippling diseases such as polio and potentially fatal illnesses such as tetanus, pneumonia, and diphtheria. Children adopted from the United States and from other countries should receive all recommended childhood immunizations. Individuals who adopt foster children should obtain a copy of their immunization record. Adoptive parents should not assume that foster children have received all the immunizations that they should have received by their current age.

Most public and private schools in the United States require proof of immunizations before a child may enter the school. There are state and federal laws about which immunizations must be received before school entry.

Parents should consult with their physicians if their children have known immune deficiencies or allergies to eggs, since some vaccines contain egg proteins.

Parental Fears about Immunizations

In recent years, some parents, including adoptive parents, have expressed concern that childhood immunizations, particularly the measles, mumps, and rubella (MMR) vaccine, may cause serious psychiatric illnesses such as autism. This unfounded fear is at least partially responsible for the under-treatment of children in the United States because parents have delayed or in some cases refused to obtain immunizations for their children.

Yet these parental fears are largely founded. For example, in 1993, the MMR injection was replaced with single vaccines in Japan. British and Japanese scientists studied the incidence of autism spectrum disorders before and after the change in the vaccines, and their findings were reported in *New Scientist* in 2005. The researchers noted that before 1993, an estimated 48 to 86 children per 10,000 in Japan were diagnosed with autism. Subsequent to the withdrawal of the MMR vaccine, the rate of autism *increased* to 97 to 161 per 10,000 children who were diagnosed with autism. They attributed the increase to possible unknown environmental factors, while other experts believe that changing diagnostic criteria were primarily responsible for the increase. The point, however, which was also confirmed in many other papers, is the belief that the MMR vaccine had somehow caused autism was now debunked.

In a study reported in the *Journal of the American Medical Association* in 2005, only 18 percent of children in the United States received their vaccines at the recommended times and more than one in three children were undervaccinated for six months or more in the first two years of life. As a result, many children were at risk for diseases as well as at risk for spreading diseases that they contracted to other children and adults.

Childhood Immunizations in the United States

If children are born in the United States, the Centers for Disease Control and Prevention recommends that they be immunized against hepatitis B, diphtheria, tetanus, and pertussis (DPT is included in one injection), *Haemophilus influenzae* type b, polio, measles, mumps, and rubella (MMR is given as one injection), chicken pox, and pneumococcal disease. New polyvalent vaccines reduce the number of required shots. (See Table I.) If children do not receive injections on time, an alternative schedule is recommended based on their ages, as shown in Tables II and III.

Older children (ages seven through 18) need fewer injections and generally need not be immunized against pneumonia or *Haemophilus influenzae*.

Children Adopted from Other Countries

Children adopted from other countries often have had at least some immunizations, but in some cases these immunizations may need to be repeated. In some cases, such as children adopted from China, Russia, and other eastern European countries, studies have shown that many children have not received sufficient immunizations, particularly with regard to diphtheria-tetanus-pertussis (DTP). Some children have not been immunized against polio, which is still a necessary step despite the stunning advances against this crippling disease since Dr. Jonas Salk created a vaccine against polio more than 50 years ago.

It may be hard to obtain the child's medical and immunization records or they may be difficult to read. The records must usually be translated from another language. (See Table IV for common terms in the foreign language characters.)

In some cases, records may have been falsified. More commonly, vaccines are administered but may not successfully induce immunity. Malnutrition, serious illness, or other factors in the child may reduce immunity, while problems with the production and/or storage of the vaccine may reduce its effectiveness. In general, the immunization records of children adopted from South Korea are generally thought to be reliable; information about the accuracy of immunization records for children from other countries is incomplete.

Some immunizations may need to be repeated. However, blood testing can usually reveal the child's level of vaccine-induced antibodies. When present in adequate amounts, these antibodies indicate that additional injections are usually unnecessary. Particularly with young children (less than 15 months of age), however, restarting vaccines may be preferable, as the presence of maternal antibodies in the child's blood may confuse interpretation of the test results.

Pediatricians should refer to *The American Academy of Pediatrics Report of the Committee on Infectious Diseases* (colloquially known as the "Red Book") to determine the most current information on which immunizations and other tests are needed when the child is adopted and subsequent to the adoption. An overview of recommendations for internationally adopted children is also available at the

RECOMMENDED CHILDHOOD AND ADOLESCENT IMMUNIZATION SCHEDULE, UNITED STATES, 2006

Vaccine ▼ / Age ▶	Birth	1 month	2 months	4 months	6 months	12 months	15 months	18 months	24 months	4–6 years	11–12 years	13–14 years	15 years	16–18 years
Hepatitis B[1]	HepB	HepB	HepB	HepB[1]		HepB					HepB Series			
Diphtheria, Tetanus, Pertussis[2]			DTaP	DTaP	DTaP			DTaP		DTaP	Tdap		Tdap	
Haemophilus influenzae type b[3]			Hib	Hib	Hib[3]	Hib								
Inactivated Poliovirus			IPV	IPV		IPV				IPV				
Measles, Mumps, Rubella[4]						MMR				MMR	MMR			
Varicella[5]							Varicella				Varicella			
Menningococcal[6]									MPSV4		MCV4		MCV4	
													MCV4	
Pneumococcal[7]			PCV	PCV	PCV	PCV	PCV		PCV	PCV				
											PPV			
Influenza[8]						Influenza (Yearly)					Influenza (Yearly)			
Hepatitis A[9]									HepA Series					

Vaccines within broken line are for selected populations

This schedule indicates the recommended ages for routine administration of currently licensed childhood vaccines, as of December 1, 2005, for children through age 18 years. Any dose not administered at the recommended age should be administered at any subsequent visit when indicated and feasible.

Indicates age groups that warrant special effort to administer those vaccines not previously administered. Additional vaccines may be licensed and recommended during the year. Licensed combination vaccines may be used whenever any components of the combination are indicated and other components of the vaccine are not contraindicated

and if approved by the Food and Drug Administration for that dose of the series. Providers should consult the respective ACIP statement for detailed recommendations. Clinically significant adverse events that follow immunization should be reported to the Vaccine Adverse Event Reporting System (VAERS). Guidance about how to obtain and complete a VAERS form is available at www.vaers.hhs.gov or by telephone, 800-822-7967.

Legend:
- Range of recommended ages
- Catch-up immunization
- 11–12-year-old assessment

FOOTNOTES, RECOMMENDED CHILDHOOD AND ADOLESCENT IMMUNIZATION SCHEDULE, UNITED STATES, 2006

1. Hepatitis B vaccine (HepB). AT BIRTH

All newborns should receive monovalent HepB soon after birth and before hospital discharge. **Infants born to mothers who are HBsAg-positive** sould receive HepB and 0.5 mL of hepatitis B immune globulin (HBIG) within 12 hours of birth. The mother should have blood drawn as soon as possible to determine her HBsAg status; if HBsAg-positive, the infant should receive HBIG as soon as possible (no later than age one week). **For infants born to HBsAg-negative mothers,** the birth dose can be delayed in rare circumstances but only if a physician's order to withhold the vaccine and a copy of the mother's original HBsAg-negative laboratory report are documented in the infant's medical record. *FOLLOWING THE BIRTH DOSE:* The HepB series should be completed with either monovalent HepB or a combination vaccine containing HepB. The second dose should be administered at age 1–2 months. The final dose should be administered at age ≥ 24 weeks. It is permissible to administer four doses of HepB (e.g., when combination vaccines are given after the birth dose); however, if monovalent HepB is used, a dose at age four months is not needed. **Infants born to HBsAg-positive mothers** should be tested for HBsAg and antibody to HBsAg after completion of the HepB series, at age 9–18 months (generally at the next well-child visit after completion of the vaccine series).

Infants born to HBsAg-positive mothers should receive HepB and 0.5 mL of hepatitis B immune globulin (HBIG) at separate sites within 12 hours of birth. The second dose is recommended at age 1–2 months. The final dose in the immunization series should not be administered before age 24 weeks. These infants should be tested for HBsAg and antibody to HBsAg (anti-HBs) at age 9–15 months.

Infants born to mothers whose HBsAg status is unknown should receive the first dose of the HepB series within 12 hours of birth. Maternal blood should be drawn as soon as possible to determine the mother's HBsAg status; if the HBsAg test is positive, the infant should receive HBIG as soon as possible (no later than age one week). The second dose is recommended at age 1–2 months. The last dose in the immunization series should not be administered before age 24 weeks.

2. Diphtheria and tetanus toxoids and acellular pertussis (DTaP) vaccine.

The fourth dose of DTaP may be administered as early as age 12 months, provided six months have elapsed since the third dose and the child is unlikely to return at age 15–18 months. The final dose in the series should be given at age four years.

Tetanus and diphtheria toxoids and acellular pertussis vaccine (Tdap: adolescent preparation) is recommended at age 11–12 years for those who have completed the recommended childhood DTP/DTaP vaccination series and have not received a Td booster dose. Adolescents 13–18 years who missed the 11–12-year Td/Tdap booster dose should also receive a single dose of Tdap if they have completed the recommended childhood DTP/DTaP vaccination series. Subsequent **tetanus and diphtheria toxoids (Td)** are recommended every 10 years.

3. *Haemophilus influenzae* type b (Hib) conjugate vaccine.

Three Hib conjugate vaccines are licensed for infant use. If PRP-OMP (PedvaxHIB® or ComVax® [Merck]) is administered at ages two and four months, a dose at age six months is not required. DTaP/Hib combination products should not be used for primary immunization in infants at ages two, four, or six months but can be used as boosters after any Hib vaccine. The final dose in the series should be administered at age ≥ 12 months.

4. Measles, mumps, and rubella vaccine (MMR).

The second dose of MMR is recommended routinely at age 4–6 years but

may be administered during any visit, provided at least four weeks have elapsed since the first dose and both doses are administered beginning at or after age 12 months. Those who have not previously received the second dose should complete the schedule by age 11–12 years.

5. Varicella vaccine.

Varicella vaccine is recommended at any visit at or after age 12 months for susceptible children (i.e., those who lack a reliable history of chicken pox). Susceptible persons ≥ 13 years should receive two doses administered at least four weeks apart.

6. Meningococcal vaccine (MCV4).

Meningococcal conjugate vaccine (MCV4) should be given to all children at the 11–12-year-old visit as well as to unvaccinated adolescents at high school entry (15 years of age). Other adolescents who wish to decrease their risk for meningococcal disease may also be vaccinated. All college freshmen living in dormitories should also be vaccinated, preferably with MCV4, although **meningococcal polysaccharide vaccine (MPSV4)** is an acceptable alternative. Vaccination against invasive meningococcal disease is recommended for children and adolescents aged ≥ 2 years with terminal complement deficiencies or anatomic or functional asplenia and certain other high-risk groups (see *MMWR* 2005; 54[RR-7]:1–21); use MPSV4 for children aged 2–10 years and MCV4 for older children, although MPSV4 is an acceptable alternative.

7. Pneumococcal vaccine.

The heptavalent **pneumococcal conjugate vaccine (PCV)** is recommended for all children aged 2–23 months and for certain children aged 24–59 months. The final dose in the series should be given at age ≥ 12 months. **Pneumococcal polysaccharide vaccine (PPV)** is recommended in addition to PCV for certain high-risk groups. See *MMWR* 2000; 49(RR-9):1–35.

8. Influenza vaccine.

Influenza vaccine is recommended annually for children aged ≥ 6 months with certain risk factors (including, but not limited to, asthma, cardiac disease, sickle cell disease, human immunodeficiency virus [HIV], diabetes, and conditions that can compromise respiratory function or handling of respiratory secretions or that can increase the risk for aspiration), health-care workers, and other persons (including household members) in close contact with persons in groups at high risk (see *MMWR* 2005; 54[RR-7]:1–21). In addition, healthy children aged 6–23 months and close contacts of healthy children aged 0–23 months are recommended to receive influenza vaccine because children in this age group are at substantially increased risk for influenza-related hospitalizations. For healthy persons aged 5–49 years, the intranasally administered, live, attenuated influenza vaccine (LAIV) is an acceptable alternative to the intramuscular trivalent inactivated influenza vaccine (TIV). See *MMWR* 2005; 54(RR-8):1–55. Children receiving TIV should be administered a dosage appropriate for their age (0.25 mL if aged 6–35 months or 0.5 mL if aged ≥ 3 years). Children aged ≤ 8 years who are receiving influenza vaccine for the first time should receive two doses (separated by at least four weeks for TIV and at least six weeks for LAIV).

9. Hepatitis A vaccine (HepA).

HepA is recommended for all children at one year of age (i.e., 12–23 months). The two doses in the series should be administered at least six months apart. States, counties, and communities with existing HepA vaccination programs for children 2–18 years of age are encouraged to maintain these programs. In these areas, new efforts focused on routine vaccination of one-year-old children should enhance, not replace, ongoing programs directed at a broader population of children. HepA is also recommended for certain high-risk groups (see *MMWR* 1999; 48[RR-12]:1–37).

CATCH-UP SCHEDULE FOR CHILDREN AGED FOUR MONTHS THROUGH SIX YEARS

Vaccine	Minimum Age for Dose 1	Minimum Interval between Doses			
		Dose 1 to Dose 2	Dose 2 to Dose 3	Dose 3 to Dose 4	Dose 4 to Dose 5
Diphtheria, Tetanus, Pertussis	6 weeks	4 weeks	4 weeks	6 months	6 months[1]
Inactivated Poliovirus	6 weeks	4 weeks	4 weeks	4 weeks[2]	
Hepatitis B[3]	Birth	4 weeks	8 weeks (and 16 weeks after first dose)		
Measles, Mumps, Rubella	12 months	4 weeks[4]			
Varicella	12 months				
Haemophilus influenzae type b[5]	6 weeks	4 weeks if first dose given at age < 12 months 8 weeks (as final dose) if first dose given at age 12–14 months No further doses needed if first dose given at age ≥ 15 months	4 weeks[6] if current age < 12 months 8 weeks (as final dose)[6] if current age ≥ 12 months and second dose given at age < 15 months No further doses needed if previous dose given at age ≥ 15 months	8 weeks (as final dose) This dose only necessary for children aged 12 months–5 years who received three doses before age 12 months	
Pneumococcal Conjugate[7]	6 weeks	4 weeks if first dose given at age < 12 mos. and current age < 24 mos. 8 weeks (as final dose) if first dose given at age ≥ 12 mos. or current age 24–59 mos. No further doses needed for healthy children if first dose given at age ≥ 24 months	4 weeks if current age < 12 months 8 weeks (as final dose) if current age ≥ 12 months No further doses needed for healthy children if previous dose given at age ≥ 24 months	8 weeks (as final dose) This dose only necessary for children aged 12 months–5 years who received three doses before age 12 months	

CATCH-UP SCHEDULE FOR CHILDREN AGED SEVEN YEARS THROUGH 18 YEARS

Vaccine	Minimum Interval between Doses		
	Dose 1 to Dose 2	Dose 2 to Dose 3	Dose 3 to Booster Dose
Tetanus, Diphtheria[8]	4 weeks	6 months	6 months if first dose given at age < 12 months and current age < 11 years 5 years if third dose given at age ≥ 7 years
Inactivated Poliovirus[9]	4 weeks	4 weeks	IPV [2,9]
Hepatitis B	4 weeks	8 weeks (and 16 weeks after first dose)	
Measles, Mumps, Rubella	4 weeks		
Varicella[10]	4 weeks		

1. **DTaP**
   The fifth dose is not necessary if the fourth dose was administered after the fourth birthday.
2. **IPV**
   For children who received an all-IPV or all-oral poliovirus (OPV) series, a fourth dose is not necessary if third dose was administered at age ≥ 4 years. If both OPV and IPV were administered as part of a series, a total of four doses should be given, regardless of the child's current age.
3. **HepB**
   Administer the three-dose series to all children and adolescents < 19 years of age if they were not previously vaccinated.
4. **MMR**
   The second dose of MMR is recommended routinely at age 4–6 years but may be administered earlier if desired.
5. **Hib**
   Vaccine is not generally recommended for children aged ≥ 5 years.
6. **Hib**
   If current age < 12 months and the first two doses were PRP-OMP (PedvaxHIB® or ComVax® [Merck]), the third (and final) dose should be administered at age 12–15 months and at least eight weeks after the second dose.
7. **PCV**
   Vaccine is not generally recommended for children aged ≥ 5 years.
8. **Td**
   Adolescent tetanus, diphtheria, and pertussis vaccine (Tdap) may be substituted for any dose in a primary catch-up series or as a booster if age appropriate for Tdap. A five-year interval from the last Td dose is encouraged when Tdap is used as a booster dose. See ACIP recommendations for further information.
9. **IV**
   Vaccine is not generally recommended for children aged ≥ 18 years.
10. **Varicella**
    Administer the two-dose series to all susceptible adolescents aged ≥ 13 years.

VACCINE TERMINOLOGY IN RUSSIAN, CHINESE, ROMANIAN, AND SPANISH

Language	Diphtheria, Pertussis, Tetanus	Polio	Measles, Mumps, Rubella	Hepatitis B	Other
Russian	Дифтерия Коклюш Столбняк ,АКДС	Полиомиелит	Корь Эпидемический паротит Краснуха	Гепатит Б	Ветряная оспа = Varicella
Chinese	白喉 百日咳 破傷風	小兒麻痹	麻疹 腮腺炎 德國麻疹	乙型肝炎	日本乙型腦炎 "Encephalitis" or "cerebrospinal meningitis" usually refers to Japanese encephalitis but occasionally refers to meningococcal vaccine
Romanian	Tetracoq	AP (although occasionally this refers to antiparotitis)	AR (anti-rubeola)	AH	
Spanish	Difteria Tos ferina Tetanós	Polio	Sarampión Parótidas Rubeóla	Hepatitis B	"Meningitis" usually indicates *H. influenzae B* (HIB)

From the *Handbook of International Adoption Medicine* by Laurie Miller, copyright Oxford University Press. Used by permission of Oxford University Press, Inc.

Web site http://www2.ncid.cdc.gov/travel/yb/utils/ybGet.asp?section=children&obj=adoption.htm&cssNav=browseoyb.

See also HEPATITIS; MEDICAL PROBLEMS OF INTERNATIONALLY ADOPTED CHILDREN; SYPHILIS; TUBERCULOSIS.

Centers for Disease Control and Prevention. "Recommended Childhood and Adolescent Immunization Schedule, United States, 2005," Department of Health and Human Services. Available online. URL: http://www.cdc.gov/nip/recs/child-schedule-bw.pdf, downloaded on April 15, 2005.

Coghan, Andy. "Autism Rises Despite MMR Ban in Japan," *New Scientist.* Available online. URL: http://www.newscientist.com/article.ns?id=dn7076, downloaded on April 15, 2005.

Luman, Elizabeth T., et al. "Timeliness of Childhood Vaccinations in the United States: Days Undervaccinated and Number of Vaccines Delayed, *Journal of the American Medical Association* 93, no. 10 (March 9, 2005): 1,204–1,211.

Miller, Laurie C., M.D. *The Handbook of International Adoption Medicine: A Guide for Physicians, Parents, and Providers.* New York: Oxford University Press, 2005.

———. "International Adoption: Infectious Diseases Issues," *Clinical Infectious Diseases* 40 (January 2005): 286–293.

incest   See SEXUAL ABUSE.

income tax law benefits for adoptive parents

Credits or exclusions to income taxes that are given to individuals when they adopt children. The federal government offers such a benefit, as do some states with state income taxes. Stepparent adoptions and surrogate parent arrangements are not considered qualifying adoption expenses for federal income tax benefits. The child must be younger than 18 years old. The tax credit is per child. Parents use IRS Form 8839 with either Form 1040 or Form 1040A to file for the federal adoption tax credit and exclusion.

The current federal adoption expense tax credit was enacted in 2001 and made the adoption tax credit permanent, which was a modification of the earlier Adoption and Promotion Stability Act in 1996.

The newer law doubled the tax benefit to over $10,000 (a maximum of $10,390 for 2004) from the former $5,000 allowed for fees spent. In addition, the current law allows for an automatic tax credit for the full amount when children with SPECIAL NEEDS from the U.S. foster care system are adopted, regardless of the amount actually spent by the adoptive parents and even if *no money* was expended by the adoptive parents. Thus, if parents adopt two siblings with special needs from foster care, they are entitled to a tax credit of over $20,000.

If children do *not* have special needs, however, then the adoption expenses must be documented, and they are limited to actual expenditures. Thus, if an adoption costs less than $10,000, then the adoption credit will be equal to that lesser amount. Children adopted from other countries may not qualify for the special needs credit, even if they have disabilities. However, families are entitled to the tax credit when they adopt children from other countries and document their expenses.

The law also allows for exclusion from income taxes of adoption benefits provided by the parent's employer. (These benefits are not taxable.) If the adoptive parent's employer provides reimbursement for adoption expenses, this reimbursement is also excluded from income taxes up to the maximum allowed for the tax credit, or $10,390 for income earned in 2004.

There are some liberal limitations on the tax credit and exclusion. For 2004, the family's adjusted gross income must be less than $195,860 to qualify for the benefit. Families whose adjusted gross income is $155,861 to $195,859 are eligible for reduced tax credit or exclusion. Families whose adjusted gross income is $155,860 or less are eligible for the full tax credit and exclusion.

For further information on the federal income tax credit for adoption and employee exclusions for adoption reimbursements, families should contact the Internal Revenue Service and ask for Publication 968, "Tax Benefits for Adoption," to find the most recent information on adoption tax credits and exclusions, or call the IRS at (800) 829-3676. They may also go to the IRS Internet Web site at http://www.irs.gov.

For information on state income tax credits for adoption, families should contact their state organization that oversees state income taxes. In addition, adoption agencies within the state should also be familiar with state adoption tax credits.

Internal Revenue Service. "Tax Benefits for Adoption," Publication 968, U.S. Department of Treasury, 2005.

independent adoption Nonagency adoption, usually handled through adoption attorneys but sometimes by physicians or other intermediaries. Independent adoption is sometimes referred to as private adoption.

Most independent adoptions are nonrelative adoptions. (In general, relative adoptions are referred to as kinship adoptions.) At least half of all infant adoptions of healthy infants born in the United States are adopted through independent adoptions. Many of these adoptions are OPEN ADOPTIONS, in which the birthparents and adoptive parents are known to each other. People who adopt independently usually adopt babies, while those who wish to adopt older children usually contact the state public agency or a private, nonprofit agency for assistance. Very occasionally, people adopt toddlers through attorneys when mothers voluntarily place them.

In international adoption, it is increasingly difficult to adopt a child through attorneys or other intermediaries, and consequently, nearly all adoptions are managed by adoption agencies. With the full implementation of the HAGUE CONVENTION ON INTERCOUNTRY ADOPTION, which should take place by 2007 in the United States, accredited adoption agencies will manage all international adoptions by citizens of the United States and other member countries.

Nonagency adoptions are sometimes called *gray market* adoptions, a term which connotes unsavory, unethical, or questionable practices; however, this is an unfair term since independent adoptions are lawful in nearly all states. In addition, many ethical attorneys handle independent adoptions, although prospective adoptive parents should always ask for information about the attorney's experience and check that no complaints have been filed about his or her adoption practices with the state bar association.

The American Academy of Adoption Attorneys, an organization of experienced adoption attorneys throughout the United States, which is based in Washington, D.C., offers a listing of adoption attorneys in each state at their Web site: http://www.adoptionattorneys.org/member_directory.htm.

Several studies of the outcome of independent adoptions have been performed over many decades. In 1963, the findings of a study of 484 children placed with 477 families in Florida were reported by Helen L. Witmer, Elizabeth Herzog, Eugene A. Weinstein, and Mary E. Sullivan in their hook *Independent Adoptions.* About two-thirds of the adoptions were rated "excellent" to "fair," while one-third were rated "poor."

A study by William Meezan, S. Katz, and E. Manoff-Russo published by the Child Welfare League in 1978 found most independent adoptions had a good outcome; however, concern was expressed about the lack of background information provided to the birthmother. In addition, some adoptive parents reported extremely high amounts paid to adopt the child.

State Laws Governing Independent Adoption

Independent adoption is legal in most states but not in Connecticut, Delaware, Massachusetts, and North Dakota. It is important to note, however, that birthparents may choose nonrelative adoptive parents for their children in all states and plan an adoption. Presuming that the laws of the states have been followed, which usually includes a HOME STUDY of the prospective adoptive parents, the adoptive parents selected by the birthparents will be approved by the court. Some states require a preliminary home study prior to the placement of a child in an independent adoption.

State laws vary considerably with regard to adoption practices, and even neighboring states may have very different adoption laws.

Supporters and Dissenters of Independent Adoptions

Many adoption agency social workers disdain independent adoption, just as some individuals who manage independent adoptions may believe that agency adoptions are inferior. Many social workers see independent adoption as a form of competition, a method to "beat the system," and an approach that often avoids important aspects of sound adoption practice, such as mandatory counseling for the birthmother. Concerns about independent adoption are part of the reason some social work organizations have called for an end to independent adoptions.

Conversely, those who support independent adoption may view agencies as antiquated, judgmental bureaucracies and may perceive agency social workers as intrusive, cold busybodies who ask far too many irrelevant or personal questions. Worse, some agencies and social workers are seen as "anti-adoption."

Note, however, that increasing numbers of adoption agencies are encouraging prospective adoptive parents to locate pregnant women interested in adoption on their own. In addition, many states require individuals who are adopting independently to have an adoption agency perform a home study, and many adoption attorneys offer the opportunity for counseling services to birthparents. Thus, the lines between independent adoption and agency adoption are far more blurred than in past years.

Reasons for the Choice

The primary reason people choose independent adoption over agency adoption is that they believe that independent adoption offers them more of a sense of control. For instance, they can actively try to find a pregnant woman themselves, instead of waiting for an agency to call them to notify them of a pregnant woman who may be interested in placing her child with them or to notify them when a child has already been born.

Individuals who choose to adopt independently may fit most adoption agencies' criteria for their own applicants: under age 45, married for at least three years, infertile, and other criteria that adoption agencies may apply. On the other hand, independent adopters may be older than 45, already have several children, and be married for a short period.

Pregnant women choose independent adoption over agency adoption for several major reasons. Many women do not have private health insurance, and they prefer the opportunity to receive private medical care rather than needing to use services provided through Medicaid and/or the state health department. Most state laws allow adoptive parents to pay for the prenatal care and the delivery of the baby. If state law allows it, the pregnant women may also receive support money (including wage replacement) from the adoptive parents through the attorney or intermediary. Many agencies cannot afford such support money or they refuse, on principle, to provide such money to the pregnant woman.

Risks of Independent Adoption

Just as independent adoption has its advantages, so does it also have its risks, including major financial and emotional disadvantages. The key risk to the adopting parents is that if the woman changes her mind before or shortly after the baby is born and before signing any formal consent papers, she has the right to parent the child. How much time the birthmother has to change her mind varies from state to state, but in many states it is two or three days subsequent to the child's birth.

Most birthmothers who change their minds about an adoption do so just before or immediately after the birth and before signing consent to the adoption. Few seek a return of the child after the placement with the adoptive family, although the risk may be somewhat higher with independent adoptions than with agency adoptions.

In one survey of 143 adoption agencies nationwide that were asked if an adoption had fallen through because of a birthparent challenge after placement, reported in *The Adoption Option Complete Handbook 2000–2001*, 81 percent of the agencies reported no such problem, while 8 percent said they had one such incident, 4 percent had two or more incidents, and 7 percent had three or more incidents. However, the author had assumed that most agencies would provide 1998 data, and some agencies reported the percentage of *ever* having such an incident; for example, one agency reported experiencing five cases out of 500 in their entire experience, while one agency said that over the course of 10 years, they had experienced four such incidents among 940 placements. Clearly, the incidence of birthparents challenging adoptions after placement with a family is less common among agencies than is popularly perceived, although further research is needed to confirm or refute this finding.

Among the 64 adoption attorneys nationwide who responded to the question of whether a birth-parent challenge had caused an adoptive family to lose a child, the majority (57 percent) said this had not occurred, while 13 percent said they had experienced one such case, and 14 percent reported two incidents.

Another key risk in independent adoption is that the financial risks to the prospective family can be high if the birthmother decides to parent her child. Any money that the prospective adoptive family may have paid will probably be lost, because most pregnant women considering adoption for their children are indigent and cannot repay money expended for medical care, food, and other necessities. In addition, most state laws preclude legal recovery of the money already spent. In past years, adoption insurance was offered to some adoptive families to mitigate their financial risk, but this option is no longer available.

Although the financial risk may be troubling, most adoptive parents agree that the emotional trauma of a birthmother changing her mind is far worse than the money they have lost, and, of course, the euphoric adoptive parents who succeed consider the emotional roller coaster well worth the ride.

In contrast, adoption agencies may not inform a prospective couple about a child until all the consent papers have been signed. Then they call and give the couple days to arrange to pick up their child. As a result, the couple avoids the stress-filled months of anxiety; conversely, they are also deprived of months of active fantasizing before the child's arrival. However, if the adoption is to be an open adoption, then the parents have met the birthmother before the baby's birth, and they too risk the emotional trauma of a potential change of heart by the birthmother.

Intermediaries

Pregnant women find intermediaries through the INTERNET, Yellow Pages advertisements, classified ads, and networking with their friends (which is also the way some prospective adoptive parents find their attorneys.)

Some physicians serve as intermediaries. A woman's obstetrician is likely to know infertile couples or can easily identify several through his or her own contacts. Adoptive parents may also find a pregnant woman on their own through networking or advertising and then contact the attorney and ask him or her to facilitate the adoption.

However a pregnant woman who is interested in adoption is identified, it is extremely advisable to rely only on experienced and ethical attorneys beforehand and throughout the adoption process, even if the adoption appears very straightforward and simple.

Neither a pregnant women nor prospective parents should accept any pressure from an attorney nor other intermediary to accept a particular situation which feels uncomfortable. One example is adoptive parents who do not sound like the type of family the birthmother was looking for. Another example is if the adopting parents feel pressured to adopt the child of a woman with emotional problems that concern them. If either party begins to feel pressured, they should leave and contact another attorney or adoption agency.

Costs

The cost of an independent adoption varies greatly from state to state, depending on the individual case and the state laws. A very approximate average figure is about $25,000. If the birthmother must have a caesarean section and the adoptive parents are paying the medical bills, this will increase the costs by several thousand dollars.

Birthmothers and pregnant women should never pay attorneys to arrange an adoption, and any attorney who asks a pregnant woman for a fee should be avoided. Adoptive parents pay all legal fees.

Before giving an attorney thousands of dollars, prospective adoptive parents should understand exactly what the lawyer is promising, the time frame involved, what losses they could incur, and so forth. State laws on adoption are available at most large public libraries, and a reference librarian can direct readers to their exact location.

In many instances because of ethical considerations and American Bar Association guidelines the adopting parents will be represented by one attorney, and they will hire a different attorney to represent the birthmother.

Interstate Independent Adoptions

Many independent adoptions occur across state lines; for example, the birthmother may reside in one state, and the adoption parents may live in a neighboring (or faraway) state. It is important to understand that the provisions of the INTERSTATE COMPACT ON THE PLACEMENT OF CHILDREN must be followed. This is a sort of treaty between states that regulates interstate adoption, and each state has a compact administrator headquartered at the state public welfare office.

Generally, the laws of the "receiving" state, or the state where the child is placed, prevail; however, compact administrators strive to ensure that the laws of both states are obeyed. Adoptive parents should not remove a child from another state without the permission of the compact administrator because by doing so they risk having the adoption overturned. This has happened, although rarely.

Most independent adoptions are lawful and probably successful, and most attorneys engaged in managing independent adoptions appear to behave in an ethical manner.

Adamec, Christine. *The Adoption Option Complete Handbook 2000–2001.* New York: Prima Publishing, 1999.
———. *The Complete Idiot's Guide to Adoption.* New York: Alpha Books, 2005.
Meezan, William, S. Katz, and R. Manoff-Russo. *Adoptions without Agencies: A Study of Independent Adoptions.* New York: Child Welfare League of America, 1978.
Witmer, Helen L., et al. *Independent Adoptions: A Follow-up Study.* New York: Russell Sage Foundation, 1963.

India, adoptions from   One of the countries from which children are adopted by Americans as well as by people from other countries. In fiscal year 2005, 323 children were adopted from India by Americans, according to statistics provided by the U.S. State Department.

In general, adoptive parents who adopt children from India receive extensive information. According to Dr. Miller in *The Handbook of International Adoption Medicine,* "This may include information about the circumstances by which the child entered care, the child's physical condition, developmental information, intercurrent illnesses and hospitalizations, x-ray reports, laboratory tests, and, occasionally, ancillary information such as electroencephalograms (EEGs) or specialized scans. Results of testing for hepatitis B, HIV, and syphilis are usually included."

Many children are low birth weight, malnourished (before or after entry into care), and carrying INTESTINAL PARASITIC INFECTIONS. Most reside in orphanages prior to adoption; in general, they receive loving and attentive care and have access to good quality medical care. Girls adopted from India are the group of internationally adopted children most likely to develop EARLY PUBERTY.

See also INTERNATIONAL ADOPTION; MEDICAL PROBLEMS OF INTERNATIONALLY ADOPTED CHILDREN.

Miller, Laurie, C., M.D. *The Handbook of International Adoption Medicine: A Guide for Physicians, Parents, and Providers.* New York: Oxford University Press, 2005.

Indian Child Welfare Act of 1978   A law enacted by Congress in 1978 that mandates special provisions for Native American children and their placement into foster or adoptive homes. Under the act, an Indian child's tribe or the Bureau of Indian Affairs must be informed before the child is placed for adoption, and preference in placement must be given first to the child's tribe and last to another culture.

Supporters of the law say that, prior to its passage, as many as 25 percent of Native American children were placed into foster or adoptive homes because of such reasons as a lack of indoor plumbing in the biological parents' home, small houses, or other conditions of poverty or social problems.

They believe TRANSRACIAL ADOPTION is not a good policy and believe placing an Indian child with a non-Indian family ultimately causes confusion in the child's sense of identity.

The law requires agencies or anyone involved with placing an Indian child to first inform the tribe or the Bureau of Indian Affairs.

There have been several cases of parents (non-Indian and Indian) fighting in court to keep a particular Indian child they have adopted. The tribe has prevailed in some cases and overturned adoptions in several cases, including one in which the adoptive parents were of the child's tribe.

Hollinger, Joan Heifetz. "Beyond the Best Interests of the Tribe: The Indian Child Welfare Act and the Adoption of Indian Children," *University of Detroit Law Review* 66 (1989): 450–501.
Lenmann, Michelle L. "The Indian Child Welfare Act of 1989: Does It Apply to the Adoption of an Illegitimate Indian Child?" *Catholic University Law Review* 38 (1989): 511–541.

infant adoption   The adoption of newborns or babies or toddlers under the age of two years.

Most people who wish to adopt an infant are seeking a healthy newborn or a child who is at most only several months in age. It is not clear how many people are actively taking steps to adopt, but for a variety of reasons, including abortion, birth control, and the rise in single parenthood, it is clear there are insufficient numbers of adoptable infants to meet demand.

Infant adoption is a relatively new phenomenon in the United States, and prior to the late 1920s, few newborn infants were adopted. Children who were adopted were primarily older children who were homeless or had lost one or both parents or whose parents were financially or emotionally unable to care for them.

When infant formula became widely available in the late 1920s, this development made it possible for pregnant women to place their babies with adoptive couples shortly after the baby's birth. Prior to the perfection of infant formula, newborn babies were breast-fed and could not survive without mother's milk. (Wet nurses were sometimes used for infants whose mothers did not nurse them, but many babies died.)

Infants who need adoptive families are placed through ADOPTION AGENCIES, ATTORNEYS, or through other intermediaries, such as physicians or even friends of the birthmother, with the counsel of a state, county, or private social worker. In some states it is legal for an adoption facilitator or intermediary who is neither an attorney or a social worker to arrange adoptions for a fee.

Ironically, it is often easier to adopt a newborn infant than it is to adopt a child of one, two, or even three years of age in the United States. The reason for this is that an adoption decision regarding a newborn infant is usually made by the birthmother, and most birthmothers make this decision during their pregnancies or shortly thereafter. Few make a voluntary decision in favor of adoption when the child is two or three years old because they then have a relationship with the child.

As a result, small children and infants who are in state custody are usually there because of ABUSE, ABANDONMENT, or NEGLECT. They are placed in FOSTER CARE, often for at least a year, with the state agency seeking to solve the problem in the biological family that required the removal of the child.

If the problem cannot be solved, for example, if a birthmother cannot resolve a problem with drug or alcohol abuse that led to the reason why the child was placed in foster care, the state will ultimately go to court to terminate parental rights. In the past, many children in foster care were at least six or seven years old, and often much older, by the time the state terminated the rights of the parents. With the passage of the ADOPTION AND SAFE FAMILIES ACT, more children are adopted at an earlier age. However, children are usually at least several years old before the parental rights are severed. As a result, few healthy toddlers are free to be adopted in the United States.

The situation is not the same with INTERNATIONAL ADOPTION, and older infants and toddlers are available to be adopted through international adoption agencies. As a result, families who wish to adopt older babies or toddlers may opt to adopt internationally. Babies adopted from other countries are generally at least four months old because of the time lag between the birth of the child and the matching with a particular couple, who must then travel to the infant's country to follow foreign and American immigration requirements. However, rarely, some infants adopted from other countries may be only a few days old, especially if the adoption has been facilitated by an attorney in the child's homeland.

Health of Newborn Infants

Most U.S.-born adopted babies are healthy, although a substantial number of those placed for adoption are of low birth weight (less than 5.5 pounds), and many are premature. The birthmother may have received little or no prenatal care and may or may not have had adequate nutrition during her pregnancy. (See PRENATAL EXPOSURES.)

Many U.S. birthmothers also smoke, which can account in part for their low-birth-weight babies.

infectious diseases, serious Bacterial, viral, and other illnesses that can be transmitted to others through the air, blood, food, skin, or water, and which may cause severe health problems if not detected and treated. It is important to identify the illness in the early stage to increase the odds of recovery and decrease the risk of contagion. Some examples of serious infectious diseases include HEPATITIS; HUMAN IMMUNODEFICIENCY VIRUS (HIV); INTESTINAL PARASITIC INFECTIONS; SYPHILIS; TUBERCULOSIS; and other SEXUALLY TRANSMITTED DISEASES.

Children and adolescents at risk for developing serious infectious diseases include those who

- Are exposed to contaminated food and/or water
- Live in impoverished environments
- Reside in institutions such as ORPHANAGES or GROUP HOMES
- Live in poor countries outside North America and western Europe
- Are sexually active with multiple partners and engage in sexual acts without the use of a condom
- Are born to mothers with certain untreated infectious diseases
- Travel to countries where infectious diseases are common
- Are malnourished
- Have immunodeficiencies

Infectious diseases are diagnosed and treated by a medical doctor. The diagnosis is made based on the patient's signs (such as chronic cough or other overt indicators of disease) and symptoms (complaints that the patient has, such as fatigue or pain). Various laboratory tests are used to diagnose infections; for example, the Mantoux test is used to diagnose tuberculosis, while a stool sample is used to diagnose an intestinal parasitic infection. The treatment depends on the type of infection but usually includes some form of antimicrobial medication.

See also HELICOBACTER PYLORI; MEDICAL PROBLEMS OF INTERNATIONALLY ADOPTED CHILDREN.

Miller, Laurie C. "International Adoption: Infectious Diseases Issues," *Clinical Infectious Diseases* 40 (2005): 286–293.

infertility The inability to create a pregnancy among people who wish to bear children. The problem may be short term, long term, or permanent. The infertility may be correctable by simple means or by modern "high-tech" and often expensive techniques. In other cases, the infertility may stem from a problem requiring surgery. The infertility may lie primarily or solely with the male (such as a low sperm count) or with the female (such as failure to ovulate). In some cases, both parties have a fertility problem. In some cases, the cause of the infertility cannot be determined, despite extensive testing.

Some women have common but undiagnosed endocrine disorders, such as hypothyroidism, hypertension, or polycystic ovary syndrome (present in about 7 percent of women of childbearing age, or about four million women in the United States), which cause their infertility. Treatment may facilitate a successful pregnancy. In some cases, the infertility may be medication-induced; for example, research published in Norway in 2005 indicated that nonsteroidal anti-inflammatory drugs (NSAIDs) interfered with ovulation, causing a reversible infertility that resolved when the drug was withdrawn. (Individuals should not stop taking medications unless they consult with their physician first.) Further research is needed to confirm this finding.

Individuals may spend months or years seeking to create a biological child. If they do not succeed, some will remain childless, while others will seek to adopt a child.

Couples who have been unable to conceive after one year should see a fertility specialist because many causes of infertility can be treated. They should also contact a support group, such as Resolve, Inc., a national organization, which can provide practical information and emotional support.

Author Brette McWhorter Sember advises that individuals with fertility problems should seek a referral to a fertility specialist from the woman's gynecologist. In addition, if there are medical schools in the area, they may be consulted for a recommendation to a fertility expert. Advises McWhorter Sember, "Before visiting a specialist or clinic, call and ask if the providers are board certified or board eligible in gynecology and obstetrics as well as in *reproductive endocrinology.* Fertility specialists should be certified in both of these areas."

According to McWhorter Sember, most assisted reproduction clinics have reproductive immunologists, embryologists, reproductive urologists, and genetic counselors on staff. She advises that patients should also inquire about the clinic's success rate in achieving a "take-home baby" as opposed to achieving pregnancies, because sometimes pregnancies end in miscarriages. Some clinics focus on very difficult cases of infertility and thus, they may have a lower success rate than other clinics, and if so, this factor should also be considered in choosing a clinic.

Common Emotions of Infertile Couples

Author Christine Adamec, in her book *Is Adoption For You? The Information You Need to Make the Right Choice,* says that the following emotions are common to infertile couples:

Denial: The doctor must have made a mistake. Someone mixed up the lab results. Something else happened.

Shock and Powerlessness: Infertile people often feel that they have been thwarted by their own bodies. They may also feel cheated.

Feelings of Inadequacy: Some women say that they feel they are defective and maybe don't even deserve a child. They may feel unfeminine and unattractive. Men may feel inadequate, in the sense of having a defective body and of not being able to give their wives what they most want. People may say such things as "he's shooting blanks!" compounding feelings of inadequacy.

Anger at Infertility in General: Adoption agencies report that many adopting couples are very angry, not only about the unfairness of their infertility, but also about the many requirements they must undergo as prospective adoptive parents. They really hate the idea that they must prove their worthiness while people they perceive as incompetent parents can bear child after child, with no one asking them for references, no one making them undergo a physical examination or talk with a social worker or take classes.

Adamec says infertile women may feel angry and upset when they see pregnant women and become angry and distraught when their menstrual period comes yet again.

Occupational Status and Success at Adopting or a Live Birth

In one unusual study that compared the success of infertile couples at becoming pregnant or adopting,

Canadian researchers found a significant link to their occupation and socioeconomic status. Specifically, they found a link between occupations that are considered in the higher echelons and success at becoming a parent. They did not find a link between income and success at becoming a parent.

The researchers studied 1,567 couples who consulted with physicians at 11 teaching hospitals in Canada. All had been infertile for more than one year. Six percent of the couples adopted a child, and professionals had a higher success rate at adoption than nonprofessionals. Researchers found the probability of adopting dropped if the infertility had lasted longer than three years.

Researchers also found that adoption was 1.64 times more likely when the male partner was a professional and 1.49 more likely when the female partner was in a professional occupation.

Said the researchers, "Partnerships in the higher occupational strata were more likely to achieve live-birth or adoption and less likely to become lost to follow-up. The effect of occupation was similar with respect to both pregnancy and livebirth; also, in repeated analyses using different occupational variables, the upper stratum of the occupation range was consistently associated with pregnancy and livebirth, and the association is independent of treatment."

Even when expensive treatments were taken into account, such as in vitro fertilization, this did not change the findings.

Although they could not identify the factors that caused the higher success rates professionals experienced with becoming pregnant, researchers speculated that individuals at higher socioeconomic levels may be less likely to smoke and more likely to be healthy.

See also ASSISTED REPRODUCTIVE TECHNOLOGY.

Adamec, Christine. *Is Adoption For You? The Information You Need to Make the Right Choice* New York: John Wiley & Sons, 1998.

Azziz, R. "Healthcare-Related Economic Burden of the Polycystic Ovary Syndrome (PCOS) during the Reproductive Lifespan," *Journal of Clinical Endocrinology Metabolism* 90, no. 8 (June 8, 2005).

Collins, John, M.D., et al. "Occupation and the Follow-up of Infertile Couples," *Fertility and Sterility* 60, no. 3 (September 1993): 477–486.

McWhorter Sember, Brette. *The Complete Adoption & Infertility Legal Guide.* Naperville, Ill.: Sourcebooks, Inc., 2004.

Skomsvoll, J. F. "Reversible Infertility from Nonsteroidal Anti-Inflammatory Drugs," *Tidsskr Nor Laegeforen* 125, no. 11 (June 2, 2005): 1,476–1,478.

informal adoption   The rearing of a child as one's own, without benefit of legally adopting the child through the courts. Ever since and even before the pharaoh's daughter chose to raise Moses as her son, informal adoption has been a constant in our society. No longer popular among whites, it appears that many blacks still rely on informal adoptions. (This may be partly a function of necessity rather than desire. See BIRTHMOTHER.)

The problem with an informal adoption is that the child has no rights to the "adoptive" parents' social security benefits, inheritance, and so forth, and the "parents" have no legal status as parents unless or until they formally adopt the child. In addition, birthparents and relatives may come back months or even years later and reclaim the child, with no recourse to the informal adopters.

See also RELATIVE ADOPTIONS.

inheritance   Money and/or property that is bequeathed to survivors subsequent to the death of a person, or in the event of intestacy (no will) inherited in accordance with state law. (See table.) Although it would seem logical that a child adopted by nonrelatives would inherit from his or her adoptive parents and not from birthparents (and indeed this is true in most cases), there are many ramifications of the laws regarding inheritances, and the statutes vary from state to state.

Generally, an adopted child inherits from his or her adoptive parents and may not also inherit from the biological parents unless the child is specifically named in a will. However, in some states, such as Colorado, Kansas, Louisiana, Maine, Rhode Island, Texas, and Wyoming, inheritance rights to the estate of the birthparents may be maintained, subject to state law, and even when no will was made. In many states, however, the adopted person is specifically excluded from inheriting from birthparents. Note that in most cases, adoptive parents may inherit from their adopted children.

STATE INTESTATE* INHERITANCE LAWS, ADOPTED PERSON TO BIRTHPARENTS AND TO ADOPTIVE PARENTS

	Birthparents	Adoptive Parents
Alabama	Not addressed in statute reviewed. However, a person may bequeath to anyone.	After adoption, the adopted person shall be treated as the natural child of the adopting parents and shall have all rights and be subject to all of the duties arising from that relation, including the right of inheritance.
Alaska	After adoption decree has been entered, the adopted person is a stranger to the birth relative for all purposes including inheritance, unless the decree of adoption specifically provides for continuation of inheritance rights.	The adopted person is entitled to inherit, in order to create a parent-child relationship between the adopting parent and the adopted person.
Arizona	The relationship of birth parent and adopted person is completely severed upon entry of the adoption decree and all legal consequences of the relationship cease to exist, including the right of inheritance.	The adopted person is entitled to inherit from and through the adoptive parent and the adoptive parent is entitled to the same from the adopted person, as though the child were born to the adoptive parents.
Arkansas	All legal relationships, including right to inheritance, are terminated between natural parents and adopted person upon entry of the adoption decree.	The adopted person is entitled to inherit, in order to create the relationship of parent and child between adopting parent and adopted person.
California	A natural parent may not inherit from or through a child on the basis of the parent-child relationship if someone, other than the spouse or surviving spouse of the natural parent, has adopted the child.	A relationship of parent and child exists between an adopted person and the persons' adopting parent or parents for the purpose of determining intestate succession.
Colorado	A birth child may inherit from a natural parent if there is no surviving heir under subsections (1) to (5) of this section and if the birth child files a claim for inheritance with the court having jurisdiction within 90 days of decedent's death. For purposes of this subsection, the term "birth child" means a child who was born to, but adopted away from, his or her natural parent. The same is true for birth parents.	For purposes of intestate succession by, through, or from a person, an adopted individual is the child of his or her adopting parent or parents and not of his or her birth parents, except for inheritance rights as specified in § 15-11-103(6) and (7).
Connecticut	The biological parent or parents and their relatives shall have no rights of inheritance from or through the adopted person, nor shall the adopted person have any rights of inheritance from or through the biological parent.	The adopting parent and the adopted person shall have rights of inheritance from and through each other. Such rights extend to adopted relatives and the heirs of the adopted person.
Delaware	Upon the issuance of an adoption decree, the adopted child shall lose all rights of inheritance from its natural parent and their relatives. The rights of the natural parent or relatives to inherit from such child shall also cease.	For purposes of intestate succession, an adopted person is the child of an adopting parent.
District of Columbia	All rights and duties, including those of inheritance between the adopted person and his or her natural parents, cease upon the final adoption decree.	A final decree of adoption establishes the relationship of parent and child between adopter and adopted person for all purposes, including mutual rights of inheritance.

(continues)

(Table continued)

	Birthparents	Adoptive Parents
Florida	The adoption decree terminates all legal relationships between the adopted person and the adopted person's relatives, except that right of inheritance shall be as provided in the Florida Probate Code.	For the purpose of intestate succession by or from an adopted person, the adopted person is a descendant of the adopting parent.
Georgia	An adoption decree terminates all legal relationships between the adopted person and his birth relatives, including rights of inheritance.	The adoptive parents and relatives of the adoptive parents shall be entitled to inherit from and through the adopted person under the laws of intestacy. An adopted person, in the absence of a will, may inherit from his or her adoptive parent.
Hawaii	All legal rights and duties between birth parents and an adopted child cease upon entry of adoption decree. Though not explicitly stated, it is implied that the right of inheritance is included.	An adopted person and his or her adopting parent shall sustain towards each other the legal relationship of parent and child, including the rights of inheritance from and through each other.
Idaho	Unless the decree of adoption otherwise provides, the natural parents of an adopted person are relieved of all parental duties toward the adopted person, including the right of inheritance unless specifically provided by will.	An adopted person and adopting parent shall sustain toward each other the legal relation of parent and child, and shall have all the rights and duties of that relation, including the right to inherit.
Illinois	The natural parent and relatives shall take from the adopted person and the adopted person's adoptive family the property that the adopted person has taken from or through the natural parent or relatives by gift, will, or under intestate laws.	An adopted child is a descendant of the adopting parent for purposes of inheritance from the adopting parent. If the adopted person is adopted after the age of 18 years and the child never resided with the adopting parent before attaining the age of 18 years, he or she will not be able to inherit (intestate) from the relatives of the adopting parents. An adopting parent and relatives of the adopting parent shall inherit property from an adopted child to the exclusion of the natural parent.
Indiana	For all purposes of intestate succession, an adopted child shall cease to be treated as a child of the natural parents.	For all purposes of intestate succession, an adopted child shall be treated as a natural child of the child's adopting parents.
Iowa	A lawful adoption extinguishes the right of intestate succession of an adopted person from and through the adopted person's biological parents and vice versa.	The adopted person inherits from and through the adoptive parents and vice versa.
Kansas	Upon adoption, all the rights of birth parents to the adopted person, including their right to inherit from or through the person, shall cease. An adoption shall not terminate the right of the child to inherit from or through the birth parent.	When adopted, a person shall be entitled to the same personal and property rights as a birth child of the adoptive parent.
Kentucky	Upon granting an adoption, all legal relationship between the adopted child and the biological parents shall be terminated. It may be inferred that the right to inheritance is included.	Upon entry of the adoption decree, the adoptee shall be deemed the child of the adoptive parents for purposes of inheritance.

(continues)

	Birthparents	Adoptive Parents
Louisiana	Upon adoption, the blood parent and relatives of the adopted person are relieved of all of their legal duties and divested of all of their legal rights with regard to the adopted person, including the right of inheritance from the adopted person. The adopted person is relieved of all similar rights and duties to the blood parents and relatives, except the right of inheritance from them.	The adopted person is considered for all purposes as the legitimate child and heir of the adoptive parent, including the right of the adopted person to inherit from the adoptive parents and their relatives. The adoptive parent and their relatives also have the right to inherit from the adopted person.
Maine	An adopted person retains the right to inherit from the adopted person's biological parents if the adoption decree so provides, as specified in § 2-109.	An adopted person has all the same rights, including inheritance rights, that a child born to the adoptive parents would have.
Maryland	The Estates and Trusts Article shall govern all rights of inheritance between the adopted person and the natural relatives.	Not addressed explicitly in states reviewed. May be inferred from Fam. Law § 5-308: After a decree of adoption is entered, the adopted person is the child of the petitioner and is entitled to all the rights and privileges of and is subject to all the obligations of a child born to the petitioner.
Massachusetts	Upon adoption, a person shall lose his right to inherit from his natural parents or family.	If the adopted person dies intestate, his property shall be distributed according to Chap. 190 and 196 among adoptive parents and family. An adopted person may inherit from adoptive parents in the same manner.
Michigan	After entry of the adoption decree, an adopted child is no longer an heir at law of the natural parent.	After entry of adoption decree, the adopted person becomes an heir at law of the adopting parent.
Minnesota	The child shall not owe the birth parents or their relatives any legal duty nor shall the child inherit from the birth parents or their family. The birth parents shall have no rights over the child's property.	By virtue of the adoption, the adopted person shall inherit from the adoptive parents or their relatives as though the adopted person were the natural child of the parents. In [the] case of the adopted person's death intestate, the adoptive parents and their relatives shall inherit the adopted person's estate.
Mississippi	The natural parents and their relatives shall not inherit by or through the adopted child.	The adopted child shall inherit from and through the adopting parents and their relatives by the laws of descent and distribution of the State of Mississippi, and likewise the adopting parents and relatives shall inherit from the adopted child.
Missouri	If for purposes of intestate succession, a relationship of parent and child must be established to determine succession by, through or from a person, an adopted person is not the child of the natural parents.	An adopted person shall be considered for every purpose the child of the adoptive parents including inheritance rights. The adoptive parents shall be capable of inheriting from their adopted child.
Montana	Inheritance from or through an [adopted] child by either natural parent or their family is precluded.	For purposes of intestate succession, a parent-child relationship exists between an adopted person and an adopting parent.

(continues)

(Table continued)

	Birthparents	Adoptive Parents
Nebraska	After an adoption decree has been entered, the natural parents of the adopted child shall be relieved of all parental duties toward and all responsibilities for such child and have no rights over or to such adopted child's property by descent or distribution.	For purposes of intestate succession, a parent-child relationship exists between an adopted person and an adopting parent.
Nevada	After an adoption decree is entered, the natural parents of the adopted child shall be relieved of all parental responsibilities for such child, and they shall not exercise or have any rights over an adopted child's property. The child shall not owe his natural parents or their relatives any legal duty, nor shall he inherit from his natural parents or family.	By virtue of an adoption, an adopted person shall inherit from his adoptive parents or their relatives as though he were the legitimate child of such parents. If an adopted person dies intestate, the adoptive parents and their relatives shall inherit his estate.
New Hampshire	Upon the issuance of a final adoption decree the adopted child and the natural parents shall lose all rights of inheritance from and through each other.	Upon the issuance of a final adoption decree, the adopted person and adopting parents shall acquire the mutual right to inherit from and through each other.
New Jersey	Upon final adoption decree, the natural parents and their family lose their right to take and inherit intestate personal and real property from and through the person adopted.	Upon adoption, the adopting parents and the adopted person gain the right to take and inherit intestate personal and real property from and through each other.
New Mexico	For purposes of intestate succession by, through, or from a person, an adopted individual is not the child of his natural parents.	The adopted person and adopting parent shall have all rights and be subject to all of the duties of the parent-child relationship upon adoption, including the right to inheritance from and through each other.
New York	The rights of an adoptive child to inheritance and succession from and through his birth parents shall terminate upon the making of the adoption decree; the rights of the birth parents over such adoptive child or his property by descent or succession will also cease.	The adoptive parent and the adopted child shall sustain toward each other the legal relation of parent and child and shall have all the rights and be subject to all the duties to that relation, including the right on inheritance from and through each other.
North Carolina	After the entry of a decree of adoption, the birth parents are relieved of all legal duties and obligations due from them to the adopted person and are divested of all rights with respect to the adopted person.	From the date of the signing of the decree, the adopted person is entitled to inherit real and personal property by, through, and from the adoptive parents in accordance with the statutes on intestate succession.
North Dakota	For purposes of intestate succession, an adopted person is not the child of the biological parents.	Upon adoption, the adopted person gains the right of inheritance from the adopting parents, to create the relationship of parent and child.
Ohio	The final adoption decree terminates all legal relationships between the adopted person and the adopted person's birth parents and relatives, for all purposes including inheritance.	The adopted person gains the right of inheritance from the adopting parent upon final decree to create the relationship of parent and child, as if the adopted person were the legitimate blood relative of the adopting parent.

(continues)

	Birthparents	Adoptive Parents
Oklahoma	After a final decree of adoption, the biological parents of the adopted child shall be relieved of all parental responsibilities for said child and shall have no rights over the adopted child or to the property of the child by descent and distribution.	From the date of the final decree of adoption the child shall be entitled to inherit real and personal property from and through the adoptive parents in accordance with the statutes of descent and distribution. The adoptive parents shall be entitled to the same.
Oregon	An adopted person shall cease to be treated as the child of the person's natural parents for all purposes of intestate succession.	An adopted person and the adoptive parents and their relatives shall take by intestate succession from each other.
Pennsylvania	An adopted person shall not be considered as continuing to be the child of his natural parents except in distribution of the estate of a natural kin, other than the natural parent, who has maintained a family relationship with the adopted person.	For purposes of inheritance by, from, and through an adopted person, he or she shall be considered the issue of his or her adopting parent or parents.
Rhode Island	The parents of the adopted child shall be deprived of all legal rights respecting the child, and the child shall be freed from all obligations of maintenance and obedience respecting his or her natural parents; except it will not deprive an adopted child of the right to inherit from and through his natural parents as provided in § 33-1-8.	A child lawfully adopted shall be deemed, for the purpose of inheritance from and through the parents by adoption and their relatives, the child of the parents by adoption the same as if he or she has been born them in lawful wedlock.
South Carolina	The mutual right of inheritance between an adopted child and his or her birth parents terminates after a final order of adoption.	After the final decree of adoption is entered, the relationship of parent and child and all the rights, duties, and other legal consequence exist between the adopted person, the adoptive parent, and the family of the adoptive parent.
South Dakota	The natural parents of an adopted child are, from the time of the adoption, relieved of all parental duties towards, and of all responsibility for the child so adopted, and have no right over the child.	For purposes of intestate succession by, from, or through a person, an adopted individual is the child of that individual's adopting parent or parents.
Tennessee	An adopted child shall not inherit real or personal property from his or her biological parents or their relatives when the relationship between them has been terminated by final order of adoption, nor shall the biological parent or their relatives inherit from the adopted child.	The adopted child and the child's descendants shall be capable of inheriting and otherwise receiving title to real and personal property from the adoptive parents and their descendants. The adoptive parents and their family shall have a right of inheritance but only as to property of the adopted child acquired after the child's adoption.
Texas	The natural parents of an adopted child shall not inherit from or through said child, but said child shall inherit from and through its natural parents.	An adopted child may, under the laws of descent and distribution, inherit from and through the adopting parents and their relatives and the adopting parents and their family may inherit from and through such adopted child.

(continues)

(Table continued)

	Birthparents	Adoptive Parents
Utah	For purposes of intestate succession by, through, or from a person, an adopted individual is not the child of the birth parents.	For purposes of intestate succession by, through, or from a person, an adopted individual is the child of the adopting parents.
Vermont	All parental rights and duties of the birth parent of the adopted person terminate, including the right of inheritance from or through the adopted person, upon final decree of adoption. The child's right to inherit from the birth parents also terminates.	The adoptive parent and the adopted person have the legal relation of parent and child and have all the rights and duties of that relationship, including the right of inheritance from or through each other.
Virginia	For the purpose of determining rights in or to property, an adopted person is not the child of the natural parents.	For the purpose of determining rights in or to property, an adopted person is the child of the adopting parents.
Washington	A lawfully adopted child shall not be considered an "heir" of his natural parents.	An adopted person shall be, to all intents and purposes, and for all legal incidents, the child, legal heir, and lawful issue of the adoptive parent, entitled to all rights and privileges, including the right of inheritance.
West Virginia	Upon the entry of the final adoption decree, the birth parents shall be divested of all legal rights, including the right of inheritance from or through the adopted child. Such child shall not inherit from any person entitled to parental rights prior to the adoption.	From and after the entry of the order of adoption, a legally adopted child shall inherit from and through the parents by adoption. If the adopted person dies intestate, all property, including real and personal of such adopted person shall pass to the adopting parents.
Wisconsin	A legally adopted person ceases to be treated as a child of the person's birth parents for the purposes of intestate succession. Rights of inheritance by, from, and through an adopted child are governed by §§ 854.20 and 854.21.	A legally adopted person is treated as a birth child of the person's adoptive parents for purposes of intestate succession by, through, and from the adopted person.
Wyoming	An adopted person is the child of an adopting parent and of both the natural parents for inheritance purposes only.	An adopted person is the child of an adopting parent and of both the natural parents for inheritance purposes only.

Source: National Adoption Information Clearinghouse, "Intestate Inheritance Rights," 2003 Adoption State Statutes Series Statutes-at-a-Glance, The Children's Bureau, Administration for Children and Families Department of Health and Human Services, 2003.
* "Intestate" means the deceased person did not leave a will, and consequently, state laws regarding intestacy will be followed. It is best for individuals to create wills stipulating their wishes, but often they do not.
Note: Because state laws are subject to change, individuals should consult with an attorney in their state to determine if changes have occurred. Note also that if the adopted person is an adult who is married and has not left a will, the laws related to his or her marital relationship and any children born in that relationship will apply. Thus, a wife will inherit ahead of an adoptive parent.

In the case of a STEPPARENT ADOPTION, in some states, the adopted child may inherit from both biological parents as well as the stepparent, but in other states, the adopted child may only inherit from the custodial parent and stepparent.

It is best for individuals interested in this issue to review current state law and consult an attorney in the event of a question or a desire to provide an inheritance for an adopted-away child. Note: Several legalistic terms are used when discussing inheritance, such as *adopted-away* and *adopted-in*. An adopted-away child is a child who is born to a family and then leaves the birthparents because of adoption. An *adopted-in* child is a child that enters a family by adoption. Another frequently used term is *natural parent* to denote the biological parent. Many individuals do not like the way these terms sound, but it is important to understand that they are terms used by some attorneys and in state laws.

If the child is adopted by nonrelatives, inheritance generally must come through adoptive parents; however, as recently as 1986, a challenge was made to this assumption in New York. Jessie Best wrote her will in 1973 and provided for her assets to be given to her "issue." Her daughter had given birth 21 years earlier to a son who had been adopted by nonrelatives. The executor of Best's will discovered the existence of the adopted grandchild. With the permission of the birthmother, who also had a child born within wedlock, the trustees asked the adoption agency for identifying information since the adopted grandchild might stand to inherit a considerable sum.

The adoption agency told the adoptive parents, who disclosed the son's legal name. When the birthmother died in 1980, the trustees asked the court to determine whether the adopted child would share in the division of assets with the child born within wedlock and not adopted.

The court decided the adopted child was "issue" and could inherit; however, the court of appeals overturned this decision.

In a very unusual case, adopted adult Cathy Yvonne Stone alleged she was the birthdaughter of Hank Williams, the late singer. Stone sued to receive part of the royalties accruing to Williams's estate. Her suit was rejected at a lower court level, but on appeal, a federal court decided she was entitled to have her case heard by a jury. In 1990, the U.S. Supreme Court affirmed this decision. In addition, the Supreme Court refused to overturn an Alabama Supreme Court decision that decreed Stone was a lawful heir to the estate of Williams.

Inheritance laws may change; however, the table starting on page 155 conveys information on state laws in relation to the adopted person and birthparents and adoptive parents, as of 2003, the most recent information available from the National Adoption Information Clearinghouse.

National Adoption Information Clearinghouse. "Intestate Inheritance Rights," 2003 Adoption State Statutes Series Statutes-at-a-Glance, The Children's Bureau, Administration for Children and Families Department of Health and Human Services, 2003.

insurance   The primary insurance concern of most adoptive parents is health insurance for the newly adopted child. State laws varied greatly in the past when an adopted child was covered by health insurance, and many companies disallowed certain claims made for an adopted child because they evolved from preexisting conditions.

The Health Insurance Portability and Accountability Act, passed in 1996, stipulated by federal law that children adopted with "preexisting" conditions could not be denied insurance coverage. Of course, this refers to cases in which families have health insurance coverage, which is probably the vast majority of adoptive parents, and it also refers to conditions that are included in their health plan.

In a few states, children are covered before arrival in the home; for example, the medical expenses of a newborn after birth and still in the hospital are covered in some states. Generally, the cost of childbirth is not covered. Adopting parents should check on what their state law mandates. Particular provisions of each state law should be checked by adopting parents to determine whether the parents comply with various requirements, such as deadlines for enrollment in insurance plans or filing claims.

Some adopted children are covered by MEDICAID, which adoptive parents may be able to use indefinitely or at least until they are able to use their own private insurance.

Because of the difficulty in obtaining health insurance coverage, many children with SPECIAL NEEDS are covered under Medicaid, a federally-funded health insurance program; however, many physicians refuse to accept Medicaid.

See also EMPLOYMENT BENEFITS.

intelligence   Children's genes set forth their basic potential intelligence; however, there are some indications that a positive adoption experience can increase IQ (intelligence quotient) levels by as much as 15 points or more.

A study by Christiane Capron and Michel Duyme, French researchers at the University of Paris, looked at the socioeconomic status (SES) of birthparents and adoptive parents and found an apparent environmental impact. All the adopted children studied were adopted before the age of six months, and the average age of the adopted person at the time of the study was 14 years.

The researchers found clear-cut differences in the adopted children's scores related to the SES of their birthparents and their adoptive parents.

"Children reared by high-SES parents have significantly higher IQs than those reared by low-SES parents," stated the researchers, referring to adoptive parents.

The highest IQs of adopted children were recorded when the SES of both the birthparents and the adoptive parents were high, and researchers found a mean IQ score of nearly 120. The lowest scores occurred when both the birthparents and adoptive parents were of low SES, and the average IQ was 92 points.

Probably the most likely actual scenario is the low SES birthparent and the high SES adoptive parent: in this case, the mean IQ score was about 104 points. (A person with an IQ score of about 100 is generally considered of "average" intelligence, and incremental increases of 10 points are significantly important.)

It appears the intelligence level of adopted children can be raised by nearly 16 points or more when the adoptive parents are of a high SES, despite the birthparents' SES. It would be fascinating to learn if the IQ differences remained constant when the adopted adults grew up and moved away from home. An IQ difference of 16 points could mean the difference between topping out educationally with a high school diploma or going on to obtain a college degree. Some researchers speculate that the effect of the adoptive parent's SES wanes as the adopted person ages.

Capron and Duyme do not explain why or how higher adoptive SES homes apparently produce children with higher IQs. Said psychology professor Matt McGue in *Nature*, "It remains unclear whether the SES effect is related to access to quality education, the variety and complexity of intellectual stimulation in the home, the parents' press for scholastic achievement, or some other factor that differentiates between high- and low-SES homes."

According to McGue, other studies have correlated the adoptive mother's encouragement, the child's attainment of self-confidence, and his or her subsequent test performance.

In his study of 300 adoptive families and the birthmothers of the adopted children, Joseph M. Horn concluded, "Adopted children resemble their biological mothers more than they resemble the adoptive parents who reared them from birth."

He found that children with higher-IQ birthmothers were more intelligent, saying, "Children from higher-IQ unwed mothers surpassed those from lower-IQ unwed mothers, even though the intellectual potential in their environments was comparable."

More recently, researchers van IJzendoorn, Juffer, and Klein Poelhuis performed a meta-analysis of 62 studies on the IQs and school performance of adopted and nonadopted children, which they reported in a 2005 issue of *Psychological Bulletin*. The researchers found that in the few studies that compared adopted children to nonadopted children who remained with the birthparents or other children left behind in the former environment, the adopted children compared significantly better in terms of their IQ as well as their school performance. The researchers said that for many adopted children "adoption involves a drastic change of environment, and this change may be an effective intervention that improves their cognitive development." In addition, the adopted children's school performance surpassed that of their biological siblings or former peers.

In considering their current school peers or their current "environmental" siblings, the adopted children lagged behind slightly. Said the researchers, "Overall, we found that studies reported a negligible difference in the IQ of adopted children and their nonadopted environmental siblings or peers. Comparing their school achievement, we documented that the adopted children did somewhat less well in school, but the effect size was small."

The third finding, according to the researchers, was that in "a small set of studies we found that the percentage of adopted children who needed special education for their learning problems was about twice as large as the percentage of nonadopted children. This minority of adopted children with learning problems is clinically important because the children suffer from these problems and need special treatment. However, their difficulties should not be confused with those experienced by the average adopted child. Most adopted children do remarkably well, certainly much better than their siblings or peers who had to stay behind in poor institutions or deprived families."

See also FETAL ALCOHOL SYNDROME; GENETIC PREDISPOSITIONS.

Capron, Christiane, and Michel Duyme. "Assessment of Effects of Socioeconomic Status on IQ in a Full Cross-Fostering Study," *Nature* 340, no. 6234 (August 17, 1989): 552–553.

Horn, Joseph M. "The Texas Adoption Project: Adopted Children and Their Intellectual Resemblance to Biological and Adoptive Parents," *Child Development* 54 (1983): 268–275.

McGue, Matt. "Nature-Nurture and Intelligence," *Nature,* August 17, 1989, 507–508.

Plomin, Robert, and J. D. DeFries. "The Colorado Adoption Project," *Child Development* 54 (1983): 276–289.

Rutter, Michael, et al. "Genetic Factors in Child Psychiatric Disorders—I. A Review of Research Strategies," *Journal of Child Psychology and Psychiatry* 31 (January 1990): 3–37.

van IJzendoorn, Marinus H., Femmie Juffer, and Caroline W. Klein Poelhuis. "Adoption and Cognitive Development: A Meta-Analytic Comparison of Adopted and Nonadopted Children's IQ and School Performance," *Psychological Bulletin* 131, no. 2 (2005): 301–316.

intercountry adoption See INTERCOUNTRY ADOPTION.

intermediary Person who facilitates or who acts to put together an INDEPENDENT ADOPTION; a "broker" as middleman in an adoption; May be an ATTORNEY or PHYSICIAN or other person, as determined by state law.

international adoption The adoption of a child who is a citizen of one country by adoptive parents who are citizens of a different country. Most of the children who are adopted from other countries are infants and small children at the time of their adoption; however, older children are sometimes

TABLE I: WORLD TOTAL OF IMMIGRANT VISAS ISSUED TO ORPHANS COMING TO THE UNITED STATES FOR ADOPTION, FY 1995–FY 2005

Year	Number of Visas/Children
2005	22,728
2004	22,884
2003	21,616
2002	20,099
2001	19,237
2000	17,718
1999	16,363
1998	15,774
1997	12,743
1996	10,641
1995	8,987

Source: U.S. State Department, http://travel.state.gov/family/adoption/stats/stats_451.html, downloaded March 4, 2005.

adopted. Most children adopted internationally are adopted by citizens of the United States, Canada, and other Western countries.

U.S. citizens adopt thousands of infants and children each year, primarily from countries in eastern Europe, Asia, and Latin America. In fiscal year 2005, 22,728 children from other countries were adopted by adoptive parents in the United States. (See Table I.) The largest proportion of this figure, nearly a third of all international adoptions, was children adopted from China, or 7,906 children in 2005. (See Table II.) Adoptions from China were followed in number by adoptions from Russia; for example, in 2005, Americans adopted 4,639 children from Russia. (See CHINA, ADOPTIONS FROM; RUSSIA, ADOPTIONS FROM.)

As can be seen from Table II, which includes data on the top 12 countries from which children have been adopted from fiscal year 1995 to 2005, many changes have occurred in international adoption. The total numbers of international adoptions more than doubled from 8,987 adoptions in 1995 to 22,728 in 2005, and there is no reason to think that adoptions will wane in the next several years. However, individual countries can suddenly "close their doors" to adoption at any time, should they wish to do so.

In most cases, the children who are adopted from other countries have been living in orphan-

TABLE II: NUMBER OF IMMIGRANT VISAS ISSUED TO ORPHANS COMING TO THE UNITED STATES FOR ADOPTION: TOP COUNTRIES OF ORIGIN, FY 1995–FY 2005

	2005	2004	2003	2002	2001	2000	1999	1998	1997	1996	1995
1	7,906 China	7,044 China	6,859 China	5,053 China	4,681 China	5,053 China	4,348 Russia	4,491 Russia	3,816 Russia	3,333 China	2,130 China
2	4,639 Russia	5,865 Russia	5,209 Russia	4,939 Russia	4,279 Russia	4,269 Russia	4,101 China	4,206 China	3,597 China	2,454 Russia	1,896 Russia
3	3,783 Guatemala	3,264 Guatemala	2,328 Guatemala	2,219 Guatemala	1,870 South Korea	1,794 South Korea	2,008 South Korea	1,829 South Korea	1,654 South Korea	1,516 South	1,666
4	1,630 South Korea	1,716 South Korea	1,790 South Korea	1,779 South Korea	1,609 Guatemala	1,518 Guatemala	1,002 Guatemala	911 Guatemala	788 Guatemala	555 Romania	449 Guatemala
5	821 Ukraine	826 Kazakhstan	825 Kazakhstan	1,106 Ukraine	1,246 Ukraine	1,122 Romania	895 Romania	603 Vietnam	621 Romania	427 Guatemala	371 India
6	755 Kazakhstan	723 Ukraine	702 Ukraine	819 Kazakhstan	782 Romania	724 Vietnam	709 Vietnam	478 India	425 Vietnam	380 India	351 Paraguay
7	441 Ethiopia	406 India	472 India	766 Vietnam	737 Vietnam	659 Ukraine	500 India	406 Romania	352 India	354 Vietnam	350 Colombia
8	323 India	356 Haiti	382 Vietnam	466 India	672 Kazakhstan	503 India	323 Ukraine	351 Colombia	233 Colombia	258 Paraguay	318 Vietnam
9	291 Colombia	289 Ethiopia	272 Colombia	334 Colombia	543 India	402 Cambodia	248 Cambodia	249 Cambodia	163 Philippines	255 Colombia	298 Philippines
10	271 Philippines	287 Colombia	250 Haiti	260 Bulgaria	407 Colombia	399 Kazakhstan	231 Colombia	200 Philippines	152 Mexico	229 Philippines	275 Romania
11	231 Haiti	202 Belarus	214 Philippines	254 Cambodia	297 Bulgaria	246 Colombia	221 Bulgaria	180 Ukraine	148 Bulgaria	163 Bulgaria	146 Brazil
12	182 Liberia	196 Philippines	200 Romania	221 Philippines	266 Cambodia	214 Bulgaria	195 Philippines	168 Mexico	142 Haiti	103 Brazil	110 Bulgaria

Source: U.S. State Department, http://travel.state.gov/family/adoption/stats/stats_451.html, downloaded March 4, 2005.

ages and/or were considered legally abandoned (or actually were physically abandoned) by their birth-parents. In some cases, adoptions have been arranged using the INTERNET; however, it is very important for prospective parents to obtain the services of a reputable licensed ADOPTION AGENCY because of complications and outright frauds that sometimes occur with international adoptions.

See FRAUD IN ADOPTION.

Origins of International Adoption

In 1918, the Displaced Persons Act was created by Congress to enable more than 200,000 European refugees to immigrate to the United States. This act also allowed 3,000 "displaced orphans" to enter the United States, regardless of their nationality. A sponsor did not have to promise to adopt the child but only had to promise that the child would be "cared for properly." The orphan provisions of the Displaced Persons Act were temporary, but they were periodically renewed by Congress, with expiration dates varying from one to three years.

From 1935 to 1948, only about 14 immigrants per year in the category of "under 16 years of age, unaccompanied by parents" entered the United States. It is unknown how many of these children were actually adopted. Nearly all adoptions in the United States were domestic adoptions during the pre–World War II years. In addition, adoption agencies at that time strongly emphasized the concept of matching the child to the adoptive parents as closely as possible so that the unknowing stranger would presume that the child was a birth child of the adoptive parents. As a result, international adoption, and the obvious racial distinctions between some children and their adoptive parents, would have been viewed negatively during those years.

After World War II, when Americans first became very interested in international adoption, it was primarily U.S. immigration laws and quotas that held them back from adopting children from other countries. Initially, the laws were changed to allow only military members to adopt limited numbers of children.

During and after the Korean War, many American servicemen became interested in adopting South Korean orphans, and in 1953, Congress allowed up to 500 special visas for orphans who would be adopted by American servicemen or by civil servants of the federal government. At this time, immigration was open to orphans from any nation: prior to that time, the immigration of orphans had been limited to the adoption of European orphans only.

The Refugee Relief Act of 1953 was subsequently passed, allowing for 4,000 orphan visas over the next three years. Yet this act, combined with the earlier provisions for special visas, was insufficient to accommodate all the orphans that service members and federal employees wished to adopt from other countries.

In 1957, Congress lifted all the numerical quotas on orphan visas, but this action too was limited in time because Congress mistakenly perceived that the need and desire to adopt orphans from other countries was a short-term situation only. Finally, in 1961, the Immigration and Nationality Act incorporated a permanent reference to the emigration of orphans from other countries to be adopted by Americans.

The Vietnamese "Baby Lift" occurred in 1975 after the fall of Saigon, South Vietnam, when thousands of Vietnamese children who were presumed to be orphans were flown to Western nations to be adopted. It was later discovered that some of those children had living parents who had not wished for their children to be adopted, and instead, they had only wanted their safe removal from the country. As a result, U.S. immigration laws were tightened.

International adoption has continued to date, and tens of thousands of children from other countries have been adopted by U.S. citizens as well as by the citizens of other countries. At least half of all the children adopted from abroad by Americans have emigrated from South Korea, and there were 1,630 adoptions of South Korean children by U.S. citizens in 2005. (See SOUTH KOREA, ADOPTIONS FROM.) However, since the early 1990s, adoptions from South Korea have been supplanted by adoptions of children from China and Russia. Many children are also adopted from Guatemala. (See GUATEMALA, ADOPTIONS FROM.)

The initial impetus to adoptions from eastern Europe in the latter part of the 20th century came with the fall of the Romanian dictatorship, and the subsequent discovery of thousands of infants and children living in orphanages under extremely deprived conditions. This situation was televised worldwide in documentaries that were seen by millions of horrified viewers. As a result, many Americans, Canadians, and other individuals from western Europe flocked to Romania to adopt children. Abuses in fraud in adoption practices eventually led to the new Romanian government essentially shutting down adoptions; however, in the meantime, many people became aware that there were other children in eastern European orphanages in other countries who needed adoptive families. (See ROMANIA, ADOPTIONS FROM.)

In the mid-1990s, partly because of the end of the cold war and also because of improved relations between the United States and Russia, Russia began allowing the adoptions of children, as did other countries in the former Soviet Union, such as Ukraine and Kazakhstan.

Factors abroad Influencing International Adoption

International adoption is changeable and highly driven by the policies of the foreign countries as well as by U.S. adoption practices and immigration law. Most of the countries that allow the immigration of their orphans to the United States have great difficulty with poverty and economic and social problems. If these problems were resolved, it is less likely that they would favor international adoption.

Some factors driving the American interest in international adoption, as Elizabeth Bartholet wrote in her 1996 article, are similar to those in other Western countries, " . . . contraception, abortion, and the increased tendency of single parents to keep their children."

In addition, many Americans who are interested in adopting children believe that it is too difficult or even impossible to adopt an infant or small child in the United States, and so they decide to adopt an infant or toddler from another country. Others know that it is possible to adopt a baby in the United States, but they do not wish to engage in an OPEN ADOPTION, which usually involves at least a meeting between the prospective adoptive parents and the birthmother, as well as the possibility of a

continuing relationship as the child grows up. Skeptical of the feasibility of this option, they may turn instead to international adoption, which is rarely an open adoption.

A General Accounting Office (GAO) report on international adoption prepared for Senator Arlen Specter in 1993 demonstrated the discomfort among American prospective adoptive families with domestic adoption, a situation that is still relevant today.

When asked why they had chosen international adoption (some families chose more than one reason), 104 of the 203 families (51 percent) said that they believed they were ineligible for domestic adoption, and 38 percent thought that an international adoption could be completed more quickly than a domestic adoption. Twenty percent said that they believed an international adoption would be easier to achieve than a domestic adoption.

In about 10 percent of the cases, the families said that they had adopted internationally because they were worried about birthparent rights in a domestic adoption. Many Americans believed (and continue to believe) that if they adopt children in the United States, the birthparents may come back to claim the children, even years later. This belief is generally driven by sensational media coverage of a handful of highly publicized lawsuits and is not a valid one, since very few birthmothers change their mind about adoption after the baby has been placed with adoptive parents. However, this perception is very persistent.

See also ATTITUDES ABOUT ADOPTION; INDEPENDENT ADOPTION.

Differing Cultural and Legal Views about Adoption

It is very important to understand that many nations do not share the philosophy or the understanding of adoption that most Americans take for granted. For example, in some countries, the birthmother of a child need not execute a written consent to relinquish her child. She may or may not receive any counseling, depending on the laws of the nation.

As a result of differing laws and requirements, it is advisable for adopting parents to work with a licensed adoption agency in the United States that is not only reputable but is also experienced with the adoptions of children in the particular country from which the family wishes to adopt the child. In addition, it is one positive indication when the agency has sent at least one staff member to the other country to meet with orphanage officials. Of course, each agency should be thoroughly screened by the prospective adoptive parent before any written or verbal agreement is reached between the parties, with checks through state social service departments as well as local Better Business Bureaus where the agency is located to determine if any complaints have been made against the adoption agency.

Federal Legal Requirements to Adopt

United States citizens cannot adopt children from other countries unless they follow the requirements of the U.S. Citizenship and Immigration Services. (Formerly called the Immigration and Naturalization Service, or INS.) Although this organization is *not* a child welfare agency, it does strive to determine if the prospective adoptive parents are suitable, based on information that has been provided in the mandated HOME STUDY prepared by an adoption agency. This home study is actually a process, and it encompasses not only several home visits but also includes checks with the applicant's personal references, verification of the prospective parent's current income, reviews of recent past income tax returns, and a check to make sure the applicant does not have a criminal record and is not listed on a state child abuse registry. (Fingerprinting is required to assist with the various checks.)

A great deal of paperwork is required to adopt a child from another country, and international adoption should never be considered an easy process to undergo; however, many adoption agencies can help ease the way for prospective parents.

In many countries, the FINALIZATION of the adoption actually occurs in the foreign court. However, even when the child is formally adopted overseas in a foreign court, some experts recommend that the adoptive parents also perform a RE-ADOPTION of their child in their home state. Many states have legal provisions for the re-adoptions of children adopted from other countries. A re-adoption in the state will provide the child with a U.S. birth certificate listing the adoptive parents as the parents,

similarly as is done with the adoption of adopted children born in the United States.

Adoptive parents may believe that a U.S. birth certificate will look less imposing and confusing to others in its appearance than would a foreign birth certificate and would avoid extra questions and bureaucracy.

Birth certificates are not needed frequently by most people, but they are used for such purposes as the child's entry into school. The child will need the birth certificate later in life, such as when he or she applies for a driver's license, wishes to marry, join military service, obtain a professional license or apply for a passport, or wishes to adopt a child.

Why People Adopt from Other Countries

Some people have asked why U.S. citizens do not adopt children from within the United States in larger numbers, rather than adopting children from other countries. As mentioned, one reason is that some adoptive parents believe that it is difficult or impossible for them to adopt from the United States or they do not wish to participate in an open adoption. In addition, families who are interested in adopting older children may believe that children in foster care in the United States are far too troubled for them to parent because of past abuse and neglect, and they may believe that children in orphanages overseas are more emotionally healthy than foster children in the United States. Sadly, however, children in foreign orphanages may also suffer from abuse and/or neglect, and some children, especially children adopted at older ages, may have the same (or worse) emotional problems as are common among children who have spent years in foster care in the United States (See FOSTER CARE.)

It is also true that some individuals wonder why more families, especially white families, do not adopt children of other races from the United States when there are so many needing families, rather than adopting children of other races from other countries. One answer is that TRANSRACIAL ADOPTION has been actively fought by some groups in the United States that view transracial adoption as a form of "racial genocide."

Although federal laws, such as the MULTIETHNIC PLACEMENT ACT, have outlawed using race as a factor in whether a particular family may adopt, statistics available on children adopted from the foster care system in 2001 revealed that most children adopted from foster care (about 93 percent) were adopted by same-race families rather than in transracial adoptions. As a result, individuals for whom race is not a major factor have turned to international adoption, and many have successfully adopted children of all races from throughout the world. Some international adoption agencies place black children from other countries, for example, Ethiopia and Haiti, with white families, believing that the children are far better off in a happy adoptive family than they would be living in an orphanage.

Note that families to whom SKIN COLOR is a very important feature of the child to be adopted should not adopt a child from another country. Some people mistakenly believe that all children adopted from eastern Europe are blue-eyed blonde children. However, children from eastern Europe could be white, Asian, or a mixture of races. In some cases, the race of the child's birth family may be unknown and can only be guessed at by the child's appearance, especially if the child was abandoned to the orphanage.

Some individuals seek to adopt children from abroad because they are seeking to adopt a child of their own cultural heritage; for example, a couple of Russian origin may wish to adopt a Russian child. It should be noted that some countries require at least one of the adoptive parents to be of the same national origin as the child.

Looking at People Who Adopt from Other Countries

Individuals of all ages and races in the United States, up to about age 55 or 60 years, adopt children from other countries throughout the world. Most adoptive parents are married, but increasing numbers are single, particularly single women.

Some adoptive parents who adopt children from other countries are OPTIONAL ADOPTERS, that is, they are fertile but believe in providing a home for a child who is "already here." (See FERTILE ADOPTIVE PARENTS.) In some cases, the adoptive parents are older than 45 years old or they do not fit the criteria of local adoption agencies and they did not realize that they could adopt using the services of agencies in other states.

Some individuals would be accepted by domestic adoption agencies, and they know it, but they choose to adopt their children from other countries because they believe that children in the United States will eventually be adopted but some children in overseas orphanages will not be otherwise adopted.

Criteria Set by Other Countries for Adoptive Parents

Some countries that allow intercountry adoption set restrictions on adoptive parents beyond those mandated by adoption agencies in the United States; for example, they may accept only married couples. Some countries ban homosexuals from adopting children, and they may also ban single people from adopting, largely because they fear that single individuals may be homosexual.

Most countries require the adopting parents to travel to their countries and stay at least a few days until the various paperwork and legal requirements are satisfied. In some cases, several trips to the country are required. Such a stay can be difficult for some Americans, particularly those who have never left their own country before that time; however, the time abroad may sensitize the new parents to the radical changes that the child will undergo. (See CULTURE SHOCK.)

The child adopted from another country will have plenty of new cultural experiences to absorb and assimilate; for example, some children who live in orphanages abroad receive sponge baths, and consequently, they may be frightened by their first sight of a tub that is full of water. They may also be initially fearful of flushing toilets, noisy vacuum cleaners, and a host of experiences common to the everyday U.S. household. Most children quickly adapt to these changes, but some children need more time than others.

It should also be noted that other countries have their own way of accomplishing bureaucratic tasks, and sometimes Americans can become very impatient and frustrated with foreign officials who they believe are not acting quickly or efficiently enough. Often paperwork is misplaced, and there are numerous frustrations to endure in dealing with foreign governments. As a result, international adoption should never be considered the "easy" way to adopt.

The International Adoption Process

Most married couples or single persons in the United States who adopt a child from another country use the services of a licensed U.S. adoption agency. Subsequent to the implementation of the HAGUE CONVENTION ON INTERCOUNTRY ADOPTION (expected by 2007), which is a treaty between "sending" and "receiving" countries, families will need to deal with accredited agencies. Some countries, such as Russia, convey accreditation on some adoption agencies in the United States, and Russian children may only be adopted through these agencies.

Subsequent to the approval of the family, the agency attempts to identify a child for the family. After the agency notifies the family of an available child, they must decide whether to adopt the child, sometimes based on very sketchy information. The agency will often attempt to obtain a photograph of the child along with social and medical information. In some cases, VIDEOTAPES of the child are available to prospective parents. Often families report that they feel that they "bond" to these photographs or videos, which is a problem if, for some reason, the adoption does not occur.

Many families obtain medical information on the child, and they may seek an opinion from an international ADOPTION MEDICINE expert as to the state of the child's health. The doctor will review translated medical records, photographs, and other information that is available on the child, and then provide an analysis to the family. Usually the doctor does not advise the family that they should or should not adopt a child, except in rare cases of extremely ill or high-risk children.

Many children from other countries have minor or more serious health problems. Some are common and correctable problems, such as INTESTINAL PARASITIC INFECTIONS or infections with lice or scabies. (See also MEDICAL PROBLEMS OF INTERNATIONALLY ADOPTED CHILDREN.) Dental decay is common, due to frequent bottle propping and lack of dental hygiene. Others have longer-term problems, such as FETAL ALCOHOL SYNDROME, DEVELOPMENTAL DISABILITIES, or ATTACHMENT DISORDER.

Once adopted, the child will attain U.S. citizenship, although the parents must prepare several forms to achieve this goal. In the recent past, attaining citizenship for their adopted children was much more difficult, and as a result, the CHILD CITIZENSHIP ACT was enacted in 2000. This law was created in part because some adoptive parents in the past did not realize that they should have applied for citizenship for their children. In some rare but sad cases, children who were adopted as infants or small children were deported as adults, in part because of their lack of citizenship. Adoption agencies should be able to assist parents with completing the now streamlined citizenship paperwork for their child.

Children adopted from other countries should receive a complete physical examination within several weeks after their entry into the United States. If physicians are unfamiliar with what laboratory tests are needed, they may consult with the "Red Book" offered by the American Academy of Pediatrics. Children's IMMUNIZATIONS should also be validated. In some cases, the physician will check the child's blood for immunity to vaccine-preventable diseases, such as tetanus, diphtheria, polio, measles, mumps, and rubella (MMR), HEPATITIS B, and varicella (chicken pox).

Sometimes the child will need additional immunizations. Some doctors repeat all immunizations, to be certain that the child has received sufficient dosages of all needed vaccines.

Adjustment Challenges for Children Born Overseas

Most experts agree that adopting parents should learn as much as possible about how their child was cared for abroad; for example, whether the child slept in a crib or on a floor mat, slept wrapped tightly in a blanket or loosely, and so on. In addition, perhaps his formula was very sweet. The child may also have been carried on the caretaker's back. The agency should be able to obtain this kind of information from the orphanage staff, in most cases. Whenever possible or reasonable, the adoptive parent should try to recreate familiar situations so that the child will feel as comfortable as possible.

It is advisable for prospective parents to learn some basic words in the child's native tongue before the child arrives home, such as "mother," "father," "toilet," "time to eat," and "I love you." When possible and appropriate for the child's age, caregivers in the orphanage should prepare the child as much as possible for the adoption, showing the child photos of the adoptive parents before they arrive in the country. (See PREPARING A CHILD FOR ADOPTION.)

Families also need to realize that an extensive stay in an orphanage can have a profound impact on a child. Over the long term (years), orphanages are bad for children, even when they are staffed by well-meaning and kind people. Often orphanages are understaffed, and children do *not* receive enough attention or care. Kim MacLean discussed the impact of institutionalization in a 2003 article for *Development and Psychopathology.*

MacLean stated that, based on numerous studies, although institutionalization is a risk factor for less optimal development of a child, it does not inevitably lead to psychiatric problems. Said MacLean, "Institutionalization is clearly a risk factor for compromised development, but it is not possible to predict developmental outcome with any certainty knowing only that a particular child has been institutionalized early in life. When institutionalization is combined with other risk factors (e.g., low IQ, behavior problems, parenting stress, low socioeconomic status), it becomes easier to predict poor development outcomes."

More recently, researchers did an analysis of studies on children adopted from other countries, reporting their findings in a 2005 issue of the *Journal of the American Medical Association.* The researchers found that for the most part, children adopted from other countries were doing well. In fact, they found that children adopted internationally experienced fewer behavior problems and were less likely to be referred to psychiatric services than children adopted domestically. (It was unclear what the ages of the children were who were adopted domestically, so the comparison is inexact.)

However, this analysis did not include large numbers of children adopted in the past eight to 10 years from eastern European orphanages. Some evidence suggests that a significant number of those children have increasingly severe behavior disturbances as they enter adolescence and young adulthood.

Overall, however, the research generally continues to reflect the findings of earlier experts, confirming that most children adopted internationally fare well. This does not mean, however, that all is rosy, and some children have serious and long-term problems.

The longitudinal research of Rita Simon and Howard Altstein, and their findings on international adoptions, have been generally positive.

The most troubling findings have come from research on children adopted from Romania, but those data are not surprising, given the horrendous conditions of that country's orphanages at the time that Ceauşescu, the former dictator, was deposed and assassinated. In many cases, however, children have experienced catch-up in growth and development.

Some authors have warned that although many challenges can be surmounted and many children adopted from other countries are resilient, it is a mistake for adoptive parents to assume that race is not an issue. The reality of racial slurs is painful, but when children hear them, whether they are Asian, Latino, African American, Chinese, or of another race, their emotions need to be heeded. Rather than brushing it off as unimportant or saying that the comment was made by a child with "low self-esteem," the parent needs to acknowledge the problem. At the same time, parents should not overreact to every situation. It can be a difficult balancing act.

Says author Cheri Register in *Beyond Good Intentions: A Mother Reflects on Raising Internationally Adopted Children,* "Color blindness is a luxury our children can't afford. Although they have been raised in our families with whatever privileges we white parents claim for ourselves—material riches, well-maintained neighborhoods, good schools—away from home they take on the color of whichever ethnic or immigrant group they most resemble."

A Study of Adopted Adults

It is also instructive to look at adopted adults to obtain outcome data on individuals adopted from other countries. In one study of adopted adults from South Korea, published by the Evan B. Donaldson Adoption Institute in 2000, the researchers reported on their responses from 163 adults adopted from South Korea, 95 percent of whom were adopted by Americans. The respondents were recruited from international adoption agencies nationwide. They were adopted between 1956 and

1985, and the median age at the time of adoption was two years old.

The majority of the respondents (62 percent) had lived in an orphanage when they were adopted and 33 percent had lived with foster families, while 4 percent lived with their birth families. Most (71 percent) were raised by their adoptive families in small towns or rural areas. About half (52 percent) had one or more siblings also adopted from South Korea.

Among the respondents, 82 percent were female and 96 percent resided in the United States. The average age of the respondents was 31 years. Most were highly educated, and only 7 percent had just a high school diploma, while 42 percent were college graduates, and 24 percent had graduate degrees. The others had some college education or some graduate work or were students.

Most of the survey respondents (58 percent) were married or reported having a significant other. Male respondents had a 50 percent rate of having spouses/significant others who were Asian; the remainder had partners who were Caucasian. In contrast, 80 percent of the female respondents had a Caucasian partner, while 13 percent had Asian partners, 3 percent had African-American partners, and 3 percent had Latino partners.

The researchers found that the adopted adults who identified themselves with the Korean or Asian culture were more likely to be highly educated. Said the researchers, "With each higher educational level (high school, some college, college degree, graduate work and graduate degree), the level of identification with Korean or Asian heritage increased."

About half the respondents said they had explored their Korean heritage as children, and female respondents (57 percent) were more likely to have done so than male respondents (40 percent).

Most of the survey respondents reported experiencing discrimination as children, and race (70 percent) was cited more frequently than adopted status (28 percent) as the problem.

With regard to searching for their birthparents, about a third (29 percent) said that they had no interest in searching, while another third (34 per-

cent) said they were interested but had not yet taken any action. Twenty-two percent had searched or were currently searching for their birthparents, and 15 percent were not sure if they wanted to search.

Of those who said that they wanted to search for birthparents, the reasons given were as follows, with some respondents giving more than one reason (and they essentially duplicate the reasons why adults who were adopted domestically say that they wish to search for their birthparents): to obtain medical information (40 percent), curiosity (30 percent), to meet individuals they closely resembled (18 percent), to discover why the adoption occurred (18 percent), to determine if they had any biological relatives, especially siblings (16 percent), to gain a sense of closure or fill an emptiness (16 percent), and to give a message to their birthparents (10 percent).

When the adopted adults reported that they wanted to give a message to the birthparents, the messages were positive, such as "I would like to thank my mother," "I am happy and not to worry," and so forth.

See also ANEMIA, IRON DEFICIENCY; ATTACHMENT DISORDER; BONDING AND ATTACHMENT; EARLY INTERVENTION; EARLY PUBERTY/PRECOCIOUS PUBERTY; EASTERN EUROPEAN ADOPTIONS; EATING DISORDERS; GROWTH DELAYS; *HELICOBACTER PYLORI*; HUMAN IMMUNODEFICIENCY VIRUS; INDIA, ADOPTIONS FROM; LANGUAGE DELAY; LATIN AMERICAN ADOPTIONS; ORPHANAGE; PSYCHIATRIC PROBLEMS OF ADOPTED PERSONS; RESILIENCE; SENSORY INTEGRATION DISORDER; SLEEP DISORDERS IN NEWLY ADOPTED CHILDREN; TUBERCULOSIS.

Adamec, Christine. *The Complete Idiot's Guide to Adoption.* New York: Penguin, 2005.

Bartholet, Elizabeth. "International Adoption: Propriety, Prospects and Pragmatics," *Journal of the American Academy of Matrimonial Lawyers* 13, no. 2 (Winter 1996): 181–210.

Carlson, Richard R. "Transnational Adoption of Children," *Tulsa Law Journal* 23 (Spring 1988): 317–377.

Freundlich, Madelyn, and Joy Kim Lieberthal. *The Gathering of the First Generation of Adult Korean Adoptees: Adoptees' Perceptions of International Adoption.* New York: Evan B. Donaldson Adoption Institute, June 2000.

General Accounting Office. "Intercountry Adoption: Procedures Are Reasonable, but Sometimes Inefficiently Administered: Report to the Honorable Arlen Specter, U.S. Senate." GAO/NSIAD-93-83, April 1993. Available online. URL: http://archive.gao/gov/t2pbat6/149161. pdf. Accessed on August 2, 2005.

Juffer, Femmie, and Marinus H. van IJzendoorn. "Behavior Problems and Mental Health Referrals of International Adoptees: A Meta-Analysis," *Journal of the American Medical Association* 293, no. 20 (May 25, 2005): 2,501–2,515.

MacLean, Kim. "The Impact of Institutionalization on Child Development," *Development and Psychopathology* 15 (2003): 853–884.

Miller, Laurie, C., M.D. *The Handbook of International Adoption Medicine: A Guide for Physicians, Parents, and Providers.* New York, Oxford University Press, 2005.

Register, Cheri. *Beyond Good Intentions: A Mother Reflects on Raising Internationally Adopted Children.* St. Paul, Minn.: Yeong & Yeong Book Company, 2005.

Simon, Rita J., and Howard Altstein. *Adoption across Borders: Serving the Children in Transracial and Intercountry Adoptions.* Lanham, Md.: Rowman & Littlefield Publishers, 2000.

Sullivan, Sharon, M.D. "Cultural and Socio-Emotional Issues of Internationally Adopted Children," *International Pediatrics* 19, no. 4 (2004): 208–216.

Internet   People interested in adoption use the Internet for a variety of reasons; for example, ADOPTION AGENCIES create Web sites so that people can read about their organization without having to call them on the telephone to request brochures and pamphlets.

Public social service organizations also use the Internet to help them find adoptive families for foster children. The National Adoption Center makes extensive use of the Internet, providing photos of "waiting children" needing adoptive families and offering information on adoption topics at their Web site: http://www.adopt.org.

The National Adoption Information Clearinghouse offers publications on numerous adoption topics at their Web site: http://www.naic.acf.hhs.gov.

Adopted adults and birthparents also use the Internet extensively. Some are searching for biological relatives, and they use the Internet to perform the search as well as to obtain advice on how to perform the search. Some adopted adults strongly favor OPEN RECORDS, and they use the Internet to convey their opinion and to share news around the nation and the world. Some birthparents use the Internet in a similar way—to locate biological children and to learn new information or share information.

Some Drawbacks of the Internet

Although the Internet has many positive features, such as access to entire government documents and an immense array of research information, there are also some potential drawbacks. For example, there are some individuals with nefarious desires or motives who seek to obtain financial advantage over others, and who use the Internet to achieve their goals. (See FRAUD IN ADOPTION.)

Another problem is that many people who purvey information on the Internet have little or no knowledge about the topics in which they claim expertise. Before assuming the information on a Web site is accurate, it is important to try to determine if the individual or organization operating the site has any professional expertise or if there is any reason to believe that he/she really understands the topic. A mere presence on the Internet does not ensure expertise.

Many people make common errors with regard to the Internet. Some common errors include the following assumptions:

- That the information on the Internet is very current and was posted today or recently. In fact, the information could be several years old or more. Sometimes the date the information was posted or updated is listed on the site.

- That the information is accurate because it was posted by a person with a degree, such as an M.D. or J.D. Information should always be double-checked, as these credentials may be fraudulent.

- That the information is valid if the Web site is impressive-looking. It is relatively easy for one person to create a Web site—or to hire someone else to create it. A fancy Web site does not indicate that the information is valid.

- That sites with pictures of babies and/or stories that appeal to prospective adoptive parents are run by good people who really understand how they feel. What they may really understand is how to manipulate others, although many sites are run by sincere individuals.

Adamec, Christine. "Adoption and the Internet," *Adoption Factbook III*. Washington, D.C.: National Council for Adoption, 1999, 405–407.

interracial   See TRANSRACIAL ADOPTION.

interstate adoption   The adoption of a child who lives in one state by adoptive parents who reside in another state. The INTERSTATE COMPACT ON THE PLACEMENT OF CHILDREN (ICPC) is an agreement between the states that delineates how interstate adoption should be handled. All states in the United States are members of the compact at the time of this writing.

State social services department in each state administer the compact and ensure compliance with state laws.

Interstate Compact on Adoption and Medical Assistance (ICAMA)   An agreement between member states that governs the interstate delivery of medical services and adoption subsidies for adopted special needs children. Adopted in 1986 by nine states, 47 states plus the District of Columbia are now members. As of this writing, only the following states are *not* members: New York, Vermont, and Wyoming. In 1996 the Association of Administrators of the Interstate Compact on Adoption and Medical Assistance (AAICAMA) established associate memberships for private agencies, individuals, tribes, and others involved with the adoption of children with special needs. The American Public Human Services Administration acts as the secretariat for the AAICAMA, providing organization and staff support.

The reason for the creation of ICAMA was to protect children with special needs who move across state lines and ensure that they continue to receive appropriate medical assistance and subsidies.

When a family moves or a child is relocated to another state, the child has a MEDICAID card from the placing state; however, medical providers are often reluctant to accept Medicaid from another state. As a result, member states will provide a Medicaid card from the state to which the child has relocated.

States may either join ICAMA by enacting legislation of their state legislature, or an executive branch official may act for the state and sign the compact. For further information on ICAMA, contact:

Secretariat to the AAICAMA
American Public Human Services Association
810 First Street NE
Suite 500
Washington, DC 20002-4205
(202) 682-0100

See also ADOPTION SUBSIDY; INTERSTATE COMPACT ON THE PLACEMENT OF CHILDREN.

Interstate Compact on the Placement of Children
An agreement between states that governs the placement of children for adoption or foster care across state lines. It was drafted in the late 1950s, and New York was the first state to join the compact. According to the American Public Human Services Association, as of this writing, all states are members of the compact.

The compact is a safeguard for children. It ensures that the laws of both states involved have been complied with and that the child will receive appropriate supervision and required home studies will be done and followed up.

Each state appoints a compact administrator, who is within the state social services arm of the public welfare department (commonly known as the human services department.)

Compact administrators need about six weeks or more from the time the receiving compact office is notified of the proposed placement to process the various papers. (Some cases may take more or less time, depending on individual situations.)

The sending agency retains financial and legal responsibility for the child until the interstate placement ends due to adoption, the child reaching the age of majority or some other change. Violations of the compact are rare, but penalties do exist and children have been returned to the sending state when they were illegally placed.

The compact includes 10 articles.

intestinal parasitic infections   Infection with microorganisms including worms, protozoans, amoebae, and other organisms that usually live in the intestinal tract. Most parasitic infections are spread through contaminated food or water by individuals who have used poor personal hygiene. Some infections are spread via person-to-person while others may enter the body through contact with soil or animals. Most parasites are microscopic, but several forms can be seen with the naked eye when passed in the stool.

Parasites are extremely common in the developing world; some are also common in some regions of the United States. For example, *Giardia* is common in wooded areas. Studies indicate that 20–99 percent of children in developing countries are infested with one or more parasites. In many countries, treatment is not even given because the likelihood of reinfection is so great, and thus treatment seems futile. Infestation with multiple types of parasites is also common in residents of developing countries.

All internationally adopted children should be screened for intestinal parasites upon their arrival in the United States. Furthermore, if they develop symptoms suggestive of infection later on, screening should be repeated, because sometimes parasites are missed in the initial screening examinations.

Internationally adopted children frequently have intestinal parasites, and published prevalence studies have shown infection rates of 0–44 percent of international adoptees, depending on the country of origin. Children adopted from South Korea rarely have intestinal parasites, while virtually all children from Ethiopia are infected. About 20–40 percent of children adopted from Russia, other eastern European countries, China, and India have one or more intestinal parasite.

Types of Parasites Commonly Found among Children Adopted from Other Countries

Giardia lamblia, a protozoan, is the most commonly identified intestinal parasite found among internationally adopted children. It is transmitted through contaminated water or food. A stool immunoassay that is specific for *Giardia* infection is widely available and can be used to supplement direct fecal examination for diagnosis.

Other parasites reported as frequently occurring in internationally adopted children include *Enta-moeba histolytica* (an amoeba), *Dientamoeba fragilis, Ascaris lumbridoides, Trichuris trichiura CK, Strongyloides stercoralis,* various forms of hookworms, and *Enterobius* (pinworms). Other nonpathogenic parasites are often found in stool samples, but they do not usually require treatment.

Symptoms and Diagnostic Path

Infection with a parasite may cause such symptoms as anemia, diarrhea, flatulence, abdominal pain, and poor growth, as well as other clinical problems. However, some infected individuals have no symptoms or they are only intermittently symptomatic.

The diagnosis is made by examining stool samples. The recommended method is to collect three samples that are each two-three days apart. An examination of a fresh sample or one that has been collected in a special preservative (polyvinyl alcohol) is the best means to identify the presence of any parasites. These samples should be submitted to an experienced microbiology laboratory for analysis.

Treatment Options and Outlook

Specific treatments (specialized antibiotics) are recommended to treat each type of parasite, thus, a child with multiple parasites may require several courses of different treatments. Internationally adopted children who are treated for parasites not common in the United States should remain parasite-free once the infestation has been cleared.

Risk Factors and Preventive Measures

Most parasites are transmitted by fecal-oral contact, person-to-person contact, or by contaminated toys or bathwater. Transmission is best prevented by thorough hand-washing after diaper changes and by hand-washing after each use of the toilet. Bathwater should not be reused for a second or third child, and each child should be bathed individually until parasites are eradicated. Careful attention to hygiene helps to limit exposure to parasites.

jargon used in adoption   See TERMINOLOGY.

judge   Elected or appointed individual, usually also an attorney, who grants the FINALIZATION of an adoption and gives the adopted child all the legal rights of a child born to the family. Usually this procedure is performed in the judge's chambers or a private waiting room, although some adoption proceedings are held in a courtroom.

When protective services social workers recommend that parental rights of an abusive or neglectful parent be terminated, it is the judge who will decide whether or not to terminate these rights.

See also CUSTODY; TERMINATION OF PARENTAL RIGHTS.

kin See BIRTH KIN.

kinship care Generally, refers to foster children cared for by biological relatives of the birthparents. Sometimes included under the definition are informal arrangements that do not involve any foster care or government involvement.

As part of FAMILY PRESERVATION, or in some cases to avoid TRANSRACIAL ADOPTION, kinship care has been seen as a way to keep children in their biological families until their birthparents can care for them again. As many as half of the children in foster care may be living with relatives. According to a 1998 article in *Social Work*, "Currently, although all states treat kinship care as a kind of family foster care guided by federal policies on out-of-home placements . . . jurisdictions vary widely in their kinship care policies and practices." For example, relative caregivers may or may not be able to receive foster-care payments, depending on state policy.

Advantages and Disadvantages to Kinship Care

A primary advantage to kinship care is that the child can continue contact with relatives, often individuals he or she has known for years, and who love and accept the child. It may also be less stigmatizing to a child to be in kinship care than to be in the foster-care system with nonrelatives.

The key disadvantage, however, is that sometimes the extended family has as many emotional or other problems as the birthparents and thus may not always provide suitable care for the children. Kinship arrangements are likely to involve caregivers who are older, in poor health, less educated, and poorer than nonrelative foster parents. Also, when the child lives with relatives, the child may have more contact with the abusive or neg-lectful parent than social workers feel is appropriate. In addition, critics argue that kinship care providers are not as thoroughly screened by state social workers as are nonrelative foster parents, nor are the children's cases monitored as closely. Adoption is also less likely, as relatives are often hesitant to move to terminate parental rights.

In most cases, the person providing kinship care is the child's grandmother, followed by the aunt. Some research has indicated that as many as 90 percent of the children in kinship care are African Americans. In some states where Latinos are the majority ethnic group in foster care, they are underrepresented among kinship care families.

As with children in nonrelative foster care, children in kinship care often do not receive adequate immunizations or routine health care or dental care. According to an article in a 1998 issue of *Pediatric Nursing*, "There are greater numbers of developmental and mental health problems in children in kinship care than in children in foster care." When health care is used, it is often the hospital emergency room, because the child has no regular physician.

According to *CQ Researcher*, problems with kinship care have led some states to establish a "subsidized guardianship" arrangement, wherein the relative receives a monthly subsidy and is recognized as the child's legal guardian, but there are serious questions about using "guardianship" as a means to deal with these problems.

Because of serious problems with children who remain in the foster care system, many of whom are in kinship care, the ADOPTION AND SAFE FAMILIES ACT was passed in 1997. This legislation was created to move children out of foster care and back to their families or to an adoptive family, but it does provide language that is flexible and can be applied by the states to kinship care. In many cases, states may avoid termination of parental rights if the child is being cared for by a relative.

A National Adoption Information Clearinghouse factsheet released in March 2005 recommends that new kin caregivers should ask the child welfare caseworker the following questions when assuming formal responsibility for the child or children:

- Who has legal custody of the children?
- What rights and responsibilities does legal custody give in this state? Physical custody?
- Will I or the children have to go to court?
- Who is responsible for enrolling the children in school, obtaining health insurance, granting permission for medical care and obtaining it, signing school permission forms, etc?
- Will someone from child welfare services visit my home on regular basis?
- What are the requirements for me and my home if I want the children to live with me?
- Are the requirements different if the children are with me just temporarily?

- What services are available for me and for the children, and how do I apply?
- Are there restrictions on the discipline I can use (such as spanking) with the children?
- What subsidies or financial assistance is available? What do I need to do to apply?
- Am I eligible to become a licensed foster parent and receive a foster care subsidy?

See also FOSTER CARE; GRANDPARENT CAREGIVERS; GRANDPARENT ADOPTIONS.

Cox, Rachel. "Foster Care Reform," *CQ Researcher* 8, no. 1 (January 9, 1998): 3–10.

Gennaro, Susan. "Vulnerable Infants: Kinship Care and Health," *Pediatric Nursing* 24, no. 2 (March–April 1998): 119–124.

National Adoption Information Clearinghouse. "Kinship Caregivers and the Child Welfare System: A Factsheet for Families." U.S. Department of Health and Human Services, Administration for Children and Families, Administration on Children, Youth and Families, Children's Bureau, Washington, D.C., March 2005.

Korea   See SOUTH KOREA, ADOPTIONS FROM.

language   See TERMINOLOGY.

language delay   Speaking words or phrases later than is expected for the child's chronological age. Such delays are common among internationally adopted children.

Many internationally adopted children have language delays related to the need to learn to speak a new language. However, delays in the child's birth language are exceedingly common. These delays hinder mastery of the new language. Many parents who adopt children from other countries seek out the assistance of speech pathologists. According to speech pathologist Sharon Glennen in her article for the *American Journal of Speech-Language Pathology*, after pediatricians and dentists, speech pathologists are the third most popular specialists sought out by adoptive parents.

Some children adopted in the United States also have language delays due to DEVELOPMENTAL DISABILITIES, PRENATAL EXPOSURES, and other problems, such as child abuse or neglect. Children may have other disabilities causing language delays, such as hearing impairments. Children adopted from other countries also often experience environmental deprivation that may lead to generalized developmental delays and compound their problem of language delays.

Adoptive parents who suspect or know that a child has language delay should seek assistance from their pediatrician as well as from school authorities. If the child is of preschool age, he or she may benefit from an EARLY INTERVENTION program.

A major dilemma in an expert evaluation of internationally adopted infants and toddlers is that most have not fully mastered age-appropriate language skills in their country of origin. These delays

hinder the transition to the new language of their adoptive parents. Yet most children do successfully master this task. Researchers have not been able to determine which children are more or less likely to have more long-lasting language delays.

If a child born in the United States has a language delay, this is a far more obvious problem than when the child is born in another country and has lived there for a year or longer. Nor is the situation of the internationally adopted infant or toddler comparable to the situation of an adolescent or adult who has fully mastered the language and then relocates to another country and subsequently becomes bilingual. The children adopted as infants or toddlers will not retain the language learned in infancy unless others continue to speak to them in this tongue, which is very unlikely.

Complicating the problem, according to Glennen, is that the child originally may have been speaking a language other than what was recorded in the official records, thus making the evaluation more difficult. Often speech experts rely upon patterns found in the native language to predict a child's possible strengths and weaknesses in English. However, Glennen points out that the language the child has learned may be very different from the language the parents assume he or she has learned. Says Glennen,

> For example, some children adopted from Latin America are from regions in which Indian languages such as Quecha are spoken. Children from China or India may be from regions in which languages other than Mandarin or Hindi are L1 [language one, or the first language]. Adoptive parents who don't speak the language may not realize what language or dialect the child was learning, and may erroneously assume that the language used on government documents was the child's birth language.

If the child is from a country with multiple languages or distinct regional dialects, families and professionals should make inquiries through the adoption agency or international adoption support groups, or consult with natives of the country to determine the likely birth language.

Some studies have shown dramatic catch up from language delays in some children. For example, in a study of 186 girls, aged 18–35 months old, who were adopted from China by Americans when they were between the ages of three and 25 months (with an average age of 11.0 months), described in *Early Childhood Research Quarterly* in 2005, the researchers found that the adopted children were fully caught up to their peers in the United States after living with their adoptive families for an average of about 16 months. Incredibly, after that point, some children surpassed the level of their peers in language development. This is encouraging information for many adoptive parents, although more research is needed.

See also INTERNATIONAL ADOPTION; MEDICAL PROBLEMS OF INTERNATIONALLY ADOPTED CHILDREN.

Glennen, Sharon. "Language Development and Delay in Internationally Adopted Infants and Toddlers: A Review," *American Journal of Speech-Language Pathology* 11 (November 2002): 333–339.

Miller, Laurie, C., M.D. *The Handbook of International Adoption Medicine: A Guide for Physicians, Parents, and Providers.* New York: Oxford University Press, 2005.

Xing Tan, Tony, and Yi Yang. "Language Development of Chinese Adoptees 18–35 Months Old," *Early Childhood Research Quarterly* 20 (2005) 57–68.

large families

Some adoptive parents have very large families, at least in terms of U.S. averages.

Those who believe some of these large families are not healthy describe adoptive parents in such large families as "child collectors" and believe that the children do not receive adequate individual attention. Scattered media stories of rare cases of children in large families feed this viewpoint.

Supporters believe the children provide each other with a great deal of attention, and a large family can be particularly nurturing for a child with SPECIAL NEEDS.

Sometimes a family is large because it adopts four or more siblings. Researchers and social workers Dorothy LePere, Lloyd Davis, Janus Couve, and Mona McDonald studied adoptions of large sibling groups and reported their findings in the booklet *Large Sibling Groups: Adoption Experiences.* The majority (87%) of the siblings studied were adopted together in groups of three or more children.

According to the researchers, parents with experience are good candidates for becoming well-functioning adoptive parents. "Those who are already parenting four or more children, or who have come from large families of origin, seem to have fewer adjustment problems."

Researchers noted that families who adopt large sibling groups sometimes cannot depend on their extended family or friends for support and should have the capacity to develop new support systems.

The authors concluded that large families can work effectively and stated, "The results of the questionnaire and the authors' research and experiences have demonstrated that the adoption of a large sibling group is rewarding and challenging both for the family and for the adoption worker."

LePere, Dorothy W., Lloyd E. Davis, Janus Couve, and Mona McDonald. *Large Sibling Groups: Adoption Experiences.* Washington, D.C.: Child Welfare League of America, 1986.

Latin American adoptions

The adoption of children in Central and South America and Mexico. According to the U.S. State Department, 4,172 orphans were adopted from Central and South America by Americans in fiscal year 2005. Most of the children (3,783) immigrated from GUATEMALA, with 291 from Colombia, and 98 children adopted from Mexico. Guatemala has been one of the top five countries of origin of children adopted from other countries since 1992.

Criteria for prospective parents wishing to adopt from Latin America, including the upper limit on age of adoptive parents and number of children already in the home, vary greatly. Some countries will allow adoptive parents as old as 55 years to adopt infants and have no limits on the number of children in the home already. Most Latin American countries require adopting parents to travel to the country and stay at least several days until legal paperwork is accomplished. In some cases, the stay may last weeks.

International adoption is very changeable, and prospective adoptive parents are urged to thoroughly investigate this form of adoption before applying to an agency or identifying a foreign attorney. An adoptive parents support group is a good start.

See also INTERNATIONAL ADOPTION; MEDICAL PROBLEMS OF INTERNATIONALLY ADOPTED CHILDREN.

Latinos   Many U.S. adoptive parents adopt children from Latin America; in addition, Latino children are also available to be adopted in such states as Texas, New York, Florida, California, and other states with large Latino populations. Most adoptive parents are probably not of Latino ancestry.

Most agencies are willing to place Latino children with non-Latino families, although some agencies make a concerted effort to place Latino children only in Latino homes of a similar culture, race, and physical appearance.

A study of transethnically adopted Latino children was undertaken by Estela Andujo. Andujo studied 30 Anglo families who adopted Mexican-American children and 30 Mexican-American families who adopted Mexican-American children, both groups in the Los Angeles, California, area. She found no differences in the self-esteem levels of the children in either group; however, she did find differences in how the children perceived themselves, with the children raised in Anglo families identifying more with their white parents and identifying less with the Mexican-American community.

See also INTERNATIONAL ADOPTION.

Andujo, Estela. "Ethnic Identity of Transethnically Adopted Hispanic Adolescents," *Social Work* 33 (November/December 1988): 531–535.

laws, federal   See ADOPTION AND SAFE FAMILIES ACT; ADOPTION ASSISTANCE AND CHILD WELFARE ACT OF 1980; FEDERAL GOVERNMENT; INDIAN CHILD WELFARE ACT OF 1978.

laws, state   Each state has its own set of laws that govern who may adopt, who may be adopted, and under what conditions adoptions may occur. Other issues, such as whether information on the adop-

tion may be made available, whether or not adoption must be confidential, and how adoptions are to be administered are also issues the state decides.

The states must follow federal rules and regulations regarding the adoption of certain children or risk losing federal funds. Probably the most important federal laws to impact adoptions have been the ADOPTION ASSISTANCE AND CHILD WELFARE ACT OF 1980 and the ADOPTION AND SAFE FAMILIES ACT of 1997.

Adoption laws are not static, and changes to state laws are common.

lawsuits   See ATTORNEYS; BLOOD TIES; INHERITANCE; SURROGACY ARRANGEMENTS; TERMINATION OF PARENTAL RIGHTS; WRONGFUL ADOPTION.

lawyer   See ATTORNEYS; INDEPENDENT ADOPTION; WRONGFUL ADOPTION.

legal custody   See CUSTODY.

legal father   The man legally recognized as the father of a child, irrespective of whether he is the biological father or not. When a couple is married, and the wife bears a child, the law generally presumes her husband is the biological father of the child, even though he may not be. (See BIRTHFATHER for more information on the 1989 challenge to this status, which the U.S. Supreme Court denied.)

In a few states, this presumption cannot be challenged, and the U.S. Supreme Court has upheld such laws (*Michael H. v. Gerald D.,* 57 U.S.L.W. 4691, June 13, 1989). In many states, however, the presumption of paternity can be legally challenged with strong evidence, such as genetic testing. If there is no challenge to the legal father's status, then it stands.

Also, in about half the states, the husband is specifically described as the legal father in the case of artificial insemination.

As a result of statutes regarding legal fathers, if a married woman wishes to plan adoption for her child, her husband, as the presumed legal father, must also sign the consent for adoption forms. Some agencies and attorneys may seek consent from the alleged biological father as well as the husband if the mother states that the child's father is someone other than her husband.

If the name of a man not married to the child's mother is listed on the birth certificate of a child with his consent and if the mother is not married to someone else, then he is the presumed father. Some states, however, permit rebuttal of this presumption by proof (usually genetic tests) showing that the presumed father is not the biological father.

Adoptive fathers become legal fathers upon finalization of an adoption when a new birth certificate is issued with the adoptive father's name appearing as the father.

See also SEALED RECORDS.

legal risk adoption   See AT-RISK PLACEMENT.

lifebook   As used in an adoption of an OLDER CHILD especially, a scrapbook documenting a child's life to date and created for and with a child with the assistance of a social worker, psychologist, foster parent, and/or other individuals. The lifebook may be one of the few possessions the child can call his own prior to his adoption.

The purpose of the lifebook is to provide meaning and continuity to a displaced child whose life may have been extremely disrupted. It is designed to capture memories and provide a chance to recall people and events in the child's past life, to allow for a sense of continuity. The lifebook can also serve as a focal point to explore painful issues with the child that need to be resolved.

Children who grow up as members of one family usually have ready access to birth certificates, baby and family pictures, and other evidences of growing up, as well as items that would be placed in a scrapbook.

Foster children often do not have tangible information about their growing up, and the lifebook can serve to help them feel important and "connected" in time. Lifebooks also may cover and explain major events and developmental milestones, such as when the child first walked, talked, and so forth.

See also PREPARING A CHILD FOR ADOPTION.

loss   A feeling of emotional deprivation that is, at some point in time, experienced by each member of the ADOPTION TRIAD.

No matter how certain a birthparent is that adoption is the right decision for a child, there will be times when the loss of the child is keenly felt. The initial loss will usually be felt at or subsequently to placement of the child. Caring social workers realize that when a birthmother goes home from the hospital, she must contend with feelings of loss and separation in addition to any hormonal imbalance she may also suffer. Birthmothers also report that they think about the child on the child's birthday.

If the birthmother was not pressured into her decision to place the child for adoption and believes it was primarily her own decision, she is more able to cope with the feelings of loss she will experience. She will also realize that whatever the resolution of a pregnancy, particularly if it is unintended, some feeling of loss is inevitable.

Adoptive parents who are infertile feel a loss as well, and their loss is their inability to bear a genetic child. Individuals who are actively seeking to achieve a pregnancy have reported feeling anger or despair when they see pregnant women in public and a terrible sense of a lack of control over their own destinies. Hopefully, they will have resolved most of their own anxiety over infertility prior to adopting a child so they can fully accept a child who does not share their genes. (See INFERTILITY.)

An adopted child may feel a sense of loss at various points in time; for example, if a child is adopted at infancy, the first time the child realizes he is adopted, perhaps at age five or six, and that this means his adoptive mother was not pregnant with him, can be painful because the child loves the mother and wants to be as close as possible to her. Another possibly difficult time for an adoptive child is adolescence, when questions of identity and questions about life become important to the average teenager, adopted or nonadopted. Although most adopted children who were adopted as infants are as well-adjusted as the average nonadopted person, if there will be an identity crisis, it will probably be during adolescence. (See ADOLESCENT ADOPTED PERSONS; IDENTITY.)

Katherine Gordy Levine, M.S.W., director of group homes, SCAN, in New York and also adjunct professor at the Columbia University School of Social Work, points out that it should not be presumed that children adopted as adolescents who are ACTING OUT are unhappy with their parents or feel their parents are inadequate. Instead, she says, "The adjustment of children to a foster home before becoming adolescents is a good barometer of whether the problem originates in parental problems or the adolescents' shifting thoughts."

In some cases, Levine says, the adolescent may blame adoptive parents for problems stemming from treatment received by birthparents. "The tendency to blame the current parents and to focus on their limitations is often simultaneously used by placed adolescents to negate biological parents' failings. If all parents are bad, biological parents are not so bad."

Levine says adolescents "need to mourn and make sense of the experiences of their lives . . . when the wounds created by placement can be closed, peace can be made with the past, and life can move forward once again."

Adopted adults may again experience a sense of loss when they marry and have children themselves, wondering about their genetic links to their birthparents. If the adopted adult is infertile, the infertility may be even more painful than for the nonadopted infertile person; however, presuming the adopted person felt positively about his or her own adoption, he or she may perceive adoption as a very good way to create his or her own family.

Older adopted children may experience feelings of loss, not only from their birthparents, if they were old enough to remember when they separated, but also from foster parents, if they are adopted by another family. Adoptive parents are advised to recognize these feelings and help the child resolve them. If possible, adopting parents should initially meet the child at the foster parents' home.

Many experts recommend the use of a LIFEBOOK, which is a special scrapbook for adopted older children, chronicling the child's life. It is also helpful to allow the child to talk about the past and reflect upon it. Talking about previous experiences need not mean the child is unhappy with the adoptive parents but is more likely to mean the child feels comfortable and safe about talking about important events in his or her life.

See also BIRTHMOTHER.

Fahlberg, Vera, M.D. *Attachment and Separation: Putting the Pieces Together.* Chelsea, Mich.: National Resource Center for Special Needs Adoption, 1979.

Jewett, Claudia. *Helping Children Cope with Separation and Loss.* Boston: Harvard Common Press, 1982.

Levine, Katherine Gordy. "The Placed Child Examines the Quality of Parental Care," *Child Welfare* 67 (July–August 1988): 301–310.

married birthparents   An estimated 6 percent or more of all infants placed for adoption were placed by their married parents, according to studies by the National Center for Health Statistics.

Married birthparents place their infants for adoption primarily because they do not believe in abortion but feel unwilling or unable to parent the child. Often they may have other children and suffer financial problems.

They may also be on the verge of a divorce or a separation and not want the child as a constant reminder of their former relationship together.

When married birthparents decide on adoption for their infants, they are often viewed with contempt and suspicion by the rest of society, who cannot understand how or why a married birthparent would do such a thing; ironically, it is perfectly understandable and acceptable to many that married people might choose to abort a fetus.

Sometimes the child who is placed for adoption is a toddler, and the reasons for placement are similar to the reasons for making an adoption decision for a newborn infant: financial problems, marital problems, child abuse or neglect, or career goals that conflict with parenting a child.

The married birthparent might also face debilitating health or personal problems that his mate also finds difficult to cope with; as a result, both feel that having the child adopted by a loving couple is a viable solution.

For married birthparents, confidentiality and anonymity may be particularly important, given the lack of understanding society often has for their dilemma.

matching   The attempt to select adoptive parents similar to the child to be adopted. The selected parents and children may be similar in appearance, interests, intelligence, personality, or other traits. This practice has also become known more recently as trying to achieve a "good fit" when choosing a family for a specific child. Other components may be included in the parent selection process, such as the ability to meet a child's unusual or specific needs (for example, if the child has a medical problem with which the parents have experience).

Religion

Some agencies attempt to match a child based on religion, although religious matching is more often based on the preference of the birthmother. (Most sectarian agencies limit applications to couples with certain religion backgrounds.)

State adoption laws prior to the 1970s were very restrictive in some states and mandated matching despite the wishes of the birthmother. (Several cases are covered in *The Law of Adoption and Surrogate Parenting* by Irving J. Sloan.)

In 1954, in the Massachusetts case of *In re Goldman*, a Jewish couple attempted to adopt twins whose birthmother was Catholic. Although the children had lived with the couple for three years, the court decreed they could not adopt the children because Catholic couples waited to adopt children. The court refused to consider the birthmother's wishes. In contrast, a birthmother today may often specify the religion of the family that will adopt her child.

In a 1957 case, the Ellis family, a Jewish couple, adopted a newborn child in Massachusetts. State officials later demanded the child be returned since the birthmother was Catholic. The adoptive parents fled to Florida. (The birthmother did not wish to revoke consent.)

Governor Collins of Florida, who received more than 9,000 calls, letters, and telegrams both pro and con, refused to extradite the couple, stating that "the controlling question . . . must be the welfare of the child."

In another case in 1971, a trial court held that a couple could not adopt because a "lack of belief in a Supreme Being rendered them unfit to be adoptive parents." The adoption agency had insisted the prospective adoptive parents were people of high moral standards and argued they should be allowed to adopt. The New Jersey Supreme Court reversed the lower court.

Ethnic Matching and Physical Appearance

If the child to be adopted is an infant, the social worker will compare the birthparents to the adoptive parents in an attempt to make a suitable match; for example, if the birthmother is very musically inclined, the social worker seeking to make a match will not place the infant in a home where both adoptive parents are tone-deaf. (Note: Some caseworkers do not believe in physical matching, and adopting parents should not depend on adopting a child who resembles them.)

When attempting to match for personality (if such matching is tried), a social worker will not place the child of a serious and bookish birthmother with a family who lives for weekend football.

Sometimes a factor to be considered in making a match is socioeconomic status: The child of a college student will probably not be placed with a blue-collar worker, particularly in the case of an OPEN ADOPTION. (On the other hand, the child of a blue-collar worker will be placed with an upper middle-class family.)

Proponents of matching point to studies that indicate similarities between the adoptive parents and their adopted offspring lead to greater harmony and happiness. Adoption experts, such as Ruth McRoy, Ph.D., say the "goodness of fit" is important, and the more closely the child fits in with the family, the more he or she will thrive. McRoy, et al., also take issue with the MULTIETHNIC PLACEMENT ACT.

Dissenters insist it is often impossible to achieve realistic matches, and just because a birthmother is musical does not mean her child will also be musi-

cally talented nor will the child's personality necessarily be anything like that of the parents. They also point out that biological children often do not resemble their parents.

Opponents of matching add that painstakingly trying to match an adopted child to an adoptive family is a form of denial and a way to make it easier for the adoptive family to pretend the child is their biological child. Other opponents of matching say the practice results in unnecessarily long stays in foster care for black and other non-Caucasian children.

See also GENETIC PREDISPOSITIONS; RELIGION.

Delaney, Robert W. "1957 Decision Puts Baby-Swapping Case in Perspective," *Florida Today,* November 17, 1988, 10B.

McRoy, Ruth G., Harold D. Grotevant, Louis A. Zurcher Jr. *Emotional Disturbances in Adopted Adolescents: Origins and Development.* New York: Praeger Press, 1988.

Sloan, Irving J. *The Law of Adoption and Surrogate Parenting.* New York: Oceana Publications, 1988.

maternity homes   Residences for pregnant women. The number of homes has decreased over the past two decades, and existing homes often have a waiting list of women.

Some organizations have recruited families who volunteer to house women in crisis pregnancies, but these are usually not licensed and are not included in the estimates.

The women who live in a maternity home usually pay no fee to live in the home, and they often apply for public assistance and MEDICAID payments to cover their medical costs.

Women who use maternity homes may be adults or adolescents. They may also be teenage foster children who are wards of the court, if the maternity home has a license for group foster care.

The services provided by a maternity home usually include counseling, aid in applying for public assistance programs such as Temporary Aid to Needy Families (TANF), food stamps and Medicaid, nutritional advice, and encouragement and assistance in continuing education or identifying career opportunities.

Most maternity homes utilize volunteers who will drive women to the physician, supermarket, welfare office, and other sites where she must go.

See also CRISIS PREGNANCY.

maternity services   See MATERNITY HOMES.

mature women planning adoption   Although most women with crisis pregnancies who choose adoption are in their late teens or early twenties, there are also women in their late twenties and thirties and even forties who choose adoption for their children.

They may be married and already have three, four, or more children. Faced with an unplanned pregnancy but morally opposed to abortion, they view adoption as a loving solution. Other mature women may be divorced or divorcing, or they may be single women.

Few adoption agencies are structured to deal with mature women; instead, their informational packets and counseling are more oriented to teenagers with crisis pregnancies. There are, however, agencies that offer separate living quarters and specially designed programs for this age group.

Social workers should realize that mature women with unplanned pregnancies also need positive support and do not desire patronizing attitudes.

Some mature women have asked agencies for help only to be turned away and told to come back in their last trimester if they still want help. Such action does not allow the woman a chance to receive counseling and other services. If she is turned away, she is deprived of needed assistance to plan for her child's future and her own future as well, and this action can severely inhibit the success of an adoption plan should the birthmother desire adoption.

Whether they are considering adoption or not, such women need information and assistance to help them gain necessary prenatal care. They may also need income and shelter to avoid the plight of homelessness or physical abuse by the father of the baby.

media and adoption   Depictions of adopted children and adults, adoptive parents and birthparents in the broadcast media (television and radio), movies and theatre, and print media. In addition, many people obtain information about adoption from media outlets available on the INTERNET.

One common complaint of adopted individuals and adoptive parents about the media's depiction of adoption is the frequent singling out of a celebrity's adopted children and children born to the family when adoption plays no role whatsoever in the story. For example, a celebrity's biological child may be simply referred to as "Mary" while his adopted son is alluded to as "Frank, his adopted son." If adoptive status is irrelevant, then it should not be mentioned. (See also ATTITUDES ABOUT ADOPTION.)

Although it is not possible to quantify the overall effect of the media on people's general views about adoption, some effect is very likely, particularly when considering the television media and its extensive reach to all segments of society. The effect of movies is also important on a smaller segment of society. Print media, albeit more selective, also has a broad impact, as does radio broadcast media. The Internet has a broad global reach, with some researchers posting studies for anyone to read, and adoption agencies or support groups providing information and advice on adoption. There are thousands of sites on the Internet that mention adoption.

Key Study of the Media and Adoption

Although performed in 1988, one study of the media and its depiction of adoption is still valuable. This study, performed by Dr. George Gerbner of the Annenberg School of Communications at the University of Pennsylvania, concentrated on television, film, and print coverage of adoption. The study was funded by the Catholic Adoptive Parents Association Inc. in New York City. According to Gerbner's report, Americans encountered vivid images of adoption, adopted children, and adoptive parents most often in television drama. Significant dramatic portrayals occurred, on the average, at least six times a year.

Television   According to Gerbner's analysis, "The treatment of adoption ranged from the highly sensitive and thoughtful to the hackneyed and stereotypic." He found the legal process of adoption as the predominant theme, appearing in nearly half of the television programs offering adoption themes.

Next most prominent, with almost one-third of the programs depicting some variation on this theme, was the "shady deal": baby buying, cheating birthmothers, and the stealing of babies.

Although illegal activities do occur in the real world of adoptions, they represent a tiny minority of all adoptions. Instead, most infant adoptions are lawful; however, a primary purpose of electronic media such as television and movies is to entertain and dramatize. The average successful adoption would probably seem very boring to a television producer.

As a result, when the public continually views stories about adoption scams, it is highly probable viewers will conclude that shady adoptions are an everyday occurrence. In addition, adoption itself is viewed more suspiciously, as are birthmothers considering adoption and prospective adoptive parents.

Films Portrayals of adoptions in 87 films from 1927 to 1987 were analyzed by Gerbner. Of these movies, 60 percent concentrated on the process of adoption, a pattern also seen in television. The researchers selected movies that seemed to typify plots over the long term. "Bad seed" themes were considered: in fact, a film entitled *The Bad Seed* was released in 1956 and depicted a child with homicidal traits, supposedly inherited from her biological grandparent.

These and similar films may have profoundly affected viewers' attitudes toward adoption, particularly the attitudes of baby boomers who were then children. Such film treatments cause concern over possible GENETIC PREDISPOSITIONS toward "evil" and inherited bad genes.

The researchers stated that film coverage appeared to be less bound to "formulas" than is television coverage in depiction of adoption.

Print Media The print media is rife with misinformation and negative information on adoption. Said Gerbner, "Litigation, rackets, abuses, and other illegalities linked to adoption, including suits over parenthood, claims of baby-switching and selling, race-related disputes, and various scandals are the most likely to make the subject of adoption—as indeed many other subjects—newsworthy," said Gerbner.

Gerbner concluded, "Adoption is depicted as a troubling and troublesome issue . . . Useful and helpful information is available to those who seek it. But images and messages most viewers and readers encounter most of the time are more likely to project than to deflect the common problems adopted persons and their families face in our culture."

A Newer Media Study

A decade after Gerbner's work, Beth Waggenspack analyzed media coverage of adoption in her 1998 article for *Adoption Quarterly* and found dismaying results. According to Waggenspack, "Unfortunately, most people hear about adoption only through popular media (news and entertainment), which skews coverage towards the dramatic, sensational, or exploitative."

She found negative media coverage in a ratio of at least 2 to 1. She said that adopted children were frequently depicted as troubled individuals, and if an adopted person committed a crime, that fact was mentioned even though it was nearly always irrelevant to the crime. Said Waggenspack, "One might even argue that if the popular press always mentioned when a criminal had red hair, the public would soon develop prejudices about redheads, given what we know about the media's ability to set our agendas and direct our cognitive patterns."

Gerbner, George B., with the assistance of Sr. Elvira Arcenas and Marc Rubner. *Adoption in the Mass Media: A Preliminary Survey of Sources of Information and a Pilot Study,* unpublished, The Annenberg School of Communications, University of Pennsylvania, Philadelphia, November 21, 1988.

Waggenspack, Beth M. "The Symbolic Crises of Adoption: Popular Media's Agenda Setting," *Adoption Quarterly* 1, no. 4 (1998) 57–82.

Medicaid Medical assistance program for individuals categorically eligible for public assistance, including low-income pregnant women, low-income parents with dependents (both are eligible under Temporary Aid to Needy Families [TANF]) and other categories. The program is funded with both federal and state money and originated with the 1965 amendments to the Social Security Act (Title XIX). It was also referenced in the ADOPTION AND SAFE FAMILIES ACT because children need services Medicaid pays for.

Adoptive parents of children with special needs are eligible to receive Medicaid for their adopted children. Problems have arisen when a Medicaid card was issued to a child in one state and the parents then moved to another state or when the child was adopted by parents from another state. Many of these problems have been resolved by issuing the parent a card from the state in which he or she lives; however, problems still occur.

See also INTERSTATE ADOPTION; INTERSTATE COMPACT ON THE PLACEMENT OF CHILDREN.

medical history Information on medical, mental, or genetic background and/or chronic diseases and conditions in birthparents as well as in their parents, siblings, uncles, aunts, and grandparents. These conditions are identified in the child, when known, and also include birth history, serial growth measurements, a record of hospitalizations and surgeries, list of medications given, physical examination findings, and a record of IMMUNIZATIONS. In addition, the medical history includes information on lifestyle choices, such as prenatal alcohol or drug use or smoking behaviors of the birthparents, their previous imprisonments, occupations, and so forth.

In some cases, particularly with an INTERNATIONAL ADOPTION, there may be little or no medical history available on the birthparents. In some cases, medical information on the birthparents of children in FOSTER CARE, and sometimes on the children themselves, may be sketchy and difficult to obtain.

It is also true that even when birthparents are willing and available to provide medical history information, sometimes they may provide only limited data. For example, they may be in good health, since most birthparents choosing adoption in the United States are in their 20s or younger and at the peak of their health, unless there is an alcohol or drug abuse problem that is present. As a result, social workers should ask birthparents to obtain and provide medical information about their own parents, since many chronic illnesses (such as arthritis, cancer, diabetes, hypertension, and heart disease) appear when individuals are in their 40s or older. These illnesses often have a genetic component, and thus the information would be useful to the adoptive parents and the adopted child.

Obtaining Available Medical Information Is Important

Adoptive parents should obtain as much medical information as reasonably possible on the child or children they adopt. Not only will this information assist their pediatrician, but it will ultimately serve to assist the adopted adult later in life. Adult adopted persons, particularly women when they are pregnant, often report anxiety about a lack of medical history information. This information could satisfy their curiosity about their heredity and the genes they may pass on to their children. However, when medical information is not available on birthparents, in some cases physicians can perform laboratory tests on children to detect the presence or likelihood of many illnesses.

Questions about Health Conditions Prospective Adoptive Parents Will Accept in a Child They Adopt

In many cases, social workers supply prospective parents with a checklist of ailments, disabilities, and other conditions they would be willing to accept in a child. For example, mental illness in the birth family, incest, the rape of the birthmother, heart disease, genetic diseases, congenital birth defects or alcohol exposure, prematurity, and a broad spectrum of possible diseases or conditions may be listed. Prospective parents may be asked to state yes, no, or maybe to each case or condition.

When parents will be adopting an infant, the caseworker will want to know if they are willing to accept an infant whose birthmother abused drugs or alcohol during her pregnancy, because such conditions can lead to permanent birth defects or long-term health problems, such as FETAL ALCOHOL SYNDROME, in the case of prenatal alcohol exposure. (See PRENATAL EXPOSURES.) Such children are considered to have SPECIAL NEEDS.

When a Particular Child Is Discussed with Prospective Adoptive Parents

The adoptive parents should be thoroughly briefed on the known health of the child they may adopt, despite their prior written acceptance of conditions: parents sometimes may be too naive about their ability to manage some conditions, or they may believe that they should tell the agency what they think the agency wants to hear.

After approval of the adoptive parents and before the child is placed with them, the parents will be presented with a "referral"—medical information, genetic background, and the personal history of the child, based on known information.

When available, the child's birth measurements (head circumference, birth weight, and length), health condition at birth and other factors will also be shared.

If it is an older child who is being adopted, the adoptive family should be provided with as much social, developmental, and medical information as available. Any serious injuries or chronic illnesses as well as learning disabilities should be explained. In addition, any history of physical or sexual abuse should be discussed as completely as the social worker's information allows. Agencies should go back to obtain all possible additional information from relatives, foster families, birthparents, schools, and others who have had contact with the child through the years.

As mentioned, in the case of an international adoption, medical history information may be sketchy, unavailable, or in some cases even falsified, and frequently only the current physical condition of the child can be provided. As a result, adoptive parents should seek out a pediatrician knowledgeable about ADOPTION MEDICINE, who is experienced in recognizing medical problems such as malnutrition or problems stemming from the lack of stimulation that is common in orphanages, among many other potential health risks. Some adoption medicine experts may be hired to provide an evaluation of a child before adoption, based on VIDEOTAPES, photographs, medical records, and information from the orphanage.

Adopting Parents Usually Must Undergo a Medical Evaluation

The adopted child is not the only person on whom medical information is gathered. The adopting parents are medically evaluated as well, and an adoptive parent must usually undergo a complete physical examination and a discussion of his or her own medical history with the doctor. This medical history information will be provided to the social worker, who will evaluate whether there are any medical conditions that would make it difficult or impossible for the prospective adoptive parent to properly care for the child and/or to live a normal life expectancy, based on current information. A psychiatric evaluation may also be included in the HOME STUDY evaluation of adoptive parents.

Recent disabling accidents, major surgery, and other serious medical problems will be thoroughly analyzed before the placement to ensure that the child's best interests are met.

Disabled parents have often found agencies prefer to match disabled children to them, especially if the disability is shared, believing they would have a certain affinity to each other. However, if a disabled prospective parent feels that he or she is capable of parenting a healthy infant or child, that person should seek an agency interested in working with them.

See also BACKGROUND INFORMATION; GENETIC PREDISPOSITIONS; MEDICAL PROBLEMS OF INTERNATIONALLY ADOPTED CHILDREN.

medical problems of internationally adopted children Children adopted from other countries are at risk for a broad range of short-term and long-range medical and developmental problems, including infectious diseases, developmental delays, and psychiatric and behavioral problems.

Sometimes these problems are readily apparent based on the child's appearance, behavior, or existing medical records, while in other cases, they are more subtle or even not evident at all until the child becomes older. In addition, a key difficulty with foreign medical records is that they may not be translated accurately into English, and they may also be incomplete or inaccurate records. In many cases, jargon that is confusing may be used.

It should be noted, however, that even children who *seem* healthy when they are adopted may later develop medical or psychiatric problems, just as children born into a family sometimes develop such problems. Physicians attempt to screen major health problems and risks, but there are no guarantees with birth or adopted children. It is also true sometimes that children who seem sickly can thrive with appropriate medical care that they did not receive in their native country.

The IMMUNIZATIONS of children adopted from other countries may not be up to date by Western standards. Some doctors choose to restart all immunizations or, alternately, obtain blood to verify immunity.

Many children adopted from other countries benefit from being treated by a pediatrician who is knowledgeable about diseases and disorders common in other countries; however, a physician who is interested and willing to learn is often a good choice as well.

Infectious Diseases

Children adopted from other countries may have serious or minor infections. Serious infections, though rare, include the HUMAN IMMUNODEFICIENCY VIRUS (HIV)/ACQUIRED IMMUNODEFICIENCY SYNDROME (AIDS), SYPHILIS, and other SEXUALLY TRANSMITTED DISEASES, such as gonorrhea. More common infections that are found among children adopted from other countries include various forms of HEPATITIS as well as TUBERCULOSIS.

Screening for these infections may be performed in the sending country, but it is often advisable to repeat these tests in the United States.

The prevalence of infections varies in different countries; for example, the rate of HIV is very high in Africa, particularly sub-Saharan Africa. HIV is also a major problem in some European countries, such as Romania and Ukraine. In Central America, HIV prevalence is high in Guatemala.

HEPATITIS B and C occur among some children adopted from other countries. Although most infected children are asymptomatic carriers of these viruses, hepatitis B and C may cause progressive liver damage and may spread to others who may suffer serious complications of infection. Parents planning an international adoption should be vaccinated against hepatitis B early in the process, as it takes six months to complete the series. (There is no vaccine against hepatitis C.)

Many children adopted from other countries are infected with INTESTINAL PARASITIC INFECTIONS, which may be treated with medications. Infections with lice and scabies are also common. Although adoptive parents may find these diseases distressing, these infections usually respond well to medication.

The American Academy of Pediatrics has established guidelines for tests that should be performed on children adopted from other countries. Colloquially known by pediatricians as the "Red Book," *The American Academy of Pediatrics Report on Infectious Diseases* has a chapter on recommended tests for children adopted from other countries. The failure to use this recommended screening tool is the most common reason why infectious diseases are not diagnosed.

Developmental Problems

Some medical problems experienced by children adopted from other countries were caused by PRENATAL EXPOSURES, such as alcohol abuse or alcoholism during pregnancy that leads to fetal alcohol syndrome in the child. As with infectious diseases, the risk for developmental problems is greater among some countries; for example, fetal alcohol syndrome is more common among children adopted from eastern Europe than children adopted from Asia.

Some children experience problems with LANGUAGE DELAY, usually because of minimal exposure to language in their preadoptive environments.

Children with developmental delays may benefit greatly from an EARLY INTERVENTION evaluation by state and local authorities, an option available at no cost for children aged zero to three. (Some states will screen and treat children up to age five.)

Growth Issues

Children adopted from other countries are often smaller than their American-born counterparts, and their growth rates may not track expected growth rates for American children. However, most adopted children show rapid catch-up growth within the first three to four months after adoptive placement. Those who do not exhibit such growth recovery deserve complete medical evaluations for failure-to-thrive.

In some cases, assessment of growth is complicated, as the child's age is unknown. An age assignment may be inappropriately young because of chronic malnutrition and small size. For children with uncertain ages, bone age and dental X-rays may help to determine an appropriate age assignment after six to 12 months of nutritional rehabilitation has occurred.

In some cases, children adopted from other countries experience EARLY PUBERTY/PRECOCIOUS PUBERTY. This has been particularly noted in some girls adopted from India. Early puberty leads to a shorter final stature than would have been attained with puberty occurring at a normal age.

Nutritional Deficiencies

In most cases, nutritional deficiencies identified among many children adopted from other countries are easily managed by the pediatrician: malnutrition, RICKETS, and iron deficiency ANEMIA.

Psychiatric and Behavioral Problems

Whether adopted children in general (or from other countries) experience a greater number of psychiatric problems than nonadopted children is an issue that is often researched and discussed by medical experts, social workers, adoptive parents, and others. In general, the level of deprivation that the child experiences in early life seems directly correlated with the development of later neuropsychiatric problems, with severe deprivation often leading to serious emotional disorders. However, some adopted children have remarkable RESILIENCE, and with loving families to help them, they are able to overcome very deprived early backgrounds to lead normal and healthy lives.

That said, however, it is still important for adoptive parents and others to understand that even the most loving and attentive parents cannot always help a child overcome emotional or psychiatric problems that develop.

Some children adopted from other countries (as well as some children adopted from FOSTER CARE in the United States) suffer from ATTACHMENT DISORDER, which may be amenable to treatment, while other times, the problem is very difficult to treat. Experts do not agree on how this problem should be treated; however, they do agree that "rebirthing therapy," or forcing a child to push his or her way through tight blankets, is not an effective treatment. (Several children have died with this treatment.)

Some children adopted from other countries have EATING DISORDERS and SLEEP DISORDERS, often related to the major cultural change from living in an orphanage to living with a family as well as the many other changes involved with relocating from another country. These problems are usually temporary and resolve within a few months after adoption.

Prenatal Exposures and Other Exposures

Some children adopted from other countries (or domestically adopted in the United States, Canada, and other Western nations) have been exposed prenatally to a variety of substances toxic to the fetus, such as alcohol, illegal drugs, and tobacco. Of these, prenatal exposure to alcohol has the most serious and pervasive long-term effects on the child. (See FETAL ALCOHOL SYNDROME.) Children born to mothers who drink excessively during pregnancy may have lifelong impaired growth, development, and neurologic function, as well as various birth defects. Children exposed prenatally to illicit drugs may have increased learning disabilities and behavior problems (such as attention deficit hyperactivity disorder).

Many people in countries outside the United States and Canada are heavy smokers, and smoking may continue throughout the pregnancy, leading to children with a lower birth weight and more respiratory and other health problems.

After birth, children may continue to be exposed to toxic substances, such as tobacco smoke. In addition, children may be at risk for lead poisoning as well as exposure to other dangerous substances that can impede their growth and development.

See also ADOPTION MEDICINE; INTERNATIONAL ADOPTION; PRENATAL EXPOSURES; SENSORY INTEGRATION DISORDER.

Miller, Laurie, C., M.D. *The Handbook of International Adoption Medicine: A Guide for Physicians, Parents, and Providers.* New York: Oxford University Press, 2005.

mental health of adopted children and adults
See PSYCHIATRIC PROBLEMS OF ADOPTED PERSONS.

military members and adoption   Adoption, especially U.S. adoption, may be challenging for active duty members of the military and their spouses who are subject to frequent transfers to other states or even other countries, particularly if they wish to adopt a healthy newborn. Many agencies have waiting lists for years; consequently, military families are often not in one place long enough to make it to the top of many agency waiting lists. In addition, the adoption HOME STUDY is usually not "transferable," thus a person in the armed forces often must start the adoption process over again in the new location. A further difficulty is that some agencies may require a criminal record check for every state the family has resided in, which can be time-consuming.

However, adoption *is* possible for military families who are willing to network actively and seek out agencies willing to work with them. In addition, some agencies will accept home studies from other agencies. Military families who live overseas may be able to have their home studies completed by a social worker approved by the agency. Some social workers travel throughout Europe to perform home studies for military and civilian families from the United States who wish to adopt children. The family services office at the base or post should be able to offer advice on adoption. In addition, the National Military Family Association, based in Alexandria, Virginia, offers information on adoption and other topics.

Because of the diverse ethnic and racial mix of the military, many military members are good candidates as adoptive parents. Military families may be more accepting of TRANSRACIAL ADOPTION and INTERNATIONAL ADOPTION than families who reside in communities that are not ethnically or racially diverse. Many military families have traveled abroad, and they have far more cosmopolitan and accepting attitudes than families who have never left their home areas.

Some adoption agencies are biased against military members; for example, because of the "macho" image of the military, some agencies may mistakenly believe that such parents may be harsh disciplinarians, authoritarian, or even physically abusive. This is an unfair stereotype.

Military members are eligible for a $2,000 reimbursement upon finalizing an adoption of a child, whether the child was adopted through a private adoption agency, attorney, international adoption agency, or any other legal means of adoption. However, stepparent adoptions and adoptions related to surrogate parent arrangements are excluded from this benefit. Military members are also entitled to the same INCOME TAX LAW BENEFITS FOR ADOPTIVE PARENTS as other citizens.

Individuals in the military are not eligible for parental leave under the Family and Medical Leave Act; however, they may request military leave from their commanders to have time to bond with the child and make any needed child care arrangements. Many military installations offer child care

centers. Military members who adopt children are excluded from deployments from home for four months, unless they waive this deferment.

National Adoption Information Clearinghouse. "Military Families and Adoption: A Fact Sheet for Families," U.S. Department of Health and Human Services, 2003.

multiethnic   A child of mixed cultures or nationality; for example, the child may have one Hispanic parent and one Anglo parent. The term is frequently misapplied to the child who is biracial and has instead a racial heritage of two different races. (Most often the term "biracial" is used to describe a child who has one black and one white parent.)

In the strictest sense, most Americans are "multiethnic" because few can trace their heritage solely to one country or culture.

Multiethnic Placement Act (MEPA)   A law prohibiting discrimination in race by adoption, initially spearheaded in 1994 by Senator Howard M. Metzenbaum (D-Ohio), who succeeded in attaching his bill, the Metzenbaum Multiethnic Placement Act, to another law moving through the Senate. His bill essentially required that those organizations receiving federal funds could not delay or deny the placement of a child in adoption or foster care because of considerations of race or ethnicity.

Two years later, frustrated by the continuing unwillingness of the U.S. Department of Health and Human Services (HHS) to issue regulations reflecting the spirit of his law, and receiving complaints about continuing discrimination, Senator Metzenbaum went back to Congress. He asked that the only bill ever to bear his name be repealed or amended to close the loopholes in the law. Senator Metzenbaum's effort was successful, and in 1996 MEPA was amended by the Removal of Barriers to Interethnic Adoption (IEP) provisions, which were attached to another piece of legislation.

The personal acceptance of the value of the act and the 1996 amendment varies among the officials and caseworkers. Some social workers have welcomed the removal of routine race-matching from the child welfare definition of best interests of a child and from placement decisions. Others believe that children—particularly minority children—should always be placed in homes that will support a child's racial identity. For some individuals, this means a home only with same-race parents.

See also TRANSRACIAL ADOPTION.

A Guide to the Multiethnic Placement Act of 1994, as Amended by the Interethnic Adoption Provisions of 1996. Washington, D.C.: American Bar Association Center on Children and the Law, 1998.

mutual aid groups   See SUPPORT GROUPS.

mutual consent registries   Registries that will provide identifying information if both the birthparent and the adopted adult are registered. Because some adopted persons and birthparents SEARCH for each other after the child has grown into adulthood, and nearly all states seal confidential adoption records, these mutual consent registries have been established.

Groups that support OPEN RECORDS, or the ready availability of identifying data to adopted adults and birthparents, do not believe mutual consent registries go far enough. However, supporters of the registries believe it is important to protect the confidentiality of both the adopted person and the birthparents, and unless they both wish to meet, then they believe that the information should not be shared.

The following states have established some form of mutual consent registry as of this writing: Arkansas, California, Colorado, Connecticut, Delaware, Florida, Georgia, Idaho, Illinois, Iowa, Kentucky, Louisiana, Maine, Maryland, Massachusetts, Michigan, Minnesota, Missouri, Montana, Nevada, New Hampshire, New Jersey, New Mexico, New York, North Dakota, Ohio, Oklahoma, Oregon, Rhode Island, South Carolina, South Dakota, Tennessee, Texas, Utah, and West Virginia.

Some states have enacted "search and consent" laws, allowing adopted adults to contact the state social services department or an adoption agency and request that the birthparent(s) be located. If the birthparent(s) are located, their consent is then sought to provide their identifying information to the adopted person. The following states have search and consent laws: Arizona, Colorado, Kansas, Montana, New Jersey, New Mexico, Oklahoma, Pennsylvania, Washington, and Wyoming. (Note that some states have both mutual consent registries and search and consent laws.)

Six states allow adopted adults to obtain their original birth certificates as of this writing: Alabama, Alaska, Kansas, Maryland, New Hampshire, and Pennsylvania.

See also ADULT ADOPTED PERSONS; REUNION; SEARCH.

naming When a child is adopted and the adoption is "finalized" in court, the adoptive parents have the legal right to change the child's entire name, including first, middle, and last names.

Often they do not know the name the birthparents gave the child on the original birth certificate, if they provided a name. However, the original birth certificate usually says "Baby Girl" or "Baby Boy" if the child was born in the United States. After the finalization, the original birth certificate becomes a SEALED RECORD in most states, and the name given by the adoptive parents is placed on a new birth certificate.

The name given to every child, adopted or not adopted, is very important to that child, because the name is an integral part of the identity. Even perfect strangers respond to a person's name with preconceived ideas of what a "Larry" or a "Francis" is like; consequently, the choice of a name should be made very carefully.

Naming an Infant

As mentioned, if the child is a newborn infant, he or she may have been given a name by the birthparents. Even if the birthparents do choose to name the child, it is unlikely a name change would be detrimental to the adopted infant.

In some cases of OPEN ADOPTION, the adoptive parents and birthparents both choose the child's name or share the naming of the child. Opponents of this practice believe it could create a problem of ENTITLEMENT for the adopting family and a false sense of control for the birthparents. Supporters believe it is a positive act of sharing and acceptance. In the majority of cases, the adoptive parents alone choose the child's name.

Adoptive parents may choose a name for the pleasant sound of it or may choose a name with biblical or religious meaning; for example, "Matthew" means "gift of God" in Hebrew.

Other parents may choose the names of a favorite relative, such as a grandparent or cousin, thus adding a sense of family belonging, not only to the adoptive parents and later to the child but also to the extended family.

Says author Cheri Register,

> Giving a family name to an adopted child also makes a statement to the extended family: The parent claims the right to share the family heritage with a child who is not a blood relative.

Occasionally, relatives will disagree with the choice of name, believing "family names" should only be reserved for blood relatives. Register describes an incident in which an adopted child was named after the adoptive parents' fathers. Later, when a child was born to the family, an uncle was angry that the names had not been "saved" for the child with the genetic link.

If the child has been adopted internationally, the family may opt to choose a name that is common or acceptable in the birth country of the child. Some families who have adopted Korean-born children have chosen to use a Korean middle name; for example, Register named her daughter "Grace" and "Keun Young" for her first and middle names. According to Register, some countries require adoptive parents to name their child with at least one name common to the country of origin. (This requirement is, however, not enforceable once the child has relocated to the United States.)

Naming an Older Child

When the child who is adopted is not an infant, the child almost invariably has been given a name by others. As a rule, if the adopting parents can retain the child's original first and middle names, it would probably be best for the child. Almost inevitably, the child's last name will be changed. To change a child's first and middle names, along with changing the child's environment, could theoretically affect the child's identity as well.

Although she was not adopted, actress Patty Duke has discussed and written about the dissonance and the dismay she felt when her original name "Anna" was replaced by "Patty" and how this name change affected her identity and feeling of selfhood. It seems likely that an adopted child whose name is changed against her wishes or desires would also feel negative or confused about her identity.

There are exceptions; for example, if the child detests his first name or normally goes by his middle name, then he may desire a legal name change. Sometimes the adoptive family will retain the child's first birth name and opt to give the child a family middle name, in an effort to retain the child's original identity and also bond the child with the new family.

One adoptive family finalized the adoption of their 10-year-old child over the summer vacation. She was very eager to have her last name changed to match the name of her parents because she wanted to go to school with the same last name as theirs.

Register, Cheri. *"Are Those Kids Yours?": American Families with Children Adopted from Other Countries.* New York: Free Press, 1990.

National Adoption Month   Celebrated in November of each year. According to the North American Council on Adoptable Children (NACAC), National Adoption Week was first proclaimed in Massachusetts in May of 1976. President Ford proclaimed the first federal National Adoption Week later that year. In recent years, adoption groups have celebrated the entire month of November as "Adoption Month."

Each year, increasing numbers of adoptive parent support groups, adoption experts, and other proponents have worked to promote adoption during National Adoption Month. The adoption of children with SPECIAL NEEDS who wait for parents to adopt them is especially promoted at this time.

Adoptive parent support groups and state social services departments celebrate National Adoption Month in different ways: holding adoption seminars, picnics, or fairs with information about special needs adoption available to the general public; coordinating letter campaigns to encourage adopted children to write about how they feel about adoption.

Celebrants of National Adoption Month do their best to obtain media coverage, although coverage is spotty, perhaps because of the time of year during which it occurs.

Native Americans   See INDIAN CHILD WELFARE ACT.

naturalization   See IMMIGRATION AND NATURALIZATION.

natural parents   The man and woman who conceived a child together; also known as "birthparents" or "biological parents," usually used when the child is placed for adoption and parental rights and obligations are transferred to the adoptive parents.

The terminology "natural parents" is out of favor with many adoptive parents and adoption professionals, who point out that the opposite of "natural" is "unnatural." As a result, many adoptive parents prefer the words *birthparents* or *biological* or *genetic* parents.

See also BIRTHPARENT.

neglect   Failure to provide adequate care and supervision for a minor child by a parent or adult caretaker. Parents or other caregivers may fail to provide food, clothing, and shelter to children. In the case of an infant or toddler, neglect may cause death or severe injury. The caregiver may also withhold needed medical attention. ABANDONMENT is a form of neglect. Neglect may be more traumatic to a child than physical abuse, and it is a serious problem in the United States and the world.

According to statistics from the National Child Abuse and Neglect Data System on abuse and neglect in the United States in 2002, an estimated 896,000 children were the victims of abuse and neglect. Most of the children (61 percent) were victims of neglect. In contrast, 20 percent were victims of physical abuse, 10 percent of the children were sexually abused, and 7 percent were victims of emotional maltreatment. About 20 percent of the children were victims of other forms of mal-treatment. (Some children were victimized by more than one form of abuse.)

Neglect may be willful on the part of a parent or other caregiver or may be unintended, such as when the parent has a severe mental illness (such as depression) or a physical illness or a develop-mental delay and consequently is unable to care for the child.

Discovery of Neglect

Sometimes the first time that the neglect of a child is noticed by others is when a parent or someone else brings a child to a hospital emergency room in severely poor health or when others report the child's plight to state protective service investigators. Long-term neglect can cause severe growth deficits, and some children who were underfed for years have appeared younger than their actual age. In some cases, neighbors were shocked to learn the children's true age.

Removal from the Home

The immediate consequence of a discovery of child neglect is that the child is often removed from the home, unless it can be ascertained that the neglect is minor and will be immediately corrected. When the child is removed, he or she will be placed in the FOSTER-CARE system and will live with a foster fam-ily or a relative or will reside in a GROUP HOME. During that time, the parent will be given an opportunity to resolve the problems that led to the child neglect, whether the problems were sub-stance abuse, mental illness, poverty, or other problems. The parent will be given specific goals to meet, such as getting a job, cleaning up a filthy house, refraining from substance abuse, and so on.

If the parent meets these goals, then the court may decide to return the child to the family. If the parent fails to meet these goals within the time frame set by the ADOPTION AND SAFE FAMILIES ACT and by state law, then parental rights may be ter-minated. The child may then be considered for an adoptive placement, depending on the individual circumstances.

Neglect in Orphanages

Children residing in many orphanages throughout the world experience neglect. Excessive child-to-staff ratios, poor staff training, and limited budgets all contribute to child neglect in orphanages. Chil-dren may suffer from both physical and emotional neglect. Some orphanages actively discourage emotional involvement of the caregivers with the children because of the misguided notion that this will make it harder for the child when he or she must be removed from that person's care. Children with special needs are especially vulnerable to neg-lect in many institutional settings.

Consequences to the Child of Neglect

The short-term consequences of neglect can be severe, depending on the age of the child when the neglect occurred, the severity of the neglect, and what happened to the child after the neglect was identified. Neglected children may have many medical problems, including severe vitamin defi-ciencies, growth delays, and other problems. They may have LANGUAGE DELAYS if the neglect occurred in infancy and early childhood. They may also have emotional disorders.

Over the long term, many medical problems due to neglect can be corrected. However, the psy-chological and emotional impact of neglect, espe-cially if it was severe, may be difficult or impossible for the child and the later adult to overcome. In addition, such factors as the individual resilience of the child, or the ability to overcome early adverse experiences, are also important.

See also ABUSE; RESILIENCE.

Administration for Children and Families, Department of Health and Human Services. *Child Maltreatment 2002.* Washington, D.C., 2004.
Clark, Robin E., Judith Freeman Clark, and Christine Adamec. *The Encyclopedia of Child Abuse.* 2nd ed. New York: Facts On File, 2001.

nonidentifying information Information provided to adopting parents, birthparents, adopted persons, or others, excluding identifying data; for example, a birthparent may be told the adopting parents are athletic and be given general information about their occupation, ethnic and racial background, and religion. Similar information about the birthparents is shared with the adopting parents.

Identifying data, such as names, city where the person lives, and other information that could help identify a person, are not revealed unless the adoption is an OPEN ADOPTION.

See also CONFIDENTIALITY; GENETIC PREDISPOSITIONS; MEDICAL HISTORY.

nonsectarian agencies　See ADOPTION AGENCIES.

notice　Information on a pending court action, for example, a hearing to place a child for adoption or to finalize an adoption, that is given to specific interested parties.

Generally, it is those parties from whom CONSENT is required who must be notified of an impending adoption. Other parties may also be designated by the state to receive notice. States differ on who must be given notice. (Also, laws change, and readers should review current state laws to ensure notice requirements have not changed.)

older child   Generally school-age children at the time of adoptive placement, who are considered to be SPECIAL NEEDS children by virtue of their age alone. The age threshold at which a child is considered hard to place varies according to the state and may be six or eight years—or older or younger.

Older children in the foster care system are usually known to and listed by the state social services department, although sometimes their adoptions are arranged through adoption agencies. Attorneys are rarely involved with adoptions of children who are not infants.

Most older children have entered the child welfare system as foster children and were removed from their parents' homes due to ABANDONMENT, ABUSE and/or NEGLECT. When attempts by a social worker to reunite the child with the family fail, the worker ultimately will request the court to terminate parental rights and place the child in an adoptive home or will find a group home for the child if adoption seems unlikely. Some older children are adopted from orphanages in other countries (and a few come to the United States for summer visits with prospective families prior to their adoptive placement), although most children adopted from other countries are infants or toddlers.

In the recent past, the prevailing feeling among many in society was that adoptive families for older children could not be found; however, many adoption professionals and adoptive parent groups believe today that older children can and should be adopted. However, the older the child is, the more difficult it is to identify a suitable family, and it is usually most difficult to find families for adolescents. Yet many experts believe that every child deserves a family to love and one to whom the young adult can return for holidays, in crises, and at other times.

Many older children are a part of a sibling group, and if the sibling group is large (three or more children), placement is further complicated. Most adoptions of older children are successful, according to adoption experts and researchers, although they do have a higher rate of problems than infant adoptions. (See DISRUPTION.)

The older adopted child may show some initial negative reactions; possible behavior problems should be discussed in advance with adopting parents. A newly adopted older child may immediately express anger and reject the adoptive family because of a fear of rejection or because of a misguided attempt to "connect" with the adoptive parent.

It is also very common for all children to test parents, whether they are biological parents or adoptive parents. A newly adopted child is often in a honeymoon phase and strives mightily to please the adoptive parents and be a perfect child, but after the honeymoon period may come a very trying time for the adoptive parents—extensive testing by the child of the limits of what is accepted behavior.

Ann Hartman describes the period after the honeymoon stage and says a minor altercation can be exaggerated in the child's mind as a fear of being sent away, driving the child to even further negative actions. She says the adoptive parent needs to know that such behavior is not a negative sign but actually symbolic of the beginnings of the attachment of the child to the family.

Adoption agency professional, teacher, and adoptive parent Grace Robinson says in *Older Child Adoption*:

"By the time most older children are removed from abusive families, their traumatic abuse has been ongoing. In these cases children have learned to expect abuse and to defend themselves against it by distancing themselves from their feelings and from other people. The problem is that their defenses are not selective—they defend themselves from the good as well as the bad. These defenses, which have served the children so well in the abusive situation, make them difficult to get close to. Have you ever tried to hug a porcupine? For children who have been traumatized by ongoing abuse, the healing of wounds and memories requires taming the porcupine."

Older children may have experienced wartime trauma, sexual abuse, and many terrible experiences. They may need therapy. Loving parents cannot wipe out all past negative experiences, although they can teach children that life can be much better.

See also PREPARING A CHILD FOR ADOPTION; RESILIENCE; SIBLINGS; SPECIAL NEEDS ADOPTION.

Hartman, Ann. "Practice in Adoption," in *A Handbook of Child Welfare: Context, Knowledge, and Practice.* New York: Free Press, 1985.

Robinson, Grace. *Older Child Adoption.* New York: Crossroad Publishing Company, 1998.

only child adoptive families There are indications that as many as 50 percent or more of all adoptive parent couples (or singles) adopt one child only. Many parents adopt only one child because the agency they dealt with will only place with childless couples. (Many agencies are moving away from this stance and will place two children in a home.) Other parents want one child only and are satisfied after the adoption. Other parents cannot afford to adopt more than one child.

When only one child is adopted and there are no biological children, the adopted child's situation is similar to the situation of an only biological child, and there may be a risk of overindulging the child or expecting too much of the child.

Adoptive parents would probably also be interested in the results of a study of BIRTH ORDER and academic achievement, although adopted children were not studied. Researcher Varghese I. Cherian studied more than 1,000 children and found a direct relationship between birth order and academic achievement, with the oldest child or the only child usually achieving the best grades.

See also ACADEMIC PROGRESS.

Cherian, Varghese I. "Birth Order and Academic Achievement of Children in Transkei," *Psychological Reports* 66 (1990): 19–24.

Glenn, Norval D., and Sue Keir Hoppe. "Only Children as Adults," *Journal of Family Issues,* September 1984.

open adoption The term *open adoption* is the most accurate term to describe an adoptive placement in which the BIRTHMOTHER and sometimes the BIRTHFATHER as well exchange specific identifying information with the adopting parents. Information such as names, addresses, and other data may be exchanged so that ongoing contact between the adopting and birth families is possible. Whether ongoing contact is monthly, annually, or sporadic depends on the parties, and most experts believe it should be decided between them rather than by an agency or attorney. The parties involved usually have some form of written agreement, although this does not always occur.

The opposite of an open adoption is a confidential adoption (sometimes called a "closed" adoption), in which identifying information is *not* shared between the adoptive parents and the birthparents. Some ADOPTION AGENCIES in the United States strongly favor open adoptions over confidential adoptions.

It is also true that some individuals use the term *semi-open* to indicate some level of openness, such as a meeting between the pregnant woman and the prospective parents, but without sharing of their last names. There are many different forms of "semi-open" adoptions, such as with pregnant women choosing adoptive parents based on informational RÉSUMÉS they have provided about their family, yet without the disclosure of identities.

The definition of open adoption to the parties involved, including the birthparents and adopting parents as well as the social worker and/or attorney, is critically important because tremendous confusion about the definition of this phrase abounds nationwide. Some adoption agencies differ in their definition of how much "openness" qualifies as an open adoption, for example, the situation in which the pregnant woman considering adoption for her child is given nonidentifying résumés to review may be considered an open adoption by some agencies, while other agencies consider a brief meeting between the parties with no exchange of identities to be an open adoption. Still others insist that only a full disclosure of identities is an open adoption. Consequently, until more universal agreement on a definition is achieved, it is very important to obtain an exact definition from the agency or attorney on specifically what is meant by "open adoption."

Most open adoptions occur with children born in the United States or Canada, while international adoptions are rarely open adoptions.

RELATIVE ADOPTIONS in the United States are generally open, and they represent a special category of adoption with unique pros and cons; for example, the child may resemble the adoptive parents. Sometimes relative adoptions are adversarial, resulting from a court battle. In some cases, there will be no counseling or social work assistance to help with the reorganization of kinship role and status and the concomitant feelings that occur. Emergent negative feelings among battling relatives can be extremely painful for the adopted child and affect him or her even to adulthood. (See KINSHIP CARE.)

It is also important to understand that a FOSTER PARENT ADOPTION is sometimes open simply because many foster parents know identifying information about the birthparents, especially if the child is over six. Some foster parents have allowed visitations in their own home during foster care, and they may continue to allow telephone or written communication with the birthparents after the adoption occurs. In other cases, contact with the birthparents is discouraged because of past abuse that has traumatized the child. When possible, children should have an opportunity to meet with their biological siblings in foster care (or who are adopted), unless the siblings themselves are abusive.

History

Open adoptions were once the norm, and in the 1920s, some women advertised their own children for adoption. Primarily indigent women, they performed their own screening and decided for themselves if the placement would occur. Social workers and others were understandably distressed by this practice, both because they felt the parents might have considerable difficulty in adequately screening the people who would adopt their children and also because they were concerned about people who might sell their children.

As a result, social workers in Massachusetts and other states actively sought to ban parents from ADVERTISING their children for adoption, and today most states that allow adoption advertising only allow adoption agencies, attorneys, or prospective adoptive parents to advertise. Some states prohibit advertising altogether, whereas other states require specific wording in the advertising.

Confidential adoptions became the norm by the 1930s. Original birth certificates became SEALED RECORDS, and they were replaced with a new birth certificate that listed the adoptive parents as the parents. At that time and up until about the 1970s, it was considered extremely shameful to bear a child out of wedlock. Some young women were sent to maternity homes in the final months of pregnancy, while their families lied to others that the woman had gone to take care of a sick relative or another excuse was manufactured.

A key reason for many agencies (and attorneys) offering open adoption is that there are fewer babies available for adoption than 20 or more years ago, thus pregnant women considering adoption have more control than in the past (although some do not realize this.) Another reason for fewer babies needing adoptive families is that out-of-wedlock births no longer carry the severe stigma of past years, when unwed pregnant women and single mothers were objects of ridicule. Today, many single women parent their infants and children with little or no stigma attached.

Some adoption agencies use open adoptions as a form of marketing to attract women to adoption. If the agency promises the woman that she will experience little or no emotional pain with an open adoption, this is deceptive. There is nearly always some pain with the relinquishment of a child, whether in an open or confidential adoption.

Arguments in Favor of Open Adoptions

Advocates of open adoptions insist that openness is best for the child, who will not spend a lifetime wondering what a birthparent looked like or why he or she was placed for adoption. Some proponents cite studies of adopted adults who have been institutionalized and/or required psychotherapy, and they have made a leap to conclude that the secrecy inherent in confidential adoption contributed to or caused the mental illness. (See PSYCHIATRIC PROBLEMS OF ADOPTED PERSONS.) However, those who oppose generalizing pathology suffered by some adopted persons to an entire population of adopted individuals cite many studies that indicate many adopted children and adolescents are well adjusted.

Open adoption proponents also state that the experience among some new adoptive parents of babies adopted in the United States, who wonder whether every young woman in the supermarket could be the birthmother, will not be a problem in an open adoption, since the adopting parents know exactly who the birthmother is. Open adoption advocates also say that the fear of the unknown birthmother coming back to "reclaim" the child by kidnapping disappears if an adoption is open. Despite the fact that a birthmother could theoretically take such action when she knows the identities of the adoptive parents, few have actually done so.

Many advocates believe that open adoption helps a child better cope with the loss of a birthparent and that it also helps birthparents and adoptive parents cope with their sense of loss.

Open adoption advocates also believe that adoptive parents gain a strong respect for the birthmother when they actually know who she is. They claim that the sense of ENTITLEMENT that adoptive parents feel toward the child is stronger when the adoptive parents are personally chosen by the birthparents.

Kathleen Silber and Phylis Speedlin, authors of *Dear Birthmother: Thank You for Our Baby*, argue against confidential adoptions, saying that birthmothers, adoptive parents, and adopted children are forced to accept whatever information an intermediary was willing to provide in a confidential adoption. Hence, adoptive parents may see birthparents as "shadowy figures," while birthparents wonder intensely whether or not their children are all right with the adoptive parents.

Arguments in Favor of Confidential Adoption

Supporters of confidential ("closed") adoptions have several major reasons for their objections to open adoptions. Many of them are the converse of the arguments used to support open adoptions.

Some say women are more likely to choose unwanted abortions or to have unwanted children

whom they may later neglect or abuse if they cannot maintain confidentiality. However, this is a theory only, ungrounded in any study.

Those who do not support open adoption may argue, as social workers argued back in the 1920s, that the pregnant woman considering adoption is often in a highly emotional state and she is not the best judge of who would make good parents. However, it should be pointed out that nearly all adoptive parents must undergo a background check in home studies, which will screen out individuals with a criminal record or who have been placed on a child abuse registry because of past abuse or neglect of a child. As a result, if the birthmother chooses naively or badly, the adoptive parents will usually be prevented from adopting as a result of the home study process.

Others argue that adopting couples may feel *less* entitlement to a child in an open adoption, rather than more, when the birthmother's identity is known. The adoptive parents may feel more like foster parents or legal guardians despite the emotional, legal, and financial commitment they incur with adoption.

It is also argued that the birthmother will not resolve her own feelings of entitlement toward the baby in an open adoption, and it may become difficult or impossible for her to disengage from the child. In addition, what she originally considered acceptable contact; for example, photographs sent every few months, may become unacceptable to the birthmother, and she may seek more involvement with the child.

Sometimes the age of the birthmother can be an important factor; for example, some experts, such as Adrienne Kraft and others, argue that adolescent birthmothers would have considerable difficulty with open adoptions, and they are unprepared to determine whether or not they should continue contact with a child through an open adoption. In addition, the adolescent birthmother may not understand that she is irrevocably transferring her parental rights, because she is not mature enough to understand this pivotal point.

Studies on Open Adoption: Birthmothers

Research appears to refute the hypothesis that the birthmother will experience less grief when she knows the identity of the adoptive parents. A study of 59 birthmothers by Terril Blanton, crisis pregnancy counselor at Buckner Baptist Benevolences in Dallas, Texas, and Jeanne Deschner, associate professor at the Graduate School of Social Work at Arlington, Texas, was reported in 1990, and their findings are still useful today.

The researchers compared birthmothers who had chosen an open adoption (defined as at least having personally met the adoptive parents) to birthmothers who had chosen confidential adoptions. These two groups were also compared to bereaved women whose children had died.

The birthmothers were an average age of 21.3 years for the 18 open adoption birthmothers and 25.6 years for the 41 confidential adoption birthmothers. The researchers found that the birthmothers who had placed their children in an open adoption suffered *more* than mothers whose children died. Said the authors, "Indications were strong that biological mothers who know more about the later life of the child they relinquished have a harder time making an adjustment than do mothers whose tie to the child is broken off completely by means of death. Relinquishing mothers who know only that their children still live but have no details about their lives appear to experience an intermediate degree of grief."

The authors hypothesized that the birthmothers in an open adoption could be compared to divorced women who may have more difficulty adjusting to their marital loss than bereaved widows. In addition, the birthmother may not fully accept the loss of her nurturing role as a parent.

Some who say that they support open adoption also reveal serious conflicts about the practice. In her lengthy article in *Law & Society Review,* adoptive mother Barbara Yngvesson describes her confusion about open adoption, as well as the ambivalence of others, both birthparents and adoptive parents.

For example, she describes the feelings of the birthmother "Cassie" as feeling as if she is on the margins of a family and says, "She can see no place for herself in the adoptive family that will be 'comfortable' and 'clear' for her son, so that he will know 'who's who and what's what' and will not be confused about who is his 'real' mother. She's worried that he will 'hate' her for giving him away. As a result—and this has come up repeatedly in other birthmother interviews—her desire to act in the best interests of her son works against her desire to forge a relationship with the adoptive parents so that she can keep in contact with him. At the same time, her desire not 'to be left out' continually reminds them, and herself, of the tenuousness that *each* experiences in the connection to the adopted child."

Yngvesson also describes a birthmother who was terribly upset when the adoptive parents did not contact her on her son's birthday or on Mother's Day. The social worker contacted them and learned that the adoptive mother felt that it might upset the birthmother to contact her, since her last contact with them had been pretty "generic," or noncommittal. A third party, the social worker, clearly intruded herself into the process, pressing the adoptive parents to make contact, and using (perhaps unknowingly) guilt and shame among her tactics.

For example, according to what the social worker told the author, the social worker said to the adoptive father, "There are people who would give their left arm for a caring, loving birthmom like Cassie," and she also stated that Cassie had chosen them because she wanted openness. Said the social worker, "You said yes although no one contracted anything, that it would be four times a year plus a personal visit. My feeling is, you've got to live that up, the way you said you were going to do it. If you agreed to send her stuff, let *her* decide if she wants to open it." And "You need to nurture her, you need to nourish her, reach out to her."

In another article in *Social Work,* a piece strongly supportive of open adoption, author Deborah Siegel described the advantages and disadvantages of this practice. One disadvantage that she felt sometimes occurred was an extreme closeness of the birthmother to the adopting parents.

Said Siegel of one case, "They lived for a while with her in her apartment, counseled her through several crises, and wiped her brow during labor. A year after the adoption, they found that she was having trouble letting go of the intimate relationship with them despite previous agreements to do so; she continued occasionally to call them when she was in crisis." As a result, the adoptive parents have become unofficial counselors and saviors of the birthmother, who they feel they "owed" for their child. She, in turn, became used to their assistance and did not want to lose it.

In another case, the birthmother confided to the adoptive mother that she learned she had become infertile. The adoptive mother had difficulty dealing with this knowledge and wanted to distance herself from it, but she did not want to hurt the birthmother's feelings.

Studies on Open Adoption: Adoptive Parents

Most studies look at the effects on either birthmothers or adopted children, but very few address how open adoption may affect or is regarded by adoptive parents. In one study on how adoptive families adjusted to open adoption, published in 2003 in *Adoption Quarterly,* researchers studied 90 families shortly after an infant was placed with them and again about 18 months later. These families had a varying degree of information about the birthparents, ranging from no information to medical information only to frequent visits and phone calls with the birthparents.

The researchers found that about a third of the adoptive parents (31 percent) later wished to change their level of openness, with 57 percent of those desiring a change seeking a more open adoption while 43 percent wished for a more closed adoption. The desire for a change in openness was often related to child-rearing problems, and adoptive mothers who reported difficulty with child rearing were more likely to wish to change their level of openness.

Another interesting finding was that some of the adoptive parents expressed a desire for more information about the birthfather, and those who wanted to change the level of openness were more likely to seek more information about the birthfather.

Other findings, according to the authors, were "Desire to change openness, *in either direction,* was related to several other factors measured in this study. Adoptive parents who were unhappy in their marriage or who were depressed were more likely to desire a change in openness."

The researchers also found that information on the birthparents positively affected the perception of the adoptive parents toward them, even when the information was negative. Said the researchers, "This is potentially reassuring for birthparents, who may fear that sharing such information would negatively influence the adoptive parents and, ultimately, their birth child's outcomes. Preliminary evidence from one-half of our sample for whom birthparent data were available suggests that the positive influence of birthparent information held *regardless* of the level of psychopathology in the birthparent."

Studies on Open Adoption: Public Attitudes

In another unique study, the researchers surveyed the general public on their attitudes toward open adoption versus confidential adoption, reporting on their findings in the *Journal of Family Issues* in 2005. In this telephone survey in Canada, the researchers initially surveyed 82 people, and then in Phase 2 they surveyed 706 individuals aged 18 years and older throughout Canada. The majority of men (58 percent) and women (65 percent) expressed support for open adoptions.

The respondents were asked about their opinions with regard to advantages and disadvantages to adoptive parents, birthparents, and adopted children, with some openness in the adoption versus a fully confidential adoption. Said the authors, "The most frequently cited advantage by female and male respondents was that adoptive parents could learn more about the medical background of the adopted child and the birth parents. This would enable adoptive parents to anticipate potential problems and assist them in understanding and assisting their adopted child." Other advantages cited were the opportunity to use the information to help their child in understanding his or her background as well as the greater ease in contacting birthparents in the future, if the child later desired to make contact.

The key perceived disadvantages to adoptive families, when there was some level of openness, were that it would make rearing the child more difficult and it might create conflict between the adoptive family and the birth family with regard to child rearing.

The key advantages seen to birthparents in some level of openness was that they would have more peace of mind knowing that the adoptive parents were good parents. Another advantage was the possibility of having a favorable influence over the child's development. The major perceived disadvantages were that the birthparents might disagree with the adoptive parents' child rearing and/or they might feel that they had made a mistake by placing the child for adoption.

With regard to adopted children and openness, the key advantages were seen as having information about themselves that would satisfy their curiosity and alleviate distress about why they were placed for adoption. The main disadvantage perceived to adopted children was seen as conflict, distress, and confusion that could be created by "two sets of parents."

Opinions on the advantages and disadvantages to confidential adoptions were also surveyed. With regard to the adoptive parents, the respondents felt that the adoptive parents would feel free of interference in raising the child with a confidential adoption and also would be more likely to regard the child as their own. With regard to the birthparents, the respondents felt confidential adoptions would better allow birthparents to get on with their lives. (This view is actively disputed by proponents of open adoptions.) The primary advantages of confidential adoptions to adopted children, according to the respondents, were a feeling of belongingness to the adoptive family and the lack of confusion that could occur if there were contact with the birthparents.

The disadvantages of confidential adoptions were a converse of the perceived advantages of open adoptions. Said the authors, "Specifically, female and male respondents felt that adoptive parents would be disadvantaged by the lack of medical and personal background information on their child and would be unable to answer questions posed by their adopted children about their origins." In addition, with regard to disadvantages to birthparents in confidential adoptions, the researchers stated that, "female and male respondents identified psychological distress engendered by lack of information about the fate of their child and what the adoptive home was like."

Finally, the key perceived disadvantages to adopted children in confidential adoptions were seen as not knowing about their background, who their parents were, or why they were placed for adoption.

The researchers concluded, "The results discussed in this article reveal that the larger community is not as conservative in its views toward adoption and openness, nor as enthusiastic about fully disclosed adoption as the professional community might believe. As such, the community in general appears more likely to accept a variety of openness arrangements, offering further support to the notion that choice should be left to the individual families themselves, in the best interests of the children they serve."

The Open Adoption Process

The first step to an open adoption may be a contact with a social worker, attorney, or a friend of the pregnant woman or adopting couple. In some cases, pregnant women find prospective parents on INTERNET sites. The pregnant woman may view photographs and résumés of prospective adoptive couples and select one or more couples she may like to meet. She may choose a family she thinks physically resembles herself, or she may simply like the way the husband and wife look in their photograph.

If she meets the couple, she may decide they appear to have good parenting skills and generally appear to offer security for the child to develop to his or her full potential. The birthmother may also think the couple's hobbies and interests are similar to her own; for example, they may have expressed a love of travel, which she shares and values.

The adoption may not start out as open during the period when the birthmother reviews résumés and/or photographs. If the pregnant woman opts to meet the couple, and especially if she meets them more than once, it becomes extremely difficult to maintain confidentiality.

Potential Problems with Open Adoption

Sometimes after placement and especially after finalization of the adoption, the adopting parents lose their eagerness to communicate with the birthmother. Perhaps they were dishonest with the birthmother in their zeal to adopt a baby, or they may have lost their enthusiasm for the previously agreed-upon open adoption, especially as the child grows older. In some cases, birthparents may contact the adopted child less and less and sometimes contact altogether ceases.

If the baby has been placed in an open adoption and the adoptive parents later "slam the door shut," this action could be very traumatic for the birthmother. In some cases, she may not have placed the child for adoption at all and would have opted to raise the child as a single parent had open adoption not been presented to her as a very positive option. Whether the law supports the birthmother in a legal action depends on the state, and some states have ruled in favor of birthmothers who sought previously promised information while others have not upheld them.

Critics also fear that a birthmother may make unreasonable financial and emotional demands on a couple she personally knows, either before the adoptive placement or in the future, playing on their guilt feelings over "taking her baby." If the couple offers or gives the birthmother any money directly before placement or even finalization, this could be construed as BABY SELLING, which should be avoided because it is illegal, immoral, and could be grounds for overturning an adoption. If it is lawful to provide financial support to a pregnant woman considering adoption, as it is in many states, the funds should be provided through a third party, such as an adoption agency or an adoption attorney. Many states require that an accounting of all financial disbursements be provided to the court before finalization of the adoption may occur.

Making Open Adoption Work

Deborah Siegel and others describe methods to make an open adoption work. For example, she recommends, "Because people's needs change over time, they should have an agreed-on mechanism for renegotiating their plan. For instance, they may agree that the person who wants a different arrangement will communicate that wish to the social worker, who will then contact the other party to begin formulating a new agreement. Leaving these issues inadequately explored before placement can arouse unnecessary anxieties and produce avoidable misunderstandings later."

Siegel and others who support open adoption insist that adoptive parents and birthparents are usually pleased with the arrangement, despite the problems that may occur. According to the authors of *The Open Adoption Experience,* open adoptions "do not require that you live without rules or by someone else's set of rules . . . An adoptive family can and should have appropriate boundaries about its relationship with the birthfamily. The difference between open adoption and confidential adoption is not that there are no longer boundaries but that there are boundaries where there used to be walls."

See also OPEN RECORDS; REUNION; SEARCH.

Blanton, Terril L., and Jeanne Deschner. "Biological Mothers' Grief: The Postadoptive Experience in Open vs. Confidential Adoption," *Child Welfare* 69 (November–December 1990): 525–535.

Hollenstein, Tom, et al. "Openness in Adoption, Knowledge of Birthparent Information and Adoptive Family Adjustment," *Adoption Quarterly* 7, no. 1 (2003): 43–52.

McRoy, Ruth G., Harold D. Grotevant, and Kerry I. White. *Openness in Adoption: New Practices, New Issues.* New York: Praeger, 1988.

Melina, Lois Ruskai, and Sharon Kaplan Roszia. *The Open Adoption Experience.* New York: HarperPerennial, 1993.

Miall, Charlene E., and Karen March. "Open Adoption as a Family Form: Community Assessments and Social Support," *Journal of Family Issues* 26, no. 3 (April 2005): 380–410.

Ramsey, Sarah H., and Douglas E. Abrams. *Children and the Law.* St. Paul, Minn.: West Group, 2001.

Siegel, Deborah H. "Open Adoption of Infants: Adoptive Parents' Perceptions of Advantages and Disadvantages," *Social Work* 38, no. 1 (January 1993): 15–23.

Silber, Kathleen, and Phylis Speedlin. *Dear Birthmother: Thank You for Our Baby.* San Antonio, Tex.: Corona, 1982.

Yngvesson, Barbara. "Negotiating Motherhood: Identity and Difference in 'Open' Adoptions," *Law & Society Review* 31, no. 1 (1997): 31–81.

"openness"   A commonly used and confusing term that refers to a wide spectrum of information-sharing practices. Such information may, at one extreme, simply refer to offering a birthmother (and birthfather) nonidentifying information to help choose adoptive parents while at the other extreme it refers to providing birthparents and adopting parents with identifying information about each other. Some adoption professionals see a sort of openness continuum.

Until the mid-1970s, birthparents were given almost no information about adopting parents.

Today most agencies offer birthparents choices; for example, the birthmother may often be able to specify the religion of the adopting couple as well as their interests, age (within certain guidelines), and other factors. Many agencies offer birthparents nonidentifying RÉSUMÉS of prospective adoptive parents, and the birthparents then select the adoptive parents for their child.

Other agencies encourage actual meetings between prospective adoptive parents and birthparents, and still other agencies would like to eliminate CONFIDENTIALITY altogether.

OPEN ADOPTION refers to a full disclosure of identities between the parties involved. Some agencies are using the word "openness" as a kind of "soft" definition of open adoption. It's very important for prospective adoptive parents and birthparents to request a clear definition of "openness" or "open adoption" when contacting an adoption agency to ensure the agency's policies are compatible with their own beliefs and desires.

See also GENETIC PREDISPOSITIONS; MEDICAL HISTORY; NONIDENTIFYING INFORMATION; OPEN RECORDS.

open records A variety of confidential and sealed adoption information that is made available to a member of the ADOPTION TRIAD, usually the adopted adult or adoptive parents. In most cases, the original birth certificate is sought in addition to adoption records. In some states, a court order must be acquired to obtain information while in other states, such as Alabama, Alaska, Kansas, New Hampshire, and Pennsylvania, adopted adults may simply request the information and it will be provided.

Some adopted adults seek their original unamended birth certificates, in order to learn their original birth surname and subsequently to search for their birthparents. If the adoption was finalized in the United States (or a child adopted from another country was readopted in the United States), a new birth certificate was issued, with the adoptive parents listed as the parents and the original birth certificate was sealed.

Some states have confidential intermediary systems, also known as a SEARCH AND CONSENT system, in which the person who is sought (usually the birthparent) is contacted and asked if he or she wishes further contact. These states include Arizona, Colorado, Montana, New Mexico, Oklahoma, and Wyoming.

Many states have MUTUAL CONSENT REGISTRIES, in which both the adopted adult and the birthparent must register their desire for identifying information to be released before such a release can occur. Most open record advocates are dissatisfied with mutual consent registries because they think they do not go far enough and they make few matches because of restrictions.

Sometimes access to identifying information depends on *when* the adopted person was born. For example, in Hawaii, if the adoption was finalized before December 31, 1990, then adopted adults or the adoptive parents must petition the court for the information. However, if the adoption was finalized *on* or *after* January 1, 1991, the adoptive parents or the adopted adult may receive the information unless there is an affidavit on file from the birthparent requesting continued confidentiality.

Age Requirements

The age requirement for the adopted adult to obtain identifying or nonidentifying information varies from state to state but usually is no younger than age 18 and may be age 21. However, in Nebraska, an adopted adult must be age 25 to obtain an original birth certificate, if neither the adoptive parents or birthparents have filed nonconsent.

Legal Challenges

In *ALMA Society v. Mellon,* 601 F2d. 1225, cert. den. 444 U.S. 995 (1979), adopted adults sued for identifying information, stating they were being unfairly denied information and treated as a special class when it did not serve the state's interests or the adopted person's interests. However, the Court found that the New York laws did not "unconstitutionally infringe upon or arbitrarily remove appellants' rights of identity, privacy, or personhood."

In a state court case, a physician's estate was successfully sued by a birthmother for revealing identifying data that enabled an adopted woman to seek out her birthmother. In the Oregon case of *Humphers v. First Interstate Bank* in 1985, the court ruled the physician had breached his professional responsibility to maintain confidentiality. Other similar lawsuits have been filed, some succeeding while others have not.

Arguments in Favor of Open Records

Most adoption search groups (usually comprised of adopted adults and birthparents who either have searched or are searching for birth relatives), are proponents of open records. They believe that birthparents and adopted persons should have access to identifying information, and that such information will make it easier to locate a triad member. They also believe that contact will help resolve the losses and pain they view as caused by adoption. Open record proponents argue that adopted adults are treated as if they were children and forced to adhere to a contract they never agreed upon when confidentiality is mandated.

An adoption search group is a group that seeks to help an adopted person or birthparent to locate birthparents or birth children, respectively, or provides them with the techniques or information to enable them to perform their own search. They may also support the searcher emotionally.

Search groups especially believe that adopted persons have an inviolable right to information concerning their genetic origins, and they have difficulty understanding why this information can or should be denied. Some adopted adults do not believe that 20 or more years ago unwed motherhood was considered reprehensible or shameful by many segments of society, who shunned unwed pregnant women. They may know many people who parent children out of wedlock in society today.

Whether meeting an adult birth child would lessen these powerfully negative feelings is a matter of much heated debate between open birth record advocates and proponents of confidentiality.

Some advocates of open records believe adoption information should not be available to an adopted person until adulthood (or the age of 18 or 21). Others believe that minor children and all the members of the adoption triad should have access to identifying information from the point of adoptive placement.

In the case of an OPEN ADOPTION, where identifying information is shared, there is less reason for adopted persons or birthparents to prepare an elaborate search strategy because this information is already known. However, it is estimated that only about 10 percent of all infant adoptions are open adoptions by this definition. (An open adoption allows for complete disclosure of identities.)

Adopted adult and attorney Heidi A. Schneider has stated that the state's efforts to protect confidential information from curious or prying eyes has also prevented adopted adults from obtaining background information, which she believes rightfully belongs to the adopted person. Schneider believes most of the courts are unreasonably restrictive to adopted adults who seek information. She adds that even when both adoptive parents and birthparents agree to open confidential adoption records, some courts will mandate an investigation as to whether the information should be released.

Some open records proponents argue that adopted people need medical information, although this reason is often used as a "front" because curiosity alone would probably not satisfy a judge deciding whether or not to release records. It is also true that records alone would not provide sufficient medical information in most cases because the birthparents' health 20 or more years ago was probably more robust, and many health problems would not yet have surfaced.

Those who favor open records include adopted persons who have begun search groups, birthparent support groups, and activist social workers. In addition, some adoptive parents favor open records, although many adoptive parents remain skeptical.

Arguments against Opening Identifying Information

Advocates of continued confidentiality are concerned that opening birth records would violate the confidentiality that was promised to most birthparents and adoptive parents in the United States in the past.

Many birthparents have married or remarried, and they may have other children. They may or may not have told their families about the child or children they placed for adoption.

Proponents of SEALED RECORDS also argue that most adopted persons do not opt to search, and instead they are satisfied with the nonidentifying medical, social, and other information provided to them by their adoptive parents or the agency. In the event of some compelling need to locate the birthparent, for example, a life-threatening problem requiring the birthparent to be contacted, an adopted person or the adoptive parents can request a court order to unseal the records.

Proponents of sealed birth records also argue that despite the joyous REUNION stories published in magazine and newspaper articles, some adopted persons who locate birthparents are devastated by the results of the search, particularly if they are rejected by the birthparent. Open birth record advocates counter that it is better to know the truth, even when the truth is very painful and does not live up to the fantasy that the adopted adult may have created about birthparents and his or her genetic origins.

Court Order to Unseal Adoption Records

When courts are asked to provide access to sealed records, the requester must usually provide a "good cause." Good cause may include a need for critical medical information.

If the adopted person is mentally stable, and the driving force appears to be curiosity, many courts would not consider that to be sufficient "good cause" to open up adoption records and court proceedings.

Carp, E. Wayne. *Family Matters: Secrecy and Disclosure in the History of Adoption.* Cambridge, Mass.: Harvard University Press, 1998.

Hollinger, Joan. *Adoption Law & Practice.* Washington, D.C.: LexisNexis, 2004.

Lifton, Betty Jean. *Lost and Found: The Adoption Experience.* New York: Harper & Row, 1988.

National Adoption Information Clearinghouse. "Access to Family Information by Adopted Persons: Summary of State Laws," State Statutes Series 2004, U.S. Department of Health and Human Services, Administration for Children and Families, 2004.

Schneider, Heidi A. "Adoption Contracts and the Adult Adoptee's Right to Identity," *Law and Inequality* 6 (1988): 185–229.

optional adopter   See FERTILE ADOPTIVE PARENTS.

orphan   A person whose parents have died or who are presumed dead; usually refers to a dependent child. Few of the infants and older children who are adopted in the United States are orphans. Instead, most are voluntarily placed for adoption by living birthparents, or parental rights are involuntarily terminated by the state (because of abuse, neglect, abandonment, or another reason), and the child is subsequently adopted.

The term *orphan* has a different meaning to the U.S. Citizenship and Immigration Services, the federal agency that oversees international adoption. To this organization, an orphan is a child from another country with no known parents or whose sole-surviving parent has signed an irrevocable consent to an adoption. There is also an upper age limit on orphans from other countries who may be adopted by U.S. citizens; the orphan petition must be filed before the child's 16th birthday.

Once the petition is approved, the child is considered as a relative of a U.S. citizen (at least one of the parents must be a U.S. citizen; in the case of a single parent, the single parent must be a U.S. citizen).

orphanage   Institution that houses children whose parents are deceased, unavailable, unable, or unwilling to provide care. The term is generally considered outmoded in the United States, although it is frequently used to describe institutions abroad.

Untold thousands of children reside in orphanages throughout the world, and many children experience extreme deprivation in these institutions. Clearly, an adoptive home would be a better environment. However, Dr. Miller points out that it is also important to consider the alternative to orphanages in many countries and says, "In some countries, infanticide, especially of females, is practiced. Unwanted children may lead stark and dangerous lives alone on the streets, may be 'sold' into servitude as laborers, servants, or even as child sex workers, or may be neglected, exploited, or abused by family members. Thus, when reviewing the ill effects of institutional life, it is important to remember the bleak alternatives that abandoned children may face if such facilities did not exist."

Dr. Miller points out that there are health risks to children living in orphanages, including poor or no medical care, exposure to respiratory and INTESTINAL

PARASITIC INFECTIONS and other health problems, GROWTH DELAYS, DEVELOPMENTAL DISABILITIES, LANGUAGE DELAY, and physical and emotional neglect. As a result, some children develop a variety of behavior problems, such as stereotypical rocking and other self-comfort or self-stimulating behaviors.

In the United States, the term GROUP HOMES is used to describe the types of institutionalized residences that usually fulfill this function; however, the group homes of today have smaller numbers of children than did the orphanages of earlier days. Group homes usually are staffed by live-in house parents. Children enter this alternative living arrangement because of a parental inability to control the child's behavior or because of abuse, abandonment, or neglect. Many group homes have a therapeutic or treatment component, although they differ from RESIDENTIAL TREATMENT CENTERS.

See also MEDICAL PROBLEMS OF INTERNATIONALLY ADOPTED CHILDREN; INTERNATIONAL ADOPTION.

Miller, Laurie C., M.D. *The Handbook of International Adoption Medicine: A Guide for Physicians, Parents, and Providers.* New York: Oxford University Press, 2005.

"orphans of the living"   A phrase to describe the many children in foster care in the late 1950s and early 1960s and before the movement for PERMANENCY PLANNING began in the mid-1970s. The phrase was also used to describe children who were stigmatized by illegitimacy in past years.

Social workers in the early 1960s became increasingly concerned that many children were remaining in foster homes throughout their childhood and never returning to their biological families or being placed in adoptive homes. Nor would they necessarily remain in one foster home. Children could be moved numerous times and never form strong attachments to parent figures.

This temporary home status of the children was perceived as a serious problem; however, little action was taken until testimony before Congress in the 1970s, and the first steps were taken to place children with SPECIAL NEEDS back with their parents, in adoptive homes, or in long-term foster care with the same caretakers or institutional care.

Orphan Train   Refers to the era of 1854–1929, when an estimated 150,000 homeless children were placed on trains and taken to rural sites concentrated in the Midwest and West in search of homes where the children could live and work. The children ranged in age from as young as about one year old to age 16 or 17.

Limited follow-ups of the children revealed that then, as now, the children who adapted the most readily were usually the younger children, and the older teenagers faced the greatest difficulty in adjusting to a radically different environment.

These homeless children came primarily from large cities on the Eastern Seaboard, such as New York City. Most were poor, and many had been involved with minor or serious infractions of the law. Many also had siblings and were separated from them for life as a result of the move. Yet most of the children made successful new lives for themselves, leaving behind them severe poverty and desolation.

The Orphan Train era was initiated by social welfare reformer Charles Loring Brace of the Children's Aid Society in New York. Brace urged that children of paupers not be left to languish in large crowded institutions but instead be given an opportunity to live and work in a family home.

Homelessness was a severe problem in Brace's time, and thousands of children often engaged in petty crimes, such as picking pockets, in order to survive. Police reports in New York City in 1852 revealed that in 11 wards, 2,000 homeless girls aged eight to 16 were arrested for theft.

Children arrested for "vagrancy" and other infractions were housed together with pauper children in large institutions, influencing each other. These children were referred to as the "dangerous classes."

Part of the problem was that there was almost no need for "honest labor" in the large cities, which was why the children had turned to dishonest labor. Large numbers of immigrants had teemed into the major Northeast cities, especially New York City, between 1847 and 1860. There was insufficient demand for the labor of this huge influx of adults, let alone children. (This was prior to the child labor movement, and at this time, everyone worked.)

At the same time, the midwestern and western farmers suffered a severe labor shortage. Brace saw the answer in Christian terms as well as in economic terms: provide children to the farmers—children who would work in exchange for a home—and get the children out of their evil urban environments and into rural America.

Brace contrasted the chance to live with a family to what he saw as the demoralizing effects of growing up in an institution, and to him, the choice was clear.

Poor children were often not taught to read and write and had little hope for a successful future. Brace envisioned the children sent out on the trains as having a better life, growing up to be farmers and farmer's wives.

He was supported in this movement by organizations within the Catholic Church and other groups; for example, the Sisters of Charity of St. Vincent de Paul and the New York Foundling Hospital were both actively involved in the Orphan Train movement.

The children were accompanied on the train by adults, often Catholic nuns, who rode with the children to their destinations and destinies.

The movement was also known as the "Placing Out" program and preceded adoption as we know it today.

The children left the train at each stop and were chosen or not chosen by people who came to the station to see them. In some cases, the match was made ahead of time, and the couple would present a number to the children's chaperone who would match the number to the child wearing the same number.

In other cases, the matches were far more informal. One train rider reported that her adoptive mother wanted a brunette girl, but the child with the right number refused to leave the nun. The red-haired and fair-skinned 18-month-old train rider happened to look at the woman and say "Mama." She was chosen.

Some of the Orphan Train riders were ultimately adopted, while others were not. Some were "indentured," which means their labor was sold to waiting farmers, but many were taken in as one of the family and raised as if they had been adopted, whether or not an adoption was ever legitimized.

Brace was opposed to indenturing children because it did not work and too often the children ran away. Instead, he believed the children should be treated with dignity and respect, and they would respond admirably.

Wrote Brace in 1859 in his book *The Best Method of Disposing of Our Pauper and Vagrant Children,*

> The children of the poor are not essentially different from the children of the rich; the same principles which influence the good or evil development of every child in comfortable circumstances, will affect, in greater or less degree, the child of poverty. Sympathy and hope are as inspiring to the ignorant girl, as to the educated; steady occupation is as necessary for the streetboy, as the boy of a wealthy house; indifference is as chilling to the one class, as to the other; the prospect of success is as stimulating to the young vagrant, as to the student in college.

The Orphan Train riders continued their treks west until about 1929. Although today the idea of sending homeless children to strangers in other states may sound cruel and inhuman, it must be remembered that diseases abounded in the almshouses and orphanages and that yesterday's orphan trains were not all that different from today's "Adoption Fairs," wherein caseworkers bring adoptable children to a picnic or party that is attended by previously approved prospective adoptive parents.

There were critics of Brace and the New York Aid Society. Brace's organization did not attempt religious matching, and often children of Catholic immigrants were placed in Protestant homes. Concern over this practice grew and ultimately resulted in attempts to place children in homes with the same religious background as their parents.

Critics also said Brace did insufficient investigations of the foster or adoptive homes and little follow-up or documentation. In Brace's defense, communications and transportation of his era had little resemblance to our society today.

Today the history of the Orphan Train era is kept alive by the Orphan Train Heritage Society of America Inc., based in Springdale, Arkansas. Members assist each other in finding birth families and in reminiscing about their shared history.

outreach An effort, usually by a human service agency, to reach out to enlist clients in the community who need services but have not yet sought such services. Individuals who need assistance may be unaware the agency exists or not know the range of the services offered by the agency.

Some agencies promote their services to the general public as well, not only educating the entire community about what the agency achieves but also reaching potential clients needing service who are unknown to the agency.

In the case of an adoption agency, outreach could include programs open to the public, articles in the newspaper, visits to clubs and high schools, and other attempts to reach particular people.

Agencies who are interested in reaching out seek to extend their services beyond the usual 9-to-5 working day, will often answer questions and provide counseling during evening hours or on weekends, and frequently utilize volunteers to supplement staff.

See also ADOPTION AGENCIES.

parens patriae The concept that the state has responsibility for a child when the parent or guardian cannot effectively continue in a parental role. As a result, if a parent abuses or neglects a child, the state has the right to remove the child from the home. If the state determines that the parent cannot or will not become an adequate parent, then the courts may terminate parental rights without the consent of the parents and place the child in an adoptive home. (See TERMINATION OF PARENTAL RIGHTS.)

Parens patriae was based on the English common law whereby the king protected children within his kingdom. According to Lela B. Costin, one of the contributors to *A Handbook of Child Welfare*, the concept of *parens patriae* was given a more liberal interpretation in America during the frontier period, when children were at great risk for being orphaned, abandoned, or neglected. As a result, *parens patriae* came to be interpreted as a rationale for the state stepping into the parent-child relationship when needed.

Parens patriae is a principle also used beyond the field of adoption; for example, the state requires children to go to school up to a certain age, and parents and children must comply with this requirement. (Some states recognize homeschooling as acceptable.)

Up to about a century ago, the parents were usually seen as the supreme arbiters of the children's fate, and it was not up to neighbors or society in general to set rules or standards for parents. Child labor laws did not exist, and many children worked long hours at low wages. Social reforms were passed, and today children occupy a special role in society.

Costin, Lela B. "The Historical Context of Child Welfare," in *A Handbook of Child Welfare: Context, Knowledge, and Practice.* New York: Free Press, 1985.

parental leave Time taken off from work by a mother or father to care for a child.

Because adopting parents often receive very little notice that a child is available—perhaps only a few days—it is impossible for employees to give their employers even two weeks notice about an impending leave. Consequently, adoption leave may be perceived negatively by employers. In the past whether parental leave was granted or not depended on state laws and corporate policies. Only 13 states mandated some form of personal leave in 1989. The Family and Medical Leave Act of 1993 changed this. The FMLA mandates an unpaid leave of up to 12 weeks for employees working at companies employing more than 50 workers. The FMLA specifically includes adoptive parents in the law.

See also EMPLOYMENT BENEFITS FOR ADOPTION; INSURANCE.

parental rights Parents have the right to choose the religion of their child, place the child in public or private schools (or homeschool), select health care providers, and make a myriad of decisions affecting a child's life. Parents do not have the right to abuse a child, and if state social service officials believe parents are abusing their children physically or sexually or are neglecting the children or have abandoned them, state workers have the right to remove the children from the home and place them in foster care or institutional care.

Parents may voluntarily choose to place their children for adoption. This involves a formal termination of rights.

States also have the right to terminate parental rights, although rights are usually only involuntarily terminated in the most extreme cases. (For a detailed discussion of voluntary and involuntary ending of rights, see TERMINATION OF PARENTAL RIGHTS.)

In most cases, if a biological parent expresses a desire to retain parental rights and appears willing and able to work toward correcting the condition that led to the child's removal, then parental rights will not be terminated.

Parents have the right to appeal when a child is removed from the home if they feel the charges of abuse or neglect were unfair; however, there are often periods of weeks or even months before a court will decide whether or not to return the child home.

If the state social services department decides to initiate action to terminate parental rights, then the parent may appeal these actions as well. If the court does terminate parental rights, the parent has no further recourse (presuming all appeals are exhausted.)

Most children needing adoptive families under the control and authority of the state social services system are over age eight, even if they entered foster care three or four years earlier, because few states comply with federal laws requiring action be taken on a child's case 18 months after entry into foster care.

Part of the problem is the difficulty in preparing a case for court to terminate parental rights, and another part of the problem is many caseworkers and/or judges who are extremely hesitant to terminate parental rights, even in the face of extreme cruelty or obvious parental abuse or neglect.

paternity testing   A technique that analyzes genetic material (DNA) to determine the father of a child. The technique of genetic fingerprinting, developed by Dr. Alec Jeffreys, a genetics professor at the University of Leicester in England, was first created in 1984. Prior to that time, it was possible to identify the likely father of a particular child, but not to prove it definitively. Genetic fingerprinting provides a certainty of paternity in an estimated 99 percent of the cases in which the biological father has been tested, and it has successfully been used in many paternity lawsuits nationwide.

The relevance of paternity testing to adoption arises if a birthmother wishes to plan adoption for her child but a man who alleges he is the father tries to block the adoption. In this situation, genetic testing can prove whether or not the man is actually the biological father.

If she is not married to the man and he is not the biological father, his claims are generally considered less valid than if he is the biological father. (In some cases, the law takes into account an existing relationship a minor has with a parent figure.)

If the birthmother is married, the law generally presumes her husband is the father of her child, although genetic testing may refute this presumption.

Paternity testing can be performed by blood or by samples of tissue from inside the cheek. In-home tests are available for the personal use of interested parties; however, most courts require that a laboratory have a chain of custody, which means that they can verify that they have maintained control of the samples and that the samples have not been tampered with. Paternity test results available through a laboratory can usually be performed within several days.

pathology and adoptive status   The theory that there are problems in a person that are related to adoptive status, either directly or indirectly. These could include problems with identity, psychiatric problems, alcohol abuse, or criminal behavior.

Some adoption writers believe adopted persons are at risk for developing certain problems. Psychologist David Kirschner has claimed that 5 percent to 10 percent of adopted children develop "adopted child syndrome," which includes such behaviors as lying, stealing, learning difficulties, and occasional violent acts. However, most adoption and psychiatric experts do not accept this theory and state that data from the Search Institute and other research demonstrates that adopted persons are not necessarily at risk for developing behavioral problems.

See also ADOLESCENT ADOPTED PERSONS; ADULT ADOPTED PERSONS; ALCOHOLISM AND ADOPTED PERSONS; IDENTITY; OPEN RECORDS; PSYCHIATRIC PROBLEMS OF ADOPTED PERSONS.

pediatricians   Physicians who specialize in treating children and adolescents. Physicians who specialize in treating children adopted from other countries are said to be specialists in ADOPTION MEDICINE.

permanency planning Refers to a movement which developed in the 1970s, to either return foster children to their biological homes or terminate parental rights and place the child for adoption. This movement led to the ADOPTION ASSISTANCE AND CHILD WELFARE ACT OF 1980, which mandated permanency planning for all states.

Prior to this time, most older children who were placed in foster care remained in the system until they "aged-out" at 18 years old. Caseworkers began to realize that they could find families for children over age eight, and there were also families for children in sibling groups, handicapped children, minority children, and other categories of children previously considered UNADOPTABLE.

Subsequent to the passage of the ADOPTION AND SAFE FAMILIES ACT in 1997, many states increased efforts to find permanent homes for foster children who could not be safely returned to their families of origin.

See also FOSTER CARE; FOSTER PARENT; FOSTER PARENT ADOPTION; SPECIAL NEEDS ADOPTION.

photolistings Refers to photographs and description of children available for adoption, who are also known as WAITING CHILDREN. Many agencies, attorneys, and organizations now offer photolistings of children who need adoptive families on their INTERNET Web sites.

Starting in 1971, the Adoption Listing Service in Illinois was the first organization to use a photolisting service to find families for older children. Subsequently, the Massachusetts Adoption Resource Exchange (MARE) and Children Awaiting Parents (CAP) also began using photolistings in 1972. In 1975, New York law ordered that all children needing adoptive families be photolisted.

State social services agencies offer a photolisting book, usually available to individuals who have completed their home study or who are considering adopting a child with SPECIAL NEEDS. How frequently updated these listings or Web sites are varies from state to state. Photolistings are used in conjunction with videotapes of children needing families, media campaigns, adoption fairs and pic-

nics, and a variety of tactics to recruit adoptive parents. Sometimes libraries have photolistings available. The reference librarian at the local public library will know if they are available or if not, if the information can be ordered through another library.

Most photolistings are of children with special needs who are black or mixed race, are over age eight, or have siblings and have some degree of emotional, mental, or physical disability.

It is clear from the efforts of the CAP book as well as the many state photolisting services that photolisting children is an effective way to recruit adoptive parents. Giving a "face" and a description to a child inspires many adopting parents to select a particular child or at least ask for further information.

Other variants on photolistings are weekly newspapers or television segments featuring a specific child, such as a WEDNESDAY'S CHILD program. Such campaigns have been successful in recruiting families into adoption, even if not for the child featured.

Some organizations have expressed reservations about photolistings on the Internet, concerned about the privacy rights of waiting children and the potential for these well-intentioned listings to be misused. A critical concern is that sexual predators could pervert the sound goals of photolisting.

See also ADVERTISING AND PROMOTION; FOSTER CARE; VIDEOTAPE.

physicians Doctors play an important and broad role in the field of adoption. They are often the first to confirm a pregnancy in a teenager. They also diagnose and treat adopted children as they grow, and attitudes of the physician toward the adopted children are important. Physicians are also critically important in INTERNATIONAL ADOPTION because children who are being adopted from other countries may suffer ailments that are unknown or highly unusual in the United States.

Crisis Pregnancies

Doctors vary widely in their opinions about adoption. As in the society at large, some physicians believe adoption is the best answer to most crisis pregnancies while others believe parenting should be chosen. Ideally, a physician will present the pros and cons of all the various options and enable a pregnant girl or woman to make her own informed decision.

Physicians are also affected by the attitudes of society at large; for example, if the average person believes an unmarried person should abort before she should consider having a baby and placing it for adoption, physicians, too, may be influenced by such an attitude.

Teen Pregnancies

Because the physician may be the first adult an adolescent talks to about the pregnancy, the physician's response is very critical, and adoption is one option that should be discussed. To properly discuss adoption with the patient, the physician should be aware of adoption agencies and counseling resources available in the community. Physicians should also be sure to talk to the pregnant adolescent in person rather than over the telephone to ensure privacy. (In some states, privacy rights cover adolescents, and diagnoses of pregnancy or other medical conditions may not be given to individuals other than the minor unless she has given her permission.)

Physicians as Intermediaries

A few physicians actually arrange independent adoptions, particularly physicians who are also obstetricians. They may have patients who are infertile couples and arrange for the woman with the crisis pregnancy to place her child with one of these infertile couples.

Social workers argue that adoption agencies are much better suited to provide objective counseling to a pregnant woman considering adoption for her child than is her physician, whose expertise lies in the medical arena rather than the social work field. (This argument is also advanced against attorneys who are involved with placing children in independent adoptions: social workers assert that lawyers are more qualified at handling legal matters than at counseling adopting parents or birthparents.)

Physicians who do provide advice should repeat information at least several times because if the pregnant woman faces a crisis pregnancy, she may be so anxious that she may have difficulty listening.

Adoptive Parents and Physicians

Adoptive parents who are adopting either an infant or older child should talk to the pediatrician they are considering to determine if he or she is generally favorable or neutral about adoption.

Studies of internationally adopted children have revealed that physicians may be unaware of medical problems foreign children may suffer. (See MEDICAL PROBLEMS OF INTERNATIONALLY ADOPTED CHILDREN.)

As a result, adopting parents should educate themselves as much as possible about necessary tests and should also seek out a physician at or near a major medical center whenever possible.

See also HOSPITALS' TREATMENT OF BIRTHMOTHERS; INDEPENDENT ADOPTION; PEDIATRICIANS.

placement The point at which a child begins to live with prospective adoptive parents. After a certain period, depending on the state in which the adoptive parents reside, the adoption may be finalized, and the adopted child will have all the rights and privileges of a biological child born to the family.

placement outcome Refers to the success or failure of an adoption, whether the adoption is disrupted or dissolved or successful. The overwhelming majority of adoptions are successful.

See also DISRUPTION.

post-legal adoptive services Also known as postadoption services, these are services provided by an adoption agency subsequent to legal finalization of the adoption. The adopted person, birthparents, or adoptive parents may have questions soon after finalization or many years later.

Adopted adults may have questions about adoption in general or their own birthparents. Adopted persons, birthparents, and/or adoptive parents may wish further information about genetic backgrounds or may wish an actual meeting to be arranged between the parties.

Families who adopt children with SPECIAL NEEDS may need further counseling and support after the "honeymoon" period ends. Even parents who adopt children as infants often find adoption issues arise later and may seek expert assistance and counseling. Those who adopt children internationally may have dual challenges. Children may have developmental needs as well as questions about culture and country-specific issues.

postplacement services The range of counseling and services provided to the adoptive parents, adopted child, and birthparents subsequent to the child's adoptive placement and before the adoption is legally finalized in court.

Birthparents may need counseling to resolve feelings of loss after they have placed a newborn infant for adoption. Older children usually need counseling after an adoptive placement, no matter how positive the child feels about the adoptive parents. Postplacement services are provided to make the adoption experience as positive and satisfying as possible to all parties.

preadoptive counseling Counseling provided to prospective adoptive parents while they are being assessed and before they are approved to adopt a child. Another phrase in common usage for this process is the HOME STUDY.

prebirth consent to an adoption Legal agreement to an adoption before a child is born. In approximately half the states in the United States, prebirth consent may be obtained from a biological father not married to the biological mother. Prebirth consent from the birthfather assures pregnant women planning adoption for their babies that the biological father has agreed to the plan.

When a man who is not married to the birthmother signs papers allowing an adoption to go forward, it is not always a "consent" to an adoption. In some instances, the statement filed says essentially, "I am not the father but if I were the father, I would have no objection to the child being adopted."

Whether or not prebirth consent may be revoked after the birth of the child depends on the laws of the state. As of this writing, the following states allow prebirth consents to be taken: Alabama, Arkansas, Delaware, Florida, Hawaii, Illinois, Indiana, Kansas, Louisiana, Michigan, Missouri, Nevada, New Mex-

ico, New York, North Carolina, North Dakota, Oklahoma, Oregon, Pennsylvania, South Dakota, Tennessee, Utah, Vermont, and Washington.

pregnancy after adoption Although the majority of adoptive parents do not have a biological child subsequent to an adoption, virtually every new adoptive parent has heard about a person with this experience. It is unknown how many adoptive mothers become pregnant after adopting but probably well less than 10 percent have biological children after they adopt a child. In many cases, the pregnancy is unplanned because the mother presumed she was infertile.

In an extensive study performed by Michael Bohman, he found 8 percent of the adoptive parents ultimately had a biological child. According to Bohman, 8 percent of the infertile couples who had applied to the agency and then withdrew before adopting also later had biological children. Bohman discussed other studies, which indicate postadoptive pregnancies at a rate of about 3 percent to 10 percent.

The act of adopting a child cannot erase a woman's or man's infertility problem, and individuals who suggest adoption as a psychological "cure" to infertility are sadly misled. What is likely to happen in those instances is that infertility caused by unknown factors was somehow diminished. Since about 20 percent of infertile couples have "unexplained infertility" for their diagnosis, this is likely to account for such a phenomenon.

Adoption experts strive to ensure that prospective adoptive parents have resolved as much of their conflicts about infertility as possible prior to adoption so the adopted child will be fully accepted.

With increasing breakthroughs in ASSISTED REPRODUCTIVE TECHNOLOGY, it may be possible for a greater number of adoptive mothers to successfully bear biological children, should they wish to do so.

See also SIBLINGS.

Bohman, Michael. *Adopted Children and Their Families.* Stockholm, Sweden: Proprius, 1970.

pregnancy counseling A service provided to women with crisis pregnancies. Counseling may be offered by social workers at adoption agencies, counselors at family planning clinics, pregnancy centers, or schools, or other individuals.

The woman with a CRISIS PREGNANCY may need assistance in resolving her immediate needs, for example, verification that she actually is pregnant, location of a place to stay (if needed), and initiation of medical care. She may be eligible for public assistance, such as Temporary Aid to Needy Families (TANF), food stamps, and Medicaid.

She may also be uncertain as to whether or not she should continue her pregnancy and may feel compelled to abort her baby because she is fearful of what her parents, friends, and others will think when she becomes visibly pregnant.

Often she may have vague and erroneous ideas about adoption that need to be clarified after her immediate needs are met. Should she consider adoption or parenting (presuming she continues the pregnancy), she needs someone who can fully explore both options with her. The agency social worker is usually the best qualified person to provide this service. Whoever provides her counseling should be sure to include the adoption option as one possible choice, whether the woman appears interested or not.

In his study of counselors, Edmund Mech found that many counselors never discussed adoption with pregnant teenagers because they were convinced teens were completely uninterested. On the contrary, when Mech surveyed pregnant teens, he found the majority were interested in learning more about adoption. Yet this omission causes a problem for the teenager (or woman) who is interested: if she brings the subject up herself, will the counselor think she is a "bad" person? By not approaching the topic of adoption, the counselor implicitly conveys the idea that adoption is not acceptable—or at least not acceptable in this person's case.

In addition, a failure to discuss adoption shortchanges the woman who might consider it if she understood what it entailed.

Jerome Smith and Franklin Miroff describe feelings the birthmother faces as she makes her decision about whether to parent or make an adoption plan in their book *You're Our Child: The Adoption Experience.*

According to the authors, the birthmother may tell herself that an infertile couple will adopt her baby, and without her, they would be unable to adopt. If she is religious, she may see herself as "God's instrument." She may also try to think of the baby as the adoptive couple's child rather than her child. By such thinking, she defends herself against maternal attachment, thereby reducing the sense of anticipatory loss.

She will also swing back and forth between deciding to parent or to delegate parenting to others more prepared for it. Smith and Miroff explain the ambivalence of the woman (or girl) as a "head-heart" response.

Smith and Miroff believe counseling is critically important and state, "A warm, supportive, nonjudgmental atmosphere will allow the woman to think through her situation and discuss the practical aspects of her planning free from coercion."

They add, "In assisting the woman in decision making, the counselor must help her to separate fact from fantasy, help her to see the realities involved with raising a child alone and with relinquishing a child she may never see again."

Most birthmothers say they have some future plan for themselves after placement; for example, they plan to return to high school or college or they expect to resume their job or career. A study by Jane Bose and Michael Resnick revealed the teenagers who made adoption plans had much higher educational aspirations than did the teenagers who chose parenting.

Women who refuse to make future plans and who have no idea what will happen to them after the baby is born are far more likely to change their mind about placing the child for adoption, either just before or after the baby is born and before consent is signed, than is a woman with a plan for her future.

Stages of Counseling

In a paper on pregnancy counseling, former vice president of the National Council for Adoption, Mary Beth Style, discussed stages of the counseling process, including assessment, decision making, making an "action plan," mourning, and acceptance and integration of the adoption experience.

According to Style, it is the initial assessment that requires the most skill on the part of the pregnancy counselor. It is at this point when the counselor must learn about the woman or teenager, her family, and her relationships and also evaluate her intellectual and emotional levels. In addition, if possible, the counselor will actually involve the birthfather and the family of the birthmother (and sometimes the family of the birthfather as well), not only to help the social worker with assessment but to involve people who are intimately connected to the crisis at hand and who can help the pregnant woman with resolution, whatever her ultimate decision is.

Style says it is dangerous to concentrate on the outcome (parenting or adoption) at this point because there are many other issues that more urgently need to be discussed (although the woman should be assured that the agency can assist with adoption, should that option be chosen).

During the decision-making phase of counseling, the pregnant woman begins evaluating the pros and cons of parenting and adoption as she explores each option and considers her own unique case.

When she is in the "action plan" stage, she is ready to formulate a plan; however, she cannot make a plan unless the counselor has fully explained both adoption and parenting to her. Says Style, "If the client knew everything she needed and wanted, chances are she would not be in the counselor's office . . . She may not know the possible repercussions of any of her choices on herself, her baby or the adoptive family unless the social worker leads her through a thoughtful decision-making process after outlining all possible options and supports available to her."

The last stage of counseling is grief counseling. Some counselors may try to shorten this phase because it is painful; however, this well-meaning action could result in even more pain because it inhibits the resolution of the loss. (See LOSS.)

As she resolves the pain associated with the loss, the birthmother can accept that adoption was the best choice for herself and her child, particularly if she feels she was not pressured to make an adoption plan but personally believed it was the best decision. Counselors should be careful not to make adoption a scapegoat if the birthmother complains of problems and should instead seek out what the problem is, whether it be family

problems, "unresolved problems of pregnancy," or other problems.

Mech, Edmund V. *Orientations of Pregnancy Counselors Toward Adoption,* U.S. Department of Health and Human Services, Office of Population Affairs, 1984.

Style, Mary Beth. "Pregnancy Counseling: Traditional and Experimental Practices," paper revised and published by the National Council for Adoption, 1999.

prenatal care   Medical care provided by a physician to a pregnant woman during the course of her pregnancy.

Many women in crisis pregnancies, particularly teenagers, do not seek prenatal care early in the pregnancy. Consequently, problems with the fetus may not be identified, or the woman herself may suffer untreated health problems.

There are several reasons women avoid prenatal care in the first trimester, including denial of the pregnancy and a conscious or unconscious desire to carry the fetus to term—a desire that is easier to realize if no one except the woman is aware of the pregnancy in the early months. Clinics have seen women in their last trimester of pregnancy who deny they are pregnant yet who are very clearly pregnant to even the most casual observer.

Poor women may not have health insurance and think they are ineligible for public assistance or Medicaid.

The lack of prenatal care contributes to the high rate of infant mortality in the United States. It is very important for every woman to see a physician for appropriate testing and care as soon as she suspects she may be pregnant.

See also PRENATAL EXPOSURES.

prenatal exposures   The use of substances during pregnancy that are often harmful to the developing fetus, such as alcohol, illegal drugs, and tobacco. Some exposures to solvents or heavy metals such as lead may also be harmful. In addition, some medications which are lawful and not harmful to the mother could be toxic to the fetus, and thus all medications and even herbal remedies should be carefully considered by the physician of the pregnant woman. Individuals who are adopting children from the United States or other countries should try to ascertain if there were any prenatal exposures to the child, although this is often difficult or impossible to determine with international adoption (unless there is clear evidence, such as the presence of FETAL ALCO-HOL SYNDROME (FAS) in a child, indicating that the biological mother was an alcohol abuser).

In the United States, the Keeping Children and Families Safe Act of 2003 added some new requirements for states, such as the requirement that states create procedures and policies by which physicians and other health-care providers will notify Child Protective Services (CPS) workers if newborn children are identified with illegal drugs or they are suffering from withdrawal symptoms caused by prenatal drug abuse by the mother. Substances such as tobacco and alcohol need not be reported under this federal law, although states may choose to do so, if they wish. As of this writing, some states have already changed their laws to comply with the new federal requirements.

Whether infants born addicted to drugs or alcohol will be removed from the home and enter the foster care system depends on state laws and policies.

Alcohol Abuse

Alcohol abuse by the pregnant woman is a problem to the fetus, and children born to alcoholic mothers may suffer fetal alcohol syndrome and other effects. In 1989, the federal government in the United States mandated public labeling of alcohol products to provide warnings to pregnant women that alcohol consumption was not recommended during pregnancy. Yet the CDC estimates that 13 percent of pregnant women in the United States continue to drink during pregnancy.

According to the CDC, rates of FAS in the United States range from 0.2 to 1.5 per 1,000 live births per year, which means that about 1,000 to 6,000 infants are born each year with FAS.

It is not known how much alcohol consumption is required to cause FAS, although some studies have shown that an amount as small as 0.5 ounces of alcohol per day consumed by a pregnant woman can lead to fetal development problems. It should be noted that binge drinking (having five or more drinks on at least one occasion in the past two weeks) is particularly dangerous to the developing fetus, and it can lead to serious problems in brain development. Because physicians cannot determine *any* safe level of drinking, doctors recom-

mend that pregnant women abstain from drinking alcohol altogether during their pregnancies to avoid any risk of FAS to their children.

If pregnant women *stop* drinking later in their pregnancies, some damage to the developing fetus may be avoided, and thus, women who have been drinkers should not assume there is no point in giving up alcohol because it is already too late and all damage has been done. For example, one of the problems caused by heavy drinking is microcephaly, a condition in which the baby has an unusually small head. However, according to information provided by Wei-Jung A. Chen and colleagues, in their article in *Alcohol Research & Health,* when pregnant women stopped drinking before the end of their second trimester, their infants had larger head circumferences than the babies of women who had kept drinking throughout their pregnancies.

According to the National Survey on Drug Use and Health in 2004, the rate of alcohol use was higher among younger pregnant women, aged 15 to 25 (5 percent) than among pregnant women who were aged 26 to 44 (2 percent).

Illegal Drugs

Illegal drugs are also very dangerous to the development of the fetus. For example, heroin use may cause a miscarriage or a premature delivery. Yet many pregnant women with substance use problems have difficulty finding a rehabilitation facility that will accept them during pregnancy. Of those who are admitted, most are cocaine abusers, compared to nonpregnant women who are admitted and whose primary substance of abuse is alcohol. (See Figure 1.)

According to the *National Survey on Drug Use and Health* in a 2004 issue of *The NSDUH Report,* in the United States about 3 percent of pregnant women aged 15 to 44 used an illegal drug in the past month, compared to 9 percent of nonpregnant women in this age group. Pregnant women aged 15 to 25 were more likely to use illegal drugs than women aged 26 to 44.

In her book *The Handbook of International Adoption Medicine: A Guide for Physicians, Parents, and Providers,* Dr. Miller notes that language, attention, behavior, and emotional regulation may all be affected by prenatal drug exposure. However, she notes that there are apparent protective effects of adoption among some drug-exposed children, although studies often fail to account for the age of the child at adoption and the care the child received prior to the adoption. With regard to internationally adopted children who were drug exposed, Dr. Miller advises:

"Language skills (including articulation), behavior, and attention span should be monitored at regular visits, and neurologic examination should be performed . . . The pediatrician should assess the child's arousal, attention, recognition memory and impulse control, with the goal of providing supportive services if needed. Although prenatal drug exposure will usually not be known with certainty, anticipatory guidance will benefit many children." In addition, children born to mothers who were intravenous drug users during pregnancy should be assessed for exposure to hep-atitis B, hepatitis C, and the human immunodeficiency virus (HIV).

Tobacco use

Mothers who smoke during pregnancy have a greater risk of delivering low birth weight babies. Low birth weight is a leading cause of infant deaths in the United States, and more than 300,000 low birth weight newborns die each year in the United States. As can be seen from Table I, smokers have about twice the rate of low birth weight babies compared to nonsmokers.

Smoking is also linked to sudden infant death syndrome (SIDS). The infants of mothers who smoke have twice the risk of developing SIDS. Babies whose mothers smoked both before and after their birth have three to four times the risk of dying from SIDS.

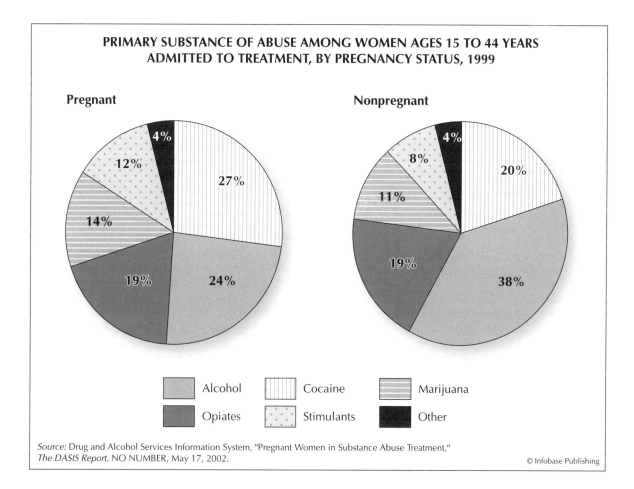

PRIMARY SUBSTANCE OF ABUSE AMONG WOMEN AGES 15 TO 44 YEARS ADMITTED TO TREATMENT, BY PREGNANCY STATUS, 1999

Pregnant

Nonpregnant

Legend: Alcohol, Cocaine, Marijuana, Opiates, Stimulants, Other

Source: Drug and Alcohol Services Information System, "Pregnant Women in Substance Abuse Treatment," *The DASIS Report,* NO NUMBER, May 17, 2002.

© Infobase Publishing

TABLE I: LOW-BIRTH-WEIGHT LIVE BIRTHS (LESS THAN 2,500 GRAMS), PERCENT OF LIVE BIRTHS ACCORDING TO MOTHER'S SMOKING STATUS, 1995–2001

	1995	1996	1997	1998	1999	2000	2001
Cigarette smokers	12.18	12.13	12.06	12.01	12.06	11.88	11.90
Nonsmokers	6.79	6.91	7.07	7.18	7.21	7.19	7.32

Source: Fried, V. M., et al. *Chartbook on Trends in the Health of Americans. Health, United States, 2003.* National Center for Health Statistics, Hyattsville, Md., 2003.

Toxic Substances

Some toxic substances such as lead are dangerous to the developing fetus and should be avoided by pregnant women. Prenatal and perinatal exposure to various substances, including methylmecury, lead, polychlorinated biphenyls (PCBs), dioxins, pesticides, and ionizing radiation, may act as developmental neurotoxicants, interfering with normal brain development and function. Some experts attribute the rise in the incidence of learning disabilities, autism, and other developmental disabilities to these and other toxic exposures in early life.

See also DRUG ABUSE/ADDICTION.

Chen, Wei-Jung A., et al. "Alcohol and the Developing Brain: Neuroanatomical Studies," *Alcohol Research & Health* 27, no. 2 (2003): 174–180.

Drug and Alcohol Services Information System. "Pregnant Women in Substance Abuse Treatment," The DASIS Report, May 17, 2002, Office of Applied Studies, Substance Abuse and Mental Health Services Administration.

Fried, V. M., et al. *Chartbook on Trends in the Health of Americans. Health, United States, 2003.* National Center for Health Statistics, Hyattsville, Md., 2003.

Gwinnell, Esther, M.D., and Christine Adamec. *The Encyclopedia of Addictions and Addictive Behaviors.* New York: Facts On File, 2005.

Miller, Laurie, C., M.D. *The Handbook of International Adoption Medicine: A Guide for Physicians, Parents, and Providers.* New York: Oxford University Press, 2005.

National Survey on Drug Use and Health. "Pregnancy and Substance Use," *The NSDUH Report,* Office of Applied Studies, Substance Abuse and Mental Health Services Administration, January 2, 2004.

preparing a child for adoption   Taking actions to ease the process for a child who will be adopted. Although no preparation of the child is needed in an infant adoption, when older children are to be adopted, caseworkers usually work together with foster parents and adopting parents to help the child get ready for the impending move. In many cases, however, children are adopted by their own foster parents, and no move is required.

Various means are employed to prepare a child for adoption. Many caseworkers use a LIFEBOOK, which is a special scrapbook describing the child's life, hobbies, and relationships. The social worker also counsels the child about what adoption will mean to him or her and makes it clear that an adoptive family is a permanent family. This explanation also necessitates the often painful realization that the biological family ties will be severed prior to the adoption.

Adopting a Child in the United States

Social workers usually arrange a meeting between the prospective adoptive parents and the child before any home visits are arranged. The child may go to a park or a fast-food restaurant with them, or they may meet in the social worker's office, or the meeting may occur at an adoption picnic. In some cases, the social worker will show the child a videotape the family has made of their home, family, and lifestyle. Social workers who use such techniques say children ask to see the videos over and over.

If the prospective parents and the child appear to be a possible "match," the caseworker will arrange a visit within their home for a day or a weekend. Many times the child and the adopting parents are anxious for visits to end and for the child to move in permanently, but caseworkers want to ensure as much as possible that the placement will work and that a DISRUPTION/DISSOLUTION will not occur, causing the child further pain.

Adopting a Child from Another Country

The preparation of children being adopted internationally is more complicated than that of a child born in the same country as the adoptive parents. Some countries such as Russia require two trips or lengthy stays (Kazakhstan) by the adoptive parents, as of this writing. This can allow the child and family to gradually accustom themselves to each other. However, in many circumstances, the child must leave a familiar environment, caregivers, and friends abruptly.

Some parents try to prepare their children for this transition by sending photos labeled in the child's language in advance of their arrival. It is helpful if the caregivers can show the child the photos before the parents arrive. Some parents find that wearing the same clothing as they wore in the photos for their first meeting with the child aids in the transition. Having a trusted caregiver explain to the child what is happening is essential for children old enough to understand.

Many internationally adopted children have resided their entire lives in institutional care, thus, riding in a car, using an elevator, eating in a restaurant, and boarding an airplane are completely unfamiliar and may be frightening if the child has not been prepared ahead of time for major changes.

See also FOSTER PARENT ADOPTION; INTERNATIONAL ADOPTION; SPECIAL NEEDS ADOPTION.

preplacement visits   Social worker visits to prospective adoptive parents before a child is placed within their home. The visits are made as a part of the HOME STUDY process, which is a preparation and evaluation of adopting parents.

private adoption   See INDEPENDENT ADOPTION.

private agencies   See ADOPTION AGENCIES.

prostitution   Providing sexual services to a variety of individuals for pay; illegal in every state except Nevada.

Few prostitutes place their children for adoption, probably because most prostitutes are aware of methods of birth control; however, with the increasing rate of drug addiction, even well-informed prostitutes may fail to use birth control and become pregnant. If an abortion is not obtained within the first two trimesters, it becomes more difficult to obtain an abortion in some states, and a prostitute may opt to place the child for adoption.

Because of the high risk of HIV and the high probability of drug use among prostitutes, few adopting parents are willing to adopt the child of a prostitute, and agencies may consider such a child to fit into the category of a child with SPECIAL NEEDS.

If a child born to a prostitute is ultimately adopted, it is likely the termination of parental rights by the state occurred after some time frame during which the child had been removed from the home and placed in foster care. In a study of children born to teenage prostitutes, 38 of 55 infants had been placed in the protective custody of the state with most of the babies being referred to protective services either prior to the child's birth or at the time of delivery. Unfortunately, according to the researchers, in many of the cases the infant was placed in the home of the prostitute's mother, "in whose home the girl may still be living while prostituting."

Motherhood did not change the girls' lifestyles. According to the researchers, "These young women usually continue with prostitution, drug involvement and a destructive lifestyle. Many return to the streets within days of delivery."

Many adopted persons who fantasize about their birthmothers imagine the birthmother at two ends of the spectrum: either a prostitute or a wealthy socialite. The reality is usually neither: most are ordinary girls or women who became pregnant as the result of a long-term relationship.

See also DRUG ABUSE/ADDICTION.

Deisher, Robert W., M.D., James A. Farrow, M.D., Kerry Hope, and Christina Litchfield. "The Pregnant Adolescent Prostitute," *American Journal of Diseases of Children* 143 (October 1989): 1,162–1,165.

protective services   Child welfare services, usually provided by state, county, or other public child welfare agencies, assigned to investigate allegations of child abuse, neglect, or abandonment. Protective service workers who believe a complaint is founded may remove a child from the home immediately and place the child in an emergency shelter home or foster home. A judge will shortly thereafter determine if continuous foster care is in the best interests of the child. Reports of suspected abuse may come from teachers, physicians, emergency room doctors, and other sources.

If the complaint was unfounded, the child will remain in the home. Unfounded complaints may come from ex-spouses, jealous neighbors, and similar other sources. Protective services workers should be trained in techniques to detect abuse and injuries most likely to have occurred from abuse.

Protective services is a high-pressure, stressful job, and many social workers working in this unit transfer to other jobs that are less stressful.

Workers report that even when they remove a child from his or her home because of severe abuse, the child is angry at the caseworker rather than at the abusive parent. In addition, the abusive parent often denies the abuse and believes the caseworker is persecuting the parent.

Often protective workers are given little time to investigate and must visit the accused person within 24 hours or 48 hours, so the pressure of time is another constraint on the worker.

Ultimately, many of the children seen by protective services workers and judged by the workers to have been abused, neglected, or abandoned will enter the child welfare system. Adoption will be the plan for some of these children. The failure of protective services to assure children's safety was a major reason Congress passed the ADOPTION AND SAFE FAMILIES ACT.

See also ABANDONMENT; ABUSE; NEGLECT.

psychiatric problems of adopted persons Serious mental disorders among children or adults who were adopted and who require treatment for these problems, which range from disorders such as attention-deficit/hyperactivity disorder to severe psychotic disorders, such as schizophrenia. Researchers actively disagree among themselves on whether adopted persons evince a greater level of mental illness than nonadopted persons. Vastly differing percentages of adopted persons have been reported in clinical studies of individuals with psychiatric problems, ranging from about 5 percent to as high as 25 percent or more, depending on the study.

One major problem with many studies on psychiatric problems among adopted children is that their age when adopted is often not reported. Yet when this information *is* provided, it is clear that in many cases, children adopted as infants or small children often have a better outcome than children adopted as older children. Another important factor is whether the children were adopted from foster care or orphanages or as infants from an agency or independent adoptions. In addition, it is important to note that many studies on psychiatric problems in children concentrate on *clinical* populations of children, as opposed to the general population of adopted children, most of whom do not need treatment.

It is irrational to generalize from a percentage of adopted children in a clinical population to the entire nonclinical population of adopted children. Yet this is what many people do, including some experts. There are individuals who assume, for example, that because a study shows that 25 percent of the children receiving treatment were adopted, this then means that 25 percent of *all* adopted children need psychiatric treatment. It makes no sense to generalize from a small group with problems to a very large group which may or may not have similar problems.

It is also very important to note that when researchers look at the nonclinical population, many studies find little or no difference between adopted people in the general population and nonadopted people in terms of the presence of psychiatric problems.

Yet understandably, some individuals continue to wonder why adopted children may represent a disproportionate percent of some clinical populations. Some possible explanations have been suggested; for example, that many adoptive parents enjoy a higher socioeconomic level than the average person and can afford to pay for psychiatric treatment for their children, including both inpatient and outpatient treatment. Adoptive parents may also be more likely than non-adoptive parents to have medical insurance coverage for such treatment. Adoptive parents may also be more educated about psychiatric problems and thus more likely to seek help, as compared to parents who are less familiar with psychiatric problems and who bring their children for treatment only if they are clearly severely disturbed.

Professionals such as teachers, guidance counselors, or pediatricians may be more likely to advise psychiatric evaluation and treatment for adopted children. There is limited recognition of what adoption researcher Joyce Maguire Pavao terms "normative crises" in adopted children and their families—that is, expected and to some extent predictable times of emotional and behavioral disturbance related to adoptive status. Moreover, there is some evidence that the incidence of mental disorders may decrease as adopted individuals grow older, possibly because they received help at an earlier age.

There are other issues that may come into play with psychiatric disorders. For example, children with PRENATAL EXPOSURES to alcohol and illegal drugs may be at a greater risk for the later development of psychiatric disorders, although much further research is needed before this conclusion can be drawn. It is not known whether adopted children are more likely to experience prenatal exposures than non-adopted children, but some researchers have speculated that this may be true.

The birthmother's emotional status during pregnancy could play a role in the development of later psychiatric problems of the child; for example, if the pregnant woman who is considering adoption (or in the case of a woman from another country, who may feel compelled to consider the abandonment of her child) is under extreme stress. The stress experienced by the fetus through the mother could translate into a risk for emotional problems in the child later on.

It is also known that there are genetic risks for many types of psychiatric disorders. For example, the rate of schizophrenia in the general population is about 1 percent; however, if a child has a parent with schizophrenia, the likelihood the child will develop schizophrenia rises to 10 percent. Yet in a study by Lowing et al. in 1983, researchers found that when the child of a schizophrenic parent was adopted, the probability of the child developing schizophrenia fell to 3 percent—still higher than the rate for the general population but much lower than the rate for the non-adopted child of a parent with schizophrenia. In this case, adoption may provide a protective effect against the development of some psychiatric disorders.

It is also true that children adopted from other countries face vastly different challenges from children adopted as infants or even older children in the United States. Sometimes adoptive parents take newly adopted children from another country to a therapist soon after the adoption because of their behavioral issues rather than consulting with a pediatrician who is experienced in international adoption. The psychiatrist may mistakenly identify attention-deficit/hyperactivity disorder, depression, or another illness in the child when what is actually needed is time for the child to adjust to the new family and new culture.

Children adopted from other countries who are older than toddlers must master a new language as well as a completely different culture and set of customs. The adjustment can take time and new adoptive parents should not be overly eager to consult with therapists because some problems will resolve themselves in the fullness of time. A good pediatrician will be able to advise parents about which problems need immediate attention and which can wait a while. Experts in ADOPTION MEDICINE may also be consulted.

Studies on Adopted Children in Clinical Populations

A clinical population is a population of subjects who are receiving treatment. One of the earlier studies on adopted persons in the United States and possible mental disturbances was reported in 1960 by psychiatrist Marshall Schechter, who concluded that about 13 percent of his psychiatric patients over age five years had been adopted. His findings were subsequently used as a basis for concluding that adoption causes or contributes to psychiatric problems. This study is still cited nearly 50 years later as proof that adopted children are more likely than non-adopted children to have emotional problems, which is why it is still an important study to discuss.

Schechter studied a very small population of adopted persons, 16 subjects of 120 patients. Of these 16 patients, at least three were over age nine at the time of adoption and had problematic experiences before the adoption. It is almost certainly unfair to include children adopted as infants with those adopted as older children with SPECIAL NEEDS, although this was not known at that time.

In addition, it is fairly evident that the practices that were prevalent at the time of the Schechter study, and which were hardly intrinsic to the institution of adoption, contributed greatly to the adopted child's problems.

For example, one of the children studied by Schechter was adopted at the age of only 14 months from a foster home and the child was not toilet trained. Today, it is extremely rare that parents would expect that a child be toilet trained at such an early age, and certainly most pediatricians would try to dissuade them from such attempts. However, at that time, it was commonly accepted by some physicians as possible and desirable to toilet train very young children. Schechter reported that a pediatrician had told the adoptive parents that they must "insist on complete control of the excretory functions immediately and forcibly. This, then, seemed to become the condition for acceptance into the family."

Understandably, the child had difficulty with this demand. In addition, it was mentioned in the article that the adoptive parents had changed the child's name. Yet even to a toddler, one's name is part of one's identity. Today social workers advise adoptive parents that children need time to adjust to their new surroundings and may actually regress in their behavior for a while. It seems likely that in this case, the trauma of relocating to a new family that was single-mindedly determined to potty train her, and also losing her name, could ultimately result in behavioral and identity problems, and it did.

In another case, Schechter described a five-year-old girl who was phobic about going to school and who had "severe temper tantrums." Schechter concluded that the child felt threatened because she had been "sent away" from her "original mother" at the age of 17 months. It would be interesting to speculate on how many non-adopted children at the age of five also experience severe difficulties surrounding entering school for the first time.

Another case cited by Dr. Schechter seems to be an obvious problem of attachment, wherein the child responded to strangers in the same way as to the adoptive parents. (At that time, little to nothing was known about ATTACHMENT DISORDER.) In yet another case, a child who was not hypothyroid had been placed on thyroid medication, which no pediatrician today would recommend. Unneeded medications can sometimes precipitate psychiatric problems.

In a later study of 57 adopted children referred to a psychiatric service in Canada, the researchers found a greater incidence of referrals to psychiatric services than would be expected for the general population. According to the researchers, adopted children "presented more with conduct disorders and less with anxiety disorders and were significantly more impaired than the controls." The researchers also discussed apparently conflicting findings of researchers on the incidence of mental problems among adopted persons.

Their explanation was that "while adopted children and adolescents may experience psychosocial problems at a relatively increased rate, these are early problems that are probably not associated with increased risk for mental illness in adulthood."

The researchers found a significant number of the adopted children came from families of a higher socioeconomic level than the control patients' families. The researchers stated, "This probably reflects the selection policy for would-be adoptive families by the adoption agencies." Other researchers have speculated that perhaps adoptive families are more likely to seek assistance when their child has a problem than non-adoptive families, in part, because they can afford it.

A much-cited study of adopted children with attention-deficit/hyperactivity disorder was reported in *Behavior Genetics* in 1982, and this study continues to be cited into the 21st century. In this study, of 200 children in a clinical population, 17 percent were adopted children. It is unknown at what age the children were adopted or what adverse experiences they may have encountered prior to the adoption, such as abuse or neglect. This study provides insufficient data to support the belief that children who are adopted are more likely to have attention-deficit/hyperactivity disorder than nonadopted children.

A 1985 study by Andrea Weiss compared the symptoms of adopted and nonadopted children who were admitted to a psychiatric hospital and found significant differences: most of the adopted children who were admitted were far *less* disturbed than were the non-adopted children. (There were no significant differences in age, gender, or social class.)

According to Weiss, the adopted children did not receive diagnoses of personality disorders at a greater frequency than the non-adopted children. In addition, they were not more likely to have been hospitalized because of exhibiting antisocial behavior. One difference Weiss did note, however, was that the adopted children were admitted to the hospital at younger ages than the non-adopted children. In addition, the adopted children were diagnosed as psychotic by physicians in significantly *fewer* cases than the non-adopted children. Weiss reported that upon discharge only 25.5 percent of the 47 adopted persons had been diagnosed with psychoses compared to 46.2 percent of the 93 non-adopted persons who had been admitted.

In an earlier report, Weiss found that psychiatrists limited visitations by adoptive parents more than they limited visitations by biological parents. They also labeled adoptive parents as "precipitants" to the hospitalization more frequently.

Said Weiss, "It was concluded that parent-child relations may be more problematic among hospitalized adopted, as compared with nonadopted adolescents. It was also suggested that psychiatric bias concerning 'typical' adoptive family dynamics might have contributed to the observed differences."

Paul Brinich and Evelin Brinich studied 113 adopted persons who had received psychiatric services from 1969 to 1978 at the Langley Porter Psychiatric Institute in San Francisco, California, and compared them to non-adopted individuals who were also registered as patients.

The authors concluded, "Adoptees are not generally overrepresented in psychiatric samples, though it is true that they may be seen somewhat more frequently in child psychiatric clinics . . . while adoption may serve as a focus for psychopathology in individual cases, adoption itself cannot be seen as specifically pathogenic."

Other Studies on Psychiatric Problems

In a study on depression in childhood, reported in a 1998 issue of the *Journal of Child Psychology and Psychiatry*, the researchers looked at a sample of 180 adopted children and 227 non-adopted children and their mothers.

The adopted children were drawn from the Colorado Adoption Project, a longitudinal study.

The researchers had information on the biological mothers, who were tested before the children were born. It should be noted however, that the data on the birthmother was obtained at only one point in time. The birthmother could have experienced depression related to the circumstances around the pregnancy and relinquishment, which were later resolved. Alternately, the birthmother may not have been clinically depressed or had other disorders at the time of the adoption but may have developed a disorder at a later time.

The adoptive mothers answered questions about the children and the children responded to questions at ages nine, 10, 11, and 12 years. The researchers also sought to find if depression was more common among males than females.

The researchers found no difference between the rate of depression between the adopted and non-adopted individuals, nor did they find any evidence of a genetic linkage of depression. They concluded, "At the very least these findings raise doubts about genetic influence on depressive symptoms in middle childhood and warrant more than usual the maxim that more research is needed." Other researchers have also found no difference in the prevalence of depression among adopted children compared to non-adopted children.

In an article in a 1998 issue of *Child and Adolescent Psychiatric Clinics of North America*, the authors said that they believed adopted children had more emotional difficulties than non-adopted children, but they also believed that too often, problems were accentuated and blown out of proportion by well-meaning but overly worried adoptive parents.

Said the authors, "Adopted children exhibit more psychopathology than nonadopted ones, but not as much as their adoptive parents think they do. Adoptive parents are predisposed to seek help regarding their children, and tend to be socioeconomically advantaged. This predisposition can be a mixed blessing. On the one hand, adoptive parents have an awareness of problems and the energy and resources to seek help when the need for help is perceived. On the other hand, their overconcern regarding problems generates some of the problems about which they are concerned."

Children Adopted Internationally v. Children Adopted Domestically

In a meta-analysis of many different studies on psychiatric problems, reported in 2005 in the *Journal of the American Medical Association,* researchers Juffer and van IJzendoorn compared studies on behavioral problems among children adopted internationally with domestically adopted as well as non-adopted children. They found that international adoptees presented with fewer behavioral problems and were less likely to be seen by therapists than children adopted domestically.

One problem with the finding may be a function of the age of the children adopted domestically, which was not reported. (Most children adopted from other countries are adopted as infants or toddlers.) As a result, the children adopted domestically may have been in foster care for years and may have suffered from past abuse and/or neglect.

As pointed out by Dr. Miller in the same issue of the *Journal of the American Medical Association,* among the children adopted domestically, "This heterogeneous group may include children placed as newborns or young infants, as well as school-age children or teenagers with extremely complex social and personal histories." Further research is needed to compare psychiatric problems among children adopted domestically to children adopted internationally.

Interestingly, the analysis of the studies indicated that adopted males did not present with greater levels of problems than adopted females, contrary to what some experts had anticipated. In addition, the researchers also found that international adoptees had *fewer* problems in adolescence compared to international adoptees in early and middle childhood. Speculated the authors, "Although it might be true in general that adoptees are questioning their identity more intensively in adolescence, international adoptees may begin struggling with identity issues much earlier because racial and cultural differences between adoptive parents and adoptees are more obvious than in domestic adoption." As a result, behavior problems may surface earlier than adolescence among some international adoptees, who may resolve these issues prior to puberty.

Time with the family was also found to be a significant factor. Said the authors, "We also found that children who had been with the adoptive family for more than 12 years showed fewer total and externalizing behavior problems than children who had been in the family for less than 12 years. This may indicate that a longer stay in the adoptive family offers children opportunities to recover from their problem behavior."

The studies combined in this meta-analysis included relatively few children from backgrounds of extreme adversity; long-term studies including such children may reveal more problematic outcomes.

It should be noted that some individual studies of internationally adopted children have found greater levels of psychiatric problems. In a study reported by Tieman, et al., in the *American Journal of Psychiatry* in 2005, the researchers found that adopted young adults (aged 22 to 32) in the Netherlands were about one and a half times more likely to have an anxiety disorder than their non-adopted peers and twice as likely to have a substance abuse or dependency. Adopted men were nearly four times as likely to have a mood disorder compared to non-adopted men, while there were no significant differences found between adopted and non-adopted women.

Problems with Finding Competent Therapists

Sometimes adopted children clearly do need therapy, and it is important to find a competent therapist. Some authors insist that mental health professionals tend to blame either the family or adoption itself as the crux of the child's problem. However, the underlying problems the child is experiencing may stem instead from earlier experiences that the child had before he came to his adopted family. In addition, the adoptive family may be struggling mightily to succeed and stay together, yet receive little credit from therapists for their efforts. It is also true that sometimes the adoptive parents are contributing to or even causing the child's problems, usually unknowingly.

In his 1994 article for the *Journal of the American Academy of Child and Adolescent Psychiatry,* psychiatrist Steven Nickman said sometimes therapists make problems worse through their own ignorance. Nickman says many therapists do not realize that children adopted as infants are a different population than children adopted as older children. Nor do they understand or acknowledge the strong bonds between child and parent. Nickman says that therapists often shut out adoptive parents from therapy and wish to see only the child, seeing the parents as the problem rather than part of the solution. He urged therapists to work with, rather than against, the adoptive parents.

See THERAPY AND THERAPISTS.

Future Research

There are many topics related to the emotional/psychiatric problems of adopted individuals that are worthy of research. In his article for *Family Relations* in 2000, adoptee and adoption care coordinator R. Don Horner identified several areas with a dearth of research, some of which follow:

- The effects of the placement of siblings in separate homes on each child in the group

- The effects of an adopted child on other children (adopted or birth children) already in the family

- The relationship between the temperament of a child and the subsequent relationship with adoptive parents

- The best method to explain to children what adoption means (there are many books on the subject but few studies)

- How to determine when acting out behaviors can be attributed to adoption

See also ADJUSTMENT; ADOLESCENT ADOPTED PERSONS; ADOPTION STUDIES; ADULT ADOPTED PERSONS; ALCOHOLISM; ATTACHMENT DISORDERS; EARLY INTERVENTION; EXPLAINING ADOPTION; FOSTER CARE; INTELLIGENCE; MEDICAL PROBLEMS OF INTERNATIONALLY ADOPTED CHILDREN; MEDIA AND ADOPTION; RESEARCH, PROBLEMS WITH; SENSORY INTEGRATION DISORDER.

Brinich, Paul M., and Evelin B. Brinich. "Adoption and Adaptation," *Journal of Nervous and Mental Disease* 170, no. 8 (1982): 489–493.

Derdeyn, Andre P., M.D., and Charles L. Grave, M.D. "Clinical Vicissitudes of Adoption," *Child and Adolescent Psychiatric Clinics of North America* 7, no. 2 (April 1998): 373–388.

Deutsch, Curtis K., et al. "Overrepresentation of Adoptees in Children with Attention Deficit Disorder," *Behavior Genetics* 12, no. 2 (1982): 231–238.

Eley, Thalia C., et al. "An Adoption Study of Depressive Symptoms in Middle Childhood," *Journal of Child Psychology and Psychiatry* 39, no. 3 (1998): 337–345.

Horner, R. Don. "A Practitioner Looks at Adoption Research," *Family Relations* 49 (2000): 473–477.

Juffer, Femmie, and Marinus H. van IJzendoorn. "Behavior Problems and Mental Health Referrals of International Adoptees: A Meta-analysis," *Journal of the American Medical Association* 293, no. 20 (May 25, 2005): 2,501–2,515.

Kotsopoulos, Sotiris, M.D., et al. "Psychiatric Disorders in Adopted Children: A Controlled Study," *American Journal of Orthopsychiatry* 58 (October 1988): 608–612.

Lowing, P., et al. "The Inheritance of Schizophrenia Disorder: A Reanalysis of the Danish Adoption Study Data," *American Journal of Psychiatry* 1400 (1983): 1,167–1,171.

Maguire Pavao, Joyce. *Family of Adoption.* Boston: Beacon Press, 2005.

Miller, Laurie C., M.D. "International Adoption, Behavior, and Mental Health," *Journal of the American Medical Association* 293, no. 20 (May 25, 2005): 2,533–2,535.

Nickman, Steven, M.D. and Robert G. Ewis. "Adoptive Families and Professionals: When the Experts Make Things Worse," *Journal of the American Academy of Child and Adolescent Psychiatry* 33, no. 5 (June 1994): 753–755.

Pardes, Herbert, M.D., et al. "Genetics and Psychiatry: Past Discoveries, Current Dilemmas, and Future Directions," *American Journal of Psychiatry* 146 (April 1989): 435–443.

Schechter, Marshall D. "Observations on Adopted Children," *Archives of General Psychiatry* 3 (July 1960): 21–32.

Shih, Regina A., Pamela L. Bemonte, and Peter P. Zandi. "A Review of the Evidence from Family, Twin and Adoption Studies for a Genetic Contribution to Adult Psychiatric Disorders," *International Review of Psychiatry* 16, no. 4 (2004): 260–283.

Tieman, Wendy, Jan van der Ende, and Frank C. Verhulst. "Psychiatric Disorders in Young Adult Intercountry Adoptees: An Epidemiological Study," *American Journal of Psychiatry* 162 (2005): 592–598.

Weiss, Andrea. "Parent-Child Relationships of Adopted Adolescents in a Psychiatric Hospital," *Adolescence* 19 (Spring 1984): 77–88.

Weiss, Andrea. "Symptomology of Adopted and Nonadopted Adolescents in a Psychiatric Hospital," *Adolescence* 20 (Winter 1985): 763–774.

Westhues, Anne, and Joyce S. Cohen. "The Adjustment of Intercountry Adoptees in Canada," *Children and Youth Services Review* 20, no. 1 (1998): 115–134.

psychological parent Also known as de facto parent; person to whom the child has bonded in a parental relationship but with whom the child does not necessarily have a biological, adoptive, or legal relationship.

This may be a person who has "informally" adopted a child; for example, a foster parent or a relative who is caring for a child but who does not have legal custody. A psychological parent could also be the live-in friend of an actual parent.

public assistance   Programs such as Temporary Aid to Needy Families (TANF) food stamps, MEDIC-AID, and other payment or in-kind programs for categorically eligible families. Indications are that unwed mothers who choose to parent their infants and children have a higher probability of applying for and receiving public assistance than do birthmothers who choose adoption for their children.

See also BIRTHMOTHER.

putative father   A man who claims to be or who is alleged to be the father of a "nonmarital" child.

After a man is proved, usually by genetic tests, to be the father of a child, he is more often known as the biological father or BIRTHFATHER.

A number of states have established putative father registries, wherein a man who believes himself to be the father of a child may register his alleged paternity with the state. Men on this registry must be notified before a child may be placed for adoption. Putative fathers are usually not married to the mother of the child nor are they named as the father on the child's birth certificate.

The registry approach in New York State's law was upheld by the U.S. Supreme Court in *Lehr v. Robertson.*

See also BIRTHMOTHER; CONSENT (TO AN ADOPTION).

race Refers to the racial heritage of a child and his or her parents. Primary races that are considered are black, Caucasian, and Asian. Latinos are sometimes inaccurately considered as a separate race, although they are actually an ethnic group. There is broad difference among Latinos who may be of Caucasian, American Indian, or black descent or various mixtures.

Some children needing adoptive families are also of mixed race or BIRACIAL. Although the term *biracial* connotes two races and includes Caucasian/Asian and Asian/black, most social workers use the term to refer to black/white children.

Whether or not race is an important aspect in the child to be adopted must be considered by adopting parents.

Studies have indicated that TRANSRACIAL ADOPTION can work very effectively for both the child and the family; however, the family must be able to tolerate criticism from family and strangers. In addition, many social workers and adoption agencies are adamantly opposed to placing a black or biracial child in a white family.

See also BLACK/AFRICAN-AMERICAN ADOPTIVE PARENT RECRUITMENT PROGRAMS; BLACK FAMILIES; SPECIAL NEEDS.

rainbow families An upbeat phrase adoptive parents sometimes use to describe their families when their children are of mixed or different races or ethnicity.

rape Forcible sexual intercourse; also includes statutory rape and "acquaintance rape" or "date rape."

Some children are conceived as the result of rape, which is one of the key arguments in favor of legal adoption. Should the woman wish to continue her pregnancy, she may opt to arrange an adoption for her child.

If the mother does not know her attacker and never identifies him, she cannot provide important medical and social information for social workers to pass on to adoptive parents.

Whether or not the circumstances of the adopted person's birth should be revealed or how it should be phrased are open to argument; however, most experts believe that this information certainly should not be shared until the child is an adolescent or an adult. If at all possible, the information should also not be provided to friends or relatives who may inadvertently leak it to the adopted person.

See also TERMINATION OF PARENTAL RIGHTS.

reactive attachment disorder See ATTACHMENT DISORDER.

re-adoption Adopting a child who was already adopted in another country. Re-adoption is not the same as the FINALIZATION of an adoption.

Re-adoption often occurs because the parents want the child to have a birth certificate issued in the United States, rather than having to rely upon an adoption decree issued by a foreign court in another language. A birth certificate that is issued in one state in the United States must be acknowledged by all other states.

Re-adoption may also protect the inheritance rights of the child, if an adoption in a foreign court is challenged by relatives as not valid, which has happened.

According to the National Adoption Information Clearinghouse, states that have re-adoption statutes include the following: California, Colorado, Connecticut, Georgia, Hawaii, Idaho, Kansas, Maine, Maryland, Minnesota, New Hampshire, North Carolina, Ohio, Oklahoma, Pennsylvania, Tennessee, and Wisconsin. For information on how to readopt a child, adoptive parents should contact their adoption agency or an adoption attorney in their state.

Some states grant full recognition of foreign adoption decrees, including some states that allow re-adoption. These states include: Alaska, Arkansas, Delaware, Florida, Georgia, Hawaii, Idaho, Illinois, Indiana, Iowa, Kansas, Maryland, Massachusetts, Minnesota, Missouri, Montana, New Hampshire, New Mexico, North Dakota, Ohio, Oklahoma, Oregon, Pennsylvania, South Carolina, Vermont, and Wisconsin.

Some states have no laws regarding international re-adoptions. These states include: Alabama, Arizona, Kentucky, Louisiana, Michigan, Mississippi, Nebraska, Nevada, New Jersey, New York, Rhode Island, South Dakota, Texas, Utah, Virginia, Washington, West Virginia, and Wyoming. However, re-adoptions may generally occur in these states, and advice on the process should be sought from the adoption agency or an experienced adoption attorney.

See also INTERNATIONAL ADOPTION; MEDICAL PROBLEMS OF INTERNATIONALLY ADOPTED CHILDREN.

National Adoption Information Clearinghouse. "Summary of Laws Regarding International Adoptions Finalized Abroad: 50 States and 5 U.S. Territories," July 2003. Available online. URL: http://naic.acf.hhs.gov/general/legal/statutes/international.pdf, downloaded March 5, 2005.
Wiernicki, Peter J. "When You Adopt under the Laws of Another Country: U.S. Readoption Explained," reprinted from *Adoptive Families* magazine (May/June 2002). Available online. URL: http://adoptivefamilies.com/pdf/readoption.pdf, downloaded March 5, 2005.

"real parents"   A phrase in wide popular use to indicate the birthparents of an adopted child. It alludes to shared genetic descent. This label is particularly disliked by most adoptive parents who feel it denigrates and verbally invalidates their relationship to the child.

The term is also technically incorrect, because parental rights, obligations, and activities have been transferred in the case of adoption.

As a result, most adoptive parents and adoption experts advise the words *birthparents* or *biological parents* (or, less frequently, *genetic parents*) be used when referring to the man and woman who conceived the adopted child.

recruitment   Adoption agencies, adoptive parent support groups, and others use a variety of means to encourage the adoption of children, particularly children with SPECIAL NEEDS. ADVERTISING AND PROMOTION, seminars, WEDNESDAY'S CHILD, PHOTOLISTINGS, and VIDEOTAPE are primary techniques.

Adoption advocates may also use bumper stickers, T-shirts, and many other creative tactics to promote adoption.

Various BLACK/AFRICAN-AMERICAN ADOPTIVE PARENT RECRUITMENT PROGRAMS have been established to help cope with the large numbers of black children waiting for adoptive parents.

Meetings

When parents are adopting an older child, agencies arrange for the parents to meet the child before committing to an adoption.

The meeting may be at a social event, such as an adoption picnic, or it may be in the agency office or at another location. Some agencies try to make the meeting appear accidental or casual, so the child will not feel threatened or feel like he or she is being examined. Many agencies use the INTERNET.

Adoption "fairs," parties, or picnics are used by some agencies to introduce children to prospective parents. Children are dressed casually and given balloons, and games and activities are planned for the children. The disadvantage of these events is that many of the children know they are on display and may feel anxious. The advantage of such events is that parents have a chance to meet kids one-on-one, and children have been adopted through this process.

If and when adopting parents are interested in an older child, the agency will often arrange for the child to spend a day or weekend with them in their home. The adoptive parents' interest in the child must be very strong before the agency will commit to such a meeting because they want to minimize the pain of rejection should the weekend not work out.

When an agency is attempting to match a particular child with a particular family, they talk to the family first to make sure the family has an interest in the child.

If there is to be a personal meeting, the social worker will usually "talk up" the family to the child and provide general and specific information about the family to whet the child's curiosity and interest in them.

If the weekend visits seem to work out well, more visits will be planned until the child is transitioned to the new home and family.

registries   See BIRTHFATHER REGISTRY; MUTUAL CONSENT REGISTRIES; PUTATIVE FATHER.

reimbursement   See EMPLOYEE BENEFITS FOR ADOPTION; MILITARY MEMBERS AND ADOPTION.

relative adoptions   Most relative adoptions are GRANDPARENT ADOPTIONS or adoptions by STEPPARENTS, although aunts, uncles, cousins, or other relatives may also adopt a child. At least half of all finalized adoptions are adoptions by stepparents or relatives, such as grandparents, aunts, etc.

Many states do not require a complete HOME STUDY if the child is adopted by a close relative, such as a stepparent, grandparent, sister, brother, aunt, or uncle.

Relative adoptions are of necessity OPEN ADOPTIONS. In some cases, however, the adoptive parents have concealed the relationship and even the adoption itself from the child.

The primary advantage of a relative adoption is the birthmother feels confident the child will be safe and loved by a family member. Such an adoption does not preclude the relative from death or divorce, and the child may ultimately end up with individuals over whom the birthmother can exert no control.

The main disadvantage of a relative adoption is that if other family members are also aware this is a relative adoption, constant comparisons may be made between the child and the birthparent, and it may be difficult for the adoptive parents to forge a strong sense of ENTITLEMENT to the child.

religion   Religion has played a strong role in the history of United States adoption from the early days of the ORPHAN TRAIN era of the late 19th century, when well-meaning Protestant reformers sent thousands of children from the Eastern Seaboard to Protestant families in the Midwest and West. Some of the children were formally adopted, but many were indentured to the families who chose them from the train platform, where they were "put up" for people to see (hence the expression, "put up for adoption").

Most of the children were orphans or immigrants of Jewish or Catholic descent, and eventually Jewish and Catholic organizations objected to these placements in Protestant homes. The ultimate result of such protests was the formation of sectarian agencies that concentrated on serving their own particular faith groups; as a result, Catholic, Jewish, and Protestant agencies evolved that accepted applications for adoption from people of these respective faiths or particular denominations.

If a child was left as a foundling on a Jewish agency's doorstep, it was presumed the birthmother wished the child to be placed with a Jewish family, and this wish was respected.

Subsequent to the legalization of abortion and with increased acceptance of single parenthood, fewer babies were placed for adoption by their birthmothers in the 1970s and to date than in past years.

With the increase of INDEPENDENT ADOPTION, designated adoption and targeted adoption, agency adoptions of healthy newborns began to decline, and the sectarian agencies became dominant among the agencies that continued to play significant roles.

The sectarian agencies and other interested individuals were also successful in passing religious matching laws in some states, requiring a child to be placed with a family of the same religion as his birthparents.

Because sectarian agencies usually have a religious requirement, prospective adoptive parents who are not of the religion of the agencies in their state may find themselves "shut out" of adoption; for example, if there are only Christian adoption agencies within a state, a Jewish family would generally only be able to adopt a child through the state social services department. (They could apply to an adoption agency in another state, which can be a complex process.)

In addition, individuals who profess no particular religious faith, or who state they believe in a deity but do not attend religious services, also could find themselves unable to adopt through a sectarian agency. Another type of family that may have difficulty is the couple wherein the wife is one religion and the husband is another; for example, the wife may be Catholic and the husband Jewish. In such an instance, they would generally be denied the opportunity to adopt a child through either a Catholic agency or a Jewish agency.

As a result of this difficulty, individuals who cannot or choose not to apply to a sectarian agency have increasingly and actively lobbied state legislatures to approve IDENTIFIED ADOPTION or designated adoptions, which are adoptions arranged by the adoptive parents themselves and subsequently approved by an adoption agency or adoption facilitator.

In some cases, individuals have sued the sectarian agency, stating that they have been discriminated against because of their religious faith. As a result, some agencies will now accept applications from individuals who are not members off the faith group the agency primarily represents. For instance, a Jewish family should not presume that Catholic Social Services will not accept their application. Policies vary from state to state and agency to agency, based on many factors, including the source of financial support of the agencies. As a result, in some cases the Jewish family would be turned down by Catholic Social Services while, in other cases, they would be served.

Although the obvious solution to religious or denominational "matching" appears to be laws requiring any otherwise suitable family to be served, there are problems.

One potential problem with requiring sectarian agencies to accept members of another faith group is that most agencies wish to give birthmothers a choice in designating the adoptive parents and how their children will be religiously reared. As a result, it is likely that a Catholic birthmother (or Jewish or Protestant birthmother) would wish her child to be raised in the same religion, and if she specifically makes this request, most agencies would do their best to honor it.

The other major problem is that birthmothers who consider religious matching important would simply do what many are already doing: they would go to an attorney or other intermediary (or to an agency in a state with different laws) who would arrange a direct placement with adoptive parents of the specified religion.

They might also decide they will need to parent the child themselves in order to carry out what they believe is in the best religious interests of the child, according to the dictates of their conscience. (See the entry on BIRTHFATHER for other reasons why birthmothers who would otherwise choose adoption decide to parent a child.)

See also ADOPTION AGENCIES.

relinquishment   Voluntarily forfeiting or terminating one's parental rights to a child for the purpose of adoption. This term is considered negative by some adoption professionals who believe it implies the birthparent has not considered the child's future when, in fact, the birthparent usually has given very serious and lengthy consideration to the child's future life. Those who are critical of the word *relinquishment* may prefer "giving consent" for an adoption or "transferring parent rights and obligations."

An involuntary forfeiture of rights is called *termination of parental rights* and usually results from the caretaker's abuse or neglect of a child and the inability of the parent or caretaker to overcome the problems that led to the child's removal from the home.

reproductive technologies   See ASSISTED REPRODUCTIVE TECHNOLOGY.

research, problems with   Although rigorously designed social science studies of adoption are fairly infrequent in the social science arena, an interest in studying members of the adoption triad (adoptive parents, birthparents, and adopted persons) and in adoption itself appears to be increasing. This is a good sign because the more valid research that is conducted on adoption, the more reliable information adoption professionals will have upon which to make sound policy decisions. In addition, such information would be very helpful to triad members.

The difficulty in studying individuals who were adopted, adoptive parents, or birthparents lies primarily in that CONFIDENTIALITY protects their identities in most cases, and thus, subjects must be recruited from adoption agencies or newspaper advertisements. Individuals who come forward in response to requests from adoption agencies or advertisements may well be significantly different from individuals who prefer to retain their privacy and anonymity. One large adoption study demonstrating problem behaviors in adopted individuals was withdrawn when researchers discovered that some of the volunteer subjects had not been adopted. The researchers termed these pseudo-adoptees *jokesters*.

Another difficulty lies in finding a way to interview young adopted persons without creating undue stress; any research involving human subjects is sensitive.

Researchers have also made errors with research, largely based on insufficient data or a lack of awareness of important factors about adoption. One common research failing of many researchers in the recent past was to include all adopted children in one sample, failing to differentiate children adopted as infants or toddlers from children who were adopted from foster care or a troubled situation at older ages. Critics say that adopted children are very diverse and to include children adopted as newborns or young infants along with those who were neglected, abused, were removed from their families and placed in foster care, and ultimately adopted at age eight or nine years old (or older) cannot provide valid results. (See PSYCHIATRIC PROBLEMS OF ADOPTED PERSONS.)

The interpretation of data may also be difficult; for example, some researchers have generalized from small groups of people to large groups of adopted individuals. In addition, some researchers have studied institutionalized adopted persons or troubled persons who were receiving therapy and generalized their results from this population to all or most adopted individuals. Information may be incomplete, especially in studies of birthparents. For example, mental health disorders in birthparents may increase or decrease over time, but researchers may only have access to information about them at the time of the adoptive placement.

Adoption research is expensive, which is why so many studies use small samples. Presuming that it would be possible to identify hundreds of adopted individuals, birthparents, or adoptive parents, it would still be expensive and time-consuming to interview and test them all. Funding must be available in order to cover this cost. Scandinavian countries maintain registries of adopted individuals and birthparents, which facilitate such research.

Another problem with research is that researchers cannot always determine causal factors; for example, if children are emotionally disturbed, are they disturbed because of an adoption issue or because of a problem that occurred before they were adopted, such as physical or sexual abuse? Or, have problems occurred in the adoptive home which have contributed to the child's problems? It is difficult to know.

Terminologies often vary, and it is important for researchers to share a common frame of reference; for example, many researchers have differing definitions of OPEN ADOPTION, varying from those who believe providing the birthmother nonidentifying information about prospective parents constitutes an open adoption to those who believe only a total disclosure of identities is open. Understanding the implications of these studies is difficult unless the researchers define their terms clearly.

Timeliness is a problem as well. Studies conducted at a single point in time do not encompass the dynamic changes that may occur. For example, some evidence suggests that behavioral problems in adopted children improve as time goes by. Because a large study may take extensive time, the information garnered may not be available for years. Some researchers undertake longitudinal studies, which study the same population at different points in time; for example, children at age three, seven, 11, and 15.

Researchers try to determine what factors have changed in the child's life, and how the child adjustment has evolved. Longitudinal studies have been performed to determine changes in ADJUSTMENT, INTELLIGENCE, and numerous other areas, such as children from TRANSRACIAL ADOPTIONS.

Although lay individuals cannot analyze the validity of any given study, they can ask themselves basic questions to determine if the research possibly could be used to generalize to a larger group of adopted children or adults. Some key points to look for within the text of the study are as follows:

- How many subjects were studied? Usually, studies with larger numbers of subjects are more valid than those with fewer subjects. Statistical analyses are more likely to yield reliable results if more subjects are included in the study. If there were fewer than 30 subjects, then generally further studies should be sought to support or refute the initial study.

- How old were the children when adopted? Were they adopted as infants or toddlers or as older children from foster care? If this information is not available, and the age range of the children is broad, such as ages six to 12, then further studies on the topic should be reviewed.

- How were the subjects for the research project recruited? Selection bias can greatly alter the results of the investigation. Research on the incidence of behavioral problems will undoubtedly yield different results if the subjects are recruited at a mental health clinic or at a school.

- Do the conclusions of the researchers support their own study? Occasionally, researchers have findings that are opposite to what they expect, and they write a great deal about why the study came out "wrong." Sometimes the study was conducted properly, although researchers did not like the logical conclusions drawn from their study.

- What precautions do the researchers cite about the interpretation of their data? Most research papers include a section where the authors describe the limitations they faced in conducting and interpreting their research results.

Miller, Laurie. "International Adoption, Behavior, and Mental Health," *Journal of the American Medical Association* 293, no. 20 (May 25, 2005): 2,533–2,535.

residential treatment centers Out-of-home placements where the child receives help with many areas of his or her life that have gone awry, particularly psychological and/or behavioral problems. Centers are funded either through public or private funds or a combination of both.

According to the book *Residential Treatment: A Tapestry of Many Therapies,* edited by Dr. Vera Fahlberg, "Residential care is usually reserved for the child who is having problems in all three major areas of his life—family, school, and peers—and even then only when the problems have not been amenable to out-patient treatment."

Residential treatment is 24-hour care and is different from a GROUP HOME, which is usually staffed by one couple and where the children are able to attend local schools. (Some children in group homes may need residential treatment or will need it in the future.)

A residential treatment center is also different from psychiatric hospitals, which are generally used for severely disturbed children who are suicidal or who are undergoing detoxification, receiving treatment for psychoses, and so forth.

Residential treatment is not a short-term solution to a problem, and the average child who needs residential treatment remains at the facility for 18 months to two years.

Says Sandra Mooney, chief clinical social worker at Episcopal Child Care of North Carolina, "Usually the child comes to the program with numerous problems which have been identified by various community agencies, police, foster families, schools, and sometimes biological parents."

Common problems of children placed in residential institutions include low self-esteem, inability or inadequacy at forming relationships with others, poor control of emotions, learning disabilities, and other problems.

Fahlberg's book also discusses a variety of children who have done well in a residential treatment center where she has had extensive experience: Forest Heights Lodge in Evergreen, Colorado. These include children with attachment problems, children who have suffered a parental loss or separation, children who are "stuck" at a childhood stage earlier than their chronological age, and children with perceptual problems. Children who are not suitable for the facility are disabled children or teenagers who are sociopathic or have other personality disorders.

It is partially the milieu as well as separation from the primary caretakers and other factors that are hoped to lead the child to recovery and an ability to function in the world. The "milieu" refers to the daily environment and its structure, and in a residential treatment center, the milieu describes a setting in which the child can grow to trust the caretakers of the center, empowering the child to change.

Children placed in residential treatment may be placed by a social worker, their biological parents, or their adoptive parents or other guardians.

According to social workers Judith McKenzie and Drenda Lakin, such children "are often youngsters for whom no other resource has been available or whose medical, cognitive, behavioral and emotional difficulties have led to residential placement usually after they have experienced many moves in the foster care system."

The children may be able, with time, to return to their adoptive or biological homes; however, therapists often have biases against adoptive parents who wish to temporarily place their children in a residential treatment facility. There may be biases against adoption on the part of the staff and an overeagerness to "rescue" the child and the adoptive parents from each other.

Children from adoptions that have disrupted or dissolved may be placed in residential treatment. It is hoped that they will learn to cope with the pain and rejection they may feel. They may have problems with attachment to adults.

Adopting parents need to be aware of the problems of the child who has previously resided in a residential treatment center. The adoption agency and the residential treatment center should both fully educate the adopting parents on the child's problems.

Adoptive parents who expect the child to be grateful he or she was "saved" from the institution will be disappointed, because the child will probably not bond readily: he or she has been disappointed too many times before.

Other issues include the capacity of the child to attach to new parents. Because of past problems forming strong relationships, the child is wary of familial-type relationships. The child may also have difficulty in attaching to both parents.

In addition, the child may have formed relationships with residential treatment center staff and suffer separation anxiety when it is time to leave the residential treatment center.

See also ADOLESCENT ADOPTED PERSONS; BONDING AND ATTACHMENT; PSYCHIATRIC PROBLEMS OF ADOPTED PERSONS.

Fahlberg, Vera, M.D., ed. *Residential Treatment: A Tapestry of Many Therapies.* Indianapolis, Ind.: Perspectives Press, 1990.

Laird, Joan, and Ann Hartman, eds. *A Handbook of Child Welfare: Context, Knowledge, and Practice.* New York: Free Press, 1985.

McKenzie, Judith K., and Drenda Lakin. "Residential Services on the Continuum of Adoption Services," *The Roundtable: Journal of the National Resource Center for Special Needs Adoption* 4, no. 1 (1989): 1–2.

McRoy, Ruth G., Harold D. Grotevant, and Louis A. Zurcher Jr. *Emotional Disturbance in Adopted Adolescents: Origins and Development.* New York: Praeger, 1988.

Mooney, Sandra. "Coordination among the Residential Treatment Center, Guardian Ad Litem, and the Department of Social Services," in *Adoption for Troubled Children: Prevention and Repair of Adoptive Failures Through Residential Treatment.* New York: Haworth Press, 1983.

resilience   The capacity of a child to adapt to and sometimes even thrive despite difficult and sometimes extremely harsh early environments. Resilience may be partly a function of temperament and partly of coping strategies the child has developed subsequent to adverse early childhood experiences. It may also be affected by the active interventions of others, such as foster parents or adoptive parents.

Interestingly, the presence of past abuse or neglect does not always equate with the decreased resilience of an individual. Some children with very difficult past lives are able to function well in an adoptive family, while others who have experienced less extreme abuse or neglect (or *no* abuse or neglect) are not as resilient.

Early adverse experiences, such as abuse or neglect, the death or loss of a parent, or extreme illness or poverty, may occur in an orphanage environment or with a biological family or foster families or relatives of the child. Even the environment of the womb can affect the child later in life, particularly when the mother abused substances such as drugs or alcohol during her pregnancy.

Some children experience many adverse experiences, and as they mount in number, the ability of the child to rebound is decreased. For example, a child may be born to a substance-abusing mother who is neglectful and lives in poverty. If the child remains in that environment and other protective factors do not emerge, such as loving family members or mentors (such as teachers or neighbors), the probability of resiliency is decreased. In general, short-term adversities are easier to overcome than chronic problems.

As might be expected, resilient children generally evince fewer behavior problems than children who have difficulty adapting to new situations. This does not mean that nonresilient children cannot transcend their difficulties. With identification of their problems and appropriate therapy as needed, many children can lead happy lives.

It is also true that some children who have undergone extremely adverse situations have, with intervention, recovered and led normal lives. Several examples of such cases are discussed in a 1998 issue of *The Psychologist.* In one case, the mother of identical twin boys died soon after they were born, and they were placed in foster care for a year and then were cared for by an aunt for six months. After that time, their father remarried a woman who was extremely cruel to the boys, confining them to the basement and beating them until the children's plight was finally identified when they were seven years old, and they were removed from the home. The twins had no language and had rickets and small stature. Doctors assumed their situation was hopeless.

The twins were eventually adopted, and their outcomes were exceptionally good. Said the authors, "Scholastically, from a state of profound disability they caught up with age peers and achieved emotional and intellectual normality." As adult males, they married and had children and were successfully employed. The authors also stated that "models of development which ascribe disproportionate long-term effects to the early years are clearly erroneous." They also added that, "an acceptance of the early years as critical can carry with it subtle lowered expectancies for psychologically damaged children and hence less than desirable interventions."

Other cases of very deprived children have shown that active intervention on the part of adoptive parents or others can enable children to obtain unforeseen or even amazing gains in intellectual and emotional development. However, in cases of severe deprivation, it is very difficult to predict which children will overcome the effects of early adversity (and are hence resilient) and which

will be unable to overcome the impact of their early damaging experiences.

Characteristics of Resilient Children

Some key characteristics of resilience as discussed in *Promoting Resilience: A Review of Effective Strategies for Child Care Services,* a 2002 report from The Centre for Evidence-Based Social Services in the United Kingdom, include the following: good social skills, feelings of empathy, a sense of humor, problem-solving abilities, personal attractiveness to others, positive peer relationships, a loving extended family, one or more mentors, academic success, involvement in extracurricular activities in school, and membership in a faith group. In addition, the ability to focus on the positive side of life rather than ruminating on past problems is another characteristic of resilience.

Situations Related to Resilience

Some researchers have studied circumstances that appear related to resilience and they have found that children who have felt the caring and support of at least one individual in their early lives are more likely to be resilient than children who have not experienced such support. The child's age at the time of adoption is also often associated with resilience: children adopted before the age of three or four years are generally more resilient than children adopted at an older age, although many children adopted when they are older than age three may flourish with their adoptive families, while some children adopted as infants may not be resilient. The individual life experiences of each child and the child's own innate personality contribute more to resilience than age alone.

Predictive Factors for Resilience

In a study of 1,343 parents who adopted foster children in Illinois, reported in 2003 in *After Adoption: The Needs of Adopted Youth,* some findings of the researchers indicated resilience among children. Most of the children had been removed from their biological families at an early age, including 50 percent before age one and 66 percent before age five. Most children were removed for severe neglect (63 percent) and prenatal exposure to drugs and alcohol (60 percent). Some children were removed for more than one reason.

Many of the adoptive parents were either foster parents (44 percent) or relatives (39 percent) of the children. Most adopters (90 percent) were of the same race or ethnicity as the child.

Some of the children had serious school problems; for example, 26 percent had to repeat a grade, usually kindergarten or first grade. Twenty-five percent of the children had been suspended or expelled. A substantial number were hyperactive; for example, 40 percent were rated as inattentive and easily distracted all the time, while 35 percent of the parents said the children were hyperactive "sometimes." It seems likely that many of the children would fit the diagnostic criteria for attention deficit/hyperactivity disorder.

More than half the children (51 percent) had behavioral problems. In terms of risk factors toward having behavioral problems, the researchers found that prenatal substance abuse among the birth-mothers was the best predictor of behavioral problems in the children. Being a male child was also a risk factor. However, the researchers also found protective factors against behavioral problems. For example, they found that the child's ability to give and receive affection (not indiscriminate affection) was the most protective factor *against* the emergence of later behavioral problems.

In general, the researchers found that a child with the highest risk for behavioral problems was "a white boy who does not give and receive affection or does so poorly. He experienced alcohol or drug exposure before birth, sexual abuse prior to placement, and was bounced back and forth between his birthfamily and other placements prior to his adoption."

In contrast, the child *least* likely to have behavioral problems fit the following profile, "an African-American girl who gives and receives affection fairly well or very well. She did not experience prenatal substance abuse or any sexual abuse. She was not moved back and forth between her birthfamily and foster care."

The researchers also found several risk and protective factors for the adoptive parents in predicting behavioral problems in the child. Risk factors were families that were white and who needed services that were not offered in the subsidy agreement that they had made with the state agency.

Protective factors were that the adoptive parents were well-prepared and were college graduates.

Comparing Resilient Children to Others in Terms of Behavior

In a study in the Netherlands of 111 children adopted from Korea, Sri Lanka, and Colombia as infants, reported in the *Journal of Child Psychology and Psychiatry* in 2004, the researchers used evaluations from the adoptive mothers and the children's teachers to determine whether children (who were all aged seven) were either resilient, overcontrollers (such as children who hold things in and have a hard time expressing themselves), or undercontrollers (such as children whose feelings are easily hurt when criticized).

The researchers identified 33 resilient children (13 boys and 20 girls), 37 overcontrolling children (17 boys and 20 girls), and 38 undercontrolling children (27 boys and 11 girls.) They also checked for externalizing problem behaviors, such as impulsivity, hyperactivity, and aggression, and found that boys were dominant. Boys and girls were equally likely to have internalizing behavior problems, such as anxious, withdrawn, and depressed behavior,.

The researchers also considered factors within the adoptive family, such as whether infertility was the main reason to adopt the child, as well as family size and whether the family had biological children as well as adopted children, and found no significant differences among the children.

Said the authors, "As predicted, flexibly operating resilient adopted children were almost without behavior problems, adopted children who too rigidly contained their emotions and impulses presented predominantly internalizing problems, and adopted children lacking adequate emotional control had mainly externalizing problems." The researchers also found that when children were peer-rated as being rejected or controversial, they were also more likely to be rated by their mothers and their teachers with higher externalizing behavior scores.

The expressed desire to be "white" was strongest among the children adopted from Sri Lanka. (Most of the Sri Lankan children had a darker skin color than the other adopted children.) Children who never expressed this wish were more likely to be classified as resilient. Interestingly, the researchers did not find much evidence of racial discrimination. Thus, it was unclear if the desire to be white, which was present among about half the children, was primarily a desire to resemble their Caucasian parents and peers or if it indicated other underlying issues.

In another study of adults who were abused and neglected as children (and who were not adopted), reported in a 2001 issue of *Development and Psychopathology,* the researchers looked at eight areas of functioning, including employment, homelessness, education, social activity, psychiatric disorders, substance abuse, and two areas of criminal behavior (official arrest records and self-reports of violent acts) among 1,196 individuals, including 676 who were abused and neglected and 520 controls. About a third of the children had been placed in foster care.

Adopted children were purposely excluded from the sample. However, this information is potentially useful to those interested in adoption since some adopted children experience abuse and/or neglect before their adoptions.

The researchers found that 22 percent of the abused and neglected adult children were resilient, and that females were more likely to be resilient than males. Among males who were abused or neglected, about 17 percent met the criteria for resilience, compared to 27 percent of abused/neglected females. (Among the control group, 33 percent of males met the criteria for resilience, as did 51 percent of females.)

It is unknown whether the percentage of resiliency would be higher among adopted children, although it seems likely that the 22 percent figure could be used as a baseline/minimum level.

Clarke, Ann, and Alan Clarke. "Early Experience and the Life Path," *Psychologist* (September 1998): 433–436.

Howard, Jeanne A., and Susan Livingston Smith. *After Adoption: The Needs of Adopted Youth.* Washington, D.C.: CWLA Press, 2003.

Juffer, Femmie, Geert-Jan J. M. Stams, and Marinus H. van IJzendoorn. "Adopted Children's Problem Behavior is Significantly Related to Their Ego Resiliency, Ego Control, and Sociometric Status," *Journal of Child Psychology and Psychiatry* 45, no. 4 (2004): 697–706.

McGloin, Jean Marie, and Cathy Spatz Widom. "Resilience among Abused and Neglected Children Grown Up," *Development and Psychopathology* 13 (2001): 1,021–1,038.

Newman, Tony. *Promoting Resilience: A Review of Effective Strategies for Child Care Services,* prepared for the Centre for Evidence-Based Social Services, University of Exeter, United Kingdom, 2002. Available online. URL: http://www.cebss.org/files/Promoting_Resilience.pdf, downloaded on January 10, 2005.

résumé   In the adoption context, a written description of a prospective adoptive family, usually written by the couple or single person wishing to adopt; also known as a "profile." Agency staff and attorneys that offer birthmothers choices in adoption often use résumés of prospective adoptive parents to assist the birthmothers in their selection of adoptive parents. A caseworker or attorney will generally review the résumé to offer suggestions for changes and improvements before showing it to a birthmother.

Some couples who wish to locate their own birthmothers will independently circulate hundreds or even thousands of résumés nationwide to obstetricians, lawyers, adoption agencies, crisis pregnancy centers, and other professionals who come in contact with pregnant women considering adoption for their babies. Increasingly, résumés are posted on the Internet, often as part of a family's home page. Couples who succeed with this method swear by it.

It is difficult to impossible to maintain confidentiality when sending out résumés to people throughout the United States; therefore, couples who do not want to take part in an OPEN ADOPTION may wish to use more traditional means to succeed at adopting their child.

Supporters of using résumés, whether in INDEPENDENT ADOPTION or agency adoption, see them as very effective and speedy while opponents believe they are costly, inefficient, and risky, and they contend that physicians and others are most interested in assisting people they already know. People can be easily targeted by confidence artists.

After the prospective parents have completed the HOME STUDY process, they may prepare their résumé. This document, sometimes accompanied by photographs of the prospective parents, will be shown with other résumés to pregnant women considering adoption. The social worker will usually show the pregnant woman three or four résumés of couples who seem most appropriate to parent the child, although some agencies open their entire file of résumés to pregnant women.

The pregnant woman will then select the family she feels most closely resembles the type of family she is seeking for her child. Some pregnant women seek childless couples while a lesser number hope to place their child with a family who already has siblings or who intend to adopt other children after this child.

In some cases, the religion of the adoptive family is important, and in other cases, it is their lifestyle that matters most, for example, if they are active, outdoorsy people, literary people, or some other patterns the pregnant woman sees as desirable.

If the prospective adoptive family has no children but has a dog or cat or other pets, this information is often included because the couple may be perceived as nurturing by the pregnant woman.

Sometimes the agency may use résumés to help the birthmother choose the adoptive parents but wait until after the birthmother has delivered to show her any of the résumés. These agencies believe it would be a form of pressure to show the woman résumés before she has her baby. The agencies that show the pregnant woman résumés, usually in her last trimester, believe it will ease her mind to know something about the adoptive family and will give her a feeling of control over a crisis situation.

Adoptive parent résumés differ from job résumés in that prospective parents believe, based on advice from adoption providers, that they need to convey both information and emotion. They have been counseled that they need to describe themselves factually as well as explain why they want to adopt a child.

Résumés usually include such information as a physical description of the couple, their hobbies and interests, whether they live in the city, country, or suburbia, whether or not they have children already, and other general information.

If the prospective adoptive mother plans to stop working outside the home in order to stay at home to provide care for the child, this information is often included. If the prospective grandparents greatly anticipate the adoption, this information is seen as valuable as well.

Many women who are considering an adoption are very concerned about how the child will be accepted by the adoptive parents' own parents and relatives; therefore, if the future extended family is very eager and anxious for the child, adoption providers say this information should be included in the résumé.

A critical portion of the résumé is why the couple or single person wishes to adopt—beyond any information about infertility. In fact, detailed information on infertility is usually unnecessary. Most pregnant women presume a couple who wishes to adopt is infertile and are not interested in details of the infertility or expenses related to infertility testing. Instead, they are most interested in why the adopting couple wants a child and what kind of home they will provide for that child.

Adoption providers advise that résumés should be no more than a page or two in length. Although résumés can be difficult to write, most social workers or attorneys provide assistance.

reunification   A currently prevailing concept in child social welfare that dictates caseworkers should do whatever is necessary to return a child to the biological home when the child or children were removed by the state due to abuse, neglect, or abandonment.

It is presumed that the biological home is the best home for a child and that the biological parents can and should be rehabilitated from whatever caused them to abuse, neglect, or abandon the child, whether causal factors were drug or alcohol abuse, psychiatric problems, homelessness, or a combination of these and other factors.

It should be noted that most children actually wish to be reunited with their biological families, even when they have been abused or neglected. This does not mean such a reunification is in the child's best interest, and caseworkers must make a determination and recommendation to the court, which will make the final decision.

While a child is in foster care, social workers attempt to arrange visits with the biological parent. If the parent appears to show improvement, caseworkers may arrange weekend visitations with the parents, and if these visits appear to go well, the child may be returned to the home. It is likely, however, that a child who enters the foster care system will remain in care for at least several months.

Although social workers are supposed to monitor parental progress to ensure children are not returned to abusive homes, severe errors occur, and sometimes children die at the hands of their abusive parents.

Sometimes it is not clear why a child is or is not returned to his birthparents. Experts recommend children be returned to their parents if the parents can properly care for the children; however, there should be clearcut evidence that the parents have the capability to care for the children and are no longer drug or alcohol dependent or abusive or no longer have the problem that led to the child's removal from the family.

According to experts, the problem with reunification as a goal is not the concept itself but the amount of time allowed to elapse before it is determined that reunification cannot occur or is not in the best interests of the child.

A major problem in the 1980s and 1990s was that many children who entered the foster care system were not legally adopted for years. Although two or three years may not seem like much time to an adult, to a six-year-old child this time span represents a significant portion of a child's life.

A child who enters the foster care system as an infant or toddler will usually become attached to the foster parents. It is very painful for the child to leave the people who are his psychological parents and return to his birthparents.

In addition, the older the child becomes, the more difficult it is to place the child in an adoptive home. Also, if the child has been in numerous foster homes, she may also have acquired a host of emotional problems as well, thus making her more difficult to adopt.

Because reunification was seen as the best solution for a foster child, adoption was perceived as the next best solution. "Permanency" is the stated goal for all children, whether through returning to their families or relatives or being placed in an adoptive family. The reality, however, is that thousands of children languish in foster homes and group homes.

Experts argue that these children who are victimized today by repeated moves will become the juvenile delinquents and criminals of tomorrow.

As a result of concern over children who were warehoused in the foster care system for years, in 1997 Congress passed the Adoption and Safe Families Act to enable children to be adopted.

See also ADOPTION AND SAFE FAMILIES ACT; ADOPTION ASSISTANCE AND CHILD WELFARE ACT OF 1980; FOSTER CARE; FOSTER PARENT; PERMANENCY PLANNING; TERMINATION OF PARENTAL RIGHTS.

reunion Term used to describe the meeting between a birthparent and an adult adopted person. Usually the adopted person was placed at an age where the person has no memory of the birthparent.

Many newspaper articles describe the fond meeting between a birthmother and adopted adult. It is hoped that most meetings are a very positive experience; however, sometimes the birthparent or the adult adopted person is opposed to the meeting and will attempt to block it. The person may not want contact or need time to adjust to the idea. In a birthparent's case, the birthparent may not have told his or her spouse or other children about the adoption.

Most original birth certificates of adopted children show the name of the birthmother and, since 1972, often the birthfather. Since these documents are sealed by the state, it may be difficult to do a SEARCH to locate a birthparent. Because of this, some SEARCH GROUPS actively favor OPEN RECORDS, which would allow an adopted person to obtain the original birth certificate upon attaining adulthood. Such groups, primarily composed of adopted adults, feel that they have the right to this information and that they have been unfairly deprived.

On the other hand, other groups believe that it is important to preserve confidentiality and protect the identities of the parties unless they mutually agree to meet, usually through a formal, state-authorized MUTUAL CONSENT REGISTRY.

Adopted adults or birthparents may seek a reunion to satisfy curiosity, but they say that they also wish urgent information. An adopted person described in a *Time* article learned that she was adopted only after she was a senior citizen. She sought her birth records to attempt to locate a genetically related kidney donor for her grandchild. Despite her medical need (which most judges would consider and accede to, providing sealed information), reportedly she has failed to obtain the information. As a result, she is a proponent of open records.

Some adopted adults wait until their adoptive parents are very elderly or even deceased before they seek to locate birthparents, fearful that the adoptive parents would feel offended. In some cases, the adoptive parents *are* offended, while others are temporarily hurt. The adoptive parents may fear their children will abandon them and love the birthparent more. Although there is no data on the subject, most adoption experts believe that these fears are seldom realized; however, there may be a period during which the adopted adult feels "torn" between the family who reared her and her biological family.

revocation When the birthparent or custodial relative formally changes his or her mind after signing a voluntary CONSENT. How long a person has to change his or her mind after signing consent and under what conditions varies from state to state.

States may allow revocation of consent if proper NOTICE has not been given to involved parties, such as the birthfather. Most states allow for revocation of consent because of fraud or duress on the part of the attorney, agency, or adoptive parents.

If proper legal procedures were not followed, revocation of consent may be allowed in many states.

It is important for pregnant women and birthparents considering adoption to understand revocation of consent is not an easy and automatic matter and will usually require the hiring of an attorney. It may also involve a long and expensive court battle.

rickets, nutritional A childhood disorder that results in a poor mineralization of the bones, and which, if untreated, may cause short stature and serious skeletal deformities. Rickets is caused by a lack of calcium or vitamin D in the diet or lack of exposure to sunlight (necessary to activate vitamin D). A proper balance of these substances is necessary to the development and growth of healthy bones.

Many people regard bones as static and unchangeable objects within the body, but instead, while a person is alive, bone is metabolically active and continually being remodeled. This process occurs throughout the course of human life but is especially active during childhood growth. The parathyroid glands, which lie behind the thyroid gland, regulate the transfer of calcium between the blood, bone, and other tissues. Because of the rapid growth of bones during childhood, children especially need calcium and vitamin D for normal and healthy growth.

Rickets is rare in the United States because needed calcium and vitamin D are commonly available in the diets of most children; much of the food in the United States is fortified with these substances. However, the problem is more prominent in some children adopted from other countries, particularly among those who have resided in orphanages. Orphanages typically provide diets that are low in calcium (dairy products) and vitamin D. In addition, a diet high in phytates (found in some grains and cereals), as is common in Asian countries, may inhibit calcium absorption. Chronic diarrhea, a common problem in many countries, may also prevent calcium absorption.

Rickets is especially common among children from northern countries outside the United States and Canada, where children may lack exposure to sufficient sunlight, particularly in the winter months.

Symptoms and Diagnostic Path

According to the Centers for Disease Control and Prevention (CDC), some symptoms of rickets are as follows:

- Bone pain or tenderness in the arms, legs, spine, and pelvis
- Skeletal deformities, such as bowed legs, or spinal deformities, such as scoliosis or kyphosis
- Thickened wrists
- Dental deformities, such as holes in the enamel of the teeth
- Impaired growth
- Decreased muscle tone
- Excessive sweating

According to Dr. Miller, a physical examination of the child with active rickets will reveal tenderness that stems from the bone rather than from the muscles or joints. Blood tests will reveal low levels of calcium and an elevated serum alkaline phosphatase level (a marker of bone turnover). X-rays of the bones will show poor mineralization and resulting changes in the structure and shape of the bones.

Treatment Options and Outlook

Treatment is oriented toward resolving the deficiency, and thus increasing sun exposure and dietary levels of calcium and vitamin D will eliminate most symptoms. Often a diet that includes calcium and vitamin D–fortified dairy products may be all that is needed. In some cases, a supplemental prescription of vitamin D and calcium is required. Skeletal deformities usually resolve over time but, rarely, may require surgery. However, most children will rapidly recover with a healthy diet and medical treatment and follow-up.

Risk Factors and Preventive Measures

If parents choose to feed their children with nondairy milks (soy, rice, etc.), they should carefully verify that these are fortified with adequate amounts of calcium and vitamin D. Otherwise, a healthy diet is the primary prevention and treatment for rickets.

See also MEDICAL PROBLEMS OF INTERNATIONALLY ADOPTED CHILDREN.

Miller, Laurie C., M.D. *The Handbook of International Adoption Medicine: A Guide for Physicians, Parents, and Providers.* New York: Oxford University Press, 2005.

Romania, adoptions from In 2004, the Romanian government placed a moratorium on adoptions, which continues as of this writing in 2006. However, this country was important in the past with regards to adoption.

Background

After the extremely repressive Ceauşescu regime was overthrown in late 1989, the world subsequently became aware of thousands of children who were warehoused in Romanian orphanages. Ceauşescu had wished to increase the population in Romania, and to that end, he had banned contraception and abortion. As a result, many families had more children than they wanted or could support, and large numbers of children were placed in orphanages. Experts estimated that between 100,000 and 300,000 children lived in baby homes, orphanages for the school-aged, or institutions for persons considered to be "irrecuperable" (unrecoverable). Most of the children experienced severe emotional and physical deprivation. The Romanian orphanage experience showed the world how cruel an orphanage environment at its worst can be.

When people from the United States, Canada, and other Western countries saw television documentaries of the appalling conditions the children suffered in the orphanages, many were eager to adopt them, and large numbers reacted emotionally, rushing to take action. Some flew to Romania knowing nothing about adoption but wishing to save a child, and they traveled to Romania without completed home studies, orphan visas, or any documentation.

There were clearly some cases of baby and child selling, when some taxi drivers and others with no social service background or training received money in exchange for giving children to Westerners. However, the immigration laws on adoption were still in effect in the United States and other countries, and as a result, many people found themselves in a difficult situation for which they were not prepared, having to back up and go through official channels to adopt. International adoption agencies assisted as much as possible, as did government officials. (International adoption requires a home study and extensive documentation of the family as well as information on the child.) In fiscal year 1991, at the height of Romanian adoptions, 2,594 children were adopted by U.S. citizens, and Romania was the number-one country from which Americans adopted that year.

Eventually, the new government stepped in to take charge, radically reducing the numbers of Romanian children adopted by parents in other countries.

In recent years, Romanian adoptions have been largely supplanted by the adoptions of children from China, Russia, and other countries. In fiscal year 2004, only 57 children were adopted from Romania because Romania severely limited the number of international adoptions and the moratorium on adoptions was set in place. It is estimated that many Romanian children continue to reside in orphanages, and some estimates are that almost 50,000 children live in Romanian orphanages. Orphanage conditions are said to be far improved over the conditions subsequent to the fall of the Ceauşescu regime.

Health of Adopted Romanian Children

Most of the children who were adopted from Romania in the initial influx of adoptions were in very poor physical health, and significant numbers of the children were malnourished, had infectious diseases such as HEPATITIS B, and severe DEVELOPMENTAL DISABILITIES. It is estimated that about 85 percent of the Romanian orphans who were adopted were not healthy, and 90 percent of the children adopted at ages older than one year had developmental delays.

Research on Romanian adopted children In 1998 British physician Michael Rutter and the English and Romanian Adoptees Study Team reported on the progress of a sample of children adopted from Romanian orphanages. They reported on 111 Romanian children adopted before the age of two years by parents in England, comparing them to 52 children of similar age who were adopted within England.

Upon entry into their new country, the Romanian children's physical health was poor. Said Rutter, "Severe malnutrition was the rule; chronic and recurrent respiratory infections were rife; chronic intestinal infections (including giardia) were common; and many of the children had skin disorders of one kind or another." The children were also found to be developmentally delayed, with an average IQ of 63.

A small subset of the Romanian children had only been in the orphanage for several weeks. These children were very different from the long-term orphanage children. Their average IQ score was nearly 97 (within the normal range), and their weights and head circumferences were significantly better than those of the orphanage children.

Romanian Children at Ages Four and Six Years

Many of the children followed in Rutter's study made astounding progress in the first few years after adoption. For example, 51 percent were below the third percentile in weight when they entered their families, but at age four, only 2 per-

cent were at this level. Catch-up growth in height was also dramatic.

Developmental and cognitive improvements were also noted and were most dramatic among the children who were adopted from the orphanage before the age of six months. In fact, researchers found that, at age four, the Romanian children adopted before six months closely resembled the growth and developmental progress of the English children who were adopted in-country. Rutter said the researchers "found no measurable deficit in those who came to the U.K. before the age of 6 months. Not only were their cognitive levels well up to U.K. norms, they did not differ from those of the within-U.K. adoptees." Neither the length of time institutionalized nor the degree of malnutrition seemed to account for the better outcome.

The mean IQ of the children improved from 63 to 107. Of the children who were adopted after the age of six months, the mean IQ doubled, increasing from 45 to 90.

Despite these improvements, however, some children adopted from Romania in the sample studied by the English and Romanian Adoptees (ERA) Study Team showed continued behavioral problems, as described in a 2002 article of *Developmental and Behavioral Pediatrics,* when the children were six years old. Many of the children exhibited quasi-autistic behaviors. For example, 47 percent of the children adopted from Romania constantly rocked themselves at the time of the adoptive placement, and by the age of six years, 18 percent continued the rocking behavior. Some parents tried to stop the rocking while others ignored it, but it did not seem to matter what the parents did.

The children most likely to exhibit the rocking behavior usually had resided in the orphanage for a longer period. For example, only 4 percent of children adopted at six months or less exhibited this behavior when adopted, and at the age of six years, none exhibited rocking behavior. Among children ages six to 12 months when adopted, 32 percent exhibited rocking. This percent of children with rocking behavior further increased to 69 percent of the children adopted at 12–24 months of age. Among children adopted over the age of 24 months, 78 percent exhibited the rocking at the time of adoption.

Among all children, the rocking behavior decreased with time. The highest percentage of rocking behaviors occurred among the six year olds who were adopted at greater than 24 months of age; 36 percent continued to evince this behavior as six year olds.

The researchers also found that 24 percent of the children engaged in self-injurious behaviors when adopted, with the greatest risk of head banging and other self-injuries occurring among older children. When the children were six years old, 13 percent continued to engage in self-injurious behaviors, and these behaviors were most common (27 percent) among children adopted when they were older than 24 months. (Among this group of older children, 42 percent had exhibited self-injurious behaviors when adopted, so many children did improve over time.)

Some of the children exhibited unusual sensory behaviors, such as a fascination with the textures of items or with light or smells. These behaviors may have resulted from the extreme deprivation experienced in the orphanage. Of the 16 children who exhibited such behaviors at the time of adoption, 10 children continued to exhibit these behaviors at the age of six years. In addition, nine children had begun developing such behaviors between their placement with the adoptive family and the age of six years.

Said the authors, "The findings in this study show that temporary sensory and social deprivation can result in a persistent pattern of behaviors, which may continue long after a child has been removed from the initial deprived environment." The authors also added, "Deciphering what vulnerability or protective influences explain the variation in response to early deprivation requires further intensive research. The further follow-up of these children, which is now under way, may provide further clues to the nature of early adversity on long-term development for developmental theory and clinical practice."

Orphanages Are Bad for Children

As noted, studies of the Romanian children as well as of children adopted from other countries have revealed that the longer that children are institutionalized, the more damage may occur, although some orphanages are more humane than others. Although the physical circumstances in Romanian orphanages have improved, psychological and developmental outcomes have not significantly changed for those children who have suffered a period of neglect.

Recommendations for the Future

Based on studies done in Canada and elsewhere, Jerri Ann Jenista, M.D., made the following recommendations in *Adoption/Medical News*:

1. All institutionalized children should be considered to have special needs at the time of adoption.

2. Efforts should be made to place children as young as possible to limit their exposure to orphanage living.

3. Parents should be thoroughly prepared for the special needs of orphanage children prior to actual adoption.

4. Children should receive a thorough medical evaluation at the time of arrival into the adoptive home.

5. All children coming from orphanages should receive remedial educational services, beginning as soon as possible.

6. Agencies and adoption facilitators should be required to provide long-term post-placement support services.

7. Research should continue to try to determine ways of improving orphanage settings to minimize the severe effects experienced by some children.

See also INTERNATIONAL ADOPTION; MEDICAL PROBLEMS OF INTERNATIONALLY ADOPTED CHILDREN; RESILIENCE.

Beckett, Celia, et al. "Behavior Patterns Associated with Institutional Deprivation: A Study of Children Adopted from Romania," *Developmental and Behavioral Pediatrics* 23, no. 5 (October 2002): 297–303.

Jenista, Jerri Ann, M.D. "Romanian Review," *Adoption/Medical News* 3, no. 5 (May 1997): 1–3.

Miller, Laurie C., M.D. *The Handbook of International Adoption Medicine: A Guide for Physicians, Parents, and Providers.* New York: Oxford University Press, 2005.

Rutter, Michael, and the English and Romanian Adoptees ERA Study Team. "Developmental Catchup, and Deficit, Following Adoption after Severe

Global Early Privation," *Journal of Child Psychology and Psychiatry* 39, no. 4 (1998): 465–476.

Russia, adoptions from   Adoptions of children from the Russian Federation (a part of the former Soviet Union). Since 1991, when only 12 children were adopted from Russia by citizens of the United States, and 1992, when 324 were adopted, thousands of children have been adopted from Russia.

Russia has been one of the top two countries of origin for internationally adopted children since fiscal year 1993. China is the other country. In 2005, 4,639 children were adopted from Russia by American parents.

It should also be noted that increasing numbers of children are adopted from other countries of the former Soviet Union; for example, in 2005, 755 children were adopted from Kazakhstan, and 821 were adopted from Ukraine.

The major reason for the increase in the number of adoptions, in addition to improved Russian-American relations, is that there are hundreds of thousands of children in about a thousand state-run orphanages, and these orphanages continue to be chronically short of funding. There is virtually no foster-care program in Russia, and thus, children who cannot remain with their parents or relatives must live in an institution. Children who are younger than age three usually live in "baby homes" (orphanages for younger children), under the jurisdiction of the regional Ministries of Health, while older children reside in orphanages under the jurisdiction of the regional Ministries of Education.

Americans and individuals from other countries who wish to adopt children from Russia must work with an adoption agency that has been accredited by the Russian government. They must provide a home study from an adoption agency. In addition, they usually must travel to Russia twice. The adoption actually occurs in a court in Russia, although some parents from the United States also seek a RE-ADOPTION after returning to their home state in the United States, so that the child may obtain a U.S. birth certificate.

Motivations of Adoptive Parents

Most people adopt children from Russia (as well as other countries in the former Soviet Union) simply because they want to a child to love. They may believe it is too difficult to adopt a child in the United States. They may wish to help any child who needs a family. They may prefer to avoid an OPEN ADOPTION, as many adoption agencies in the United States encourage with infant adoptions. They may believe that children in the foster care system in the United States are too emotionally damaged by abuse or neglect and thus may turn away from adopting a foster child. Many adopting parents are Caucasian and believe that a child of similar ethnic appearance will be easier to integrate into their family and community. Some parents assume that all Russian children are blue-eyed blondes; however, children from Russia may be of many different races.

Health Issues among Russian Children

Children adopted from Russia may be healthy, but some have serious health problems.

Russia has the highest alcohol consumption in the world, and there is a serious alcoholism problem in Russia. Mothers who feel that they are unable to parent their children may also be heavier drinkers than the average Russian woman, although this has not been studied in depth. Some children who are later adopted suffer from FETAL ALCOHOL SYNDROME. In addition, many people in Russia are smokers, and it is estimated that as many as 30 percent of adult females in Russia smoke. Most of the cigarettes that they smoke are very strong unfiltered cigarettes. The mother's smoking is harmful for the developing fetus. (See PRENATAL EXPOSURES.)

Some health problems that children from Russia (and other countries in the former Soviet Union) may experience include as follows:

- TUBERCULOSIS
- HEPATITIS
- GROWTH DELAYS
- DEVELOPMENTAL DISABILITIES
- LANGUAGE DELAY
- INTESTINAL PARASITIC INFECTIONS
- SYPHILIS (usually treated adequately prior to adoptive placement
- Behavior problems

CHILDREN ADOPTED FROM RUSSIA FROM FISCAL YEAR 1991 TO FISCAL YEAR 2005 BY U.S. CITIZENS

Year	2005	2004	2003	2002	2001	2000	1999	1998	1997	1996	1995	1994	1993	1992	1991
Number adopted	4,639	5,865	5,209	4,939	4,279	4,269	4,348	4,491	3,816	2,454	1,896	1,087	746	324	12

Source: Derived from information from the United States Department of State

Comprehensive outcome studies of children adopted from Russia have not yet been reported. However, some research suggests that many of these children have learning disabilities and emotional and behavioral problems, probably reflecting their difficult early life experiences.

Summer Trips for Russian Children from Orphanages

Some organizations sponsor summer trips to the United States and other countries for children from orphanages in Russia. Most of these programs are designed to promote the adoption of older children. Some experts are concerned by the depression experienced by children who are not selected for adoptive placement and then are compelled to return to the orphanage in Russia.

See also ADOPTION MEDICINE; INTERNATIONAL ADOPTION; MEDICAL PROBLEMS OF INTERNATIONALLY ADOPTED CHILDREN.

Miller, Laurie C., M.D. *The Handbook of International Adoption Medicine: A Guide for Physicians, Parents, and Providers.* New York: Oxford University Press, 2005.

S

school Public or private elementary, middle school, or high school, which is an environment that may have a profound impact on children, including adopted children. It is important for teachers and other school staff to seek to maintain a balanced attitude toward adopted children, not assuming that they are invariably troubled individuals, but at the same time realizing that some adopted children have come from difficult backgrounds, and they may have experienced past abuse and deprivation and thus may have learning disabilities and other problems that make it difficult for them to perform well in school.

Says Patricia Swanton in her article for *Journal of Family Health Care,* "Teachers, health professionals and educational psychologists should guard against having negative expectations of adopted children. Many children at school have troubled backgrounds of one kind or another and many professionals have known adopted children who thrive both at school and at home. However, each adopted child and set of personal circumstances is different."

As to whether the school should be told by the adoptive parents that the child was adopted (if this is an option, which it sometimes is not, since the adoptive parents are clearly of another race, as with white parents who adopt Chinese children), the decision needs to be made by the parents with regard to what is best for their own child. Some parents worry that their child could be stigmatized if the adoption were known, while others believe that telling the teacher about the adoption at the beginning of the school year is a good idea. Swanton says that "children need to know about this decision and if possible, be involved in making it. They should not be left to feel that things have been discussed or arranged behind their back."

In some cases, school projects involving family trees or family pictures are planned, and these projects may sometimes confuse children who were adopted at older ages, not knowing if they should depict their birth family, foster family, or adoptive family. It is best if the teacher explains in a nonjudgmental way that families are formed in many different ways. Teachers should never, however, single out a specific child as an example of an adopted child, unless permission was given from both the child and the parent.

In one meta-analysis of 62 studies of adopted children, reported in a 2005 issue of *Psychological Bulletin,* the adopted children were compared to their nonadopted birth siblings and their peers who they left behind, and the adopted children scored significantly higher in intelligence tests than the other two groups and had a better school performance. However, some catch-up was needed for the adopted children to perform as well as the children already in the school.

The researchers did find a small number of children who needed extra help in school and said that "the percentage of adopted children who needed special education for their learning problems was about twice as large as the percentage of nonadopted children. This minority of adopted children with learning problems is clinically important because the children suffer from these problems and need special treatment. However, their difficulties should not be confused with those experienced by the average adopted child. Most adopted children do remarkably well, certainly much better than their siblings or peers who had to stay behind in poor institutions or deprived families."

See also TEACHERS AND ADOPTED CHILDREN.

Swanton, Patricia. "The Adopted Child at School," *Journal of Family Health Care* 12, no. 6 (2002): 155–157.

Van IJzendoorn, Marinus H., Femmie Juffer, and Caroline W. Klein Poelhuis. "Adoption and Cognitive Development: A Meta-Analytic Comparison of Adopted and Nonadopted Children's IQ and School Performance," *Psychological Bulletin* 131, no. 2 (2005): 301–316.

screening   See HOME STUDY.

sealed records   The original birth certificate of an adopted person, usually born in the United States, which may also include records of court proceedings, adoption agency reports, and other matters surrounding a confidential adoption. After an adoption is finalized in the United States, the adopted child's original birth certificate is "sealed," or made inaccessible to all persons, and a new birth certificate is created. The new birth certificate indicates that the adoptive parents are the actual parents, as if the child were born to them. The practice of sealing adoptions began in the 1920s in New York, and other states passed laws creating sealed adoption records up to about the 1940s and 1950s. If a child is adopted in another country, and the parents readopt the child in their home state, the adoption records are sealed and a new birth certificate is issued, as when the child was born in the United States and then adopted.

The purpose of sealing the original birth certificate and other related records is to protect the confidentiality of the birthparents, adoptive parents, and adopted child.

Some groups and individuals challenge whether this practice should continue, stating that being born out of wedlock is no longer considered a shameful secret, as it was in long past years, and that it is not necessary to "protect" adopted children, since many adoptions in the United States are open adoptions in which the identities of the birthparents and adoptive parents are known to each other. Others believe that it is still important to seal original adoption records and the birth certificate, to avoid pain to all parties involved, particularly the adopted child.

The circumstances under which the original birth certificate may be obtained by adopted adults vary according to the state; however, most states require the adopted person to be at least 18 years old and might also require a court order before the original birth certificate may be released.

Some groups have sought to change the law to one of OPEN RECORDS. As of this writing, adopted adults in some states may obtain some or all of their adoption records or their original birth certificate on request and without a court order: Alabama, Alaska, Kansas, Maryland, New Hampshire, and Pennsylvania. In some states, adopted adults may obtain a copy of their birth certificate if the birth parent has not filed an affidavit of nondisclosure or a similar form. Such states include the following: Delaware, Hawaii, Indiana, Minnesota, Mississippi, Nebraska, Ohio, and Washington.

In states that do not have an open records law, adopted adults can often obtain their birth certificate and/or adoption records if they have a compelling reason, and they obtain a court order signed by a judge. In most cases, simple curiosity and a desire to meet the birthparents are not considered compelling reasons. Some adopted adults cite medical or psychiatric reasons for their desire to identify their birthparents. They may append a letter to their request that was written by their physician, psychologist, or psychiatrist to support their case.

See also MUTUAL CONSENT REGISTRIES; REUNION; SEARCH; SEARCH AND CONSENT LAWS.

Hollinger, Joan. *Adoption Law & Practice*. Washington, D.C.: LexisNexis, 2004.

National Adoption Information Clearinghouse. "Access to Family Information by Adopted Persons: Summary of State Laws," State Statutes Series 2004, U.S. Department of Health and Human Services, Administration for Children and Families, 2004.

search   A search in relation to adoption describes an attempt, usually by an adopted person, birthparent, or adoptive parent, but sometimes by volunteers or paid consultants, to make a connection between the birthparent and the biological child such that the two can meet. Usually one person initiates the search, but occasionally both individuals (most commonly, the birthmother and the adopted adult) are seeking each other out at about the same time.

Most adopted adults who seek their birthmothers may then follow up and seek out their birthfathers. Sometimes searches occur when the adopted person is a minor, but most searches do not occur until the adopted person is at least 18 years old. Some states will provide identifying information to adopted adults who are older than age 18 or 21, while other states will only provide such information under court order.

Each state has its own laws on the types of identifying information that may be disclosed. (See Appendix VII.) For example, some states, such as Montana and Nebraska, will provide identifying information if the adopted adult is (or may be) a Native American and is seeking information to become an official member of a tribe.

Although it is unknown how many adopted individuals or birthparents search, searching may be on the increase, at least based on the number of SEARCH GROUPS that exist nationwide and their activities on the INTERNET, although reliable statistics are not available. In addition, a great deal of media attention has focused on this issue, and numerous newspaper features about "reunions" of individuals adopted at birth and their birthmothers have been published, and many television programs about reunions have also been aired.

It should be noted, however, that some adopted adults have little or no interest in searching for their birthparents. It is also true that some adopted adults who are interested in searching delay the search until the adoptive parents' death because they fear offending them.

This can be a risky strategy for those who wish to find their birthparents, because the odds of the birthparents' death also increase with each passing year. However, sometimes adopted adults are correct in their belief that the adoptive parents may become upset or alarmed about the search. Some adoptive parents may feel a sense of abandonment when their children search for their birthparents, and they may wonder if they were "not good enough parents" in the child's eyes, which they perceive as the true impetus for the search. Yet most adopted adults say that they love their adoptive parents and that searching is not a repudiation or rejection of them. Studies seem to bear out this perception.

Some adopted adults seek out (or are sought by) their biological siblings. Some states allow birth siblings to access nonidentifying or even identifying information on siblings.

The Process of Searching

If the adopted adult knows the birthparent's name or the birthparent knows the adopted child's first name and new surname after the adoption is finalized, the search is usually much easier, especially with the use of the Internet and online telephone directories and other records. However, in many cases, the adoption was *not* an open adoption, and thus the first piece of information searchers need to recover is the name of the other party.

If they can obtain identifying information from adoption records, as is allowed in some states, information on the name as well as other data will be revealed. If the adopted adult can obtain a copy of the original birth certificate before it was sealed, this too will provide important information, that is, the name of the birthmother. Even if a birthmother has married or remarried since the adoptive placement, it is easier to locate someone when a former name is known.

Some adopted adults extensively search on the Internet to locate their birthparents while others advertise in a newspaper in the general area where they were born, with an advertisement that states their birth date and any other general information that may be noticed by the birthparent or others who are familiar with the adopted adult's birth date, such as birth grandparents or birth siblings. Some hire private detectives to assist them. However, many reference librarians at public libraries may be familiar with information on searching for birth relatives. Some adopted adults and birthparents seek out information on genealogical databases, particularly the extensive database provided by the Church of the Latter-day Saints (Mormons).

Some adopted adults seek information from old hospital records. This information is generally not provided to the public but sometimes sympathetic records clerks or physicians will "look the other way" or even actively assist the adopted person. However, some individuals who have released such information have been fired from their jobs for violating confidentiality. In a few cases, individuals who have done multiple illegal searches of government databases have been charged with crimes of illegal access and subsequently imprisoned.

There are many different organizations that help adopted adults and birthparents connect. One long-standing such organization is the International Soundex Reunion Registry in Carson City, Nevada. With this international registry, if both the birthparent and adopted adult register, the information will be released. Adoptive parents may also register their minor children who were adopted. This type of database is very useful because many people move from state to state or even to another country, and it can be cumbersome to search for information in many different states.

Some organizations charge a great deal of money for information that may be readily obtained at low or no expense from a state database or other source. Adopted adults or birthparents seeking each other should not assume that every organization that offers help with searches is an ethical organization, and they should obtain references and check with organizations such as the Better Business Bureau in the local area.

Searchers v. Non-Searchers

Many experts believe that curiosity about their origins and why they were adopted are the primary motivations for adopted adults who search. Adopted women in their childbearing years, especially women who are pregnant or who have recently had a child or adopted a child, may be most likely to wish to connect with their birthmothers. They may also seek out birthparents if they or their child has a serious medical problem that may have a genetic basis, although nonidentifying medical information is often available from an adoption registry or other source. Court orders to open adoption records and reveal the identity of the birthparents may also be sought if medical or genetic information is needed on an urgent basis.

Researchers Kowal and Schilling, in surveying adopted adults on their reasons for searching, found that 75 percent said they were seeking medical information while 71 percent said they wanted information on their birthparents' personalities. Sixty-eight percent sought a physical description of their birthparents. More than 50 percent said they wanted the following types of information: the marital status of their birthparents and information on the hobbies and careers of their birthparents.

Birthparents may search to verify that the children they bore are well and happy, and they may wish to explain why the adoption occurred. They may also wish to establish a new relationship with their adult children.

Some adults who were adopted from other countries also seek out their birthparents, but it may be difficult or even impossible to locate their birthparents. Many children adopted from other countries were abandoned to orphanages, and the identities of the birthparents are unknown. The language barriers, as well as legal obstacles in the birth country, also impede searching. Some children adopted from other countries choose to visit the orphanages and towns where they resided in their birth countries; a few seek out their foster families.

Several studies have compared and contrasted adopted adults who search for their birthparents with adopted persons who have no desire to search. The more the adopted person remembered about the information provided about the adoption and the more negative early feelings about adoption were, the higher the probability the adult adoptee would search for a birthparent.

A study by J. Triseliotis reported in 1973 discussed 70 adopted adults who used the open records available in Scotland and compared these individuals with nonsearchers. His findings were: "Adoptees who have experienced a happy home life and to whom the circumstances of their adoption has been made available by the adoptive parents, and who have not experienced a recent intense crisis, are less likely to feel the need to seek reunions." A surprising finding by Michael Sobol and Jeanette Cardiff in a Canadian study was that the greater the amount of information provided to the adopted adult on the birthparent, the *higher* the probability that the adult adopted person would initiate a search. This finding conflicts with other studies, which have found that it is a lack of information given to adopted individuals that is correlated with a desire to search. Possibly greater information gives the adopted adult a greater feeling of connection to and curiosity about the birthparent.

A study reported by Miller Wrobel, Grotevant, and McRoy in a 2004 issue of the *Journal of Adolescent Research* validated the findings of Sobol and

Cardiff in that adolescents who were interested in searching (or who had already searched for birthparents) were more likely to have been a part of an open adoption or there was some openness in their adoptions compared to the situation with non-searchers. This study was comprised of 173 adoptive mothers, 162 adoptive fathers, and 156 adopted adolescents (including 75 boys and 81 girls), and the average age of the adolescents was about 16 years. Adolescents already in contact with their birthmothers were excluded from the study. Said the researchers, "Those adolescents who had information about their birthparents as a part of their adoption were more likely to state that they intended to search or had actually searched. Having information did not reduce curiosity. Providing even partial information can create a climate in which adopted children can act to satisfy their curiosity."

The researchers found positive family dynamics among the adolescents who wished to search for their birthparents as well as those who did *not* wish to search. Said the researchers, "Contrary to popular speculation, we found no evidence that the desire to search or searching behavior is the result of poor adoptive family relationships or adolescent maladjustment."

The researchers considered adolescents who did not wish to search for their birthparents and found that they were less curious about them than the teenagers who wished to search. In contrast, those who did wish to search were more curious and wanted more openness with their birthparents.

Considering Open Adoption Records v. Sealed Records

Most adoption records are held confidential or are "closed," while in some cases, adoption records may be opened. Some adopted adults seek only their original birth certificate before it was sealed subsequent to the adoption. The information on the birth certificate will reveal their birth name and the last names of the birthparents, making a search for them easier.

Adoption records extend beyond the birth certificate and may also include highly personal information that was gathered by the agency about the birthparents, adopted child, and adoptive parents.

The following states will allow adopted adults to obtain their original birth certificates, with varying stipulations depending on state law: Alabama, Alaska, Kansas, Maryland, New Hampshire, and Pennsylvania. However, it should be noted that some states have laws in which the adopted adult may obtain an original birth certificate as long as the birthparent has not filed an affidavit denying the release of confidential records.

Mutual Consent Registries

Many states in the United States have established MUTUAL CONSENT REGISTRIES, wherein if both the birthparent and the adopted person agree that information should be shared, then identifying information shall be provided. Note that some states have several different systems, such as both a mutual consent registry and a search and consent search option.

As of this writing, the following states have established some form of a mutual consent registry or other means to provide information if both the adopted adult and the birthparents consent to the information release: Arkansas, California, Colorado, Connecticut, Delaware, Florida, Georgia, Idaho, Illinois, Iowa, Kentucky, Louisiana, Maine, Maryland, Massachusetts, Michigan, Minnesota, Missouri, Montana, Nevada, New Hampshire, New Jersey, New Mexico, New York, North Dakota, Oklahoma, Oregon, Rhode Island, South Carolina, South Dakota, Tennessee, Texas, Utah, and West Virginia.

Search and Consent/Confidential Intermediary Options

In some states, the adopted adult (and sometimes the birthparent) may request that a confidential intermediary locate the other party and determine whether he or she would be willing to have identifying information disclosed. This is referred to as a search and consent option and/or as a confidential intermediary system. In this type of system, the intermediary contacts the sought person and if he or she agrees to the release of identifying information so that contact may be made, then the information is provided to the other party. Some states which offer this option as of this writing include Arizona, Colorado, Kansas, Montana, New Jersey, New Mexico, Oklahoma, Pennsylvania, Washington, and Wyoming.

Affidavits or Notices Precluding Search (or Not)

In some states, identifying information related to the adoption may be given to the adopted adult if the individual sought has *not* filed an affidavit or other form of notice that specifically requests that the information be withheld. In this case, inaction is tantamount to consent. One problem with affidavits, however, is that unless birthparents are told about this option, they may not realize that they must act in order to maintain their confidentiality. It is also true that the child may be born in one state with one set of laws, and the birthparent may relocate to another state with very different laws. Most people are unfamiliar with their own state laws, let alone the laws of a state where they no longer reside.

Examples of states with laws on no-contact affidavits or other forms include Delaware, Hawaii, Indiana, Minnesota, Mississippi, Nebraska, Ohio, and Washington.

In some states, adoptive parents can block the release of information; for example, an adopted person age 25 or older in Nebraska may request an original birth certificate, but the adoptive parents or birthparents may file nonconsent forms to block the release of the birth certificate.

Some states have extra provisions for the release of information. For example, in Mississippi, the adopted adult must have counseling before any identifying information will be released. Mandatory counseling is also required in South Carolina before identifying information may be provided.

Court Orders Only

In some states, only by obtaining a court order may an adopted adult obtain identifying information and/or an original birth certificate. States which require court orders for the release of identifying information and/or the original birth certificate include the following: Arizona, Arkansas, California, Colorado, Connecticut, District of Columbia, Florida, Georgia, Hawaii, Iowa, Kentucky, Louisiana, Maine, Massachusetts, Nevada, New Jersey, New York, North Carolina, North Dakota, Ohio, Oregon, South Dakota, Texas, Utah, Virginia, and Wyoming.

Differing Laws Depending on When the Child Was Born

Some states base their law on providing information based on when the child was born. If the child

was born before a certain date, then one set of laws applies. If the child was born after that date, another set of laws apply, such as in Michigan, Montana, Ohio, Vermont, and Washington. For example, in Michigan, if an adoption was finalized before September 12, 1980, identifying information will be released to an adult adopted person if both birthparents have a statement consenting to the release on file with the central adoption registry. However, for adoptions finalized on or after September 12, 1980, the identifying information will be given to an adult adopted person unless a birthparent has a statement on file denying consent to release of the information.

Another example: in Montana, for adoptions finalized before October 1, 1997, the adopted adult may receive a copy of the original birth certificate only with a court order. However, for adoptions finalized on or after October 1, 1997, the adopted person may receive the original birth certificate with a written request unless the birthparent requests in writing that it not be released without a court order.

In general, the trends in changes to adoption information seem to be toward providing more information to adopted adults than in past years. Increasingly, if birthparents wish the information withheld, they must take active steps to block the release of the information.

Laws Related to Birth Siblings

In some states, identifying information will be provided to the adopted person on adult biological siblings and may also be released to the adult siblings who are searching for the adopted person. Often the mutual consent option is used, wherein both the adopted person and the adult sibling consent to identifying information being shared with the other party. States with laws regarding the release of information on siblings include the following: Idaho, Indiana, Iowa, Kentucky, Louisiana, Maine, Maryland, Michigan, Mississippi, New Mexico, New York, Oklahoma, Rhode Island, South Carolina, Utah, Vermont, and Wyoming.

See also ADOPTIVE PARENTS; BIRTHFATHER; BIRTHMOTHER.

Kowal, Katherine A., and Karen Maitland Schilling. "Adoption through the Eyes of Adult Adoptees,"

American Journal of Orthopsychiatry 55 (July 1985): 354–362.

Miller Wrobel, Gretchen, Harold D. Grotevant, and Ruth G. McRoy. "Adolescent Search for Birthparents: Who Moves Forward?" Journal of Adolescent Research 19, no. 1 (January 2004): 132–151.

National Adoption Information Clearinghouse. "Access to Family Information by Adopted Persons: Summary of State Laws," State Statutes Series 2004, U.S. Department of Health and Human Services, Administration for Children and Families, 2004.

Triseliotis, J. In Search of Origins: The Experience of Adopted People. London: Routledge and Kegan Paul, 1973.

search and consent laws State laws that specify that an adopted adult born in the United States (and sometimes, a birthparent, biological sibling, or half-sibling) may request, usually through a social services department, that an intermediary, either a social worker or other designated person, will search for and contact the birthparent to determine if she/he is willing to be identified and communicate with the adopted adult. This law is also known as the confidential intermediary law.

As of this writing, these states have passed search and consent laws: Arizona, Colorado, Kansas, Montana, New Jersey, New Mexico, Oklahoma, Oregon, Pennsylvania, Washington, and Wyoming. Note that some states have both a mutual consent registry system, in which both the adopted adult and birthparent must first register their desire for contact before the identities are disclosed to each other by a third party, as well as a search and consent law. Also note that state laws change periodically. The state social services office located in the capitol should be most familiar with current adoption laws, as are many adoption attorneys.

If the birthparent or adopted adult is found, the agency is to ask the adopted adult or birthparent if she or he wishes to release identifying information. (Most adopted adults are more eager to locate their birthmother and may later seek out their birthfather.) If the birthparent consents, then the information will be given to the adopted person, and if she or he declines, it will be withheld. Many SEARCH groups strongly believe that adopted adults are entitled to this information, regardless of the laws of the state. Others believe that intermediaries who contact birthparents as a result of search and

consent laws may pressure birthparents into unwanted contact.

See also MUTUAL CONSENT REGISTRIES; OPEN RECORDS; SEALED RECORDS; SEARCH.

Hollinger, Joan. Adoption Law & Practice. Washington, D.C.: LexisNexis, 2004.

National Adoption Information Clearinghouse. "Access to Family Information by Adopted Persons: Summary of State Laws," State Statutes Series 2004, U.S. Department of Health and Human Services, Administration for Children and Families, 2004.

search groups Organizations that assist adopted people, birthparents, adoptive parents, and others in identifying and locating birth relatives.

The first search group was Orphan Voyage and was founded by adopted adult Jean Paton in 1953.

Some search groups actively seek to change state laws; for example, many search groups are in favor of OPEN RECORDS. Groups vary in their policies.

Most groups will only help adult adopted persons seek birthparents or help birthparents seek adopted adults. Other groups assist adoptive parents who wish to seek birthparents when their adopted children are still minors.

Each group's policies and procedures should be considered before joining a particular organization. Most groups provide helpful hints on searching and recommended readings as well as emotional support from successful searchers. Others charge extensive fees and perform the actual searches. They may charge high fees for finding information that is relatively inexpensive to identify.

It is also true that some adoption agencies charge searchers. Whatever the source, adopted people, birthparents, or adoptive parents considering the use of such a search should find out what the fee (or estimated fee) will be. If agencies provide an hourly rate, then the inquirer should request an estimated number of hours the search will take as well as estimated length of time. The customer should also state that she or he expects the search service to comply with federal and state laws, not only because it is important to abide by laws but also because customers should not become entrapped.

sectarian agencies See ADOPTION AGENCIES.

self-esteem An individual's regard and respect for himself or herself and his or her sense of identity and self-worth. Individuals with high self-esteem perceive themselves as valuable, and those with low self-esteem denigrate themselves, their self-worth, and their achievements.

A person with high self-esteem has a realistic view of his strengths and weaknesses and accepts himself as he is. It is often difficult for the average person to develop a healthy self-esteem and is especially difficult for the child who was adopted at an older age—difficult, but by no means impossible.

Self-esteem is not only important to the individual but also affects his family, his friends (and whether or not he has friends), and his entire life. Most criminals have very low self-esteem. People who never fulfill their potential often hold themselves back from fear of failure traceable to a lack of self-esteem.

Adopted children who were adopted at an older age are particularly prone to low self-esteem in the early stages of their adoption. According to family counselor and author Claudia Jewett, "Low self-esteem is one of the most common characteristics in newly adopted older children."

Often these children have been abused or neglected by their biological parents who may also have verbally abused them, and the children have internalized the negative feedback.

Opponents of TRANSRACIAL ADOPTION have stated that low self-esteem is a key reason they disapprove of such adoptions, particularly involving whites adopting black or biracial children. Studies of Korean and black children adopted across ethnic lines have not borne out this prediction, and children who are transracially adopted appear to have a positive self-esteem for the most part.

When a child (or an adult) has a very low opinion of herself, then she may have exhibited a variety of behavior, including ACTING OUT in frustration, or underachieving in school. The child may find it difficult to understand or even be suspicious that someone would want to adopt and love her. To paraphrase an old Groucho Marx saying, she's not sure she'd want to live with any people who would find her acceptable.

Self-esteem can be encouraged and built up, but it also comes from within. If a child has a very low self-esteem, the parent (adoptive or biological) must strive to bring the child's self-esteem level up to a realistic point.

Jewett says praise may not work well with the child adopted at an older age, particularly generalized praise, "You're a good girl" or "You're a wonderful boy." Instead, Jewett recommends praising actions and tasks that are performed well.

She also recommends the parent teach the child self-praise. "Teaching the child to engage in self-praise not only reinforces his positive behavior, it also teaches him a new set of self-referent ideas . . . This skill of praising oneself can be nurtured by asking the question, 'Don't you think you did well on that?' The child's response can then be linked with a statement of praise, such as, 'I think you did a tremendous job, too' or 'You must feel good about that.' When the child becomes more accustomed to giving self-referent verbal reinforcement, the adult can ask, 'What do you think you should say to yourself?' If the child replies that he doesn't know, the adult can ask, 'What do I say to you?' or a similar question to help involve the child in the evaluative, praising process and to give him permission and encouragement to feel pride in himself."

Therapists should also be able to provide many helpful hints. It is important to note, however, that some therapists presume a person is disturbed for the sole reason that she is adopted when in fact other issues may be causing the problems. The child may not have low self-esteem because he wonders why his mother "gave him up" or physically abused him—his difficulty with math or reading may make him feel stupid, and tutoring can help.

Sometimes it *is* an adoption issue that disturbs a child and lowers his self-esteem. Author Stephanie Siegel described a 12-year-old boy who ran away from home because he could not resolve a conflict in his mind. He could not understand why his birthmother had chosen adoption for him and concluded that he must have been a defective child. He reasoned that his adoptive parents, then, must also have something wrong with them, or they would not have adopted a defective child.

With therapy, the child was able to resolve his anxiety, accept his adoption, and improve his self-esteem and self-worth.

One possible way to handle such a situation is for the adoptive parents to bring up the subject of adoption and ask the child if he has any questions about his birthparents. The child may have questions but be afraid to ask the adoptive parents for fear they will feel offended or unloved.

See also EXPLAINING ADOPTION.

Donovan, Denis M., and Deborah McIntyre. *Healing the Hurt Child: A Developmental-Contextual Approach.* New York: W. W. Norton, 1990.

Jewett, Claudia L. *Adopting the Older Child.* Boston: Harvard Common Press, 1978.

Siegel, Stephanie E. *Parenting Your Adopted Child.* New York: Prentice Hall, 1989.

self-help   See SUPPORT GROUPS.

sensory integration disorder   A disorder that causes difficulty with integrating the information received from the senses and significantly affects the behavior and daily life for individuals with this problem. Sensory integration (SI) disorder is also known as sensory integration dysfunction.

Most people are familiar with the senses that enable them to see, hear, smell, and taste. The tactile sense (touch) is also a known important sense. However, in addition to these five senses, there is also a sense of movement (vestibular) and a sense of one's body position in space (proprioception). Individuals with SI disorder have problems with one or more of these seven different senses.

Children with SI problems may be hyperreactive to stimuli or they may be underreactive and seek out particular stimuli, whether they are sounds, sights, and so forth. Some children alternate from being overresponsive to stimuli to being underresponsive, which can be very frustrating to parents and physicians, as well as to the child.

Children who are adopted from other countries after long stays in orphanages are at risk for sensory integration disorder, possibly because of the extreme deprivation that they have experienced in such an environment. In one study of 60 adopted children, aged four to nearly nine, reported in *The American Journal of Occupational Therapy* in 2005, the researchers compared children who had spent 18 months or longer in an orphanage to children who had spent less than six months in orphanages.

Thirty children were in the group that had been institutionalized for 18 months or longer, and 30 children were in the group that was in the orphanage for less than six months. The researchers found that the long-term group had significant problems in the areas of touching, movement, and also with audition (hearing perception). Said the researchers,

"The results of this study suggest that longer lengths of institutionalization are associated with more atypical sensory integration (sensory modulation and praxis) in children adopted from Eastern European orphanages." They added, "Occupational therapists working with children who have been exposed to early environmental deprivation may wish to consider assessing sensory integration functioning of these children if they are experiencing difficulties with their occupational performance and/or participation in school, home, and community contexts."

Symptoms and Diagnostic Path

Patients with sensory integration disorder may show varying types of symptoms. Some behavioral symptoms are extreme sensitivity to loud noises or to certain smells or even to light touch. For example, a child who is hypersensitive to tactile sensation may actively resist having his hair washed or wearing certain types of clothing which do not feel "right" to him. A child who is oversensitive to oral stimulation may refuse to eat foods with certain types of textures, such as foods that seem greasy or slimy to her. (A small child who is a "picky eater" may or may not have SI, and only an evaluation can determine this.)

Some children are very sensitive to noises. Said Biel and Peske in their book, *Raising a Sensory Smart Child: The Definitive Handbook for Helping Your Child with Sensory Integration Issues,* "Some children are oversensitive to low frequency sounds such as a lawn mower, air conditioner, or vacuum cleaner. On the other hand, some children underreact to sound. They need a lot of sound: animated voices or loud, vigorous music 'wakes up' their ears."

Some children with SI disorder have trouble with their balance and with tasks such as tying their shoes beyond the age when other children have mastered this skill. They may seem clumsy to others who observe them. They may also seem to be "accident prone," because children with SI often suffer from injuries caused by frequent falls or other accidents. Some children with SI disorder will actually walk into objects, seemingly not seeing what is before their eyes, although they have normal vision. In this case, they are not recognizing the difference between where they are and where the other object is in relation to their bodies.

Some children are distractible and disorganized. They may have great difficulty adapting to new situations and transitioning from one activity to another. In some cases, children with these symptoms may appear to have attention deficit/hyperactivity disorder (ADHD) rather than the lesser-known SI disorder. Complicating matters further, it is possible for a child to have both SI and ADHD.

Some children with SI disorder may actively seek out sensory experiences, rather than wishing to minimize them or screen them out. For example, such children may spin around over and over until they fall down. (This behavior may also occur in healthy toddlers and is not necessarily an indicator of SI disorder.)

Some children with SI disorder appear impervious to painful experiences. When other children scream when the doctor gives them the injection, the child with SI disorder may be "good," because they are oblivious to pain. Yet it is important to react to painful stimuli, and the failure to react is an indication of a problem.

Children with SI disorder may avoid other children, preferring to play alone rather than with others. Other children may seem too loud, too rough, and too demanding to deal with for the child with SI disorder. In addition, the child with this disorder may not understand *how* to deal with other children, having difficulty reading their body language cues.

Treatment Options and Outlook

If a parent or another caregiver suspects that SI disorder may be present in the child or knows that there is some as yet unknown problem, the pediatrician should be consulted first, in most cases. The doctor may recommend that an evaluation be performed by the school system as part of the EARLY INTERVENTION program. This is a program for preschool children to identify a variety of problems, including SI disorder.

If SI disorder is identified as a result of the testing process, a therapist can design a program that is specific to the child's individual needs. Note that evaluations of newly adopted children who have arrived in the country within the past month or so should be interpreted with caution. Until they adapt to the challenges of a new environment, children may exhibit behaviors that may seem abnormal but will abate with time.

Children diagnosed with SI disorder are treated by occupational therapists, who teach them techniques and skills to function better in the environment. They may also receive help from a physical therapist and a speech language pathologist. Children may also need to obtain extra help when they are older and begin to attend school.

Risk Factors and Preventive Measures

As mentioned, children who have lived in orphanage environments are at risk for SI disorder. Other children who are at risk are those who were exposed prenatally to alcohol or illegal drugs. There may be a genetic cause of SI disorder. However, sometimes the biological mother did not abuse any substances, and no identifiable reason can be found for the existence of the SI disorder.

See also INTERNATIONAL ADOPTION; MEDICAL PROBLEMS OF INTERNATIONALLY ADOPTED CHILDREN; ORPHANAGE; PRENATAL EXPOSURES; PSYCHIATRIC PROBLEMS OF ADOPTED PERSONS.

Biel, Lindsey, and Nancy Peske. *Raising a Sensory Smart Child: The Definitive Handbook for Helping Your Child with Sensory Integration Issues.* New York: Penguin Books, 2005.

Klass, Perri, M.D., and Eileen Costello, M.D. *Quirky Kids: Understanding and Helping Your Child Who Doesn't Fit In—When to Worry and When Not to Worry.* New York: Ballantine Books, 2003.

Lin, Susan H., et al. "The Relation between Length of Institutionalization and Sensory Integration in Children Adopted from Eastern Europe," *The American Journal of Occupational Therapy* 59 (2005): 139–147.

Miller, Laurie C., M.D. *The Handbook of International Adoption Medicine: A Guide for Physicians, Parents, and Providers.* New York: Oxford University Press, 2005.

Smith, Karen A., and Karen R. Gouze. *The Sensory-Sensitive Child: Practical Solutions for Out-of-Bounds Behavior.* New York: HarperResource, 2004.

Stock Kranowitz, Carol. *The Out-of-Sync Child: Recognizing and Coping with Sensory Integration Dysfunction.* New York: Perigee, 1998.

separation and loss   See LOSS.

sex of child, preference of adoptive parents   See GENDER PREFERENCE.

sexual abuse, childhood   Sexual intrusion of a child's body, which may include penile penetration or oral or anal molestation, among other forms of sexual activity. In general, sexual abuse includes any type of maltreatment that involves the child in sexual activity to provide sexual gratification or financial benefit to the perpetrator, including contacts made for sexual purposes, molestation, statutory rape, child pornography, prostitution, exposure, incest, or other sexually exploitative activities. Each state has its own definition of acts that are sexually abusive to children.

Childhood sexual abuse may have lifelong effects. Sexually abused children are significantly more likely to abuse alcohol and illegal drugs as adolescents and adults than individuals who were not abused in childhood. They are also more likely to commit suicide.

Sometimes children deny that proven sexual abuse has occurred. In one study of children who were sexually abused and in which the incidents were videotaped by the perpetrator, some of the children denied the abuse, despite the evidence, according to a study in the *American Journal of Psychiatry.* The reasons for the denial were unknown, but it may be that the children did not wish to remember the abuse or they had trouble remembering it.

Statistical Data

According to statistics from the National Child Abuse and Neglect Data System on abuse and neglect in the United States in 2003, an estimated 787,156 children were the victims of abuse and neglect. Of these, 78,188 children, or about 10 percent of the victims, were sexually abused. (Note that not all victims of sexual abuse are known.) An estimated 1.2 percent of all children in the United States were sexually abused in 2003. Other forms of abuse or neglect are more common; for example, 7.5 percent of all children were neglected in the United States in 2003, and 2.3 percent were physically abused. Less than 1 percent of children who were sexually abused died of the abuse.

Incidents involving girls who are sexually abused are far more likely to be reported than incidents with boys. It is thought that boys may be victimized less often or that they are less likely to come to medical or social attention. In addition, boys who are sexually abused may be ashamed or fearful of reporting the abuse, even more so than are girls.

The perpetrator of sexual abuse is usually someone familiar to the child. However, in very few cases (about 3 percent) are the child's parents the abusers. Instead, in most cases of sexual abuse (76 percent) the perpetrator is a family friend or a neighbor. In 11.5 percent of the cases, the perpetrator is an unmarried partner of the parent.

According to federal statistics for 2003, sexual abuse victims were 38 percent less likely to be placed in foster care than were children who were physical abuse victims. The reason for this difference is unknown.

Children Who Were Sexually Abused and Are Later Adopted

Social workers have an ethical and moral responsibility to report incidences of sexual abuse that have happened to a child being considered for adoption, so that the family can be fully aware of whether they still wish to adopt the child as well as how they can formulate plans to help the child. The social worker need not tell the adoptive parent who was the perpetrator (although this information may be revealed by the child, once he or she trusts the adopting parents) but should describe what happened to the child in as much detail as confidentiality will allow.

Unfortunately, in many instances the social worker may be entirely unaware of incidents of sexual abuse that have happened to the child, and it may not be revealed until much later by children when they feel comfortable enough with the parents to tell them what happened.

One reason that the child may not tell others about the sexual abuse is because the child presumes that he or she deserved to be abused. Says author Marian Sandmaier in her book, *When Love Is Not Enough: How Mental Health Professionals Can Help Special-Needs Adoptive Families,* "This is particularly true of sexually abused children, some of whom also have learned to equate love with sex and may not consciously feel they were maltreated." In many cases, the abuser told children that the abuse was their fault, and they internalized this guilt.

Behavior of Sexually Abused Children

Sandmaier says a child who has been sexually abused in the past may exhibit seductive behavior that can cause "outright panic among family members. Although the child may be looking for the only form of nurturance he or she knows, the parents are likely to view the child's behavior as a profound threat to family stability."

Not all sexually abused children exhibit provocative behavior and other symptoms of previous sexual abuse. Joan McNamara of the Family Resources Adoption Program in Ossining, New York, wrote an informative pamphlet for prospective adoptive parents and adoptive parents entitled *Tangled Feelings: Sexual Abuse & Adoption,* which is still relevant in the 21st century.

McNamara describes symptoms common to sexually abused children, including "sexual knowledge or behavior beyond the child's age level, aversion to touch, or, conversely, seductive or clinging behavior, marked sensitivity to body exposure (aversion or excessive interest), self-exposure and excessive masturbation."

According to McNamara, sexually abused boys are confused about their identity and act out, but girls internalize the guilt of the abuse. In addition, the child may be emotionally "stuck" at the developmental stage that he or she was in at the time of the abuse.

Counseling the Family Is Important before and Sometimes after Adoption

Counseling prospective parents before an adoptive placement occurs is a good idea because sexual abuse is an extremely emotional topic and some people may need help to decide whether they can deal with it. After the adoption, counseling may be necessary for the family as well as for the abused child. Says Sandmaier, "Without counseling to help them [the family] understand the emotional and behavioral consequences of sexual abuse, a family may declare the child incorrigible and prematurely disrupt the placement."

It is also important to note that no matter how well-prepared adoptive parents feel they are, if a beloved child suddenly describes sexual abuse from the past, many parents would understandably feel enraged. The danger in this case is that the child could internalize the guilt for what happened to him or her as well, further damaging an already battered ego. It is very important that the child realize that what happened was not his fault. Even if he or she enjoyed some of the sexual activities that occurred, it was the perpetrator's fault for introducing the child to sex, and it was the perpetrator's fault for inducing his or her will on the child.

False Accusations of Abuse Sometimes Occur

Sometimes the foster child who was abused in the past may falsely accuse someone who did *not* actually abuse him sexually or in any other way, such as a former foster parent. The child may not be lying on purpose but instead may be confused and insecure. Perhaps admitting that he was abused by a person who was supposed to protect him, such as a relative, is too painful. However, false accusations of sexual abuse are occasionally intentional in children who are acting out, and the family and the social worker should be prepared for the possibility. Sometimes this behavior is the only way the child has learned to gain power over the people around her.

Children need a safe environment where the rules are known. They need a great deal of positive reinforcement, and they may have a very difficult time accepting that they are intrinsically worthy to the parent.

McNamara concludes, "When hurt children enter a new family through adoption, past events and feelings are fused with current realities for these children and families. To help heal the hurt takes time, loving commitment, and willingness to be open to another person's pain."

Adoption Disruptions

Sexually abused children have a high risk for adoption DISRUPTION. In a study reported in *Social Work* in 1994, researchers compared problem behaviors of 33 adopted children who had been sexually abused to behaviors of 135 adopted children who were not sexually abused. The average age for the sexually abused children was 10 and for the non-sexually abused children was nine years.

The researchers found a disruption rate of 74 percent for the sexually abused children, compared to a rate of about 43 percent for the other older children who were adopted. The higher disruption rate was attributed in part to problematic behaviors that either did not get better after placement or, in some cases, worsened. For example, 40 percent of the sexually abused children had a problem with lying before placement (compared to about 23 percent of the other children). After placement, the lying behaviors increased to 45 percent for the sexually abused children, while the percentage decreased from 23 percent to about 16 percent in the other children.

Although sexual acting out decreased among the sexually abused children who were adopted (from about 43 percent before placement to 34 percent after placement), this behavior was still very troubling to many adoptive parents. The researchers noted that in many cases previous sexual abuse had not been identified until after the adoption.

The researchers also found that the sexually abused children had a much greater problem with attaching to adoptive parents than the other children who were adopted. For example, 34 percent of the sexually abused children had trouble attaching to the mother, compared to only 14 percent of the other adopted children. "Hostile acting out by child" was another problem associated with attachment difficulties, and this problem was exhibited by about 43 percent of the sexually abused children versus about 10 percent of the other children.

Said the researchers, "To facilitate a healthy adjustment in adoptive placement, children who have been traumatized by sexual abuse need help in identifying this trauma, as well as other traumas or losses that are a part of their experience, so they can heal."

Advice to Prospective Adoptive Parents

Adoptive parents and foster parents should suspect that sexual abuse may have occurred to a child who has been in many placements or lived in dysfunctional homes in the United States or other countries, or has resided for many years in an institution, such as an orphanage in another country. They should also suspect sexual abuse when an older foster child's behavior becomes much worse after placement or the child exhibits sexually precocious behavior.

See also ABUSE; NEGLECT.

Administration for Children and Families. *Child Maltreatment 2003.* Washington, D.C.: Department of Health and Human Services, 2005.

Clark, Robin E., Judith Freeman Clark, and Christine Adamec. *The Encyclopedia of Child Abuse.* 2nd ed. New York: Facts On File, 2001.

Keck, Gregory, and Regina M. Kupecky. *Parenting the Hurt Child: Helping Adoptive Parents Heal and Grow.* Colorado Springs, Colo.: Pinon Press, 2002.

Livingston Smith, Susan, and Jeanne A. Howard. "The Impact of Previous Sexual Abuse on Children's Adjustment in Adoptive Placement," *Social Work* 39, no. 5 (September 1994): 491–501.

McNamara, Joan. *Tangled Feelings: Sexual Abuse & Adoption.* Ossining, N.Y.: Family Resources Adoption Program, 1988.

Sandmaier, Marian. *When Love Is Not Enough: How Mental Health Professionals Can Help Special-Needs Adoptive Families.* Washington, D.C.: Child Welfare League of America, 1988.

Sjoberg, Rickard L., and Frank Lindblad, M.D. "Limited Disclosure of Sexual Abuse in Children Whose Experiences Were Documented by Videotape," *American Journal of Psychiatry* 159 (2002): 312–314.

sexually transmitted diseases   Infectious diseases that are contracted through direct sexual contact. The term is occasionally used to refer to these diseases when they are contracted by the fetus of an infected mother, either during the pregnancy or during delivery. The presence of one sexually transmitted disease increases the probability of other such diseases.

See also HUMAN IMMUNODEFICIENCY VIRUS; SYPHILIS.

showing of the child   See RECRUITMENT.

siblings   People who are brother or sister to one another, either through a birth or an adoptive relationship (by sharing the same birthmother or through adoption). An adopted child who is unrelated to children already in a family or who follow him through birth or adoption does *not* refer to these children as his "half" brothers or sisters: they are his brothers or sisters.

A child who is adopted may be placed with his or her other full or half siblings or may be placed in a family that already has adopted children or children by birth. In addition, the parents may adopt more children in later years or may have additional children by birth. (It is a myth that a good way to cure infertility is to adopt children. See PREGNANCY AFTER ADOPTION.)

Many children who are adopted are only children because the adoptive parents do not already have children and do not adopt again. Consequently, these children will not have siblings in the adoptive family. They may, however, have full- or half-genetic siblings within their birth family. (See ONLY CHILD ADOPTIVE FAMILIES.)

In other cases, sibling groups are placed in an adoptive family, and the consensus among adoption professionals is that siblings should be adopted together whenever possible. In a paper on siblings, social worker Kathryn Donley has said, "Only under the most extraordinary circumstances should prospective parents consider the placement of just one of the children from a family group."

She also urges that existing sibling relationships should be considered and their meanings fully explored. Children's wishes should also be considered. Donley says it is important to remember that sibling relationships can be lifelong and often when adopted adults search, they search for a sibling.

Margaret Ward, an instructor at Cambrian College in Ontario, Canada, describes several key characteristics adoption workers should look for when fitting sibling groups into their new families. One is administrative ability and the capability of juggling Boy Scout meetings with dance classes, doctor appointments, and so forth, along with the basics of running a home.

The ability to cope with emergencies was also seen as important, and the more children in the family, the greater the probability there will be emergencies. According to Ward, "Parents need to possess, or to develop, a relative unflappability. If they become too excited or panicky, the crisis will be escalated by an additional behavioral or emotional chain reaction in the rest of the family."

The ability to promote healthy family interaction and cope with sibling rivalry and group dynamics is also important when siblings are newly added to a family. Parents must be sensitized to existing relationships between children.

Other characteristics Ward identified as important included the "ability to survive in the community" and deal with the school system and other institutions; the availability of support systems, such as adoptive parent support groups, relatives, friends; the ability for the wife and husband to provide each other mutual support and not heap all parental tasks on one person; and the ability to adapt.

When children are adopted into an already existing family, the BIRTH ORDER is altered, and the former child who was the "baby" of the family may well find himself the "middle child," while the oldest child could lose his authority and become a middle child.

Adopting parents should prepare children already in the home as much as possible for the inevitable changes, whether the child to be adopted is an infant or an older child. The whole family needs to understand that there will be frustrations and stresses, particularly when adopting an older child.

Many people who adopt older children already do have children in the home, or they may have raised a family at a relatively young age and opted to parent another family through adoption.

When parents adopt a school-age child, siblings in the home may have unreasonable expectations placed on them; for example, they may be told of the deprived conditions the child lived under and may be urged to be understanding.

This may be difficult when the new child moves out of the honeymoon stage of the initial phase of adoption, when she is on her best behavior, to the testing stage when misbehavior is very common.

In addition, the newly adopted child may not feel very grateful about her adoption, which can annoy the "old" siblings who are trying to feel sorry for her and expect her to appreciate it. When a newly adopted child or a sibling group is placed in a home with children, there is a great deal of adjustment to be made by everyone.

Social worker Carole Depp says sometimes one or more of the siblings in an adoption of siblings may have severe problems. In such a case, she advises, "the best plan may be to stagger the placement of the children with the family . . . visits of a sibling with the child or children not yet placed should be arranged. If the most needful child is placed first, then some of the healing process can begin before the family assumes responsibility for additional siblings."

Adolescence

As with most other facets of adoption and indeed with life in general, adolescence appears to be the most difficult stage for both adopted persons and siblings of adopted persons. (See ADOLESCENT ADOPTED PERSONS for a further discussion of adopted teenagers.)

Margaret Ward and John H. Lewko studied families adopting school-age children after they already had existing adopted or biological children, concentrating on adolescents.

Using a questionnaire for adolescents who already lived in the home, the researchers identified several problem areas. According to Ward and Lewko, "Difficulties with all siblings were seen primarily as hassles. The adoptee was, however, reported as creating more problems than 'old' siblings."

The respondents complained the most about the newly adopted child's lying, interfering with privacy, and failing to obey rules. "Old" siblings were also rated by other old siblings, and sisters were accused of using bad language while brothers were "more likely to practice inadequate hygiene" and not "pay attention to the rules" more than the new adopted child.

According to the researchers, "The appropriate behavior for a resident adolescent is to teach the new child the rules of the family game. Yet the behavior of the new child can upset the adolescent. The daily hassles can add up to severe stress, as indicated by the respondent who stated that she wanted no children at all as a result of the adoption . . . instead of establishing a helpful attitude toward the new child, the adolescent may become alienated."

Adopting Sibling Groups

Although once it was considered acceptable or necessary to separate siblings and to place them into different adoptive families, agencies now make strenuous attempts to place sibling groups together into the same family so they will not undergo a further trauma of separation.

When sibling groups are small, with two siblings of a relatively young age, placement is far easier than when sibling groups of three or more need to be placed. (Groups may be as large as seven or more!)

Sometimes siblings are separated when one wishes to be adopted and the other does not wish to be adopted or is unready to make a commitment. If it is felt by the social worker to be in the child's best interests, then the children may be physically separated. Of course if siblings are abusive to one another, they will be separated.

Twins

In the past, particularly during the Depression era (the early 1930s), it was deemed acceptable to separate twins into different adopting families. Usually this was done because the couple could not handle the stress and financial cost of raising twins.

Social workers today believe it is cruel and unreasonable to separate twins and actively seek to identify adoptive families willing and able to rear both children.

Birth and Adopted Children

Some people have hypothesized that when adopted children join birth children already in the family (also known as a BLENDED FAMILY), the adopted child is the "odd man out," while the birth children are the favored ones.

Studies of such families have not borne out this fear, and instead, adopted children in families with birth children seem to have a higher self-esteem than adopted children whose siblings in the family are also adopted.

According to a study by Janet Hoopes and Leslie Stein, adopted children may feel more positive. They said, "The presence of biological siblings was viewed advantageously, i.e., as confirmation of own self-worth enhanced by the realization of their egalitarian treatment within the family."

In other words, if the adopted child felt as well-treated as the biological child(ren), self-esteem was high. Conversely, the adopted child in a family with only other adopted children does not know how his adoptive parents would treat biological children and may imagine that they would treat them better.

When the adopted child precedes the birth child, people may make disturbing remarks, such as "At last! Now you have a child of your own!" If the child is old enough to understand, this is a painful message, indicating the other child is more important, when in most cases the adoptive parent loves both children very much.

Disabled New Siblings

If the newly adopted child is disabled, the stress on the "old" children may he even greater than otherwise because there is more than just a new child to get used to.

Susan Maczka, director of Project S.T.A.R., a licensed adoption agency for children with developmental disabilities in Pittsburgh, Pennsylvania, wrote "A Head Start" for *OURS* magazine on how to prepare a sibling already in the home for the new child who is disabled.

According to Maczka, it is important to provide "old" siblings with information about the disability. As a result, the child will be more prepared for new needs that must be met or for disturbing behavior that may occur. Maczka also recommends adopting parents take the child to a Special Olympics or visit with a family whose child is disabled.

In addition, she advises discussing with the child ahead of time any changes that may need to be made. "Figure out ways that your children can signal you about frustrations they may feel over those changes. Ask for your children's help in making adjustments," she advises.

Maczka says parents must not place too heavy a burden on their children when the newly adopted child arrives.

"Girls notoriously 'overdo it' in the helping area, and sometimes feel angry about it later," she says.

Sibling Rivalry

Whether siblings are genetically related or are related by adoption, it is virtually inevitable that they will disagree and argue.

Sometimes the sibling rivalry can be very intense. Although caseworkers generally strive to place biological siblings together, if the rivalry is very strong, the children may be separated.

The authors of *Large Sibling Groups* argue with this policy and believe such separation teaches a child that the way to resolve conflict is to leave or to separate the individuals involved rather than actually dealing with the problems surrounding the conflict.

See also SPECIAL NEEDS.

Depp, Carole. "Placing Siblings Together," *Children Today* 12 (March–April 1983): 14–19.

Donley, Kathryn. "Sibling Attachments and Adoption," paper available from the National Resource Center for Special Needs Adoption, Chelsea, Michigan.

Fodge, Gwen. "Bringing Home Joy," *OURS*, January/February 1989, 14–15.

Havel, Pam. "The Geometric Component of Two," *OURS*, January/February 1989. 12–13.

Le Pere, Dorothy W., Lloyd E. Davis, Janus Couve, and Mona McDonald. *Large Sibling Groups: Adoption Experiences.* Washington, D.C.: Child Welfare League of America, 1986.

Maczka, Susan. "A Head Start," *OURS*, January/February 1989, 10–11.

National Council for Adoption. "Adolescent Adoptees' 'Identity Formation' Is Normal, Study Says," *National Adoption Reports* 6 (March–April 1985): 6.

Rutter, Michael, Patrick Bolton, Richard Harrington, Ann Le Couteur, Hope Macdonald, and Emily Smirnoff. "Genetic Factors in Child Psychiatric Disorders-I. A Review of Research Strategies," *Journal of Child Psychology and Psychiatry and Allied Disciplines,* (January 1990): 3–37.

Ward, Margaret. "Choosing Adoptive Families for Large Sibling Groups," *Child Welfare* 66 (May–June 1987): 259–268.

Ward, Margaret, and John H. Lewko. "Problems Experienced by Adolescents Already in Families That Adopt Older Children," *Adolescence* 23 (Spring 1988): 221–228.

single adoptive parents Because of much media attention to single biological parents, many of whom are low-income and struggling, single adoptive parents have found they have often been mistakenly categorized with this group. Yet this stereotype is unfairly applied to the average single adoptive parent, according to the National Council for Single Adoptive Parents, a support group that says most single adoptive parents familiar to the organization are middle-class females and nearly half are members of the "helping professions": teachers, social workers, nurses, and other career fields.

Many are very well-educated, according to the group, which says that the overwhelming majority of the people it surveyed are college graduates with many having earned postgraduate degrees. Most of the single adoptive parents adopt their children while they are in their 30s or 40s, although some are older. (Single adoptive parents are still in the minority, and most adoptive parents are couples.)

Until the 1980s, it was difficult to impossible for the average single woman or man to adopt a child of any age. If the single person was considered as a prospective adoptive parent, she or he was usually considered only for the most difficult to place children, often children needing extensive care and attention, for whom no other options were available. Yet single individuals usually were (and are) employed full time and may find it very difficult to care for children with severe physical or developmental disabilities.

Some experts believe couples should still he given priority in adopting children. They argue that just because a single woman or man wants a child does not mean they are automatically entitled to a child or would make a good parent.

Yet it is important to note that many single adoptive parents adopt older children, disabled children, and children who are considered to have SPECIAL NEEDS. Even when single parents choose to adopt an infant, it is usually an infant from another country and often an infant urgently needing a family and yet considered hard to place because of race, medical problems, or other factors. As a result, the child gains a much-needed parent.

Single Fathers

It may still be difficult for a single man to adopt an unrelated child, either in the United States or internationally. Experts hypothesize that women are perceived as nurturing and adoption is a nurturing act, but the motivations of a man who wishes to adopt may be suspect. In addition, some overseas nations will accept applications from single adoptive women but not single adoptive men.

Mary Ann Curran of Adoption Services of WACAP in Seattle, Washington, explained the problem:

"Not many countries accept men. We have had some very successful placements with single men, but unfortunately our options are very limited" (by the necessity of complying with the criteria of the overseas nation.)

Agencies and Support Groups

Although some agencies refuse to accept applications from single adoptive parents, other agencies concentrate on working with singles, because of very positive experiences with single adoptive parents.

Motivations

The primary motivation of a single person wishing to adopt is congruent with the primary motivation of a married couple who wishes to adopt: the desire for a child to love and cherish. The difference is that most couples who adopt are infertile, whereas the single person may or may not be infertile.

Singles may be given support from their families and friends, or they may be treated with incredulity.

Agencies cannot presume couples will stay married, nor should they presume singles will forever remain single. Instead, say singles, what should be looked at is the individual person and his or her potential parenting capacity.

Adamec, Christine. *There ARE Babies to Adopt.* New York: Kensington, 2002.

skin color   Children who need permanent, loving families through adoption come in all colors. Many adopting parents prefer to adopt children with a skin color similar to their own, although skin color and/or ethnicity is immaterial to other parents.

When people plan to adopt children internationally, they may imagine the children will be Caucasian in appearance. However, many children from other countries, including those in eastern Europe, range from light-skinned to dark-skinned, and many are ethnically mixed.

As a result, prospective adoptive parents who are sensitive to the issue of skin color should carefully evaluate their position before adopting a foreign child.

See also TRANSRACIAL ADOPTION.

sleep disorders, in newly adopted children   Difficulty with getting to sleep and/or staying asleep, which is a common problem among newly adopted children. Children adopted from other countries may have difficulty with bad dreams during naptime or evening sleeping hours, and this problem may persist for several weeks or longer after the child enters the new family.

Painful experiences of separation and loss often manifest as sleep disturbances.

Some children are alarmed at the idea of sleeping alone, having been accustomed to sleeping with others in the same room. This is particularly true of children adopted from Cambodia or South Korea, who are used to close physical contact with their caregivers during the night. Says Dr. Miller, "Many parents find that co-sleeping for the first few weeks or months after adoption greatly reduces the child's anxiety. Transition to more conventional sleep arrangements is easily accomplished when bonding to the family is more firmly established. Repeated expressions of love and provision of needed attention and security are key methods to manage sleep problems in newly adopted children."

See also INTERNATIONAL ADOPTION; MEDICAL PROBLEMS OF INTERNATIONALLY ADOPTED CHILDREN.

Miller, Laurie C., M.D. *The Handbook of International Adoption Medicine: A Guide for Physicians, Parents, and Providers.* New York: Oxford University Press, 2005.

sliding scale fees   Some ADOPTION AGENCIES peg their fees to the prospective adoptive parent's income, for example, 10 percent of their gross income with a minimum fee and a maximum "ceiling" fee.

The purpose of this policy is to enable individuals who are not wealthy to adopt, while people who are more affluent offset the difference with their greater fee. Whether to charge a flat rate fee or a sliding scale fee is left up to the policy of each agency.

Sliding scale fees are lawful in every state but Pennsylvania, whose Supreme Court decided such fees were unlawful in a 1986 court case that equated sliding scale fees with a form of baby selling. The Pennsylvania state legislature subsequently banned sliding scale fees.

social workers   Men and women trained in the field of social sciences, usually social work specifically, although college graduates in sociology, psychology, and other fields may be employed as social workers. (Some social work graduates take umbrage when a person without a social work degree is referred to as a "social worker"; this definition is given in its broadly understood sense.)

Adoption social workers may counsel birthparents, prospective adoptive parents, older children who will be adopted, birth grandparents, and other individuals involved and actively interested in adoption.

Social workers perform home studies of individuals who have applied to adopt a child or children. A HOME STUDY may include group classes, depending on the agency and the situation. The social worker will also visit the home of the prospective parents to interview the adopting parents and verify they would make suitable parents for the child and to ensure the home is safe and hygienic. After the child is in the family, follow-up visits to the home are made.

The primary goal of the social worker involved in adoption is to find good families for children and to protect the rights of the children. If a SPECIAL NEEDS adoption is planned, the social worker wants to fully educate the adopting parents so they will understand the needs and problems of the child. The social worker will also often arrange for the adoptive parents to meet the child and will prepare the child prior to the meeting.

Social workers work for both public and private agencies, as well as for lawyers and others doing independent adoptions. Some social workers are self-employed individuals who perform home studies on demand in states that allow it. (Many states require adoption agencies to administer home studies.)

Social workers are also involved in other aspects of child welfare. Protective services social workers remove children from families that are abusive or neglectful; foster care social workers oversee children in foster care; other social workers oversee the cases of individuals receiving Temporary Aid to Needy Families (TANF) and Medicaid, and there are other types of social workers.

Pay in the professional field of social work is generally modest, and most people who remain in this field are self-motivated and dedicated people who want to make a positive difference in society and people's lives by their help.

socioeconomic status   Many adopted people are adopted from families with a lower socioeconomic status than the families who adopt them; for example, the birthparents may be both blue-collar and lower middle-class people whereas the adoptive family is middle class or even upper class.

Not all birthparents are lower middle class, however, and not all adoptive parents wear "white collars." Many foster parents opt to adopt their foster children, and the average foster parent is a working-class person.

Some birthparents are middle-class or upper-class girls in high school or college who do not wish to parent a child and instead opt to place it for adoption. It is likely they will seek out an agency they feel would place their child with a socioeconomic background similar to their own, and many agencies do such socioeconomic matching.

When agencies allow birthparents to choose adoptive parents from nonidentifying RÉSUMÉS or to meet them, birthparents generally choose a family that is more affluent than their own, wanting "something better" for their child. They are not necessarily seeking a rich family, but they do not want their children to suffer any economic privation.

Studies indicate that socioeconomic status and criminality of adopted individuals are linked inversely: the higher the socioeconomic status of the birthparent and/or the adoptive parent, the lower the probability the child will commit any criminal violations.

Many agencies inadvertently screen out poor or working-class applicants for adoption by virtue of the fees they charge. As a result, many working-class families give up altogether, while others work two jobs and save their money for years in order to pay for the adoption.

Some agencies, however, will allow these families to make payments on a regular schedule. Still other agencies offer SLIDING SCALE FEES, which are dependent on a percentage of the adopting parents' income.

SPECIAL NEEDS adoptions are usually less costly than adoptions for healthy white infants, and many agencies are especially willing to work with families in these situations. In addition, state agencies charge minimal or no fees, and often offer SUBSIDIES for adopting special needs children.

Consequently, it is more likely that blue-collar workers will adopt older children or children with special needs and white-collar and middle-class workers will adopt healthy infants by virtue of the economics of adoption.

See also COSTS TO ADOPT.

South Korea, adoptions from For many years, South Korea was the most common country of origin for internationally adopted children arriving in the United States. Nearly 100,000 Korean children have been adopted by U.S. citizens since 1953. In fiscal year 2005, 1,630 children were adopted from South Korea by Americans, somewhat down from the 1,716 children adopted in fiscal year 2004. Most children adopted from South Korea are born in a hospital or a maternity home and live with a foster family prior to their adoption as infants, rather than living in an orphanage.

The adoption of a Korean child by a non-Asian family is a TRANSRACIAL ADOPTION.

U.S. servicemen began adopting Korean orphans after the Korean War, and later Americans within the United States began adopting Korean infants and children.

In 1956, Harry and Bertha Holt founded the Oregon-based Holt International Children's Service, and they ultimately placed thousands of children in the United States.

Health Information on Children Adopted from Korea

In contrast to children adopted from most other countries, a great deal of information is often available on both birthparents, including their height and weight and the presence of any medical problems as well as information on their occupations, interests, and hobbies. Information on the child's birth grandparents is also sometimes available, along with family social history. Many children are vaccinated for hepatitis B within 48 hours of birth. The children are usually placed before they are nine months old.

Says Dr. Miller in *The Handbook of International Adoption Medicine,* "Physical and developmental examinations are performed at least monthly, and results are sent to prospective adoptive parents." She also says, "Korean children are among the healthiest and most developmentally normal adoptees at arrival." However, some children have gross motor delays, possibly because they have been excessively carried by their foster mothers, and some are overweight.

Miller, Laurie C., M.D. *The Handbook of International Adoption Medicine: A Guide for Physicians, Parents, and Providers.* New York: Oxford University Press, 2005.

special needs adoption   In general, the term *special needs* refers to conditions or characteristics that make a child difficult to place by the state adoption unit or an adoption agency, some of which have nothing to do with the physical or emotional health of the child. There are children with special needs throughout the world. In many states in the United States, the majority of foster children who are adopted are considered to have special needs. (See the table.)

Note that the average American who hears the term "special needs" thinks of a child who is profoundly retarded or who is severely disabled, such as a quadriplegic or blind child. Yet most WAITING CHILDREN are physically healthy, although some have emotional problems. Some children with special needs have one or more DEVELOPMENTAL DISABILITIES and may need assistance in school and elsewhere.

Types of Special Needs

Race, age, and the number of siblings to be placed together are all key factors in the determination of whether a child has special needs, as well as the presence of medical, developmental, and psychological problems. For example, most public (state and county) and private agencies consider children and infants who are African-American or biracial or other nonwhite children to have special needs by virtue of their race alone, regardless of the child's age. (White children may be regarded as having special needs for other reasons, such as being older than a certain age, being part of a sibling group, or having a disability.)

Many agencies consider children older than age five or six years to have special needs. It is also particularly difficult to find adoptive families for adolescents.

Children with developmental disabilities, such as FETAL ALCOHOL SYNDROME, cerebral palsy, or mental retardation are often difficult to place with adoptive families.

When a child has a behavioral, emotional, or psychiatric disability, it is often very difficult to find an adoptive family. The more severe the disability, the more difficulty there usually is in finding a family for the child.

Sometimes abused children are difficult to place because of the type of abuse that they have experienced; for example, many people have trouble dealing with the idea that some children have suffered from SEXUAL ABUSE and they are not willing to consider adopting children with such past problems.

Definitions of "Special Needs" Vary

The designation of "special needs" varies among private adoption agencies, as well as among social service organizations administering the care of foster children in various states. In some cases, a child who is viewed as having a special need in one adoption agency may be described as a healthy child by another agency. For example, some agencies may consider a child who needs minor surgery to have a special need, while others would not.

Private and public (government) agencies often list categories they consider to be special needs on an adoption application, asking prospective parents to indicate their willingness to accept specific special needs by checking yes, no, or maybe to each condition.

Parents Who Adopt Children with Special Needs in the United States

Some parents adopt children with special needs from private adoption agencies in the United States, but most children with special needs are adopted from the foster care system.

Parents who adopt children with special needs are most likely to have positive relationships with their children if the agency has provided complete background information on the child, so that there are few or no surprises. The purposeful withholding of health information so that parents would assume that the child they were adopting was healthy has led to some landmark lawsuits. (See WRONGFUL ADOPTION.)

In general, families who adopt children with special needs are frequently older, and if they are married, they have been married longer than the infant adopters. Many families who adopt children with special needs already have children, and this experience is seen as a plus by numerous agencies. In contrast, a large number of adoption agencies who work with infant adoptions restrict their applications to childless couples or couples with only one child.

Single people (usually women) are usually approved to adopt children in foster care or through adoption agencies; however, some singles are offered children with special needs first, which they may resent, believing that a single person would have a harder time caring for a child with serious problems than caring for a healthy infant.

Researchers have found several key factors pivotal to parents who have adopted children with special needs. For example, in a study of 1,343 foster children who were adopted, reported in *After Adoption: The Needs of Adopted Youth*, the researchers found that the major risk factor in predicting a behavioral problem was the prenatal substance abuse by the birthmother, and because of this, the parents wished they had been given more information. (See PRENATAL EXPOSURES.)

The researchers also found that the major problem area for the children was their school functioning: 40 percent of the children had been placed in special classes in school. According to the information provided by the parents, a large number of the children had problems with paying attention and distractibility.

Note that the broad majority of adoptive parents in this study were happy that they had adopted their children, and 93 percent said that, knowing what they now knew about the child, they would definitely or probably adopt again. Also note that most of the children (92 percent) were reported in good or excellent health.

In another study that looked at the self-reported feelings of their parents' preparedness to adopt, researchers questioned 368 parents who adopted children with special needs from the foster care system. The children were an average age of 5.4 years at the time of adoption. The results were reported in a 2004 issue of *Child and Adolescent Social Work*. Researchers Susan C. Egbert and Elizabeth C. La-Mont found that such factors as the child's ability to attach to the parents and the parents' relationship with the agency were important factors.

The researchers also found that low levels of self-perceived preparedness were associated with particular factors in the children, such as the child

having experienced many foster placements before the adoption, as well as known physical, sexual, or emotional abuse or neglect that occurred prior to the adoption.

According to the researchers, among the parents who self-rated themselves as less prepared to adopt, several made such a comment as:

"We were told they were children who did not have many problems. We found out that we faced attachment disorder, sexual abuse, children who had been taught to fight and shoplift. We were in no way prepared for that."

In contrast, parents who said that they were well-prepared made such comments as, "After having the girls for a year and working with the doctors, we knew what we were getting ourselves into. We have no regrets," and, "I think what prepared us the most was that we had adopted before. [With] Our first adoption, we were totally unprepared for the problems of abuse even after hearing some stories from other parents."

Said the researchers, "Adopted children's ability to attach to their adoptive parents emerged in this study as the most significant factor in predicting whether or not adoptive parents felt prepared for their adoption experience. Problems with attachment were associated with children's abuse and neglect histories, along with their current emotional and behavioral problems. While attachment is an issue related to the child and is beyond the direct control of the parent, adoptive parents indicated that they often were uninformed about the realities of their child's background. This lack of information contributed to a lack of preparation for the severity of the behaviors that occurred after placement."

Some experts say that college-educated individuals may have a more difficult time in parenting children with special needs because of their ingrained high expectations that children could have trouble achieving, while other studies indicate that educated parents have a good level of success.

What seems to be most important in the successful parenting of children with special needs from the foster care system are parents who are flexible and who expect and accept that their children may have some problems because of their background of abuse or neglect. If there are two

PROPORTION OF ADOPTED CHILDREN MEETING SPECIAL NEEDS CRITERIA
(DOMESTIC ADOPTIONS), BY STATE, FY 2001

State	Total Percentage with Special Needs	Ages 0 to 5 Percentage with Special Needs	Ages 6 to 12 Percentage with Special Needs	Ages 13 to 17 Percentage with Special Needs
Alabama	46.8	42.7	51.4	46.2
Alaska	100.0	100.0	100.0	100.0
Arizona	83.2	75.3	90.5	93.8
Arkansas	96.1	95.5	98.1	91.5
California	97.6	96.6	98.8	99.2
Colorado*	61.7	50.7	81.0	92.9
Connecticut	0.0	0.0	0.0	0.0
Delaware	97.4	96.8	97.9	100.0
District of Columbia	97.8	91.8	100.0	100.0
Florida	96.0	94.7	97.3	98.0
Georgia	48.2	43.6	50.2	59.8
Hawaii	94.6	94.8	96.6	81.3
Idaho	91.9	89.6	97.6	86.7
Illinois	98.0	95.1	100.0	100.0
Indiana*	75.5	62.5	82.6	90.9
Iowa	56.8	39.7	71.7	69.6
Kansas	74.2	69.3	74.3	88.5
Kentucky	51.7	46.9	53.4	59.5
Louisiana	80.0	69.7	82.9	100.0
Maine	43.8	45.5	46.6	25.6
Maryland	98.0	95.5	100.0	100.0
Massachusetts	99.0	99.5	99.1	95.0
Michigan	83.7	81.1	86.4	82.5
Minnesota*	82.4	66.7	91.4	90.9
Mississippi	82.2	59.5	98.3	100.0
Missouri	80.3	76.3	83.9	85.5
Montana	84.0	64.2	100.0	100.0
Nebraska	92.5	89.1	93.8	100.0
Nevada	96.3	96.0	96.3	100.0
New Hampshire	100.0	100.0	100.0	100.0
New Jersey	89.8	88.5	91.9	88.0
New Mexico	95.4	92.9	97.4	94.3
New York	95.8	91.6	98.0	98.6
North Carolina	93.2	91.8	94.4	95.6
North Dakota	69.7	49.4	100.0	100.0
Ohio	99.9	99.8	100.0	99.5
Oklahoma	95.5	90.8	98.4	100.0
Oregon	98.9	99.0	98.7	98.7
Pennsylvania	55.1	58.0	53.2	51.8
Rhode Island	46.1	38.3	55.6	57.9
South Carolina	92.5	90.8	92.9	97.8
South Dakota	100.0	100.0	100.0	100.0
Tennessee	80.9	56.6	93.8	100.0
Texas	90.3	83.6	99.6	100.0
Utah	94.3	93.5	95.6	94.1

(continues)

	Total	Ages 0 to 5	Ages 6 to 12	Ages 13 to 17
	(Table continued)			
State	Percentage with Special Needs	Percentage with Special Needs	Percentage with Special Needs	Percentage with Special Needs
Vermont	100.0	100.0	100.0	100.0
Virginia	65.3	50.8	74.4	78.6
Washington	70.8	71.8	69.7	67.3
West Virginia	100.0	100.0	100.0	100.0
Wisconsin	94.8	91.1	98.5	100.0
Wyoming	91.3	85.7	96.3	80.0
Puerto Rico	27.0	12.9	36.4	60.0
Total	87.6	84.5	90.5	90.6

*These states had missing or invalid special needs data for more than 30 percent of their cases.
Source: Adapted from Office of the Assistant Secretary for Planning and Evaluation, *Understanding Adoption Subsidies: An Analysis of AFCARS Data.* U.S. Department of Health and Human Services, Washington, D.C., 2005.

adopting parents, it is also important that both are active in parenting roles.

Social workers say that adoptive parent groups can be very helpful to families who adopt children with special needs, although it may be difficult to find an appropriate group.

Children with Disabilities, Delays, or Diseases

Some children with special needs suffer from permanent or temporary disabilities, for example, the child may have cerebral palsy or a clubfoot. If the birthmother was a drug or alcohol abuser, her child may have been affected in utero. A baby or child born to a mother with acquired immunodeficiency syndrome (AIDS) and who tests HIV-positive at birth is definitely considered a child with special needs. (See HUMAN IMMUNODEFICIENCY VIRUS.)

Some social workers consider the background of the birthmother in evaluating a child as having potential special needs, but if the pregnant woman abused alcohol or drugs during her pregnancy, the caseworker may wait until the child is born before making a determination on whether the baby will be categorized as having special needs or not.

In other cases, if the birthmother or birthfather or their parents were known to have schizophrenia or other severe psychiatric illnesses or were alcoholics, criminals, drug addicts, or abusers, or they exhibited other diseases or maladaptive syndromes, the social worker may automatically categorize the child as one with special needs, based on suspected GENETIC PREDISPOSITIONS.

Siblings

Children with special needs may be healthy physically and mentally, but if they belong to a sibling group, this is considered a special need. (See SIBLINGS.) Most social workers strive to keep siblings together, believing that the trauma they experienced in separating from their birthparents could be unbearably complicated if they are forced to separate from each other. However, if siblings are sexually or physically abusive with each other, this guideline is relaxed, and siblings are separated.

Many children with special needs are siblings, and consequently, a 10-year-old female and her 12-year-old brother would usually be categorized as having special needs because they are siblings as well as because they are over age eight. (Children over age six or eight are considered to have special needs by many states; others raise the age level to age 10 or older, depending on the difficulty in placing the children.)

Preadolescents and Teenagers

Children around the ages of 10–12 years and teenagers are the most difficult categories of children to place with an adoptive family, yet often a suitable family can be found, and many social workers are very successful at finding good homes for adolescents. For example, in 2001, children aged 13–17 represented about 9 percent of all the children adopted from foster care. (See table.)

Older children often remember their biological parents and may initially resent being adopted. In fact, in some states children older than 12 or a similar age may refuse to be adopted. Even if they agree to be adopted, sometimes older children may exhibit reclusive behavior or may be unusually clingy with the adoptive parents. They may shun affection or demand it. They will often exhibit behavior considered inappropriate for their age, either too childlike or too adult.

The adoptions of older children are considered a greater risk than the adoptions of infants. Studies have revealed, however, that older children who are adopted can adapt very successfully to their new homes. Studies have also found a strong correlation between large families and successful placements.

According to psychologist David Brodzinsky et al. in the book *Children's Adjustment to Adoption: Developmental and Clinical Issues,* there are key areas that are important to the outcome of the adoption of a child with special needs. One key issue, according to the authors, is "integrating the child into the family; forming attachments and supporting the grief process; maintaining realistic expectations regarding child behavior and family functioning; managing troublesome child behavior; and utilizing supports and social services."

For example, in the area of "integrating the child into the family," Brodzinsky and his colleagues say that parents can ease the way for the child by taking into account their previous routines and adapting them for the new family. Identifying and concentrating on the similarities between family members and the child is another good way to help the child become an integral family member.

Behavioral Problems

The child's own behavior, for example, precocious sexual behavior, aggressive or abusive behavior, chronic bedwetting, or other actions that would require a great deal of understanding and adjustment on the part of adoptive parents, could categorize the child as one with special needs. Some children with severe attention deficit/hyperactivity disorder may be considered to have special needs. Children who have serious psychiatric problems are also considered to have special needs.

Experts report that children who have experienced previous sexual abuse are the most challenging for adoptive parents, largely because they have learned inappropriate behaviors that confuse and embarrass the parents if they are not prepared in advance by the agency.

Foster Children and Developmental Delays

Children who are developmentally delayed may or may not "catch up," depending on the specific situation, such as the child's age, intelligence level, and so forth. Social workers should provide as much information as possible to adopting parents; however, social workers and physicians cannot always predict how a child will respond and whether or not a child's behavior will significantly change. In addition, very often social workers do not have access to information about the child.

African-American and Biracial Children

Black and biracial infants and children who need adoptive families are considered to have special needs even when they are physically normal and of a normal intelligence. Unfortunately, ethnicity alone is often a sufficient criterion to categorize these children as having a "special need." Race becomes a double-edged issue in this case because the policies of nearly every state seem to be saying, by virtue of inclusion in this category of "special needs," that being nonwhite makes a child less appealing to prospective adoptive parents, and the equivalent of a child born with severe physical and mental problems. This policy seems to some experts to reflect the worst sort of racism.

For demographic and other reasons, and despite more than a generation of active efforts to recruit minority adoptive applicants, there are apparently still not enough black families aware of the need for parents for many black and biracial children. It is also true that African-American children are disproportionately represented in foster care. For example, although African-American children represent about 15 percent of all children, they account for about 47 percent of all children in foster care who need adoptive families.

As a result, many African-American children remain in foster homes until they "age out" in adulthood. Some social workers have strongly suggested that adoptive recruitment efforts in black communities have been woefully inadequate, and they hypothesize instead that greater numbers of

CHARACTERISTICS OF CHILDREN ADOPTED FROM FOSTER CARE, FY 1999–2001

	1999		2000		2001	
	Number	Percent	Number	Percent	Number	Percent
Number of adopted children	46,391		50,472		50,703	
Gender						
Female	23,236	50.1	25,250	50.0	25,192	49.7
Male	23,149	49.9	25,216	50.0	25,501	50.3
Age at adoption						
Under age 1	833	1.8	921	1.8	1,018	2.0
1–5 years	20,951	45.2	22,974	45.5	23,397	46.2
6–8 years	10,969	23.6	11,383	22.6	10,864	21.4
9–12 years	9,698	20.9	10,729	21.3	10,705	21.1
13–17 years	3,940	8.5	4,465	8.9	4,719	9.3
Race						
White	20,620	44.5	24,941	49.4	27,320	54.3
African-American	19,576	42.2	20,588	40.8	19,226	38.3
American Indian/Alaskan Native	553	1.2	926	1.8	1,177	2.4
Asian/Pacific Islander	477	1.0	602	1.2	658	1.3
Unknown	5,165	11.1	4,386	8.7	4,004	8.0
Ethnicity						
Hispanic	6,552	14.2	7,184	14.2	8,253	16.3
Non-Hispanic	39,755	85.9	43,287	85.8	42,450	83.7

Source: Adapted from Office of the Assistant Secretary for Planning and Evaluation, *Understanding Adoption Subsidies: An Analysis of AFCARS Data.* U.S. Department of Health and Human Services, Washington, D.C., 2005, page 3-2.

black families would be interested in adoption if they had information on the need and the children. Other black social workers say the problem is not recruitment efforts, the race of staff, or inappropriate requirements. They believe there are simply too many children and not enough African-American families.

Many social workers do not wish to place children in TRANSRACIAL ADOPTIONS; however, increasing numbers of adoption agencies and even state agencies are beginning to make these types of placements, especially in the face of the MULTIETHNIC PLACEMENT ACT. Transracial adoption is a hotly disputed topic in the field of social work today, and some families have sued agencies for violating their civil rights by refusing to allow them to adopt across racial or nationality lines.

Children with Special Needs from Other Countries

Children adopted through international adoption agencies or private sources may also have medical or mental problems and be classified as children with special needs by a private adoption agency. Some experts deem nearly all children adopted from other countries as having special needs, due to their complicated backgrounds, unknown medical histories, and difficult early lives.

A child with ailments readily correctable in the United States may be considered a child with special needs. A child needing corrective surgery would also be considered to have special needs; for example, a child with a clubfoot or a cleft palate. If the child remained in the foreign land, this condition might never be corrected, yet the birth defect might be relatively simple for U.S. doctors to correct. The preadoptive medical records of children with physical special needs are usually more detailed than those provided for children without these problems. In addition, it is often possible to obtain additional medical reports or tests to clarify the condition of the child prior to adoption. Moreover, the cost of adopting children with physical challenges and specific medical needs is sometimes reduced by the adoption agency.

A child from overseas might have minor problems that are readily resolved, such as lice or scabies, or might suffer from chronic diarrhea or other medical problems, but these problems would usually not be considered to give the child a categorization as a child with special needs because they are regarded as temporary and correctable.

Children adopted from other countries may also be categorized as children with special needs for the same reasons as U.S. children are so labeled: over age six to eight years old, member of a sibling group, mixed-race child, and so on. However, they are generally not eligible for an ADOPTION SUBSIDY, nor are they eligible for the tax credit that is automatically available in the United States for children with special needs adopted from the foster care system regardless of the expenses incurred. However, families who adopt children from other countries and who pay adoption fees are eligible for tax credits. In contrast, when children are adopted from the foster care system, where there are no fees, the tax credit is specifically allowed. Congress made this provision as an inducement and a reward to individuals adopting children with special needs from the foster care system.

See also ATTACHMENT DISORDER; DOWN SYNDROME; EARLY INTERVENTION; FOSTER CARE; INCOME TAX LAW BENEFITS; MEDICAL PROBLEMS OF INTERNATIONALLY ADOPTED CHILDREN; PSYCHIATRIC PROBLEMS OF ADOPTED PERSONS; SUPPORT GROUPS.

Barth, Richard, and Marianne Berry. *Adoption and Disruption: Rates, Risks and Responses.* New York: Aldine de Gruyter, 1988.
Brodzinsky, David M., et al. *Children's Adjustment to Adoption: Developmental and Clinical Issues.* Thousand Oaks, Calif.: Sage Publications, 1998.
Egbert, Susan C., and Elizabeth LaMont. "Factors Contributing to Parents' Preparation for Special-Needs Adoption," *Child and Adolescent Social Work Journal* 21, no. 6 (2004): 593–609.
Howard, Jeanne A., and Susan Livingston Smith. *After Adoption: The Needs of Adopted Youth.* Washington, D.C.: CWLA Press, 2003.
Nelson, Katherine A. *On the Frontier of Adoption: A Study of Special-Needs Adoptive Families.* Washington, D.C.: Child Welfare League of America, 1985.
Office of the Assistant Secretary for Planning and Evaluation. *Understanding Adoption Subsidies: An Analysis of AFCARS Data.* U.S. Department of Health and Human Services, Washington, D.C., 2005.

Stanley v. Illinois   See BIRTHFATHER.

state laws   See LAWS, STATE.

state social services department   The public welfare agency responsible for children in foster care and also responsible for finding adoptive parents for waiting children. Each state has a central social service department that oversees various local or county divisions. Generally, the headquarters of the state social services department is in the state capitol.

It should also be noted that the state social service department's recommendations for changes to adoption law are considered very important by legislators.

See also PROTECTIVE SERVICES.

statistics on adopted children   Quantitative data, usually on children under age 18 who have been adopted from the United States or other countries. For many years, there has been a dearth of statistical data on children adopted in the United States, in part because the federal government had stopped collecting this information and also in part because the confidentiality that is present in many adoptions makes data collection difficult. It is also true that amassing statistical data can be expensive. However, the exact number of international adoptions by U.S. citizens is known because of the visa applications that are processed by the federal government. (See INTERNATIONAL ADOPTION and CANADA AND ADOPTION.)

However, in recent years, statistical data, especially about children adopted from the foster care system, has become available because funds have been allocated due to increased interest at the federal level. In addition, the U.S. Census Bureau and the National Adoption Information Clearinghouse have both provided statistical data on all adopted children.

According to the National Adoption Information Clearinghouse, there were 127,407 children adopted by parents in the United States in 2001, the most recent data as of this writing. (See Table I for state by state adoption statistics.) This statistic does not include children adopted from other countries.

Among all children younger than age 18 in the United States, 1,586,004 were adopted, according to

TABLE I: TOTAL ADOPTIONS OF CHILDREN IN 2001

State	Total
Alabama	1,857
Alaska	616
Arizona	1,642
Arkansas	1,698
California	9,202
Colorado	2,877
Connecticut	1,164
Delaware	225
District of Columbia	548
Florida	8,435
Georgia	3,499
Hawaii	766
Idaho	1,048
Illinois	6,673
Indiana	3,588
Iowa	1,116
Kansas	1,880
Kentucky	2,086
Louisiana	1,391
Maine	957
Maryland	4,384
Massachusetts	3,259
Michigan	6,274
Minnesota	2,094
Mississippi	866
Missouri	2,554
Montana	600
Nebraska	939
Nevada	764
New Hampshire	630
New Jersey	2,384
New Mexico	680
New York	10,209
North Carolina	2,328
North Dakota	368
Ohio	5,564
Oklahoma	1,533
Oregon	2,029
Pennsylvania	4,748
Rhode Island	617
South Carolina	1,648
South Dakota	399
Tennessee	2,633
Texas	7,957
Utah	1,387
Vermont	407
Virginia	2,301
Washington	2,748

State	Total
West Virginia	908
Wisconsin	2,515
Wyoming	412
Total	127,407

Source: Adapted from U.S. Department of Health and Human Services. *How Many Children Were Adopted in 2000 and 2001?* Washington, D.C., National Adoption Information Clearinghouse, 2004.

the Census Bureau (or 2.5 percent of all children). The Census Bureau also estimated that there were about 473,000 adopted adults ages 18 and older in the United States in 2000 living with the householder. Thus, there are more than two million adopted individuals in the United States, based on the census data. (See Table IV.) Note that many adopted adults have established their own households, and thus they were not included.

Nationwide in the United States, about 40 percent of the adoptions that occurred in 2001 were managed by private adoption agencies, independent adoptions, or kinship (adoptions by relatives) or tribal adoptions. Stepparent adoptions represented about 42 percent of all kinship adoptions.

An estimated 39 percent of all adoptions in 2001 were public adoptions, or adoptions of children from the FOSTER-CARE system, more than double from the 18 percent in 1992 of children adopted from foster care before the passage of the ADOPTION AND SAFE FAMILIES ACT in 1997. (See Table II.)

Looking at all minor adopted children The U.S. Census Bureau looked at the total number of adopted minor children of all ages in 2000, compared to the total number of children. As can be seen from Table III, some states, such as Alaska (3.9 percent of the total children were adopted), Montana (3.2 percent), and Oregon (3.1 percent), had the highest percentages of adopted children of all states in the United States.

See also ADOPTION SUBSIDY; EMPLOYMENT BENEFITS; INCOME TAX LAW BENEFITS; SPECIAL NEEDS; TERMINATION OF PARENTAL RIGHTS.

Kreider, Rose. "Adopted Children and Stepchildren: 2000," *Census 2000 Special Reports*, U.S. Census Bureau, October 2003.

TABLE II: PUBLIC AGENCY ADOPTIONS AS A PERCENTAGE OF TOTAL ADOPTIONS OCCURRING IN 2001

State	AFCARS*	Percentage of Public Adoptions
Alabama	237	13
Alaska	278	45
Arizona	931	57
Arkansas	353	21
Colorado	607	21
Connecticut	444	38
Delaware	117	52
District of Columbia	177	32
Florida	1,466	17
Hawaii	244	32
Idaho	110	10
Illinois	4,079	61
Indiana	871	24
Iowa	661	59
Kansas	416	15
Kentucky	546	26
Louisiana	463	33
Maryland	806	18
Massachusetts	778	24
Michigan	2,979	47
Minnesota	567	27
Mississippi	265	31
Missouri	1,061	42
Montana	264	44
Nebraska	283	30
Nevada	243	32
New Hampshire	94	15
New Jersey	1,030	43
New Mexico	369	54
New York	3,934	39
North Carolina	1,222	52
North Dakota	127	35
Ohio	2,002	36
Oklahoma	938	61
Oregon	1,071	53
Pennsylvania	1,668	35
Rhode Island	267	43
South Carolina	384	23
South Dakota	92	23
Tennessee	555	21
Texas	2,319	29
Utah	349	25
Vermont	98	24
Virginia	490	21
Washington	1,153	42
West Virginia	360	40
Wisconsin	693	28
Wyoming	46	11

*AFCARS stands for Adoption and Foster Care Analysis Reporting System, which is data collected from all states on the numbers of foster children who are adopted.

Source: Adapted from U.S. Department of Health and Human Services. *How Many Children Were Adopted in 2000 and 2001?* Washington, D.C., National Adoption Information Clearinghouse, 2004.

TABLE III: NUMBER OF ALL CHILDREN AND PERCENT OF ADOPTED CHILDREN, UNDER AGE 18, STATE BY STATE, 2000

	Total Number of All Children under Age 18	Number of Adopted Children under Age 18	Percent of Adopted Children of Total Children
United States	64,651,959	1,586,004	2.5
Alabama	995,282	24,944	2.5
Alaska	175,315	6,910	3.9
Arizona	1,197,953	28,966	2.4
Arkansas	604,462	15,973	2.6
California	8,027,573	167,190	2.1
Colorado	1,006,573	29,438	2.9
Connecticut	775,214	19,239	2.5
Delaware	172,427	3,452	2.0
District of Columbia	87,890	2,649	3.0
Florida	3,204,362	82,179	2.6
Georgia	1,903,475	49,194	2.6
Hawaii	238,287	6,941	2.9
Idaho	344,494	9,562	2.8
Illinois	2,886,152	73,638	2.6
Indiana	1,441,338	37,004	2.6
Iowa	688,589	18,569	2.7
Kansas	662,249	19,733	3.0
Kentucky	906,933	20,661	2.3
Louisiana	1,051,564	22,827	2.2
Maine	280,763	7,137	2.5
Maryland	1,197,553	32,269	2.7
Massachusetts	1,383,945	35,647	2.6
Michigan	2,356,202	61,232	2.6
Minnesota	1,215,739	31,378	2.6
Mississippi	660,190	16,300	2.5
Missouri	1,300,281	33,156	2.5
Montana	212,401	6,803	3.2
Nebraska	421,429	11,812	2.8
Nevada	452,493	10,588	2.3
New Hampshire	290,564	6,864	2.4
New Jersey	1,881,428	42,614	2.3
New Mexico	447,024	11,764	2.6
New York	4,153,245	100,736	2.4
North Carolina	1,753,973	42,911	2.4
North Dakota	152,943	3,647	2.4
Ohio	2,643,807	62,653	2.4
Oklahoma	798,929	23,518	2.9
Oregon	770,173	23,901	3.1
Pennsylvania	2,659,562	62,328	2.3
Rhode Island	229,017	5,496	2.4
South Carolina	881,583	22,027	2.5
South Dakota	186,772	5,691	3.0
Tennessee	1,244,838	30,980	2.5
Texas	5,178,912	110,275	2.1
Utah	664,965	19,430	2.9
Vermont	139,324	4,181	3.0

(continues)

TABLE III (Continued)

	Total Number of All Children under Age 18	Number of Adopted Children under Age 18	Percent of Adopted Children of Total Children
Virginia	1,567,983	38,289	2.4
Washington	1,392,445	38,879	2.8
West Virginia	365,657	9,849	2.7
Wisconsin	1,278,901	30,583	2.4
Wyoming	118,786	3,997	3.4
Puerto Rico	937,408	10,696	1.1

Source: Kreider, Rose. "Adopted Children and Stepchildren: 2000," *Census 2000 Special Reports,* U.S. Census Bureau, October 2003, page 4.

Office of the Assistant Secretary for Planning and Evaluation. *Understanding Adoption Subsidies: An Analysis of AFCARS Data.* U.S. Department of Health and Human Services, Washington, D.C., 2005.

U.S. Department of Health and Human Services. *How Many Children Were Adopted in 2000 and 2001?* Washington, D.C., National Adoption Information Clearinghouse, 2004.

stepparent adoptions At least half of all the finalized adoptions that occur each year are adoptions by stepparents and relatives, although the number of stepparent adoptions is unknown. When stepparents adopt their spouse's children, a HOME STUDY may not be required, depending on state laws.

There has been a surprising lack of research performed on stepparent adoptions despite the increasing numbers of stepparent relationships.

A 1987 study of 55 stepparents who had adopted their stepchildren indicated three primary reasons for the adoption. These were to change the name of the child, or a result of the adopted child's positive relationship with the stepparent, or a desire for stability.

subsidies See ADOPTION SUBSIDY.

substance abuse Excessive use of alcohol and/or illegal drugs or prescribed drugs. Substance abuse may lead to child abuse. Substance abuse during pregnancy is dangerous and may be fatal to the developing fetus. It may also cause serious birth defects or long-term neurodevelopmental disabilities. It is recommended that pregnant women avoid all alcohol and illegal drugs during pregnancy and take only medications approved by their obstetricians.

See also PRENATAL EXPOSURES.

success rates The other side of the coin to rates of DISRUPTION or adoption failures. The overwhelming number of adoptions are successful, particularly placements of infants.

The adoption of children with SPECIAL NEEDS is successful in the majority of cases as well.

TABLE IV: NUMBER OF CHILDREN OF HOUSEHOLDER BY TYPE OF RELATIONSHIP AND AGE: 2000

Relationship	Total, All Ages	Under Age 18					18 Years+		
		Total	Under Age 6	6 to 11	12 to 14	15 to 17	Total	18 to 24	25 and Older
Total children of householder	83,714,107	64,651,959	20,120,106	22,803,985	11,200,237	10,527,631	19,062,148	11,185,934	7,876,214
Adopted children	2,058,915	1,586,004	389,296	598,326	316,636	281,746	472,911	273,957	198,954
Stepchildren	4,384,581	3,292,301	328,378	1,271,122	847,130	845,671	1,092,280	778,441	313,839
Biological children	77,270,611	59,773,654	19,402,432	20,934,537	10,036,471	9,400,214	17,496,957	10,133,536	7,363,421
Percent of age group	100.0	100.0	100.0	100.0	100.0	100.0	100.0	100.0	100.0
Adopted children	2.5	2.5	1.9	2.6	2.8	2.7	2.5	2.4	2.5
Stepchildren	5.2	5.1	1.6	5.6	7.6	8.0	5.7	7.0	4.0
Biological children	92.3	92.5	96.4	91.8	89.6	89.3	91.8	90.6	93.5

Source: Kreider, Rose. "Adopted Children and Stepchildren: 2000," *Census 2000 Special Reports,* U.S. Census Bureau, October 2003, page 2.

According to a 1988 article in *Child Welfare* by Joan Ferry DiGiulio, one important criterion agencies should consider in selecting adoptive parents, because it does affect the success of an adoption, is the ability of the adopting parents to accept the child as a separate person. In addition, DiGiulio hypothesizes that a prospective adoptive parent's own self-acceptance is an important criterion in determining whether or not the parent can recognize the child's separateness. She further hypothesized that the higher the score of an adoptive parent on a self-acceptance scale, the correspondingly higher the score on a parental acceptance of child scale.

Researchers administered the tests to 80 couples who had adopted children under age three and whose children averaged nine years at the time of the study.

The conclusion: "The study discovered that high self-acceptance of adoptive parents influenced high parental acceptance of the child."

The author concluded, "The importance of self-acceptance of adoptive parents can be stressed in the training of adoption professionals, who might then be more aware of the existence or absence of this trait in potential adoptive families."

DiGiulio, Joan Ferry. "Self-Acceptance: A Factor in the Adoption Process," *Child Welfare* 67 (September–October 1988): 423–429.

support groups Groups formed to help others with a similar interest or problem; also called mutual aid groups. There are adoptive parent support groups, adopted adult support groups, and birthparent support groups. It is impossible to determine the exact number of support groups nationally, but virtually every state in the United States has at least one ongoing and active group.

A few of the support groups are nonprofit organizations that number their membership in the thousands or hundreds, but most are made up of a handful of individuals who come together to form their group.

Adoptive Parent Groups

Some adoptive parent groups concentrate on the adoption of children with special needs, others are oriented more toward intercountry adoption or infant adoption, and still others attempt to cover all ages and types of adoption. Some organizations concentrate on children adopted from particular countries, such as China or Russia.

Adoptive parent groups can be extremely helpful as information providers to prospective adoptive parents. People who have already adopted can advise them on agencies, attorneys, and such issues as what a home study is really like and can also allay many of their fears about adoption.

The average person considering adoption has no idea where to turn for information, and usually friends and relatives are equally uninformed or baffled by the subject. As a result, support groups fill critical information voids.

After the adoption has taken place, other adoptive parents can provide advice and information to assist new adoptive parents through adjustment problems they may face.

Some groups are very aware of adoption issues and current federal and state legislation on adoption and keep their members informed on the latest adoption current events.

Actual lobbying of their state and federal legislators on adoption issues is another goal of some support groups, and groups have succeeded in convincing legislators at every level to pass a broad array of bills supporting adoption.

Most adoptive parent groups maintain a regular contact with their local adoption agencies and attorneys and build up a camaraderie between social workers and adopting parents. Groups invite social workers and attorneys to speak at meetings, and many plan an annual informational meeting when a variety of child-placing experts attend and explain their policies and the guidelines to follow in applying for a child.

Another goal of many adoptive parent support groups is to assist adoption agencies in recruiting adoptive parents for children with SPECIAL NEEDS. Some also raise money to buy food and clothing for overseas orphanages and Christmas presents for foster children, and they perform other charitable activities.

Groups that concentrate on the adoption of children with special needs or larger groups that attempt to encompass all forms of adoption may assist local social services departments; for example, some groups will drive foster children who are legally ready to be adopted to a photographer to have their pictures taken for the state's PHOTOLIST-

INGS of WAITING CHILDREN. Others actually VIDEO-TAPE waiting children, and tapes are shown to prospective parents.

Support Groups for Adopted Adults or Birthparents

Support groups composed primarily of adopted adults or birthparents are also interested in legislation, and some actively lobby for OPEN RECORDS. Members generally are interested in doing a SEARCH for an adopted adult or birthparents or have already accomplished such a search and wish to share this information with others. They may desire the moral support and camaraderie of people who share a common bond of adoption.

Adopted adults may wish to have a voice in lobbying state and federal legislators on a variety of adoption issues.

Reasons for Joining Support Groups

People who are in the process of adopting primarily join an adoptive parent group to learn and to obtain information and moral support. They often feel very anxious about identifying a good agency or attorney.

If they are in the midst of their HOME STUDY, they may be concerned about whether or not they will ever "pass" the home study and be able to successfully adopt a child. Other members who have successfully adopted build their confidence and hope.

The relatives of an adopting family may be very nonsupportive and urge them to drop the idea of adoption altogether; consequently, the support group serves as a kind of family.

Members who already have adopted may join a support group because they want to adopt more children via a different method than they previously used; for example, they may wish to adopt through an agency although their first child came to them through an INDEPENDENT ADOPTION. Or they may wish to adopt internationally after already adopting an American-born child.

Some members join because they believe in adoption as a positive concept, and they wish to help others. They may also wish for their children to have the chance to meet and socialize with others who were adopted.

Support groups can be a good resource for adopted children, giving them an opportunity to meet other adopted children. This is especially important for families who have adopted children from other cultures, although all children can gain reassurance from learning that adoption is a good way to form a family. In addition, support groups can provide information on adoption issues, thus helping both adoptive families and their children.

Most parent groups produce a monthly, bimonthly, or quarterly newsletter offering information on children newly adopted by members and articles written by adoptive parents or adoption experts. The newsletter serves to inform and also to reinforce the importance of adoption to its members.

To locate the nearest adoptive parent support group, individuals should contact their state adoption office. Adopted adults should also contact their state social services office or adoption agency as well as national organizations, such as the American Adoption Congress or Adoptees' Liberty Movement Association. Birthparents may wish to contact the state social services office and local agencies as well as national organizations, such as Concerned United Birthparents.

A Healthy Skepticism Is a Good Idea

Whether the group is for adoptive parents, adopted adults, or birthparents, members and visitors should keep in mind that group members' information and opinions may not be based on research or expert advice. Instead, the advice from support group leaders or other members may be based on a negative or positive experience that they generalize to all adopted people or to all adoptive parents. Thus, members should retain a healthy skepticism about information that does not sound authoritative or accurate. Individuals should be sure that they seek legal advice from attorneys and professional advice on adoption from experienced social workers.

surrender Refers to the voluntary act of TERMINATION OF PARENTAL RIGHTS to an agency or a court. Once the parental rights of a person are officially transferred to either an agency, attorney, or other intermediary as allowed by state law, the child may be placed into an adoptive family within the limits of state laws.

This term has fallen out of favor with adoption advocates, who believe it has a negative connotation.

Some adoption critics, however, purposely use the word to stress a negative message, for example, "I surrendered a child to adoption" rather than "I planned adoption" or the more neutral, "1 placed a child for adoption."

surrogacy arrangements The practice of hiring a fertile woman who agrees to become impregnated, usually with sperm from the intended father and using her own egg to create the pregnancy. The surrogate agrees ahead of time to transfer the child after birth to the infant's biological father and his wife, according to terms of a contract that was signed before the woman becomes pregnant. Some experts refer to this practice as "contractual parenting." In some cases, the surrogate is a *gestational surrogate*, which means that a donated egg, either from the intended mother or from an anonymous donor, has been used, and the surrogate has no genetic link to the fetus that she carries to term.

The sperm and the egg both come from anonymous donors. In this case, none of the parties involved in the contractual arrangement have a genetic link to the child.

Most surrogate mothers are women who are married or living with their partners. They have usually already borne children, and they often still have children in the home. They are generally working-class women, and nearly all are white.

Most intended parents who use surrogates earn in excess of $100,000 per year, probably because only more affluent individuals can afford the fees that are involved, including surrogate fees, clinic fees, physician fees, attorney fees, and so forth. Note that adoption expenses may be eligible for an income tax credit or exclusion; however, this benefit is not available to the intended parents in surrogate parenting arrangements or stepparent adoptions, according to the Internal Revenue Service.

The late Michigan attorney Noel Keane developed the first contracts for surrogacy in 1976, and by 1988 Keane had purportedly arranged 302 births from surrogates. Keane also handled the first embryo transfer surrogacy, wherein a woman carried the genetic child of another woman and man. That child, implanted by Dr. Wolf Utian of the Mt. Sinai Medical Center in Cleveland, was delivered in 1986. Some evidence indicates that Dr. Utian did not realize the mother was a paid surrogate.

According to attorney Brette McWhorter Sember in her book *The Complete Adoption & Fertility Legal Guide*, it is illegal to pay a surrogate in some states, including Michigan, New Mexico, New York, Utah, and Washington. She says that surrogacy contracts are not illegal, but they are unenforceable in some states, including the District of Columbia, Indiana, Louisiana, Nebraska, New York (where unpaid agreements may be made, but not paid ones), North Dakota, and Virginia. Some states, however, recognize the validity of surrogacy agreements, including Arkansas, Florida, New Hampshire, Nevada, Tennessee, Texas, Washington (where surrogates may not be paid), and West Virginia.

McWhorter Sember says surrogacy agreements are important, and they are also usually complicated contracts. She says, "The most important feature of a surrogacy agreement is that it revokes all rights and responsibilities the surrogate and her husband have to the child. The intended parents are the legal parents to the child."

Anyone intending to enter into a surrogacy contract should be sure to work with an attorney who is experienced in such contracts. If a surrogacy clinic offers their own contract, it may be advisable for the intended parents to seek their own legal advice to ensure that their best interests are protected.

Multiple Births

In some cases, surrogate mothers have had multiple births; for example, in one extremely unusual case in 2005, a woman gave birth to quintuplet boys that were placed with the intended parents. In several cases, the surrogate has been found to be carrying twins, and the intended parents only wanted one child. In at least one case like this, the surrogate successfully prevailed in court to retain custody of the twins.

Surrogacy v. Adoption

There are many differences between surrogacy and adoption; however, the primary difference is that in nonrelative adoptions, neither parent is biologically related to the child, nor have the prospective parents contracted with a woman in advance to create a pregnancy. Instead, actions to adopt did not commence until after the child was conceived.

With surrogacy, the pregnancy was created only because of an agreement that was made ahead of time so that the intended parents would have a child.

However, adoption does play a role in most surrogacy cases. If one of the individuals is a biological parent, usually the other partner must adopt from the surrogate mother, as in a stepparent adoption although state laws vary.

Motivations of Intended Couples Who Use Surrogates

Many infertile couples who choose surrogacy say that they do not wish to adopt because they seek a "genetic link" to their child, even if it is with only one of them (usually the intended father). It also appears that these couples may seek more control than any adoption agency would allow. For example, some surrogacy contracts stipulate that the surrogate mother may not smoke, drink alcohol, or engage in other behaviors of which the intended parents disapprove. Such stipulations cannot be made to a pregnant woman who is considering placing her baby for adoption, although it is hoped that she acts in a healthy manner during her pregnancy.

Psychological Issues

There are some key psychological issues related to surrogacy that must be overcome by both the intended parents and the surrogate. Psychologists Janice C. Ciccarelli and Linda J. Beckman in their 2005 article in the *Journal of Social Issues* say that the relationship between the surrogate mother and the intended mother creates a situation of cognitive dissonance, wherein both are supportive of motherhood and yet both are also violating cultural norms. (Cognitive dissonance refers to the difficulty involved with believing two seemingly opposing concepts at the same time. This requires a further rationalization.) In addition, the intended father often feels awkward when he is the genetic father of a child created with a woman who is not his wife, yet she is the biological mother of his child (and his wife is agreeable to this), another form of cognitive dissonance.

The psychologists say that couples may resolve this dissonance in two ways. First, the man's role may be de-emphasized, and the pregnancy and birth is then relegated to a concern for women.

Second, the biological link is also downplayed. Say the authors, "The intended mother often justifies the lack of genetic ties to the child through development of a mythic conception of the child that emphasizes her intentionality in the process (it is her desire that ultimately brings the child into being) . . . Moreover, she develops a relationship with the surrogate mother and experiences pregnancy by proxy (e.g., attending Lamaze classes, being present in the delivery room, going to medical appointments)."

Motivations of Surrogate Mothers

Although most people assume that the primary or sole motivation of surrogate mothers is to receive money, Ciccarelli and Beckman say this is untrue. Instead, say the authors, "The women have empathy for childless couples and want to help others experience the great joy of parenthood. Also, some want to take a special action and, thereby, gain a sense of achievement . . . or enhance their self-esteem."

The researchers also state that her relationship to the intended parents is pivotal to the surrogate mother, who forms a relationship with the couple rather than with the developing child. The relationship with the intended mother is especially important to many surrogates.

The authors also state that when the surrogate mother is given the opportunity to see and hold the newborn baby, she is more likely to feel respected and valued, and thus her satisfaction level with the experience will be high.

Surrogacy Fees

The fees that a surrogate may receive vary according to state laws and the arrangement made by the intended parents with the surrogate. Fees to the surrogate may be about $20,000. Surrogates who are related to the intended parents usually charge no fee. For example, sometimes sisters of the intended parents, other relatives, or one of their own mothers is willing to serve as a surrogate. Of course the intended parents must also pay medical and legal fees as well.

If the surrogate does not become pregnant, she usually receives nothing. If the surrogate becomes pregnant but miscarries, she may receive a partial payment, depending upon the agreement. Some unrelated surrogates take little or no money; for example, in 2005 the surrogate mother who bore quintuplets announced she was forgoing her fee so that the couple could use the money for the babies.

Attitudes of Others

Although the surrogate's husband or partner is usually supportive about the pregnancy and about the surrogate's intentions to place her child with the intended parents after the birth, the extended family may be opposed to the surrogacy arrangement, and some surrogate mothers have been shunned by disapproving relatives and friends. Some research indicates that less than a third of the extended family support the surrogate's decision.

As well, the intended couple may also face disapproval from their extended family and others, although some others, specifically infertile women, are more likely to be supportive of the couple, perhaps identifying with the couple's need to have a child.

Surrogacy Lawsuits

Numerous lawsuits have been filed in surrogacy cases, involving many diverse issues. In some cases, the intended parents have prevailed, while in others, the surrogate has prevailed. The most famous and the first lawsuit on a surrogacy issue was the "Baby M" case between surrogate mother Mary Beth Whitehead and the people to whom she originally arranged to give her baby, William and Elizabeth Stern. This case, *In the Matter of Baby M,* was resolved in 1988.

In this case, the Sterns hired Mary Beth Whitehead to be a surrogate mother. Mr. Stern's sperm and Ms. Whitehead's egg were used, thus Ms. Whitehead was the genetic mother. After Ms. Whitehead bore the child, she changed her mind about giving the baby to the Sterns and asked for the child. She was given the child, and she disappeared with the baby to Florida. Private detectives for the Sterns found Ms. Whitehead, and she was returned to New Jersey.

A lower court awarded custody of the child to the Sterns and made Mrs. Stern an adoptive mother. However, the New Jersey Supreme Court overturned the adoption in May 1988 but left custody of the child with the Sterns. Whitehead, the surrogate mother, was allowed visitation rights.

According to attorney John K. Ciccarelli and psychologist Janice C. Ciccarelli in their article in 2005 in the *Journal of Social Issues,* when the surrogate is both genetically connected to the child as well as actually carrying the pregnancy, "the courts have had little trouble reaching the conclusion that she is the legal mother of the child. Therefore, the logical extension of this conclusion is that she is in an analogous position to a birth mother in a traditional adoption." As a result, since a pregnant woman considering adoption can change her mind about the adoption after the child's birth, in most cases, so may a surrogate mother who has a genetic link to the child.

Advocates of Surrogacy

Supporters of surrogacy believe it is unfair for the government to interfere with individuals on private matters, and some argue that surrogacy and procreation should not be restricted in any way. They also argue that even if surrogacy were completely banned, individuals would still arrange such contracts, albeit illegally.

In addition, supporters of surrogacy believe that if a person strongly desires a genetic link to his child and a fertile woman agrees to bear the child, then the surrogacy should proceed. They believe that the surrogate mother is well-compensated for her services, and thus they see the situation as a "win-win" experience for both sides.

Arguments against Surrogacy

Critics of surrogacy sometimes argue that rich people are buying babies from poor women, and if the hourly rate were computed as a wage, the woman earns far less than the minimum wage. She also experiences the discomforts and the risks of pregnancy.

Traditional religious groups oppose surrogacy because they believe it is not in concert with the traditional role of a mother.

Feminists appear to be split on this issue. Some feminists believe that wealthy individuals misuse working-class people by hiring surrogates to bear them children. Other feminists believe surrogacy should *not* be banned because they believe that a woman has a right to use her body for childbearing for others, and they also fear that a ban on surrogacy could mean an ultimate return to a ban on abortions.

Ciccarelli, Janice C., and Linda J. Beckman. "Navigating Rough Waters: An Overview of Psychological Aspects of Surrogacy," *Journal of Social Issues* 61, no. 1 (2005): 21–43.

Ciccarelli, John K., and Janice C. Ciccarelli. "The Legal Aspects of Parental Rights in Assisted Reproductive Technology," *Journal of Social Issues* 61, no. 1 (2005): 127–137.

Keane, Noel, and Dennis L. Breo. *The Surrogate Mother.* New York: Everest House, 1981.

McWhorter Sember, Brette. *The Complete Adoption & Fertility Legal Guide.* Naperville, Ill.: Sphinx Publishing, 2004.

syphilis A disease that is caused by the *Treponema pallidum* bacterium. Most cases of syphilis are sexually transmitted. Babies can contract the disease from their pregnant mothers, either before or during birth. Routine screening for syphilis is standard for women in the United States and Canada during pregnancy. Test results should be verified in mothers of children placed for adoption or, preferably, the newborn is tested. All children adopted from countries outside the United States and Canada should be tested for syphilis as a precaution. In addition, children who have been or may have been sexually abused or who have had consensual sex with others should also be tested. Syphilis is not a common disease in infants and children, but in those who contract it, the disease can have devastating long-term consequences if it is not identified and untreated.

Cases of children born with syphilis contracted through the mother (congenital syphilis) are rare in the United States. There were 441 cases in 2001 in the United States, reflecting a steady decline from a high of 2,416 cases of congenital syphilis in 1960.

Most children adopted from other countries are tested for syphilis before arrival in the United States, but some cases of untreated congenital syphilis infections are found each year. In general, children from China and Central American countries are at greatest risk. About 15 percent of children adopted from Russia and countries that comprised the former Soviet Union have been treated for congenital syphilis prior to adoptive placement.

Symptoms and Diagnostic Path

From one-half to two-thirds of newborns infected with syphilis have no symptoms. Babies may have failure to thrive and hepatitis or enlarged liver. They may also have skin rashes.

Children who were younger than three months of age at the time of adoption should be screened for syphilis upon arrival and again between 10 and 12 weeks of age. When syphilis is present in the first two years of life, the child may have an enlarged liver and/or pancreatitis. They may also have abnormal X-rays, as with about 90 percent of children who are symptomatic and about 20 percent who are asymptomatic. They may have seizure disorders, hydrocephalus, mental retardation, and other neurological abnormalities, such as abnormal cerebrospinal fluid. An elevated serum alkaline phosphatase level may sometimes indicate the presence of syphilis.

Some older children and even some small children who are adopted have contracted syphilis due to sexual abuse they have suffered. If sexual abuse is known or suspected, the child should be screened for syphilis. One primary symptom of syphilis in an older child (not an infant or toddler) is a sore (chancre) in the genital area or in the mouth. Other symptoms may include fever, sore throat, and joint pain.

There are several stages of syphilis, including primary syphilis, secondary syphilis, latent syphilis, and tertiary syphilis. If untreated, the disease will progress. (These stages do not relate to babies with congenital syphilis.)

With primary syphilis, the typical chancre sore appears within two to six weeks. It is typically located in the infected person's vagina, penis, or vulva. The chancre may also appear on other parts of the body such as the tongue or lips.

With secondary syphilis, the patient experiences a rash of brown sores, each about the size of one penny. The rash often occurs from about three to six weeks from when the chancre first appeared. The rash may be body-wide or it may be localized, but it is nearly always present on the soles of the feet and palms of the hand.

Some patients have latent syphilis, in which the disease is not active, nor is the patient infectious to others. However, about a third of patients with secondary syphilis will become sicker and develop the complications of tertiary or late-stage syphilis. In this stage, the bacteria damages the brain, nervous system, bones, heart, eyes, joints, and other parts of the body. Late-stage syphilis can cause mental illness, blindness, and death. Coinfections with other sexually transmitted diseases, including the human immunodeficiency virus, hepatitis B, and hepatitis C, may occur in individuals with syphilis.

Tests for syphilis include the Venereal Disease Research Laboratory (VDRL) microscopic slide test or the rapid plasma reagin (RPR). A positive finding on either test is then confirmed with highly specific tests, such as fluorescent treponemal antibody absorption and microagglutination-*T. pallidum*.

Treatment Options and Outlook

When detected in the early stages, syphilis is easily treated with antibiotics, usually given as intramuscular or intravenous injections. Children with congenital syphilis should also receive eye examinations performed by an ophthalmologist, as well as hearing tests performed by a specialist, because syphilis can damage the eyes and ears. Dental evaluation is indicated because even treated syphilis can lead to dental malformations. Children diagnosed with congenital syphilis should also be screened for developmental and neurological abnormalities, although they do not appear to be common.

Risk Factors and Preventive Measures

Mothers who were recently infected with syphilis and are untreated have the highest risk of passing on syphilis to their fetus, about 70–100 percent.

The best way to avoid syphilis is to not have sex or to have sex with few partners. Since children who were sexually abused and contracted syphilis or who were born to mothers with syphilis had no choice, they could not take measures to prevent contracting the disease.

See also MEDICAL PROBLEMS OF INTERNATIONALLY ADOPTED CHILDREN; SEXUALLY TRANSMITTED DISEASES.

Miller, Laurie C., M.D. *The Handbook of International Adoption Medicine: A Guide for Physicians, Parents, and Providers.* New York: Oxford University Press, 2005.

Miller, Laurie C. "International Adoption: Infectious Diseases Issues," *Clinical Infectious Diseases* 40 (2005): 286–293.

teachers and adopted children The relationship of private and public school educators to the children they teach is often a very important one for adopted and nonadopted children. Some adoptive parents feel teachers, as part of society, may be biased for or against adopted children and recommend teachers not be told children are adopted unless absolutely necessary. They also resist filling in any "adopted" information block on a form for school registration, because they do not want the child to be singled out, in either a positive or negative way.

Others disagree, particularly when older children are adopted. They believe a teacher needs to understand if a child has had problems in the past. Of course, if the child is of another race than the parents, the adoptive status is usually readily apparent.

Some people say that adoptive parents can "practice" while their child is in preschool by talking to teachers about adoption and perceiving how they react. Parents can also bring or donate children's books about adoption to the child care center, such as *Tell Me Again About the Night I Was Born*, by Jamie Lee Curtis. Researchers and authors Ruth G. McRoy and Louis A. Zurcher Jr. reported that sometimes teachers bend over backward to be overly nice to transracially adopted children. Said the authors,

"Overenthusiastic acceptance of the black child into the classroom has been characterized as discriminatory by some transracial adoptive parents. In such instances, the teacher has reduced performance demands for the black child while keeping those standards high for the white child. This behavior is likely to occur in situations in which the teacher has had very little, if any, experience teaching black students."

Psychologist Janet Hoopes believes adopted children may exhibit behavioral problems in school. She based her opinion on teacher ratings.

"In the course of my longitudinal research on adopted children, it became apparent to me that although adopted children, compared to a matched sample of biological children, did not manifest significantly more emotional problems or identity problems, they did manifest some subtle problems in school according to teacher ratings." (Hoopes did not think teachers were biased in their ratings.)

Studying 100 adopted children aged 10 to 15 and comparing them to biological children, she found no significant differences in IQ, personality, or achievement. The one significant area of difference was in the ratings by teachers. Her findings: "The adopted child did not quite measure up to the comparison child, or, in other words, was not doing as well in school as might be expected on the basis of ability."

Early parental expectations were also negatively related to the child's later performance in school. "These findings clearly suggest that unduly high expectations of adoptive couples for the intellectual endowment of the adopted child are associated with later negative attitudes toward school (as rated by teachers) on the part of the adoptive child."

On the plus side, Hoopes found adopted children were accepted by peers. In addition, the rates of children referred for special class (learning-disabled) placement was similar to that of the non-adopted population, respectively about 10 percent versus 10–14 percent.

Hoopes also discussed the societal bias against adoption. "Reflecting upon the attitude of the general public toward adoption, one 15 1/2 year old boy in my recent study with Stein . . . on identity in the adopted adolescent poignantly stated, 'It's not adoption that is the problem, but what other people think of adopted kids. They're always shown in movies as "the druggie." ' "

Although adopted children may be treated more forgivingly, such leniency is still unequal, an aspect children quickly pick up on. Dr. Hoopes said adoptive parents' expectations might be too high, and perhaps in some cases, teachers' expectations of adopted children are too low.

There is also the issue of positive bias among teachers; for example, many expect every Asian-born child to excel at math and science, based on stereotypical attitudes often presented in the U.S. media.

It is clear more research needs to be conducted on this issue to determine if there are other factors that may affect teachers' perceptions of adopted children.

It is also important to note that many segments of society have evinced biases toward adopted children, and teachers are by no means unique if they are indeed biased. In addition, it is highly likely that as society becomes more understanding and accepting of adoption, so will teachers and other categories of professionals.

When Children Are "Late Adopted": Advice to Teachers

Some experts have provided specific advice to teachers on working with adopted children. In her essay, "Helping Late Adopted Children Make It in the Classroom," therapist Anna M. Jernberg, Ph.D., offered guidelines directed toward teachers of adopted children or foster children. For example, she recommended that a child be moved back in grades in accordance with the level of his or her emotional maturity. She also urged teachers to be sensitive rather than blaming toward adoptive or foster parents and realize that sometimes late-adopted children take out their anger and frustration on their new parents. Jernberg cautioned teachers to set limits on a child but in a positive and nurturing way.

Jernberg, Anna M. "Helping Late Adopted Children Make It in the Classroom," newsletter, Council on Adoptable Children, Knoxville, Tenn., January/February 1999.

Hoopes, Janet L. "Psychologist Sees Adopted Children at Risk for Learning Disabilities," *Hilltop Spectrum,* Hill Top Preparatory School, Rosemont, Pa., June 1986, 1–4.

McRoy, Ruth G., Louis A. Zurcher Jr. *Transracial and Inracial Adoptees: The Adolescent Years.* Springfield, Ill.: Thomas, 1983.

teenage adopted persons   See ADOLESCENT ADOPTED PERSONS.

teenagers, adopted   See ADOLESCENT ADOPTED PERSONS.

termination of parental rights   The ending of all the rights and obligations of a parent, usually a biological parent, in most cases with the goal that other individual(s) will adopt the child. Some terminations are made as a result of the willing and voluntary consent to an adoption, given by the birthparents. In other cases, the parents' rights are involuntarily terminated by the court, often because of abuse and neglect and after the child has been in foster care for an extended period. In the case of abandoned infants, however, the court may terminate parental rights more quickly than with older children.

It should also be noted that although many children who are adopted from other countries were abandoned by their birthparents, in some cases, the children were removed by the government because they were physically or sexually abused and/or neglected prior to placement in an orphanage. Sometimes this information is not known prior to adoptive placement.

Voluntary Terminations of Parental Rights

The overwhelming majority of adoptions require the voluntary or involuntary termination of the biological parental rights before the adoptive parents may formally and legally adopt a child. In some unusual cases, a child may be adopted without either a voluntary or involuntary termination of the parental rights of the biological parents, such as with a second parent adoption. In this case, the parent does not give up parental rights, and another person is also given parental rights as well. Second parent adoptions are usually (but not always) performed in a gay or lesbian relationship.

If the birthparents are deceased and their relatives have custody of the child, then the relatives may provide voluntary consent to an adoption, or, in some cases, a court may terminate custodial legal rights at the request of the relatives.

Most birthparents who voluntarily make an adoption plan for their children do so when their children are infants or toddlers; however, some parents feel compelled to take this voluntary action when the child is older. If the child has been in foster care for many years, the social worker may ask the parents if they wish to transfer parental rights willingly so that the child may be adopted.

Involuntary Terminations of Parental Rights

Sometimes children are legally separated from their parents when the parental rights are involuntarily terminated. This action is not taken lightly and usually only occurs after it has been proven to the court's satisfaction that the parents are unable and/or unwilling to assume a proper parental role. Parents who have been physically or sexual abusive, neglectful, drug-addicted, or alcoholic may lose custody of their children permanently in a termination of parental rights, after the children have been in foster care. Parents who are mentally ill or who are incarcerated for felonies may also have their parental rights terminated.

Courts understandably take the genetic ties of the children to the biological parents very seriously, and judges insist (or should insist) on strong supporting evidence before terminating any parental rights. At least one court hearing (and usually several hearings) will precede any involuntary termination of parental rights.

The ADOPTION AND SAFE FAMILIES ACT (ASFA) provides additional guidelines for when parental rights should be terminated involuntarily. Many states have changed their laws in response to ASFA, and some states have set other specific circumstances under which termination of parental rights must be initiated. (See Appendix V.)

Concerns over Terminations

Some experts worry that terminations of parental rights may occur too quickly because of ASFA and the child protective services system. Attorney Paul Chill, in his article for *Family Court Review,* argues that once children are removed from a home in an emergency proceeding, even if the removal was unwarranted, often the inexorable outcome is a termination of parental rights. Chill writes:

"Once a child is removed, a variety of factors converge to make it very difficult for parents to ever get the child back. One court has referred to this as the 'snowball effect.' The very focus of court proceedings changes—from whether the child should be removed to whether he or she should be returned. As a practical matter, the parents must now demonstrate their fitness to have the child reunited with them, rather than the state having to demonstrate the need for out-of-home placement. By seizing physical control of the child, the state tilts the very playing field of the litigation. The burden of proof shifts, in effect, if not in law, from state to the parents."

Chill argues that judges may agree to the initial child removal, fearful of past cases in which judges have not removed a child and then the child died. In addition, in many cases, the accused parents either have no legal representation or they have court-appointed lawyers who have very little time to review the case and assist them.

Some natural outcomes of the child's removal may also work against the parent. For example, says Chill, "A parent's suspicious or hostile attitude toward caseworkers may be construed as evidence of clinically significant paranoia. A parent's disclosure to a court-appointed psychologist or psychiatrist that she is experiencing depression, hopelessness, anxiety, or grief from being separated from her child may become the basis for retaining custody of the child until treatment succeeds in alleviating those symptoms."

Chill argues that emergency removal causes severe trauma to children, who may develop psychiatric illnesses that were not present beforehand. He also says that states should not remove children from families in an emergency manner unless the child is in imminent risk of serious physical injury or death.

Grounds for Termination of Parental Rights

Each state has its own laws regarding grounds for termination of parental rights. For example, some states specifically state that if the child was conceived as a result of rape, then the rapist father has no parental rights.

The Adoption and Safe Families Act requires state agencies to seek terminations when *either* of the two following conditions has been met:

- A child has been in foster care for 15 of the most recent 22 months.
- A court has determined that either:
- A child is an abandoned infant.
- The parent has committed murder or voluntary manslaughter of another child, or the parent or aided, abetted, attempted, conspired, or solicited to commit a murder of manslaughter of a child of the parent, or the parent has committed a felony assault that resulted in serious bodily injury to the child or another child of the parent.

There are also exceptions to the ASFA requirements to terminate parental rights, in some circumstances. (Some state laws include these circumstances and some do not.) These circumstances may include

- When the child has been placed in the care of a relative
- If there is a compelling reason to believe that terminating the parent's rights is not in the best interests of the child
- If the parent has not been provided with services required in the plan for reunification of the parent with the child.

Rehabilitation of Abusive Parents: It Does Not Always Work

One problem is the common view among some social workers that child abuse is a temporary stepping over the line. Unfortunately, there are a few parents who repeatedly abuse their children, and treatment by social workers, psychologists, and others will not change their behavior.

The image of the abusing parent as one who periodically loses his or her temper does not explain such cases as parents ritualistically torturing their children—binding, gagging, and beating them and performing other actions with premeditation. In addition, not all parents who harm or neglect their children do so for reasons of poverty or for reasons that social workers could help them to resolve.

Author David P. H. Jones contends that some families are "untreatable" and says factors particularly indicative of poor outcome to treatment are

"parental history of severe childhood abuse, persistent denial of abusive behavior, refusal to accept help, severe personality disorder, mental handicap complicated by personality disorder, parental psychosis with delusions involving the child and alcohol/drug abuse."

In addition, says Jones, "Severe forms of abuse (fractures, burns, scalds, premeditated infliction of pain, vaginal intercourse or sexual sadism) are more likely to prove untreatable."

Jones adds, "The idea that some families do not respond appears to be anathema to some practitioners and researchers alike. Yet the reality for those who work in the field of child abuse is that some families cannot be treated or rehabilitated sufficiently to offer a safe enough environment in which children can live."

See also ABANDONMENT; ABUSE; PARENTAL RIGHTS; REUNIFICATION.

Chill, Paul. "Burden of Proof Begone: The Pernicious Effect of Emergency Removal in Child Protective Proceedings," *Family Court Review* 41, no. 4 (October 2003): 457–470.

Jones, David P. H. "The Untreatable Family," *Child Abuse and Neglect,* 11 (1987): 409–420.

therapy and therapists As increasing numbers of children with SPECIAL NEEDS are adopted, it is likely there will be a need for adopted children and their families to receive some ongoing assistance and, in some cases, therapy. In addition, some number of adopted persons who were adopted at birth or an early age will also need counseling, although the estimated percentages of adopted adults needing counseling is open to wide dispute.

Because therapists are susceptible to hearing and believing the same prejudices and myths as the layperson, it is crucial that adoptive parents and adopted persons identify a therapist who does not presume adoption is the sole reason or the preeminent reason for an adopted person to experience emotional difficulties. Nor should the therapist automatically presume the adoptive family is the primary cause of the child's problem.

It is also important that a therapist be knowledgeable and sensitive to the unique issues that adoption does have for the child and the parents. To say that adoption plays no role is often just as damaging as it is to say it is the sole reason for a child and parents to have difficulties.

According to Marian Sandmaier, author of *When Love Is Not Enough,* therapists are particularly suspicious of adoptive parents who have adopted children with special needs, presuming that a healthy family would not wish to take on the "burden" of such a child. As a result, the therapist may instead presume that the adopting family is masochistic or has a desperate desire to be needed. Social workers strive mightily to screen out any individuals with such motives, and in fact most adoptive parents are motivated by a sincere love for children and a desire to share their love. Unless a therapist enters into a therapeutic relationship with a positive orientation toward the parents, time and energy will be wasted trying to find the hypothetical "causes" of the problems rather than focusing on the solutions.

It is also important to note that the family situation has greatly deteriorated by the time the family seeks out a counselor, and the family may be very discouraged. Often they have received little or no support from extended family members. Sandmaier says the family's urgent first need is support and validation that problems exist but there may well be a way to work them out.

In some cases, a therapist inexperienced with adoption may unfairly presume that the child's problems have been caused by the adoptive family when, in fact, the child entered the family with problems that occurred before he or she ever met family members. The family may have extended heroic efforts to help the child and a blaming attitude will confuse them and will only exacerbate the problem. The parents need to be respected for being part of the solution and not be blamed for being the cause of the problem. It is also possible that the family is contributing to the child's problems, for example, overreacting to negative behavior that may be common to a child at a certain developmental stage.

How does a parent know if and when a child needs therapy? This is a difficult question to answer because much depends on the child's age, behavior, and many other factors. There are, however, some basic guidelines to consider.

For example, if the child's overall academic performance has deteriorated, and teachers are expressing concern about the child, this is one indicator of a possible need for counseling. In addition, if the child's relationships with peers have changed, for example, the child no longer wishes to see friends or share activities with friends (or if the child has no friends), this is another indicator of a potential problem.

One of the best indicators of a child's healthy adjustment is to observe the spontaneity and frequency of a child's smile and laughter. If a child looks and acts depressed, a professional evaluation is recommended.

Finally, if the child has gained or lost a great deal of weight, the basis for weight change may be physical or psychological, and both possibilities should be explored.

As a result, the child should see a physician to rule out medical problems and subsequently see a qualified psychologist or social worker to determine any psychological problems. An ethical therapist will reassure parents if the child's behavior is essentially "normal."

If the school-age child is behaving in a secretive reclusive manner, in contrast to earlier behavior, or is hearing imaginary voices or hallucinating, the parents should seek professional help immediately. In addition, if the child is expressing suicidal thoughts, such ideas must be taken seriously.

Information on the birthparents' personality traits is a valuable source of information in understanding and accepting a child's development, and medical and psychological experts will request such information. (For example, was there a history of depression, emotional illness, or other problems in the birthfamily.) *Note:* Just because a birthparent may have had such a problem does not necessarily mean the child has inherited a predisposition to mental illness.

An effective therapist can help family members work through the pain of separation and loss, for example, the loss of birthparents and foster parents faced by the child or the loss of fertility still felt by the adoptive family. The therapist might need to help the child overcome the anguish and confusion resulting from physical or sexual abuse or help the parents deal with their frustration at being unable to reach the goal of being perfect parents.

In addition, siblings who were already in the family will need to receive counseling as the jockeying for position occurs and the relative BIRTH ORDER among family members changes and evolves. Unfortunately, some counselors choose to exclude siblings and address only the adopted child or the adopted child and adoptive parents together, despite strong evidence that the bonds of siblings can be very intense.

Another important aspect of brief therapy sessions is to find exceptions to the problem—when negative behavior (such as bedwetting) does not occur, when a child is not hostile—to get away from the presumption that the behavior always happens and cannot be rectified. One problem that adoptive parents face in finding a good therapist for their child (should the child need therapy) is that some therapists will assume the underlying problem is an "adoption issue." Adoption may or may not be part of the problem the child faces.

See also PSYCHIATRIC PROBLEMS OF ADOPTED PERSONS; SIBLINGS.

Sandmaier, Marian, and Family Service of Burlington County, Mt. Holly, N.J. *When Love Is Not Enough: How Mental Health Professionals Can Help Special-Needs Adoptive Families.* Washington, D.C.: Child Welfare League of America, 1988.

transracial adoption Generally refers to the adoption of African-American or biracial children by white adoptive families, although the term *transracial adoption* properly refers to any adoption across racial or ethnic lines, including what are probably the most frequent transracial adoptions in the United States—adoptions of Asian children from other countries by white parents in the United States. Transracial adoptions also include most adoptions from Guatemala (usually Latino children adopted by white parents), South Asia, and the small but increasing number of adoptions from Ethiopia. (See INTERNATIONAL ADOPTION.) However, because of the overwhelming emphasis on transracial adoption as a term that concentrates on the adoption of African Americans by Caucasians, most of this entry is devoted to such adoptions.

It is unknown how many adoptions nationwide in the United States are transracial adoptions, but about 15 percent of adoptions, through public agencies (foster care) were transracial adoptions in 2001, up from 11 percent in 1995. This does not include adoptions arranged by private adoption agencies or attorneys, nor does it include international adoptions.

It should however, be noted that the INDIAN CHILD WELFARE ACT OF 1978 restricts the transracial adoption of Native American children. However, if the tribe agrees to such an adoption, it may then occur. Problems arise when birthparents refuse to divulge their Native American ancestry. If there is any suspicion that birthparents may be Native American, they should be asked directly if they are Native American, so that the provisions of the Indian Child Welfare Act may be observed.

Sometimes transracial adoption involves the foster care system in the United States. African-American and biracial children in foster care who need adoptive families are considered children with SPECIAL NEEDS by most professionals in the adoption field for the simple reason that it is difficult to recruit sufficient numbers of adoptive parents willing to consider such children. In addition, adoption agencies outside the foster care system usually have difficulty finding sufficient numbers of families to adopt biracial or African-American children.

Many social workers and other experts believe that a family of the same race is the best family for a child to grow up in despite federal laws prohibiting choosing an African-American adoptive family ahead of a white family to adopt an African-American child. (See MULTIETHNIC PLACEMENT ACT.) Because African-American children in foster care (and with private adoption agencies) usually wait longer than white children for an adoptive family, many experts believe that it is permanency, rather than racial matching, that should be the paramount consideration in adoption. As a result, they believe that when an African-American family is not available for a child, then adoptive parents of another race should be considered. Still others believe in complete "color blindness," or that no consideration at all should be given to race when considering who may adopt an African-American child.

Background of Transracial Adoption

Initially considered a liberal and positive act in the late 1960s and early 1970s, adoptions of black children by white parents plummeted after the National Association of Black Social Workers issued a strong position against transracial adoption in 1972, comparing it to racial genocide.

In the past, some lawsuits were filed by white foster parents wishing to adopt their African-American foster children, but who were denied this opportunity by the state social services department because of their race. In the current environment, foster parents are generally given first preference to adopt their foster children, regardless of their race.

In general, courts have decreed that race should not be a determining factor in deciding who shall have custody of children; for example, *Palmore v. Sidot* (1984) was a U.S. Supreme Court case that disallowed racial considerations. In this case, a white father tried to take custody of their child away from his ex-wife, who lived with her black boyfriend in a black neighborhood. The mother prevailed.

Recruitment of Black Adoptive Parents

Some people have concluded that African Americans are not interested in formal adoptions or that they adopt at a much lower rate than whites. Census Bureau data reveals this is not valid, but African Americans would need to dramatically increase their rate of adoption to "absorb" all the WAITING CHILDREN who need families, because blacks are so heavily overrepresented in the foster care system. On the other hand, some opponents of transracial adoption allege that there are plenty of African-American families available to adopt but they are dissuaded by heavy-handed and racially biased criteria, a claim that may be valid but is not backed up by research.

Some black social workers insist that the active recruitment of African-American adoptive parents is inadequate, and that white social workers impose standards or criteria that are used for whites on black prospective parents in terms of age, marital status, family income, education, and other criteria; consequently many blacks are ineligible to adopt because they do not fit these criteria.

These critics argue that, in contrast, there are abundant African-American infants, toddlers, and older children needing adoptive families, and thus, age, marital status, and income criteria for black prospective adoptive parents should be reexamined.

In their book *Adoption across Borders,* a book about transracial and international adoption, Simon and Altstein discussed reasons for the discrepancy between the numbers of African-American children needing families amid insufficient numbers of approved African-American families.

Said the authors, "First of all, blacks have not adopted in the expected numbers because child welfare agencies have not actively recruited in black communities, using community resources, the black media, and churches. Secondly, there is a historic suspicion of public agencies among many blacks, the consequence of which is that many restrict their involvement with them. Third, many blacks feel that, no matter how close they come to fulfilling the criteria established for adoption, the fact they reside in less-affluent areas makes it unlikely that they would be approved."

Organizations including One Church, One Child, founded in 1981 by Rev. George Clements, a black Catholic priest who was also the adoptive parent of four children, were created to recruit qualified black adoptive parents. These organizations have successfully recruited numerous, although not enough, black parents. Dr. Clements's model was that one member of each church could adopt at least one child and be supported in this choice by the rest of the congregation.

Many states have created their own modeled programs based on One Church, One Child. The national office for One Church, One Child is located at 805 King Street, Suite 400, Alexandria, VA 22314; (703) 548-9790.

Arguments in Favor of Transracial Adoption

Supporters of transracial adoption state that virtually all studies show that children adopted by individuals of another race—most specifically, African-American children adopted by white parents—function well in society, and most are emotionally healthy compared to their peers. In the overwhelming majority of cases, the children are aware of their racial heritage, and they have a positive self-esteem and a good outlook for the future.

This may be largely because the parents who adopt transracially are usually more aware of the challenges that lie ahead as well as the potential for discrimination, although some parents are still apparently surprised when their children suffer from discriminatory remarks or treatment.

Arguments against Transracial Adoption

One argument against transracial adoption is that African Americans are supplying healthy black children to childless white couples. In addition, fears for the children themselves include the idea that the child will feel different and unaccepted when reared in a largely (or solely) white neighborhood. It is also feared that the child will be unable to relate to members of the African-American community, identifying instead with whites.

Racial Identity

A major issue with regard to transracial adoption is that of racial identity and the concern that a white family cannot give an African-American child an appropriate sense of racial identity. The argument is that the child will feel inferior, alienated, and different from other members of the same race and will suffer from low self-esteem. Studies have not borne this view out, yet many social workers continue to oppose transracial adoption.

As Simon, Altstein, and Melli reported in their article, ". . . we found that, both during adolescence *and later as adults* [emphasis added] the TRAS [transracially adopted individuals] were aware of and comfortable with their racial identity."

In a test measuring racial identity, children in both race-matched adoptive families (black children in black families) and transracial families were tested at age four and again at eight to determine if they felt a positive sense of their racial identity. Researchers Joan F. Shireman and Penny R. Johnson used the "Clark Doll Test" to determine the level of racial identity in transracially adopted children.

The preschool transracially adopted children showed a marked positive identification as black: 71 percent of them identified as African American compared to 53 percent of the race-matched adopted preschoolers. By age eight, the groups were virtually identical. Researchers concluded that racial identity was constant for the transracial

group and a later development for the race-matched group.

Because the majority of transracial adopters lived in primarily Caucasian neighborhoods, the researchers speculated on whether or not racial identity would remain the same or might change as the transracially adopted children grew older and into adolescence.

Longitudinal studies have provided the best vindication for transracial adoption. Simon, Altstein, and Melli are not the only researchers to find good adjustments among transracially adopted children. Writing in the *Albany Law Review* about adoption research published by the Search Institute, Barbara McLaughlin noted that, "in one recent study of transracial adoptees, children placed in families of a different race in most of the emotional indicators scored similar to or higher than children of racial adoptions. On a host of measures, African-American and Asian children adopted across racial lines do as well and often better than non-adopted peers."

In another study of 51 adults who had been transracially adopted and were aged 19 to 36, reported in the *Journal of Social Distress and the Homeless* in 2002, researcher Amanda Baden considered whether the adopted adults differed in terms of their knowledge of and comfort with culture of their racial group compared to the culture of their adoptive parents. These adults were adopted from birth to 144 months of age, with an average of 22 months at the time of adoption. Baden also looked at several other issues, such as the psychological adjustment among transracially adopted adults in terms of their own perceptions of their racial and cultural identity.

Baden found broad differences among the adopted adults, with no consistent cultural or racial self-definitions. She also found that psychological adjustment was unrelated to cultural or racial identity, and that adopted adults who identified more with their parents' race were at the same level of psychological adjustment as adopted adults who reported feeling more comfortable with individuals of their own racial group.

Said Baden, "The findings of this study can also greatly inform the view of transracial adoption among opponents of and proponents to transracial adoption, First, because heterogeneity exists among transracial adopters and because a particular way or ways of identifying [by race] was not associated with better or worse psychological adjustment, neither proponents nor opponents can purport a 'best way' to identify as a transracial adoptee. Second, racial differences between parents and adoptees have been targeted as the primary source of potential problems in transracial adoption. This expectation can be problematic because many other factors (e.g., parenting, reasons for adopting, hardiness, ego strength, and trauma) have been virtually forgotten and their impact has yet to be examined with respect to transracial adoptees. Although these other factors continue to deserve empirical and theoretical attention, they often do not."

Adolescence Can Be Difficult for Transracially Adopted Teens

When there are problems related to transracial adoption, they are most likely to appear in adolescence. According to findings from the Minnesota Transracial Adoption Study, reported in a 2004 issue of *Adoption Quarterly,* adopted adolescents of all races had higher rates of school problems, behavioral problems, general health problems, and delinquency. For example, in the category of school problems, the white biological children of the families had a rate of 9 percent, compared to 22 percent among white adopted adolescents, 26 percent for biracial/multiracial adopted adolescents, and 26 percent among African-American adopted adolescents. The adoptive parents were white.

Behavioral problems occurred in adolescence at different rates depending on the child's adoptive status. For example, the biological children had a rate of 20 percent in adolescence, compared to 33 percent for the white adoptees, 45 percent for the biracial/multiracial adoptees, and 67 percent for the African-American adoptees. General health problems occurred in 9 percent of the biological children, compared to 17 percent of the white adoptees, 22 percent of the biracial/multiracial adoptees, and 25 percent of the African-American adoptees.

Finally, delinquency in adolescence occurred in 4 percent of the biological children, compared to 22 percent of the white adoptees, 31 percent of the biracial/multiracial adoptees, and 29 percent of the African-American adoptees.

As can be seen from this data, there were fewer differences between the types of adopted adolescents than between adopted adolescents in general versus children born to the family. It will be interesting to see if, at a later date, these differences diminish during adulthood.

Research Studies

In their 1990–1991 study, discussed in *Adoption across Borders,* researchers Simon and Altstein asked the parents of the now-adult transracially adopted children (which included 86 children who were African American adopted transracially as well as 17 children of other races adopted transracially), if knowing what they knew now, they would have still adopted a child of another race.

Ninety-two percent said "yes," 4 percent were unsure, and 4 percent said "no." Of the three families who said "no," two said that the child had preexisting physical or emotional problems that they did not know about when the child was adopted, and the other family said it was "not a successful experience." When the parents were asked if they would recommend that other white families adopt a child of another race, 80 percent said "yes," 17 percent were unsure, and 3 percent said "no."

The researchers also located some of the transracially adopted adults from their long-term study, and they surveyed 41 African Americans who had been adopted transracially, 14 of other races adopted transracially (mostly Korean adopted adults), and also 13 white adopted adults and 30 white birth children. The median age for the transracially adopted adults was 22 years, while the white adoptees' median age was 25 and the birth children's was 26 years.

They asked the adults to describe their relationships with their parents in adolescence and in adulthood. All of the adopted children showed significant improvements in their relationships with their parents in adulthood. For example, to the question "How would you describe your relationship with your adopted mother during adolescence and at the present time?" Twenty-nine percent of the transracially adopted adults said they were very close to their mothers during adolescence, but at present, 46 percent said they were very close. In addition, 15 percent described their relationship as "very distant" in adolescence, but only 2 percent used this descriptor in adulthood.

Among the adopted white adults, none chose "very close" for their relationship with their mother during adolescence, while in adulthood 62 percent made that choice. Among this group, 23 percent described their relationship as "quite distant" in adolescence, and this percentage remained the same in adulthood.

Similar results were found with respect to their relationships with their adoptive fathers. For example, among the transracially adopted adults, 31 percent said they were very close in adolescence, and that percentage increased to 44 percent in adulthood. In response to those who described their relationship with their father as "quite distant," 15 percent reported this was true in adolescence but this percentage declined to 4 percent in adulthood.

William Feigelman reported on his study on the adjustments of transracially adopted children compared to "inracially" (same race) adopted children in *Child and Adolescent Social Work* in 2000 based on information provided by adoptive parents.

He compared adopted young adults, including 37 whites, 151 Asians, 33 African Americans, and 19 Latinos. Feigelman found that some groups experienced more discrimination than others. For example, more than half (53 percent) of the parents of African-American adults said their children had been discriminated against sometimes or often, compared to Asian adopted children (32 percent) and Latino adopted children (11 percent).

Feigelman also found that parents who lived in predominantly white neighborhoods reported that their children had more problems than did the parents who lived in racially mixed neighborhoods. He said,

"One of this study's most striking findings showed transracial adoptive parents' decisions on where to live had a substantial impact upon their children's adjustments. Transracial adoptive parents residing in predominantly White communities tended to have adoptees who experienced more discomfort about their appearance than those who lived in integrated settings. Adoptees feeling more

discomfort, in turn, were more likely to have adjustment difficulties."

Feigelman said that living in culturally heterogeneous neighborhoods was most important for African-American and Asian children adopted transracially.

In an article on what he calls the "transracial adoption paradox," in *The Counseling Psychologist,* author Richard Lee defines the paradox in this way: "Namely, adoptees are racial/ethnic minorities in society, but they are perceived and treated by others, and sometimes themselves, as if they are members of the majority culture (i.e., racially White and ethnically European) due to adoption into a White family."

Lee discussed research on transracial adoption and made several key observations. Says Lee, "Some researchers found that the variability in racial/ethnic identify development for transracial adoptees may be attributable to different extrinsic factors, such as age at adoption, race, and geography. Transracial adoptees placed at a later age, for example, identified more strongly with their ethnicities and races than did adoptees placed at a younger age."

Lee also noted that research indicates that racial identity seemed to be weaker among transracial adoptees living in racially homogeneous neighborhoods (such as African-American children living in an all-white community).

Lee also discussed research which indicates that African-American adopted children whose parents encouraged them to learn about their race had a more positive racial identify as well as a more positive adjustment.

Said Lee, "Adoptive parents who deny or overlook racial and ethnic differences between parents and child, for example, may be more likely to engage in cultural assimilation parenting strategies, which in turn, may contribute to poorer mental health." In contrast, says Lee, parents who are more accepting of racial differences and who do not rely upon the child assimilating into the culture may have children with a more positive racial identity and better mental health.

Lee advises counselors that they need to understand that transracially adopted children may have varying outlooks toward themselves and how they regard their role. Says Lee, "For example, some transracial adoptees may be more likely to identify as racial minorities than members of a specific ethnic group, whereas other adoptees may perceive race and ethnicity as synonyms." He added, "Perhaps most important, practitioners should view transracial adoptees and families as active agents of change in their personal and family lives—that is, transracial adoptees and adoptive parents likely engage in a variety of cultural socialization strategies to manage the complexities of the transracial adoption paradox."

In a unique study of family leisure activities in relation to family functioning, researchers Zabriskie and Freeman found that there was a proven relationship between family leisure activities and successful families. In other words, the family that "plays together, stays together." They decided to study family leisure involvement in families who had adopted transracially, as well as studying family functioning, and compare adoptive families to those with biological children. Their sample of respondents to their study was comprised of 197 adoptive parent respondents and 56 adopted children respondents, as well as a control group. Most of the adoptive parents were female (81 percent) and Caucasian (98 percent). Most were married (90 percent).

The researchers found that the adoptive families scored higher than the biological families in terms of family functioning, cohesion, and adaptability. They also found the adoptive families had higher scores on total family leisure and other key measures. The researchers also found a direct relationship between family leisure and family functioning, and they said that "when considering other family characteristics such as race, family size, religion, history of divorce, and annual family income, the only significant predictor of higher family functioning was family leisure involvement."

They also said that "family leisure involvement clearly must be recognized as one of the many possible factors that contribute to healthy adoptive families."

Advice for Adoptive Parents

In a small study of parents in Illinois and their transracially adopted children, there were several interesting findings of value to adoptive parents. In this study, 20 children and their families were interviewed. Fourteen of the 20 children (70 percent) were African-American biracial (African-American/White). Of the remainder, 15 percent were Latinos and the remaining 15 percent were biracial but not African-American (15 percent). Most of the adoptive parents (95 percent) were college graduates and 35 percent held graduate degrees.

The researchers noted that the adoptive parents of children of other races were very sensitive that the researchers were biased against transracial adoption and according to the researchers, "They were very protective and cautious because they often felt unsupported and had to explain their family and correct erroneous assumptions." Some of the families said their lack of support began with African-American social workers who were opposed to transracial adoption.

According to the researchers, the parents had many suggestions for agencies that placed children transracially, such as to offer parents a list of resources where they could purchase clothing, artwork, magazines, and other items that provided positive images of African Americans. They also recommended that caseworkers be educated to view transracial adoption as a viable option and learn how they can help families who do adopt African-American children. In addition, they recommended that parents be given parenting classes on raising a child of color as well as learning how to recognize and deal with racism in schools and in other situations.

The parents also had recommendations for those who plan to adopt transracially, such as making friends with people of color before adopting, rather than waiting until after the adoption and connecting with other adoptive parents who have adopted children of other races.

The adopted children (aged eight to 14 at the time of the interview) also raised issues that were of concern in transracial adoption; for example, some of the children said their white parents did not see racism when it occurred or, if they were aware of it, they tried to minimize its importance. Some of the children had experienced name-calling in their predominantly white schools.

Experts report that it is important that families are aware, even before they adopt, of the potential

WHAT ARE YOU WILLING TO DO?

Child's Challenges	Are You Willing to
Transplanted from his biological home and placed with your family—a new home, new family, new neighborhood, etc.	Visit your child's old neighborhood or extended relatives? Move to a neighborhood that reflects the child's background?
Expected to make friends with the children of your friends.	Develop close, positive relationships with persons of your child's race or culture?
Expected to attend your place of worship.	Regularly attend a religious institution familiar to your child? Join a religious institution with a diverse population?
Attend school, day care, or a community center in your neighborhood.	Participate in activities at a community center in a neighborhood that reflects the child's background? Drive your child to a day care center in the child's neighborhood?
Asked to eat food common to your culture.	Include your child in the choice and preparation of ethnic foods for your family?
Endure prejudiced comments from neighbors, classmates, and relatives.	Respond constructively when you hear prejudiced comments from colleagues, acquaintances, and loved ones?
Expect to fit in and be grateful for being adopted.	Incorporate the child's culture into your family?
Asked to take vacations with your immediate or extended family.	Plan trips to places that reflect the child's heritage or are familiar to the child?

Source: North American Council on Adoptable Children (NACAC), St. Paul, Minnesota. Available online. URL: http://www.nacac. org/transracial_willing.html, downloaded August 5, 2005. Reprinted with permission of NACAC from "Self Awareness Tool, Transracial Parenting Project," 1998.

difficulties that their children and their families will face in a transracial adoption, because society has not yet become "color blind."

Say Gail Steinberg and Beth Hall in their book, *Inside Transracial Adoption,*

> Transracial adoption means that your family becomes "public" because the differences between family members are obvious to others. As a parent, you are on display. If you enjoy being different and standing out from the crowd, as a transracial parent you will get chances every day. On the other hand, if you are shy and like to blend in with others, being out and about with your child is bound to be laborious for you because you will always be noticed.

It is important for parents who adopt transracially to realize the challenges that lie ahead. To that end, the North American Council on Adoptable Children (NACAC) has created a helpful chart comparing the child's personal challenges to what the parents may be willing to do to help the child meet these challenges.

According to NACAC, "Parents who bring a racially or culturally diverse child into their world often forget the challenges the child must face."

See also BLACK/AFRICAN-AMERICAN ADOPTIVE PARENT RECRUITMENT PROGRAMS; FOSTER CARE.

Baden, Amanda. "Psychological Adjustment of Transracial Adoptees: An Application of the Cultural-Racial Identity Model," *Journal of Social Distress and the Homeless* 11, no. 2 (April 2002): 167–191.

Banks, R. Richard. "The Color of Desire: Fulfilling Adoptive Parents' Racial Preferences through Discriminatory State Action," *Yale Law Journal,* January 1998.

De Haymes, Maria Vidal, Shirley Simon, and Jerome Blakemore. *Children of Color in Foster Care and the Multiethnic Placement Act: The Experiences of Families Involved in Transracial and Same Race Adoptions in an Illinois Sample: Final Report,* May 10, 2000. Available online. URL: http://cfrcwww.social.uiuc.edu/pubs/pdf.files/childofcolor.pdf, downloaded on August 5, 2005.

Eschelbach Hansen, Mary, and Rita J. Simon. "Transracial Placement in Adoptions with Public Agency

Involvement: What Can We Learn from the AFCARS Data?" *Adoption Quarterly* 8, no. 2 (2004): 45–56.

Feigelman, William. "Adjustments of Transracially and Inracially Adopted Young Adults," *Child and Adolescent Social Work* 17, no. 3 (June 2000): 165–184.

Lee, Richard M. "The Transracial Adoption Paradox: History, Research, and Counseling Implications of Cultural Socialization," *Counseling Psychologist* 31, no. 6 (November 2003): 711–744.

McLaughlin, Barbara. "Transracial Adoption in New York State," *Albany Law Review* 60, no. 2 (1996).

Rosnati, R., and E. Marta. "Parent-Child Relationships as a Protective Factor in Preventing Adolescents' Psychosocial Risk in Inter-Racial Adoptive and Non-Adoptive Families," *Journal of Adolescence* 20 (1997): 617–631.

Shireman, Joan F., and Penny R. Johnson. "A Longitudinal Study of Black Adoptions: Single Parent, Transracial, and Traditional," *Social Work* 31 (May–June 1986): 172–176.

Simon, Rita, and Howard Altstein. *Adoption across Borders: Serving the Children in Transracial and Intercountry Adoption.* Lanham, Md.: Rowman and Littlefield, 2000.

Simon, Rita, and Howard Altstein. *Transracial Adoptees and Their Families: A Study of Identity and Commitment.* New York: Praeger, 1987.

Simon, R., H. Altstein, and M. Melli. *The Case for Transracial Adoption.* Washington, D.C.: American University Press, 1994.

Steinberg, Gail, and Beth Hall. *Inside Transracial Adoption.* Indianapolis, Ind.: Perspectives Press, 2000.

Triseliotis, John, Joan Shireman, and Marion Hundleby. *Adoption: Theory, Policy and Practice.* Herndon, Va.: Cassell, 1997.

Weinberg, Richard A., et al. "Minnesota Transracial Adoption Study: Reports of Psychosocial Adjustment at Late Adolescence," *Adoption Quarterly* 8, no. 2 (2004): 27–44.

Zabriskie, Ramon B., and Patti Freeman. "Contributions of Family Leisure to Family Functioning among Transracial Adoptive Families," *Adoption Quarterly* 7, no. 3 (2004): 49–77.

tuberculosis   A serious potentially life-threatening chronic infection with *Mycobacterium tuberculosis.* This infectious disease is more common among children and adults in poor countries, although some individuals in the United States, Canada, and other developed countries have contracted tuberculosis. About 95 percent of the cases of tuberculosis occur in individuals in developing (poor) countries, such as India, China, Indonesia, Peru, the Philippines, Romania, Russia, Thailand, and Vietnam. Worldwide, about eight million people develop the active form of tuberculosis per year and three million people die annually of the disease. Nearly 99 percent of the deaths from tuberculosis occur in developing countries.

Within the United States, an estimated 15 million people are infected with tuberculosis and an estimated half of those who are infected were born in other countries.

Foster Children

Some studies have shown that children in FOSTER CARE have an increased risk for testing positive for tuberculosis, although it is unknown how prevalent the illness is among foster children. However, in a study of foster children and medical problems, reported in 1998 in *Pediatrics,* the researchers found that 12 percent of adolescents tested positive for tuberculosis. Interestingly, many people who wish to become foster parents or adoptive parents are required to undergo testing for tuberculosis, HIV, and other illnesses, but many foster children are not screened by physicians for these illnesses.

In one sad story reported by the Centers for Disease Control and Prevention (CDC) in 2004, a 15-year-old female foster child died of tuberculosis in Detroit. The girl had been under the care of a physician, who had noted her weight loss, night sweats, and chronic coughing but failed to test the girl for tuberculosis, despite her symptoms. When the autopsy was performed, the medical examiner found that "the lungs were completely replaced by infection and were adhered to the chest lining and diaphragm. The lung damage could possibly have been evident on a chest X ray at least 6 months prior to the death." Other findings indicated the pervasiveness of the child's tuberculosis within her body.

Individuals with whom the girl had been in contact were subsequently tested for tuberculosis and several tested positive.

Children Adopted from Other Countries

Children who are adopted internationally have an elevated risk of a tuberculosis infection. Children who are internationally adopted have at least a four to 20 or more times greater risk of a tuberculosis infection than children born in the United States.

Some children adopted from other countries have a positive reaction to tuberculin skin tests because they have received the Bacillus Calmette-Guérin (BCG) vaccine in their native country. This vaccine is not given to children in the United States or Canada, and North American doctors sometimes mistakenly believe that prior BCG vaccination is a contraindication to testing for tuberculosis.

Active and Latent (Inactive) Tuberculosis

Most cases of tuberculosis that are detected are the inactive form of the disease; only about 10 percent of patients have an active infection. However, both patients with a latent (inactive) form of tuberculosis and patients with active disease are treated. The reason for treatment of a patient with latent tuberculosis is that the disease may suddenly become active, and this is a situation that patients should seek to avoid. Disease activation may occur in young children as well as adults.

Patients with active tuberculosis sometimes have minimal symptoms; however, despite the lack of symptoms, they may transmit the disease to others.

Some active cases and their consequences have been reported. For example, in one case in 1999, described in the *The New England Journal of Medicine,* a nine-year-old child from the Republic of the Marshall Islands transmitted the active form of tuberculosis to his adoptive mother in North Dakota. Two years later, she developed tuberculous osteomyelitis (a severe bone infection), as well as arthritis, and a pelvic abscess before the tuberculosis was finally diagnosed.

Of the 276 people who had been in contact with the child up to that time in the United States and who were then tested for tuberculosis, 56 people (20 percent) had a positive tuberculin skin test result. A total of 118 of the people who had been in contact with the child were given preventive antituberculosis therapy, to be on the safe side.

In retrospect, this spread of tuberculosis and the serious illnesses of the adoptive mother could have been avoided. The child was tested for tuberculosis soon after he arrived in the United States, but the test was never read.

Symptoms and Diagnostic Path

Tuberculosis is spread through the air by infected individuals who are coughing. Contrary to old Hollywood movies depicting heroines coughing up blood because of their tuberculosis, patients may have no symptoms in the early stages of the disease, and many patients never have symptoms.

When symptoms exist in the first stage of tuberculosis, they may include the following vague indicators of disease:

- Chronic fever
- Lack of appetite
- Weight loss
- Lethargy
- Night sweats
- Chronic cough
- Poor growth (for children)

After about 12 months or longer from the time of an exposure, the disease may become evident in the lungs, lymph nodes, bones, skin, or kidneys. A chest X-ray is commonly used to evaluate the lung for the presence of tuberculosis.

Tuberculosis is primarily diagnosed with the Tuberculin Skin Test (TST), sometimes also called the Mantoux test. In this test, the patient's skin is injected with a purified protein derived from the tuberculosis microbe, and 48 to 72 hours later, the skin is checked for a reaction. A positive reaction is indicated by a bumpy area on the skin that is greater than 10 mm in size (even when a prior BCG vaccine was given). If a patient has a positive TST, then a chest X-ray should be ordered. If abnormal findings are seen on the chest X-ray, sputum samples or gastric aspirates are collected to obtain a culture, which will confirm tuberculosis if the bacteria is present.

Although reliable comparison studies have not yet been done, many physicians suggest that the TST should be repeated about four to six months after a child at risk for tuberculosis is adopted (whether the child was adopted from another country or from foster care), because the initial test only measured exposure that occurred more than

12 weeks before the test. If children had recently been exposed to tuberculosis prior to the adoption and it was not detected in the first test, then the repeat test will detect the presence of the disease. Also, various factors such as malnutrition can interfere with the accuracy of the TST.

Treatment Options and Outlook

Patients diagnosed in the early stages of tuberculosis have a good prognosis. Children and adults with latent tuberculosis are usually treated with a single medication, isoniazid (INH), which is given for nine months. This drug can be given to children either as a syrup or in the form of crushed pills, although the tablets are often better tolerated.

The medications used to treat tuberculosis may cause a medication-induced hepatitis. For this reason, adults who are treated for tuberculosis should avoid all alcohol during their treatment. Once treatment is over, the liver should return to normal in most cases. However, if the liver was additionally damaged by alcohol consumption, it is less likely that the liver will recover. Children are not as susceptible to liver problems from this medication as are adults.

Children and adults who are diagnosed with an active form of tuberculosis must be treated by an expert in infectious diseases. These patients require a variety of medications for an extended period, to be determined by their physicians. They may be given a combination of such medications as isoniazid, rifampin, pyrazinamide and ethambutol.

According to S. Jody Heymann et al., in an article in *Pediatrics* in 2000, it is vital to treat children who are infected with tuberculosis, not only for their own sakes but also to decrease the spread of the disease. Said the authors, "A 5% increase in the number of children who enter treatment leads to a 25% decline in the number of TB cases among children and a 16% decline in the number of TB deaths after 10 years."

For similar reasons, it is also vital to treat adults who are diagnosed with either the latent or active forms of tuberculosis.

Risk Factors and Preventive Measures

Children who are at the greatest risk for tuberculosis include those who

- Reside now or have lived in an institutional setting, such as an orphanage or a group home
- Have been in close contact with individuals who are infected with tuberculosis
- Were born in a country with a high prevalence of tuberculosis
- Are infected with the human immunodeficiency virus (HIV)
- Are malnourished

In addition, children who have the greatest risk of developing an active form of tuberculosis include the following:

- Children infected with HIV
- Children with malnutrition
- Children with other chronic diseases, especially those requiring immunosuppressive treatment

Adults who should be tested for tuberculosis include the following groups:

- Those who adopted a child from a country with a high prevalence of tuberculosis
- Those with symptoms of tuberculosis
- Employees of facilities that treat patients with tuberculosis
- Those with HIV
- Those with kidney failure
- Those on immunosuppressive drugs, such as patients with organ transplants or cancer

See also MEDICAL PROBLEMS OF INTERNATIONALLY ADOPTED CHILDREN.

Centers for Disease Control and Prevention. "Missed Diagnosis Leads to the Death of a 15-Year-Old in Detroit," *TB Notes* 1 (2004) 4–5.

Chen, Lin H., M.D., Elizabeth D. Barnett, M.D., and Mary E. Wilson, M.D. "Preventing Infectious Diseases during and after International Adoption," *Annals of Internal Medicine* 139 (2003): 371–378.

Heymann, S. Jody, M.D., et al. "Pediatric Tuberculosis: What Needs to Be Done to Decrease Morbidity and Mortality," *Pediatrics* 106, no. 1 (2000): 1.

Mandalakas, Anna M., M.D., and Jeffrey Starke, M.D. "Tuberculosis Screening in Immigrant Children,"

Pediatric Infectious Disease Journal 23, no. 1 (2004): 71–72.

Miller, Laurie C., M.D. "Tuberculosis," in *The Handbook of International Adoption Medicine: A Guide for Physicians, Parents, and Providers* and the *Annals of Internal Medicine.* New York: Oxford University Press, 2005: 215–229.

Minocha, Anil, M.D., and Christine Adamec. *The Encyclopedia of the Digestive System and Digestive Disorders.* New York: Facts On File, 2004.

Pickering, L. K, ed. "Section 3. Summaries of Infectious Diseases," in *Red Book: 2003 Report of the Committee on Infectious Diseases.* 26th ed. Elk Grove Village, Ill.: American Academy of Pediatrics, 2003, 642–660.

Takayama, John I., M.D., et al. "Relationship between Reason for Placement and Medical Findings among Children in Foster Care," *Pediatrics* 101, no. 2 (February 1998): 201–207.

twins   See SIBLINGS.

unadoptable   Until the late 1970s, society considered older children (over age 10) and children with serious physical or emotional handicaps as "unadoptable," presuming no one would desire to adopt such a child. It was believed that most people prefer to adopt a healthy infant.

Today many social workers believe that the majority of children can successfully attain family membership, and some adoption experts claim no child is unadoptable.

It is difficult to find appropriate families for teenagers or children who have psychiatric problems, are abusive, and exhibit other behavioral problems. Yet there are people who will volunteer to adopt children who are retarded and even children who have AIDS. As of this writing, there is a waiting list of people who wish to adopt children with DOWN SYNDROME or spina bifida. The challenge appears to be largely in identifying the right family for a specific child.

In some cases, a child may not wish to be adopted, and many states permit a child over a certain age (usually 14) to reject adoption as an option. The child may be used to the foster home or group home and unwilling to transfer her affections to an adoptive family.

It is important to understand that children who were once considered unadoptable may often require extensive therapy, and adoptive parents and social workers must not assume that love will conquer all barriers.

See also ADOPTION ASSISTANCE AND CHILD WELFARE ACT OF 1980; OLDER CHILD; PSYCHIATRIC PROBLEMS OF ADOPTED PERSONS; SPECIAL NEEDS.

updated home study   Aspects of a home study that must be updated. Often when parents wish to adopt another child from an agency that has already studied them, approved them, and placed a child with them, the updated home study need not be as comprehensive as the original home study. The social worker may request new physicals if six months or a year has passed since their last physical or may request other information.

The agency may not have placed a child with the couple yet, although they have been studied. If a child becomes available who appears would fit into this family setting but a year or more has elapsed, the agency may require an update, and additional fees may be required.

videotape Videotape (or more commonly these days, DVDs) can be used very creatively in adoption to recruit prospective adoptive parents and share information about a child with prospective parents without the child's awareness of being screened in advance. Some adoption agencies use a videotape of a family to provide information on the family to an older child who hopes to be adopted. Some agencies videotape prospective adoptive families in their own home and show the tapes to children, who, experts say, eagerly watch the tapes over and over, helping them a great deal with the preparation process.

Television stations that offer "WEDNESDAY'S CHILD" or similar formats on children in foster care needing adoptive families usually videotape the child and show the tape during a news program in an effort to recruit adoptive parents. This effort is geared toward the general public; however, individual agencies may also create their own videotapes, showing them to families who might be suitable for particular children.

Videotapes can also be used to help separated siblings keep in touch with each other or to help them prior to planned reunions.

The primary disadvantage of videotape is that it requires some labor and training to do well. An amateurish "home video," while helpful for some purposes, may not give a full picture of the child.

In recent years, the use of videotapes has become common in certain types of INTERNATIONAL ADOPTION. Medical records for children from eastern Europe and the countries of the former Soviet Union are often scanty, incomplete, inaccurate, or completely uninterpretable, because of differing terminology. In such cases, a videotape may be very helpful in confirming or refuting the written medical report.

In some countries outside the United States, videotapes are primarily used to recruit families for children with SPECIAL NEEDS, just as they are used in the United States.

Videotapes may sometimes be revealing while other times they are very concealing. For example, if an infant is closely swaddled, it is hard to draw many conclusions about the child's physical or developmental condition. If the child is videotaped on a "bad day" or when he is ill, he may exhibit atypical behavior and thus be rejected for adoptive placement. Videotapes sometimes enable physicians to discern FETAL ALCOHOL SYNDROME or other physical abnormalities. Parents who adopt the child will be far more prepared to provide the care that the child needs.

The best videotapes are those which show the child demonstrating his best skills (motor, language, etc.) in a familiar setting with the usual playmates and caregivers.

See also ADOPTION MEDICINE.

waiting children The thousands of children with SPECIAL NEEDS who are in need of families to adopt them and wait for parents to be located or identified.

waiting lists Rosters of couples or single people waiting for a HOME STUDY or, more commonly, a roster of people already studied and selected and waiting for a child who will need them as parents.

Waiting lists vary greatly from agency to agency and exist primarily as a function of the imbalance between the numbers of infants in need of families and the much larger numbers of couples and single persons who are interested in adopting children, especially infants. (Waiting lists are much shorter for individuals interested in adopting older children or children with SPECIAL NEEDS.)

Some agencies require individuals to wait for at least a year before they may be studied while others will not accept applications after a certain number of applicants have registered and until they believe they will be able to do a home study and place a child with the applicant within a reasonable length of time.

Virtually all agencies maintain waiting lists of people who have been approved to adopt. Most agencies consider a group of approved families for the next child to be adopted. Many of these agencies also offer the birthmother the opportunity to choose the adopting family from a group of nonidentifying résumés of previously approved families.

Most prospective adoptive parents do not like the prospect of spending several years' time on a waiting list, even if they understand the main reason for the wait to be an imbalance in numbers. Social workers believe that one good by-product of waiting lists is they may give applicants time that is often needed to seriously reflect on adoption and to work through any final infertility conflicts the family may have.

Parents interested in adopting a child with special needs usually are specifically matched to a child in terms of being able to deal with these special needs, and therefore, their wait may be very brief or very lengthy depending on the type of child the family feels they can accept and also depending on the suitability of their family for the child.

waiting period The time a family spends waiting to adopt a child, from the point of application to the time of placement.

Many families may state that they have waited years and years when they are actually considering the time from when they first thought about adopting a child until when the child came to them. Although numerous couples do wait years for their child, it is only reasonable to consider the waiting from the point in time when they actually took action to adopt the child by formally applying to an agency or retaining an attorney.

Studies have revealed that the most stressful time for adopting parents is that period spent in searching for an appropriate adoption agency or attorney and subsequently being accepted as a prospective parent. (See HOME STUDY.)

Although the waiting time after approval of the home study is also stressful, it is less anxiety-provoking than the time before approval because the family believes they will eventually be chosen for a child and they have done everything possible to make the adoption happen.

Wednesday's Child Recruitment program for foster children needing adoptive families, primarily relying on broadcast media as well as the INTERNET. *Wednesday's Child* is the common term for children listed on the weekly Wednesday time slots, while some television stations provide information on other days of the week, hence they have a "Tuesday's Child, "Thursday's Child," etc., program. Television programs show VIDEOTAPES of a waiting child, providing telephone numbers of social workers who can offer interested viewers further information.

Waiting child recruitment programs are very effective tools to identify families for older children and other children with special needs. They are cumbersome for social workers, because many people who call are only mildly interested, and they are unwilling to spend the time needed for classes and counseling. However, most social workers believe that even one potential prospect makes the program well worth the effort involved.

In addition, although families who contact the social worker may not be suitable for the particular Wednesday's Child of the week that they have called to inquire about, they could be a very good match for another child needing a family.

Critics of Wednesday's Child programs charge that corporations could not engage in such "bait and switch" advertising and promotion, and social service agencies should not engage in a similar practice. They also allege that often the child's problems are minimized in an attempt to effect an adoptive placement.

The National Adoption Center has an online Wednesday's Child page of video clips of children that have been shown to viewers in six cities, including Atlanta, Chicago, Los Angeles, New York, Philadelphia, and Washington, D.C., and who still need adoptive parents. It is sponsored by the Freddie Mac Foundation in Washington, D.C. Further information is available at the following Web site: http://adopt.org/wednesdayschild/home/wed-child-page.htm.

See also ADVERTISING AND PROMOTION IN ADOPTION; FOSTER CARE; PHOTOLISTINGS.

working mothers Although the majority of mothers today are in the workforce, many adoption agencies specify at least one parent must be willing to stay home with a newly adopted child for some length of time, ranging from weeks to months. Such acquiescence is a condition of application that is pointed out to prospective adoptive parents.

Which parent stays home is not always specified, but because of economic disparities, the wife is usually the individual selected. In the case of a single parent adoption, the time frame may be cut back or eliminated altogether, since the income of the single parent is what will support the child.

Parental leave policies vary from company to company, and attempts to create a national parental leave policy for new parents of biological and adoptive children have been made in recent years by members of Congress. If a company does not have a paid parental leave policy or if the time allowed for leave is shorter than the adoption agency requires, the adoptive parent may have to take a leave without pay or quit work altogether.

Some adoptive parents have found it ironic and unfair that one is expected to leave work at least temporarily and insist extra income is needed more than ever to support a child. They also say biological parents are not required to stay home with a child and believe such arbitrary judgments are unfair.

Others believe it is important for at least one parent to spend an intensive period with the child to facilitate bonding. This is true even when the child is an older child, although it is less likely a lengthy period at home would be required in the adoption of a school-age child.

When agencies request input from birthmothers on the type of adoptive parents they are seeking, most birthmothers have stated their preference for a mother who is not employed outside the home. Their attitude is if they had opted to parent the child, they would have been forced to work. They believe a full-time mother is a better situation than they could provide.

A similar attitude is evinced by birthmothers who prefer couples over single parents.

See also ADOPTIVE PARENTS; BIRTHMOTHER; EMPLOYMENT BENEFITS; PARENTAL LEAVE.

wrongful adoption A legal term for an adoption that should not have occurred or would not have occurred had all the relevant facts about the child been made available to the adoptive parents. Instead, information was deliberately misrepresented and/or withheld by the agency, and as a result, the adoptive parents were essentially defrauded.

Adoption agencies and, many times, other adoption providers such as attorneys, are not required to provide identifying information to adopting parents and in fact are precluded by most state laws from violating the birthparents' confidentiality. However, they are ethically (and often legally) bound to tell the truth about a child's medical and psychiatric status. Today, only six states do not mandate that adoptive parents must be given all known non-identifying medical information. As of this writing, these states are: Alaska, Arkansas, Florida, New York, Rhode Island, and South Carolina.

The first reported successful case of wrongful adoption occurred in 1986 in *Burr v. Board of County Commissioners of Stark County in Ohio*. Prior to this case, the only recourse for adoptive parents was to seek the dissolution of the adoption, a remedy often denied by courts, despite the circumstances. However, in this case, the parents did not seek to set aside the adoption but instead sought to receive monetary payment from the adoption agency.

The Burrs had adopted a 17-month-old boy in 1964. They had been told he was a healthy normal child born of an 18-year-old mother.

The child suffered numerous diseases and physical problems, and the Burrs opened the sealed adoption records with a court order in 1982. They sought this information because they believed the information might help them with the child's numerous physical problems.

They learned the child's birthmother was not 18 but was actually a 31-year-old inmate of a psychiatric institution, and the birthfather was probably another inmate. They also learned that psychological evaluations of the child indicated the child was subnormal intellectually and further evaluations were recommended. In addition, the social worker had not revealed that the child had been in two foster homes prior to his adoptive placement.

A jury awarded the Burrs $125,000 for medical and emotional damages. The decision was appealed to the Franklin County Court of Appeals of Ohio and later the Ohio Supreme Court, which both upheld the decision of the jury.

In a later case, withholding of information was deemed important and actionable. In *Michael J. v. Los Angeles County, Department of Adoptions*, a single adoptive mother prevailed in 1988. In this case, the child had an extensive birthmark and a physician refused to provide a prognosis. The agency told the mother that the child was in good health, and she adopted him. The agency did not tell the adoptive mother about the doctor's refusal to provide a prognosis. It later became known that the port-wine stain was a symptom of a rare disease, Sturge-Weber Syndrome. Although agency staff did not know about the child's illness or the significance of the birthmark, the court held that the adoptive mother should have been told that a doctor would not make a prognosis on the child's future health.

In another case, *Meracle v. Children's Services Society* (1989), a wrongful adoption suit was filed against a Wisconsin agency for inaccurate information that led to an adoption. In this case, the agency told the family that the child's birthfamily had a history of Huntington's disease but that the birthfather had tested negative and thus the child was not at risk. The family later learned that there was no test at that time to determine predisposition to Huntington's disease. The disease manifested later in the child. (The Huntington's gene was not isolated until 1993.)

The court ruled for the adoptive parents, stating that the agency was wrong when it told the family the child was not at risk for the disease and thus negligent in providing erroneous medical information.

In *M. H. & J. H. L. v. Caritas Family Services* (1992), the agency told the Minnesota family that there was a "possibility of incest" in the birth family, although they provided no further details. The couple adopted, and the child had severe emotional problems. Upon investigation, it was learned that the child's birthparents were a 13-year-old girl and her 17-year-old brother. The agency knew this but did not disclose the information. The adoptive parents prevailed.

In *Gibbs v. Ernst* (1994), the Pennsylvania court held "an adoption agency has a duty to disclose fully and accurately to the adopting parents all relevant nonidentifying information in its possession concerning the adoptee." In this case, the family was told that the five-year-old boy they were interested in adopting had lived with one family for two years after removal from his birthfamily for neglect. He was said to be hyperactive but with no other problems. The family had stated that they did not want to adopt a child who had any history of physical or sexual abuse.

Later, the child became severely mentally ill and was hospitalized and diagnosed with schizophrenia. It was determined that the child had been both physically and sexually abused in the past, and he had had many foster placements before the family adopted him. The agency was aware of these facts but did not disclose them.

These wrongful adoption lawsuits should not imply to readers that adoptive parents always prevail. Nor does it mean that an agency, adoption attorney, or other provider can ever "guarantee" lifelong mental and physical health for any child.

In *Harper and Johnson v. Adoption Center of Washington* (1995), a family lost their wrongful adoption case in the District of Columbia. They learned that the child they had adopted from Russia had FETAL ALCOHOL SYNDROME, a condition they would not have accepted, but the information had been disclosed to the family, in Russian, just before the adoption. The adoptive father signed a document stating that he would accept the child. He later argued that he could not understand Russian, but the court held against him, since he could have had the document translated.

Even when adoptive parents win their lawsuits, they do not necessarily recover the costs or expenses that they seek. For example, in February of 1998, the Washington (State) Supreme Court upheld a jury ruling that an agency erred in not providing information about previous abuse and the birthmother's drinking problem to a couple who later discovered their daughter had fetal alcohol syndrome.

Although they won their case, no damages were awarded, in part because the couple received some public assistance for the child's problem and also because the couple allegedly knew the child had problems. However, the adoptive mother said that social workers had told her the child would be fine with love and attention. (Children with fetal alcohol syndrome can benefit greatly from love and attention; unfortunately, it will not make the disease go away.)

In other cases, adoptive parents have lost their lawsuits because of contractual language that they had signed when they applied to adopt, which released the agency from all legal claims. This was the finding in *Ferenc v. World Child* in the District of Columbia in 1997.

Why Information Was Withheld in the Past

One explanation for why some adoption agencies, attorneys, and other adoption providers in the past failed to provide information on serious psychiatric or physical illnesses of birthparents—or of the child to be adopted—was the prevailing view at the time that environment was all and heredity was unimportant. The general viewpoint was that a "good home" could rectify any potential problems a child might have or even already exhibit.

Another reason for nondisclosure was misplaced altruism: some social workers feared that no one would adopt a child born to mentally ill parents. Or, if anyone did adopt the child, workers feared the adoptive parents would constantly watch for signs of illness in the child and would not treat him as a normal person.

This does not justify lies, evasions, and omissions that some agencies committed in the past but is only offered as an explanation for seemingly incomprehensible behavior.

Wrongful Adoption Lawsuits May Serve to Improve Adoption Practice

In her law article, Danielle Saba Donner summed up wrongful adoption in this way: "The recent emergence of the tort of wrongful adoption, with its ever-widening scope of liability, as well as its endorsement in the final draft of the UAA [Uniform Adoption Act], has tremendous implications for agency practice. Indeed, child welfare authorities, anticipating the extension of liability based on a duty to investigate, have strongly recommended that agencies implement written disclosure policies and conduct more extensive worker training . . . Whether this preference for the private remedy of wrongful adoption is attributed to market forces, even child welfare authorities agree that this reversal in agency practice, with regard to disclosure, benefits not only the adoptive parents, but the adopted child as well."

Adamec, Christine. *The Complete Idiot's Guide to Adoption.* New York: Alpha Books, 2005.

Belkin, Lisa. "What the Jumans Didn't Know about Michael," *New York Times Magazine,* March 14 1999.

Croft, Jay. "Mother's Doctor Hurt Baby, Jury Says $2.7 Million Awarded to Adoptive Parents of Child Born with Deformities after Birth Mother Took Accutane," *Atlanta Journal-Constitution,* March 14, 1998.

Donner, Danielle Saba. "The Emerging Adoption Market: Child Welfare Agencies, Private Middlemen, and 'Consumer' Remedies," *University of Louisville Journal of Family Law* (Summer 1996–1997): 473–535.

Freundlich, Madelyn, and Lisa Peterson. *Wrongful Adoption: Law, Policy and Practice.* Washington, D.C.: CWLA Press, 1998.

Gibeaut, John. "Disclosing Birth Secrets," *ABA Journal* 84 (July 1, 1998): 34.

Grandpre Combs, Claire. "Wrongful Adoption: Adoption Agency Held Liable for Fraudulent Representations," *Cincinnati Law Review* 56 (1987): 343–359.

Maley, John R. "Wrongful Adoption: Monetary Damages as a Superior Remedy to Annulment for Adoptive Parents Victimized by Fraud," *Indiana Law Review* 20 (1987): 709–734.

"Medical Liability: Interview with Sam Totaro, Attorney" *Adoption Medical News* 4, no. 9 (October 1998): 1–6.

Schiffer, Michele. "Fraud in the Adoption Setting, *Arizona Law Review* 29 (1987): 707–723.

Y, Z

youths   Minor children. In adoption, youths could be adolescent birthparents or adopted teenagers or children.

zero population growth   The concept, popularized by a group called Zero Population Growth (ZPG), that individuals should only reproduce themselves at the replacement rate; for example, a man and a woman should have no more than two children. The reason for this concern is the alleged overpopulation of our entire planet, which, zero population growth advocates believe, would be resolved if they and many others bore fewer children.

Others allege that poverty and hunger are primarily the result of an inequitable distribution of available resources, not overpopulation.

Zero population growth advocates may be actively involved in the group that formally promotes their philosophy, or they may be informal believers in this concept.

If some people were zero population growth advocates, then the alleged worldwide overpopulation problem would probably be resolved; however, many people believe in bearing many children or do not believe in using any family planning method, with the end result being that they bear many children whether they planned the births or not.

Some proponents of zero population growth, because they may enjoy raising children very much, have opted to adopt children rather than to bear more children themselves. They reason that there are already children in the world needing homes, which they can provide.

Few adoption agencies in the United States will accept an application for a healthy nonminority infant from a family that continues to be fertile, as are many zero population growth advocates, and so such people often adopt older children or minority or handicapped infants, or children from other countries, again, reasoning that the children need families to belong to and loving parents.

Social workers are (or should be) careful to ensure that the adopting family realizes they are adopting a child, not a social cause.

APPENDIXES

307

APPENDIX I
STATE ADOPTION/SOCIAL SERVICES OFFICES IN THE UNITED STATES

ALABAMA

Family Services
Department of Human Resources
50 Ripley Street
Montgomery, AL 36130
(334) 242-9500
http://www.dhr.state.al.us

ALASKA

Adoptions
Office of Children's Services
Department of Health and Social Services
P.O. Box 110630
Juneau, AK 99811-0630
(907) 465-3209
http://www.hss.state.ak.us

ARIZONA

Administration for Children, Youth, and Families
Division of Children and Family Services
Department of Economic Security
Site Code 940A
P.O. Box 6123
Phoenix, AZ 85005-6123
(602) 542-2277
http://www.azdes.gov/tp/portal.asp

ARKANSAS

Adoption Unit
Division of Children and Family Services
Department of Human Services
P.O. Box 1437, Slot S565
Little Rock, AR 72203
(501) 682-8460
http://www.arkansas.gov/dhs

CALIFORNIA

Adoption Services Bureau
Children and Family Services Division
Department of Social Services
Health and Human Services Agency
744 P Street, MS 3-31
Sacramento, CA 95814
(916) 651-8089
http://www.childsworld.ca.gov

COLORADO

Division of Child Welfare Services
Office of Children, Youth, and Families Services
Department of Human Services
1575 Sherman Street
Denver, CO 80203
(303) 866-4365
http://www.cdhs.state.co.us

CONNECTICUT

Office of Foster and Adoption Services
Department of Children and Families
505 Hudson Street
Hartford, CT 06106
(860) 550-6350
http://www.state.ct.us/dcf

DELAWARE

Division of Family Services
Department of Services for Children, Youth, and Their Families
Delaware Youth and Family Center
1825 Faulkland Road
Wilmington, DE 19805
(302) 633-2655
http://www.state.de.us/kids

DISTRICT OF COLUMBIA

Adoption Services Division
Child and Family Services Agency
400 Sixth Street SW, 3rd Floor
Washington, DC 20024
(202) 727-4550
http://cfsa.dc.gov

FLORIDA

**Child Welfare and Community-Based Care
  Program Office**
Department of Children and Families
1317 Winewood Boulevard
Tallahassee, FL 32399
(850) 488-8762
http://www.dcf.state.fl.us/adoption

GEORGIA

Office of Adoptions
Department of Human Resources
2 Peachtree Street
Suite 8-407
Atlanta, GA 30303
(404) 657-9384
http://dhr.georgia.gov

HAWAII

Child Welfare Services Branch
Social Services Division
Department of Human Services
810 Richards Street
Suite 400
Honolulu, HI 96813
(808) 586-5667
http://www.state.hi.us/dhs

IDAHO

Division of Family and Community Services
Department of Health and Welfare
P.O. Box 83720
Boise, ID 83720-0036
(208) 334-0641
http://www.healthandwelfare.idaho.gov

ILLINOIS

Department of Children and Family Services
310 South Michigan Avenue, 4th Floor
Chicago, IL 60604
(312) 793-2003
http://www.state.il.us/dcfs

INDIANA

Division of Family and Children
Family and Social Services Administration
W364 Government Center South
402 West Washington Street
Indianapolis, IN 46204
(317) 232-4622
http://www.in.gov/fssa

IOWA

Adoption Unit/Foster Care
Division of Behavioral, Developmental, and
  Protective Services
Department of Human Services
Hoover Building, 5th Floor
1305 East Walnut Street
Des Moines, IA 50319
(515) 281-5358
http://www.dhs.state.ia.us

KANSAS

Children and Family Policy
Department of Social and Rehabilitation Services
Docking State Office Building, Room 551-S
915 SW Harrison Street
Topeka, KS 66612
(785) 296-4653
http://www.srskansas.org

KENTUCKY

Division of Protection and Permanency
Department for Community-Based Services
Cabinet for Health and Family Services
275 East Main Street
Frankfort, KY 40621
(502) 564-2147
http://chfs.ky.gov/dcbs/dpp

LOUISIANA

Office of Community Services
Department of Social Services
333 Laurel Street
Baton Rouge, LA 70801
(225) 342-4086
http://www.dss.state.la.us

MAINE

Bureau of Child and Family Services
Department of Health and Human Services
11 State House Station

Augusta, ME 04333
(207) 287-5060
http://ww.maine.gov/dhs

MARYLAND

Social Services Administration
Department of Human Resources
Saratoga State Center
311 West Saratoga Street
Baltimore, MD 21201
(410) 767-7506
http://www.dhmh.state.md.us

MASSACHUSETTS

Foster Care and Adoption Services
Department of Social Services
Executive Office of Health and Human Services
24 Farnsworth Street
Boston, MA 02210
(617) 748-2248
http://www.eec.state.ma.us

MICHIGAN

Division of Adoption Services
Children's Services
Family Independence Agency
P.O. Box 30037
Lansing, MI 48909
(517) 373-3513
http://www.michigan.gov/fia

MINNESOTA

Adoption and Guardianship
Child Safety and Permanency Division
Department of Human Services
444 Lafayette Road
Saint Paul, MN 55155
(651) 296-3636
http://www.dhs.state.mn.us

MISSISSIPPI

Division of Family and Children's Services
Department of Human Services
750 North State Street
Jackson, MS 39202
(601) 359-4323
http://www.mdhs.state.ms.us

MISSOURI

Children's Division
Department of Social Services
615 Howerton Court
P.O. Box 88

Jefferson City, MO 65102
(573) 522-8024
http://www.dss.mo.gov

MONTANA

Child and Family Services Division
Department of Public Health and Human Services
P.O. Box 8005
Helena, MT 59604
(406) 444-5927
http://www.dphhs.state.mt.us

NEBRASKA

Office of Protection and Safety
Department of Services
Health and Human Services System
301 Centennial Mall South
P.O. Box 95044
Lincoln, NE 68508
(402) 471-8404
http://www.hhs.state.ne.us

NEVADA

Family Programs
Division of Child and Family Services
Department of Human Resources
711 East Fifth Street
Carson City, NV 89701
(775) 684-4407
http://www.hr.state.nv.us

NEW HAMPSHIRE

Division for Children, Youth, and Families
Department of Health and Human Services
129 Pleasant Street
Concord, NH 03301
(603) 271-4837
http://www.dhhs.state.nh.us

NEW JERSEY

Adoption Operations
Division of Youth and Family Services
Department of Human Services
P.O. Box 717
Trenton, NJ 08625
(609) 292-4441
http://www.state.nj.us/humanservices

NEW MEXICO

Policy/Procedures Bureau
Protective Services Division
Children, Youth, and Families Department
P.O. Drawer 5160

Santa Fe, NM 87502
(505) 827-8419
http://www.cyfd.org

NEW YORK

Adoption Services
Office of Children and Family Services
Department of Family Assistance
Capital View Office Park, Room 323N
52 Washington Street
Rensselaer, NY 12144
(518) 474-9406
http://www.ocfs.state.ny.us

NORTH CAROLINA

Family Support and Child Welfare Services
Division of Social Services
Department of Health and Human Services
325 North Salisbury Street
2409 Mail Service Center
Raleigh, NC 27699
(919) 733-9464
http://www.dhhs.state.nc.us

NORTH DAKOTA

Adoption Services
Children and Family Services Division
Department of Human Services
State Capitol, Judicial Wing
600 East Boulevard Avenue, Dept 325
Bismarck, ND 58505
(701) 328-4805
http://www.state.nd.us/humanservices

OHIO

Protective Services Section
Bureau of Family Services
Office for Children and Families
Department of Job and Family Services
50 East State Street, 3rd Floor
Columbus, OH 43215
(614) 466-9274
http://jfs.ohio.gov

OKLAHOMA

Swift Adoption Services
Children and Family Services Division
Department of Human Services
P.O. Box 25352
Oklahoma City, OK 73125
(918) 588-1730
http://www.okdhs.org

OREGON

Children, Adults, and Families
Department of Human Services
500 Summer Street NE, E-71
Salem, OR 97301
(503) 945-5677
http://www.oregon.gov/DHS

PENNSYLVANIA

Pennsylvania Adoption Exchange
P.O. Box 1441
Harrisburg, PA 17105
(800) 227-0225
http://www.dpw.state.pa.us

RHODE ISLAND

Department of Children, Youth, and Families
101 Friendship Street
Providence, RI 02903
(401) 528-3799
http://www.dcyf.ri.gov

SOUTH CAROLINA

Department of Social Services
P.O. Box 520
Columbia, SC 29202
(803) 898-7161
http://www.state.sc.us/dss

SOUTH DAKOTA

Child Protection Services
Division of Program Management
Department of Social Services
700 Governors Drive
Pierre, SD 57501
(605) 773-3227
http://www.state.sd.us/social

TENNESSEE

Child Permanency
Department of Children's Services
Cordell Hull Building, 8th Floor
436 Sixth Avenue North
Nashville, TN 37243
(615) 253-4359
http://www.state.tn.us/youth

TEXAS

Department of Family and Protective Services
Mail Code E-557
P.O. Box 149030
Austin, TX 78714

(512) 438-5646
http://www.dfps.state.tx.us

UTAH

Division of Child and Family Services
Department of Human Services
120 North 200 West, Suite 225
Salt Lake City, UT 84103
(801) 538-4364
http://www.dhs.utah.gov

VERMONT

Division of Child Welfare
Department for Children and Families
Agency of Human Services
103 South Main Street
Waterbury, VT 05671
(802) 241-2131
http://www.ahs.state.vt.us

VIRGINIA

Division of Family Services
Department of Social Services
7 North Eighth Street
Richmond, VA 23219
(804) 726-7530
http://www.dss.virginia.gov

WASHINGTON

Placement and Permanency Services
Division of Program and Policy Development
Children's Administration
Department of Social and Health Services

P.O. Box 4571
Olympia, WA 98504
(360) 902-7953
http://www1.dshs.wa.gov

WEST VIRGINIA

Division of Children and Adult Services
Bureau of Children and Families
Department of Health and Human Resources
350 Capitol Street, Room 691
Charleston, WV 25301
(304) 558-7980
http://www.wvdhhr.org

WISCONSIN

Bureau of Programs and Policies
Division of Children and Family Services
Department of Health and Family Services
1 West Wilson Street, Room 527
P.O. Box 8916
Madison, WI 53708
(608) 266-6799
http://dhfs.wisconsin.gov

WYOMING

Adoption/Foster Care
Protective Services Division
Department of Family Services
Hathaway Building, 3rd Floor
2300 Capitol Avenue
Cheyenne, WY 82002
(307) 777-3570
http://dfsweb.state.wy.us

APPENDIX II
PROVINCIAL SOCIAL SERVICES OFFICES IN CANADA

ALBERTA

Adoption Services
11th Floor, Sterling Place
9940-106 Street
Edmonton, Alberta T5K 2N2
(780) 422-0178
http://www.child.gov.ab.ca

BRITISH COLUMBIA

Ministry of Children & Family Development
P.O. Box 9770 Station Provincial Government
Victoria, British Columbia V8W 9S5
(250) 356-1720
http://www.mcf.gov.bc.ca/adoption

MANITOBA

Central Adoption Registrar
Child Protection Branch
Family Services & Housing
201-114 Garry Street
Winnipeg, Manitoba R3C 4V5
(204) 945-2983

NEW BRUNSWICK

Family and Community Services
Sartain MacDonald Building
P.O. Box 6000
Fredericton, New Brunswick E3B 5H1
(506) 453-2001
http://www.gnb.ca/0017/index-e.asp

NEWFOUNDLAND AND LABRADOR

Health and Community Services
Department of Health and Community Services
P.O. Box 8700
St. John's, Newfoundland A1B 4J6
http://www.health.gov.nl.ca/health

NORTHWEST TERRITORIES

Department of Health & Social Services Authority
4702 Franklin Avenue
Yellowknife, Northwest Territories X1A 2N5
(887) 873-7276
http://www.yhssa.org

NOVA SCOTIA

Department of Community Services
P.O. Box 695
Halifax, Nova Scotia B3J 2T7
http://www.gov.ns.ca/coms

NUNAVUT

Health & Social Services
(867) 975-5714
http://www.gov.nv.ca/hss.htm

ONTARIO

Ministry of Children and Youth Services Adoption Unit
80 Grosvenor Street, 87th Floor Hepburn Block
Toronto, Ontario M7A 1E9
(416) 327-4742
http://www.children.gov.on.ca/CS/en/programs/Adoption

PRINCE EDWARD ISLAND

Health and Social Services
Second Floor, Jones Building
11 Kent Street
P.O. Box 2000
Charlottetown, Prince Edward Island CIA 7N8
(902) 368-4900
http://www.gov.pe.ca/hss

QUEBEC

Secrétariat à l'adoption internationale
201, boulevard Crémazie Est, bureau 1.01
Montreal, Quebec H2M 1L2
(514) 873-5226
http://www.adoption.gouv.qc.ca/site/fr_contact.phtml

SASKATCHEWAN

**Saskatchewan Community Resources and
Development**
12th Floor, 1920 Broad Street
Regina, Saskatchewan S4P 3V6
(306) 787-5698

YUKON

Health and Social Services
Government of Yukon
Box 273
Whitehorse, Yukon Y1A 2C6
(867) 667-3673
http://www.hss.gov.yk.ca

APPENDIX III
ADOPTION-RELATED ORGANIZATIONS

Adoption Exchange Association
8015 Corporate Drive, Suite C
Baltimore, MD 21236
(410) 933-5700
http://www.adoptea.org

The ALMA Society
P.O. Box 85
Denville, NJ 07834
(973) 586-1358
http://www.almasociety.org

American Academy of Adoption Attorneys
P.O. Box 33053
Washington, DC 20033-0053
(202) 832-2222
http://www.adoptionattorneys.org

American Academy of Child and Adolescent Psychiatry
3615 Wisconsin Avenue NW
Washington, DC 20016
(202) 966-7300
http://www.aacap.org

American Academy of Pediatrics
141 Northwest Point Boulevard
Elk Grove Village, IL 60007-1098
(847) 434-4000
http://www.aap.org

American Adoption Congress
P.O. Box 42730
Washington, DC 20015
(800) 888-7970 or (202) 483-3399
http://www.americanadoptioncongress.org

American Bar Association
321 Clark Street
Chicago, IL 60610
(312) 988-5000
http://www.abanet.org

American Foster Care Resources, Inc.
P.O. Box 271
King George, VA 22485
(540) 775-7410
http://www.afcr.com

American Medical Association
515 North State Street
Chicago, IL 60610
(312) 464-5000
http://www.ama-assn.org

American Psychiatric Association
1000 Wilson Boulevard, Suite 1825
Arlington, VA 22209-3901
(703) 907-7300
http://www.psych.org

American Psychological Association
750 First Street NE
Washington, DC 20002
(202) 336-5500
http://www.apa.org

American Public Human Services Association
810 First Street NE, Suite 500
Washington, DC 20002
(202) 682-0100
http://www.aphsa.org

American Society for Reproductive Medicine
1209 Montgomery Highway
Birmingham, AL 35216
(205) 978-5000
http://www.asrm.org

American Society of Human Genetics
9650 Rockville Pike
Bethesda, MD 20814
(301) 571-1825
http://www.ashg.org

Association of Administrators of the Interstate Compact for the Placement of Children (ICPC)
American Public Human Services Association
810 First Street NE, Suite 500
Washington, DC 20002
(202) 682-0100
http://icpc.aphsa.org

Association of Administrators of the Interstate Compact on Adoption and Medical Assistance (AAICAMA)
American Public Human Services Association
810 First Street NE, Suite 500
Washington, DC 20002
(202) 682-0100
http://aaicama.aphsa.org

Association of Jewish Family & Children's Agencies
620 Cranbury Road, Suite 102
East Brunswick, NJ 08816
(800) 634-7346
http://www.ajfca.org

Black Administrators in Child Welfare, Inc.
440 First Street NW, 3rd Floor
Washington, DC 20001
(202) 662-4284
http://www.blackadministrators.org

Catholic Charities USA
1731 King Street, Suite 200
Alexandria, VA 22314
(703) 549-1390
http://www.catholiccharitiesusa.org

Centers for Disease Control and Prevention (CDC)
1600 Clifton Road
Atlanta, GA 30333
(404) 639-3311
http://www.cdc.gov

Children Awaiting Parents, Inc.
595 Blossom Road, Suite 306
Rochester, NY 14610
(888) 835-8802
http://www.capbook.org

Child Welfare League of America
440 First Street NW, 3rd Floor
Washington, DC 20001
(202) 638-2952
http://www.cwla.org

Concerned United Birthparents, Inc.
P.O. Box 503475
San Diego, CA 92150-3475
(800) 822-2777
http://www.cubirthparents.org

Council on Accreditation of Services for Families and Children, Inc.
The Association Center
120 Wall Street, 11th Floor
New York, NY 10005
(212) 797-3000
http://www.coanet.org

Dave Thomas Foundation for Adoption
4150 Tuller Road, Suite 204
Dublin, OH 43017
(800) 275-3832
http://www.davethomasfoundationforadoption.org

Evan B. Donaldson Adoption Institute
525 Broadway, 6th Floor
New York, NY 10012
(212) 925-4089
http://www.adoptioninstitute.org

Hepatitis Foundation International
504 Blick Drive
Silver Spring, MD 20904
(800) 891-0707
http://www.hepfi.org

Institute for Black Parenting
1299 East Artesia Boulevard
Carson, CA 90746
(310) 900-0930
http://www.instforblackparenting.org

International Soundex Reunion Registry
P.O. Box 2312
Carson City, NV 89702-2312
(775) 882-7755
http://www.isrr.net

Joint Council of International Children's Services
117 South Saint Asaph Street
Alexandria, VA 22314
(703) 535-8045
http://www.jcics.org

Learning Disabilities Association of America
4156 Library Road
Pittsburgh, PA 15234

(412) 341-1515
http://www.ldanatl.org

National Adoption Center
1500 Walnut Street, Suite 701
Philadelphia, PA 19102
(800) 862-3678
http://www.adopt.org

National Adoption Information Clearinghouse
330 C Street, SW
Washington, DC 20447
(703) 352-3488
http://naic.acf.hhs.gov

National Association of Social Workers
750 First Street NE, Suite 700
Washington, DC 20002
(202) 408-8600
http://www.naswdc.org

National Black Child Development Institute
1101 15th Street NW, Suite 900
Washington, DC 22005
(202) 833-2220
http://www.nbcdi.org

National Center for Adoption Law and Policy
Capital University Law School
303 East Broad Street
Columbus, OH 43215
(614) 236-6730
http://www.ncalp.org

National Clearinghouse for Alcohol and Drug Information
11426 Rockville Pike, Suite 200
Rockville, MD 20852
(800) 729-6686
http://www.health.org

National Conference of Commissioners on Uniform State Laws
211 East Ontario Street, Suite 1300
Chicago, IL 60611
(312) 915-0195
http://www.nccusl.org

National Conference of State Legislatures
7700 East First Place
Denver, CO 80230

(303) 364-7700
http://www.ncsl.org

National Council for Adoption
225 North Washington Street
Alexandria, VA 22314
(703) 299-6633
http://www.adoptioncouncil.org

National Dissemination Center for Children and Youth with Disabilities
P.O. Box 192
Washington, DC 20013
http://www.nichcy.org

National Foster Parent Association
7512 Stanich Avenue, Suite 6
Gig Harbor, WA 98335
(253) 853-4000
http://www.nfpainc.org

National Institute of Mental Health
Public Inquiries
6001 Executive Boulevard
Room 8184, MSC 9663
Bethesda, MD 20892
(301) 443-4513
http://www.nimh.nih.gov

National Resource Center for Special Needs Adoption
16250 Northland Drive, Suite 120
Southfield, MI 48075
(248) 443-0306
http://www.nrcadoption.org

North American Council on Adoptable Children (NACAC)
970 Raymond Avenue, Suite 106
St. Paul, MN 55114
(651) 644-3036
http://www.nacac.org

U.S. Department of Health and Human Services, Administration for Children and Families (ACF/HHS)
370 L'Enfant Promenade SW
Washington, DC 20201
(877) 696-6675
http://www.acf.hhs.gov

APPENDIX IV
STATE LAWS IN THE UNITED STATES ON PLACEMENT OF CHILDREN WITH RELATIVES FOR ADOPTION

Note: This appendix applies to the adoption of children by relatives. Some children are in state custody, while in other cases children have been left in the care of relatives. In some cases, parents voluntarily place the child for adoption directly with relatives.

Some states include "degrees" of kinship in their laws when defining the relationship of a child to a prospective caretaker relative, and may refer to first, second, third, and fourth degrees or even fifth degrees of kinship. In most cases, the relationship may be by "blood," (genetic/biological) or be formed by marriage or adoption.

A first-degree relative of a child is the parent, while a second-degree relative is a grandparent or sibling. (The sibling must be an adult in order to be a caretaker relative of a minor child.) Third-degree relatives include great-grandparents, uncles and aunts, and nieces and nephews. Fourth-degree relatives are great-great grandparents, great-uncles and great-aunts, and first cousins. Fifth-degree relatives are great-great-great grandparents, great-great uncles and great-great aunts, or first cousins once removed. (A first cousin once removed is the child of a first cousin).

ALABAMA

Relative(s) Who May Adopt: Grandparents, great-grandparents, great-uncle or great-aunt, siblings, half-siblings, aunts or uncles of the first degree, and their respective spouses

Requirements for Adoption by Relatives:

- The adopted person must reside for one year with the relative. The court may waive this provision.

- The relative is exempt from the preplacement investigation (including a criminal background investigation) unless one is requested by the court.

- No report of fees or charges is required, unless ordered by the court.

ALASKA

Relative(s) Who May Adopt: Not addressed in statutes reviewed

Requirements for Adoption by Relatives: Not addressed in statutes reviewed

ARIZONA

Relative(s) Who May Adopt: Not addressed in statutes reviewed

Requirements for Adoption by Relatives: Not addressed in statutes reviewed

ARKANSAS

Relative(s) Who May Adopt: In all custodial placements by the Department of Human Services, preferential consideration shall be given to an adult relative over a nonrelated caregiver.

Requirements for Adoption by Relatives:

- The relative must meet all relevant child protection standards.

- A criminal background check must be performed on all household members age 16 years and older.

- A child abuse registry check must be performed on all household members age 10 years and older.

- The placement must be in the child's best interest.

CALIFORNIA

Relative(s) Who May Adopt:

- A relative is an adult who is related to the child or the child's half-sibling, or the spouse of any relative, even if the marriage was terminated.
- A relative is an adult who is related to the child or the child's half-sibling by blood or affinity, including all relatives whose status is preceded by the words "step," "great," "great-great" or "grand," or the spouse of any of these persons, even if the marriage was terminated by death or dissolution.

Requirements for Adoption by Relatives:

- The relative must have an ongoing and significant relationship with the child.
- A home study or assessment must be conducted that includes:
  - A determination of the financial stability of the relative
  - A determination that the relative can address any racial or cultural issues that may affect the child's well-being
  - A determination that the relative has not abused or neglected the child or will likely abuse or neglect the child in the future
- A criminal records check must be conducted.
- A report of a medical examination and testing for tuberculosis shall be included in the assessment.

COLORADO

Relative(s) Who May Adopt: A kinship adoption refers to the adoption of a child by a grandparent, brother, sister, half-sibling, aunt, uncle, or first cousin and the spouses of such relatives.

Requirements for Adoption by Relatives:

- The relative is eligible to adopt the child if he or she has had physical custody of the child for a period of one year or more.
- The adoption petition shall contain a statement informing the court whether the relative was ever convicted of a felony or misdemeanor in one of the following areas:

- Child abuse or neglect
- Spousal abuse
- Any crime against a child
- Domestic violence, violation of a protection order, any crime involving violence, rape, sexual assault, or homicide
- Any felony physical assault or battery

- The relative must undergo a criminal background check.
- In the petition, the relative shall state that he or she has consulted with the appropriate departments to determine eligibility for Temporary Aid to Needy Families (TANF), Medicaid, and subsidized adoption.

CONNECTICUT

Relative(s) Who May Adopt: Not addressed in statutes reviewed

Requirements for Adoption by Relatives: Not addressed in statutes reviewed

DELAWARE

Relative(s) Who May Adopt: Family members by blood, marriage, or adoption, including grandparents, brothers, sisters, half-siblings, aunts, uncles, first cousins, great-grandparents, step-grandparents, great-aunts, and great-uncles, may adopt the child.

Requirements for Adoption by Relatives:

- A social study shall be completed that includes information regarding the background of the child, the adoptive parents and their home, the physical and mental condition of the child, and the suitability of the placement.
- The petition shall be filed only after the child has resided in the home of the petitioner for at least one year.
- The child does not have to be legally free prior to the filing of the adoption petition.

DISTRICT OF COLUMBIA

Relative(s) Who May Adopt: Not addressed in statutes reviewed

Requirements for Adoption by Relatives: Not addressed in statutes reviewed

FLORIDA

Relative(s) Who May Adopt: A child's grand-parent has the right to petition to adopt the child.
Requirements for Adoption by Relatives:

- The child must have lived with the grandparent for at least 6 months within the 24-month period immediately preceding the filing of a petition for termination of parental rights.

- This section shall not apply if the placement for adoption is a result of the death of the child's parent and a different preference is stated in the parent's will.

- This section shall not apply to stepparent adoptions.

GEORGIA

Relative(s) Who May Adopt: A child may be adopted by a relative who is related by blood or marriage to the child as a grandparent, aunt, uncle, great-aunt, great-uncle, or sibling and any spouse of such relatives.
Requirements for Adoption by Relatives:

- Adoption may occur after the voluntary surrender in writing of all rights to the child by the parent or guardian. The child, if age 14 or older must consent to the adoption.

HAWAII

Relative(s) Who May Adopt: Not addressed in statutes reviewed
Requirements for Adoption by Relatives: Not addressed in statues reviewed

IDAHO

Relative(s) Who May Adopt: Not addressed in statues reviewed
Requirements for Adoption by Relatives: Not addressed in statutes reviewed

ILLINOIS

Relative(s) Who May Adopt:

- A relative is any person, 21 years of age or older, who is related to the child by blood or adoption such as a grandparent, sibling, great-grandparent, uncle, aunt, nephew, niece, first cousin, sec-ond cousin, godparent, great-aunt, great-uncle, and the spouse of any such relative.

- A relative may also include a stepparent or adult stepbrother or stepsister.

Requirements for Adoption by Relatives:

- The relative must have the ability to adequately provide for the child's safety and welfare.

- A criminal record check and history of child abuse check are required of all members of the household.

INDIANA

Relative(s) Who May Adopt: Not addressed in statutes reviewed
Requirements for Adoption by Relatives: Not addressed in statutes reviewed

IOWA

Relative(s) Who May Adopt: A relative within the fourth degree of relationship may adopt the child.
Requirements for Adoption by Relatives:

- If a relative within the fourth degree assumes custody, a preplacement investigation may be completed at a time established by the juvenile court or may be waived.

- A criminal background and child abuse and neglect history check are required.

KANSAS

Relative(s) Who May Adopt: When making a placement for adoption, preference may be given first to a relative of the child, and second to a person with whom the child has close emotional ties.
Requirements for Adoption by Relatives:

- The relative must be willing and be a reputable person of good moral character.

- The placement must be in the best interest of the child.

KENTUCKY

Relative(s) Who May Adopt: A relative is a person related to the child through blood, marriage, or adoption, including a stepparent, grandparent, sister, brother, aunt, or uncle.

Requirements for Adoption by Relatives:

- The adoption of a child by a relative does not require placement by an agency or the permission of the Secretary as other adoptions do.
- Before a child can be placed in the home the Secretary will require a criminal background check.

LOUISIANA

Relative(s) Who May Adopt: A stepparent, step-grandparent, great-grandparent, grandparent, aunt, great-aunt, uncle, great-uncle, sibling, or first cousin may petition to adopt the child.

Requirements for Adoption by Relatives:

- The relative wishing to adopt must meet all the following conditions:
  - The petitioner must be related to the child by blood, adoption, or affinity through a parent having parental rights.
  - The petitioner is a single person over age 18 years or a married person whose spouse is a joint petitioner.
  - The petitioner has had legal or physical custody of the child for at least six months prior to filing for adoption.
- The sheriff will conduct a federal and state criminal background check.
- The department will conduct a records check for allegations of child abuse or neglect.
- A home study is not required unless the court orders one.

MAINE

Relative(s) Who May Adopt: A relative may petition to adopt the child.

Requirements for Adoption by Relatives:

- If the petitioner is a blood relative of the child, the court may waive the requirement of a home study and report.
- Each petitioner who is not a biological relative must undergo a Federal and State criminal records check that includes a screening for child abuse cases.
- Expense payment limitations do not apply when one of the adoptive parents is a relative.

MARYLAND

Relative(s) Who May Adopt: A relative of the birthparent may adopt the child.

Requirements for Adoption by Relatives: The provision of counseling to the birth mother and accounting of payments in connection with adoption are not applicable in an adoption by a relative.

MASSACHUSETTS

Relative(s) Who May Adopt: A person may adopt another person who is younger than him or herself, unless that person is his or her spouse, sibling, uncle, or aunt.

Requirements for Adoption by Relatives: A review of the criminal offender record information shall be made to assist in evaluating the suitability of the adoptive parent.

MICHIGAN

Relative(s) Who May Adopt: A relative is a person related to the child within the fifth degree through blood, marriage, or adoption. This also includes a stepparent.

Requirements for Adoption by Relatives: Nonidentifying and other relevant information do not need to be provided in adoptions by relatives.

MINNESOTA

Relative(s) Who May Adopt:

- Each authorized child-placing agency shall make special efforts to recruit an adoptive family from among the child's relatives.
- A relative is a person related to the child by blood, marriage, or adoption, or an individual who is an important friend with whom the child has resided or had significant contact.
- For an Indian child, relatives includes members of the extended family as defined by the law or custom of the Indian child's tribe or, in the absence of law or custom, nieces, nephews, or first or second cousins.

Requirements for Adoption by Relatives: Adoptive families should reflect the ethnic and racial diversity of the prospective adoptive child.

MISSISSIPPI

Relative(s) Who May Adopt: A relative is a person related to the child within the third degree, according to civil law.

Requirements for Adoption by Relatives:

- For a child who is in the legal custody of the Department of Human Services, the department may pay the costs of adoption proceedings initiated by relatives if they are unable to pay such costs.
- A 90-day residency requirement does not apply to an adoption by a relative.
- A six-month waiting period for the final decree is not required for an adoption by a relative or a stepparent.

MISSOURI

Relative(s) Who May Adopt: A relative is any grandparent, aunt, uncle, adult sibling of the child, or adult first cousin of the child.

Requirements for Adoption by Relatives: Any subsidies available to adoptive parents shall also be available to the qualified relative of a child who is granted legal guardianship of the child in the same manner as such subsidies are available for adoptive parents.

MONTANA

Relative(s) Who May Adopt: A parent or guardian may make a direct parental placement of his or her child for adoption with an extended family member.

Requirements for Adoption by Relatives: In a direct parental placement, the court may waive the requirement of a preplacement and postplacement evaluation.

NEBRASKA

Relative(s) Who May Adopt: In any adoptive placement of an Indian child under State law, a preference shall be given, in the absence of good cause to the contrary, to a placement with:

- A member of the child's extended family
- Other members of the Indian child's tribe
- Other Indian families

Requirements for Adoption by Relatives: Not addressed in statutes reviewed

NEVADA

Relative(s) Who May Adopt: A relative is a person related to the child through blood, marriage, or adoption within the third degree of relation.

Requirements for Adoption by Relatives: If one petitioner or the spouse of a petitioner is related to the child within the third degree of relation, the court may, at its discretion, waive the preplacement investigation by the agency that provides child welfare services.

NEW HAMPSHIRE

Relative(s) Who May Adopt:

- *Related child* means a child who is related within the second degree of kinship either by blood or affinity.
- Relatives within the second degree include stepparents, sisters, brothers, grandparents, aunts, or uncles.

Requirements for Adoption by Relatives:

- In the adoption of a related minor child, the court may, for good cause shown, proceed to a hearing and a decree without an assessment when both of the following circumstances are met:
  - The parents of the minor child have surrendered their parental rights.
  - The minor child has resided with the petitioners to whom the child is related for at least three years prior to filing the petition for adoption.
- The court shall require a background check in all adoption proceedings if there has not been an assessment. The background check will include both a criminal records check conducted by the New Hampshire State police and a search of the abuse and neglect registry maintained by the department.

NEW JERSEY

Relative(s) Who May Adopt: A child may be placed for adoption with a brother, sister, aunt, uncle, grandparent, birthfather, or stepparent.

Requirements for Adoption by Relatives:

- Whenever a petitioner is a brother, sister, grandparent, aunt, uncle, or birthfather of the child, the order may limit the investigation to an inquiry concerning the status of the parents of the child and an evaluation of the petitioner.

- A home study that includes a State and Federal criminal history records check is required.

NEW MEXICO

Relative(s) Who May Adopt: Any relative within the fifth degree of relation to the adoptee or that relative's spouse may seek to adopt the child.

Requirements for Adoption by Relatives:

- The child must have lived with the relative for at least one year prior to filing of the petition.

- Unless directed by the court, a preplacement study is not required in cases in which a child is being adopted by a stepparent, a relative, or a person named in the child's deceased parent's will.

NEW YORK

Relative(s) Who May Adopt: Subject to relinquishment by a parent, the court shall accept all petitions for the adoption of a child by any relative of the child.

Requirements for Adoption by Relatives: A home study is required.

NORTH CAROLINA

Relative(s) Who May Adopt: A relative, including a grandparent, sibling, first cousin, aunt, uncle, great-aunt, great-uncle, or great-grandparent, may adopt the child.

Requirements for Adoption by Relatives: A pre-placement assessment is not required if the child is placed directly with a relative.

NORTH DAKOTA

Relative(s) Who May Adopt: A relative is any person related to the minor by marriage, blood, or adoption, including a grandparent, brother, sister, stepbrother, stepsister, uncle, or aunt.

Requirements for Adoption by Relatives:

- An investigation and report is not required in cases in which a stepparent is the petitioner or the person to be adopted is an adult.

- The court may waive the home study requirement if the petitioner is a relative other than a stepparent, the minor has lived with the petitioner for at least nine months, and no allegations of abuse or neglect have been filed against the petitioner or any member of the petitioner's household.

OHIO

Relative(s) Who May Adopt: The agency shall consider giving preference to an adult relative over a nonrelative caregiver when determining an adoptive placement for the child.

Requirements for Adoption by Relatives:

- The relative must satisfy all relevant child protection standards.

- The placement must be in the best interests of the child.

OKLAHOMA

Relative(s) Who May Adopt: An adult relative related to a child within the third degree may accept the permanent care and custody of the child.

- A preplacement home study is not required if a minor is directly placed with a relative for purposes of adoption, but a home study of the relative is required during the pendency of a proceeding for adoption.

OREGON

Relative(s) Who May Adopt: Not addressed in statutes reviewed

Requirements for Adoption by Relatives: Not addressed in statutes reviewed

PENNSYLVANIA

Relative(s) Who May Adopt: Not addressed in statutes reviewed

Requirements for Adoption by Relatives: Not addressed in statutes reviewed

RHODE ISLAND

Relative(s) Who May Adopt: Not addressed in statutes reviewed

Requirements for Adoption by Relatives: Not addressed in statutes reviewed

SOUTH CAROLINA

Relative(s) Who May Adopt: Any person may adopt a child who is related by blood or marriage.
Requirements for Adoption by Relatives:

- No investigation or report is required unless otherwise directed by the court.
- No accounting of all disbursement is required unless ordered by the court.

SOUTH DAKOTA

Relative(s) Who May Adopt: Not addressed in statutes reviewed
Requirements for Adoption by Relatives: Not addressed in statutes reviewed

TENNESSEE

Relative(s) Who May Adopt:

- A relative may petition to adopt a child.
- If the child becomes available for adoption while in foster care, the foster parents shall be given first preference to adopt the child if the child has resided in the foster home for 12 or more consecutive months immediately preceding the filing of an adoption petition.

Requirements for Adoption by Relatives:

- In the case of an adoption by relatives, the residency requirement shall not apply if the petitioner is an actual resident of this State at the time the petition is filed.
- In becoming adoptive parents, the foster parents shall meet all requirements otherwise imposed on persons seeking to adopt children in the custody of the department.

TEXAS

Relative(s) Who May Adopt: The following relatives have standing to adopt a child:

- A grandparent
- An aunt or uncle by birth, marriage, or former adoption
- A stepparent

Requirements for Adoption by Relatives:

- The report on health, social, educational, and genetic history of the child is not required.
- The court shall order each person seeking to adopt a child to obtain his or her own criminal history record information. The person must request the information from the Department of Public Safety.

UTAH

Relative(s) Who May Adopt: The following relatives may adopt the child:

- A stepparent
- A sibling or half-sibling by birth or adoption
- A grandparent, aunt, uncle, or first cousin

Requirements for Adoption by Relatives:

- A person adopting a child must be at least 10 years older than the child.
- A preplacement report is not required if the prospective adoptive parent is related to the child as listed above, unless the evaluation is otherwise requested by the court.
- The relative must submit to a criminal background check and to a neglect and/or abuse history check. This requirement is applicable to all adult members of the household.

VERMONT

Relative(s) Who May Adopt:

- A relative is a grandparent, great-grandparent, sibling, first cousin, aunt, uncle, great-aunt, great-uncle, niece, or nephew of a person, whether related to the person by the whole or the half blood, affinity, or adoption.
- The term does not include a person's stepparent.

Requirements for Adoption by Relatives:

- A preplacement evaluation is not required if a parent or guardian places a minor directly with a relative for purposes of adoption, but an evaluation of the relative is required during the pendency of a proceeding for adoption.

- The preplacement evaluation shall indicate whether the person has been:
  - Subject to an abuse prevention order
  - Charged with or convicted of domestic assault
  - The subject of a substantiated complaint filed with the department
  - Subject to a court order restricting the person's right to parental rights and responsibilities or parent-child contact with a child
  - Convicted of a crime other than a minor traffic violation

VIRGINIA

Relative(s) Who May Adopt: The child's grandparent, adult brother or sister, adult uncle or aunt, or adult great-uncle or great-aunt may adopt the child.

Requirements for Adoption by Relatives:

- The court may omit the probationary period and the interlocutory order and enter a final order of adoption when a child has been placed by the birthparent with the prospective adoptive parent who is a relative named above, and the court has accepted the written consent of the birthparent and is of the opinion that the entry of an interlocutory order would otherwise be proper.
- If the court determines the need for an investigation prior to the final order of adoption, it shall refer the matter to the local director or a licensed child-placing agency for an investigation and report that shall be completed within such time as the court designates.

WASHINGTON

Relative(s) Who May Adopt: Not addressed in statutes reviewed

Requirements for Adoption by Relatives: Not addressed in statutes reviewed

WEST VIRGINIA

Relative(s) Who May Adopt: Generally, a relative is a person related to the child through blood, marriage, or adoption.

Requirements for Adoption by Relatives: Not addressed in statutes reviewed

WISCONSIN

Relative(s) Who May Adopt: Relatives include grandparent, great-grandparent, stepparent, brother, sister, first cousin, nephew, niece, uncle, or aunt by blood, marriage, or adoption

Requirements for Adoption by Relatives:

- A parent may place a child in the home of a relative for adoption without a court order.
- If the child's parent has not filed a petition for termination of parental rights, the relative with whom the child is placed shall file a petition for the termination of the parents' rights at the same time the petition for adoption is filed.
- The court may hold the hearing on the adoption petition immediately after entering the court to terminate parental rights.

WYOMING

Relative(s) Who May Adopt: Not addressed in statutes reviewed

Requirements for Adoption by Relatives: Not addressed in statutes reviewed

Source: Adapted from the National Adoption Information Clearinghouse, *State Statutes Series 2005: Placement of Children with Relatives: Summary of State Laws Adoption State Laws.* Washington, D.C.: The Children's Bureau, Administration for Children and Families, U.S. Department of Health and Human Services, 2005. Available online at http://naic.acf.hhs.gov/general/legal/statutes/placementall.pdf. Downloaded on July 30, 2005.

APPENDIX V
INVOLUNTARY TERMINATION OF PARENTAL RIGHTS IN THE UNITED STATES: CIRCUMSTANCES THAT ARE GROUNDS FOR TERMINATION OF PARENTAL RIGHTS

Many states have similar grounds for the involuntary termination of parental rights, such as child abandonment, the murder of another child in the family or of the child's other parent, or the inability of the parent to discharge parental duties due to mental illness, incarceration, or chronic drug or alcohol abuse. Some states terminate the father's parental rights if the child was conceived as a result of rape or incest.

Each state has exceptions to these laws, such as when a child is living with a relative, the child objects to being adopted, and so forth. State laws are subject to change, and an attorney or the state social service office should be able to provide information on the most recent state law.

ALABAMA

- The parent has abandoned the child.
- The parent is unable to discharge his or her parental duties due to:
  - Emotional illness, mental illness, or mental deficiency
  - Use of alcohol or controlled substances
  - A conviction and incarceration for a felony
- The parent has tortured, abused, or severely maltreated the child.
- The parent's conduct or neglect has resulted in serious physical injury to the child.
- The parent has subjected the child to an aggravated circumstance, including, but not limited to, abandonment, torture, chronic abuse, substance abuse, or sexual abuse.
- Reasonable efforts to rehabilitate the parent have failed.
- The parent has been convicted of:
  - Murder or voluntary manslaughter of another child of the parent
  - Aiding, abetting, attempting, or soliciting to commit murder or voluntary manslaughter of another child of the parent
  - A felony assault that resulted in serous bodily injury to the child or another child of the parent
- The parent has failed to support the child when financially able to do so.
- The parent has failed to maintain regular visitation, contact, or communication with the child.
- Parental rights to another child have been involuntarily terminated.

ALASKA

- The parent has abandoned the child.
- The parent is unable to discharge his or her parental duties due to:
  - Emotional illness, mental illness, or mental deficiency
  - Use of alcohol or controlled substances
  - A conviction and incarceration for a felony
- The parent has subjected the child to circumstances that pose a substantial risk of harm,

including, but not limited to, abandonment, torture, chronic mental injury, chronic physical harm, or sexual abuse.

- The parent's conduct or neglect has resulted in serious physical or mental injury to the child.

- When the child has been in foster care for 15 of the most recent 22 months, and reasonable effort to rehabilitate the parent have failed

- The parent has been convicted of:
  - Homicide of a parent of the child or a child
  - Aiding, abetting, attempting, or soliciting to commit a homicide of a parent of the child or a child
  - A felony assault that resulted in serious bodily injury to a child

- The child has been sexually abused as a result of the parent's conduct or failure to protect the child.

- The parent has willfully failed to provide the child with needed medical treatment.

- The child has committed an illegal act as a result of pressure, guidance, or approval from the parent.

- Parental rights to another child of the parent have been involuntarily terminated, and conditions that led to the termination have not been corrected.

ARIZONA

- The parent has abandoned the child.

- The identity of the parent is unknown even after diligent efforts to identify and locate the parent.

- The parent is unable to discharge his or her parental duties due to:
  - Emotional illness, mental illness, or mental deficiency
  - Chronic abuse of dangerous drugs, alcohol, or controlled substances
  - A conviction and incarceration for a felony

- The parent has neglected or willfully abused the child.

- The parent's conduct or neglect has resulted in serious physical or emotional injury to the child.

- The child has been in out-of-home placement for a total of nine months, and the parent has refused to participate in services that could remedy the circumstances the caused the placement.

- The child has been in out-of-home placement for a total of 15 months, and the parent has participated in services but has been unable to remedy the circumstances that cause the placement.

- The parent has been convicted of:
  - Murder or manslaughter of another child of the parent
  - Sexual abuse, sexual assault of a child, sexual conduct with a minor, or molestation of a child
  - Commercial sexual exploitation of a minor, sexual exploitation of a minor, or luring a minor for sexual exploitation
  - Aiding, abetting, attempting, or soliciting to commit murder or manslaughter or any of the crimes listed above

- A putative father has failed to establish paternity or respond to notice.

- Parental rights to another child of the parent have been involuntarily terminated within the preceding two years, and conditions that led to the termination have not been corrected.

ARKANSAS

- The parent has abandoned the child.

- The parent is unable to discharge his or her parental duties due to:
  - Emotional illness, mental illness, or mental deficiency
  - A conviction and incarceration for a felony

- The parent has neglected or willfully abused the child.

- The parent's conduct or neglect has resulted in serious physical or emotional injury to the child.

- The child has been out of the parent's custody for 12 months, and reasonable efforts to rehabilitate the parent have failed.

- The parent has been convicted of:
  - Murder or voluntary manslaughter of any child
  - Aiding, abetting, attempting, or soliciting to commit murder or voluntary manslaughter of any child
  - A felony battery of assault that results in serious bodily injury to any child

- The parent has subjected the child to aggravated circumstances, which can mean:

- The child has been abandoned, chronically abused, subjected to extreme or repeated cruelty, or sexually abused.
- A judge has determined that there is little likelihood that services to the family will result in successful reunification.
- The child has been removed from the custody of the parent more than three times in the last 15 months.
- The parent has willfully failed to provide significant material support in accordance with the parent's means.
- The parent has failed to maintain meaningful contact with the child. A presumptive legal father is not the biological father of the child.
- Parental rights to another child of the parent have been terminated involuntarily.

CALIFORNIA

- The parent has abandoned the child.
- The parent is unable to discharge his or her parental duties due to:
  - Mental disability
  - Extensive, abusive, and chronic use of alcohol or drugs
  - Incarceration or institutionalization
- The parent has physically or sexually abused the child.
- The parent's conduct or neglect has resulted in serous physical injury to the child.
- The parent has refused reunification services.
- The parent has been convicted of a violent felony, indicating parental unfitness.
- The child has been left without any provision for his or her support.
- The parent has failed to visit or contact the child for six months.
- The whereabouts of the parent have been unknown for six months.
- Parental right to another child of the parent have been involuntarily terminated.
- The parent has caused the death of another child through abuse or neglect.
- The parent has subjected the child to severe or repeated sexual or physical abuse.

- The child was conceived as a result of a sexual offense against a child.
- The parent willfully abandoned the child, and the abandonment itself constituted a serious danger to the child.

COLORADO

- The parent has abandoned the child.
- The parent has been found to be unfit due to:
  - Emotional illness, mental illness, or mental deficiency
  - A single incident of serious bodily injury or disfigurement to the child
  - Use of alcohol or controlled substances
  - Long-term incarceration
- The parent has caused serious bodily injury or death to a sibling of the child due to abuse or neglect.
- The parent's conduct or neglect has resulted in grave risk of death or serious physical injury to the child.
- The parent has subjected the child to an aggravated circumstance, including, but not limited to, abandonment, torture, chronic abuse, substance abuse, or sexual abuse.
- Reasonable efforts to rehabilitate the parent have failed, or the parent has failed to reasonably comply with a treatment plan.
- The parent has been convicted of:
  - Murder or voluntary manslaughter of another child of the parent
  - Aiding, abetting, attempting, or soliciting to commit murder or voluntary manslaughter of another child of the parent
  - A felony assault that resulted in serious bodily injury to the child or another child of the parent
- The parent has neglected the child, and is unable or unwilling to provide nurturing and safe parenting.
- The parent has failed to maintain regular visitation with the child.
- Parental rights to another child of the parent have been involuntarily terminated, unless the prior sibling termination resulted from a parent delivering the child to a firefighter or hospital, pursuant to the provisions of § 19-3-304.5.

CONNECTICUT

- The parent has abandoned the child.
- The parent has inflicted sexual abuse, sexual exploitation, or severe physical abuse on the child, or has engaged in a pattern of abuse of the child.
- The parent is unable or unwilling to benefit from reunification efforts.
- The parent was convicted of a sexual assault that resulted in the conception of a child. The court may terminate the rights of the parent to such child at any time after the conviction.
- A court has found that the parent has:
  - Killed, through a deliberate, nonaccidental act, a sibling of the child
  - Requested, attempted, conspired, or solicited to commit the killing of the child or a sibling of the child
  - Assaulted the child or sibling of the child, and such assault resulted in serious bodily injury to the child
- The parent has failed to maintain a reasonable degree of interest, concern, or responsibility as to the welfare of the child.
- Parental rights to another child of the parent have been involuntarily terminated.

DELAWARE

- The parent has abandoned the child.
- The parent has abandoned a baby in accordance with Tit. 16 § 907A and failed to manifest an intent to exercise parental rights within 30 days.
- The parent is unable to discharge his or her parental duties due to:
  - Mental incompetence
  - Extended or repeated incarceration
- The parent's conduct or neglect has resulted in serious physical injury to the child.
- The parent has subjected the child to torture, chronic abuse, sexual abuse, or life-threatening abuse.
- Reasonable effort to rehabilitate the parent have failed.
- The parent has been convicted of
  - A felony-level offense against the person, and the victim was the child or any other child

- Aiding, abetting, attempting, or soliciting the commission of such offense
- The offense of dealing in children
- The felony-level offense of endangering children
- The parent has failed to support the child when financially able to do so.
- The parent has failed to maintain regular visitation, contact, or communication with the child.
- Parental rights to another child of the parent have been involuntarily terminated.

DISTRICT OF COLUMBIA

- The parent has abandoned the child.
- Drug-related activity continues to exist in the child's home environment after intervention and services have been provided.
- The parent has been convicted of:
  - Murder or voluntary manslaughter of a child sibling or another child
  - Aiding, abetting, attempting, or soliciting to commit such murder or voluntary manslaughter
  - A felony assault that has resulted in serious bodily injury to the child, a child sibling, or another child
- The child has been subjected to intentional and severe mental abuse.
- Parental rights to another child of the parent have been involuntarily terminated.

FLORIDA

- The parent has abandoned the child.
- The parent is unable to discharge his or her parental duties due to extended incarceration or there has been a finding that the parent is a:
  - Violent career criminal
  - Habitual violent felony offender
  - Sexual predator
- The parent has subjected the child to egregious conduct, including abuse, abandonment, or neglect that is flagrant or outrageous by a normal standard of conduct.
- The parent has subjected the child to an aggravated child abuse, as defined in § 827.03, that includes sexual battery, sexual abuse, or chronic abuse.

- Reasonable efforts to rehabilitate the parent have failed.
- The parent has been convicted of:
  - Murder or voluntary manslaughter of another child of the parent
  - Aiding, abetting, attempting, or soliciting to commit murder or voluntary manslaughter of another child of the parent
  - A felony assault that resulted in serious bodily injury to the child or another child of the parent
- Parental rights to another child of the parent have been involuntarily terminated.

GEORGIA

- The parent has abandoned the child.
- The parent is unable to discharge his or her parental duties due to:
  - A medically verifiable deficiency of his or her physical, mental, or emotional health
  - Excessive or chronic use of alcohol or controlled substances
  - A conviction and incarceration for a felony
- The parent has physically, mentally, or emotionally neglected the child, or there has been past neglect of the child or another child.
- The parent's conduct or neglect has resulted in serious physical injury to the child or in the injury or death of a sibling.
- The parent has subjected the child to egregious conduct, or there has been past egregious conduct toward the child or another child, of a physically, emotionally, or sexually cruel or abusive nature.
- Reasonable efforts to rehabilitate the parent have failed.
- The parent has been convicted of:
  - Murder or voluntary manslaughter of another child of the parent or the child's other parent
  - Aiding, abetting, attempting, or soliciting to commit murder or voluntary manslaughter of another child of the parent or the child's other parent
  - A felony assault that results in serous bodily injury to the child or another child of the parent
- The parent has failed to comply with a court order to support the child for a period of 12 months or longer.

- The parent has failed to develop and maintain a parental bond with the child in a meaningful, supportive manner.
- The child has been in foster care for 15 of the the past 22 months.
- Parental rights to another child of the parent have been involuntarily terminated.

HAWAII

- The parent has abandoned the child.
- The parent is unable to discharge his or her parental duties due to mental illness or mental deficiency.
- The parent has tortured the child.
- The parent has subjected the child to an aggravated circumstance.
- Reasonable efforts to rehabilitate the parent have failed.
- The parent has been convicted of:
  - Murder or voluntary manslaughter of another child of the parent
  - Aiding, abetting, attempting, or soliciting to commit murder or voluntary manslaughter of another child of the parent
  - A felony assault that resulted in serious bodily injury to the child or another child of the parent
- The parent has failed to provide care and support for the child for at least one year.
- The parent has failed to communicate with the child for at least one year.
- The parent has voluntarily surrendered care and custody of the child to another person for at least two years.
- The parent is not the child's natural or adoptive father.
- Parental rights to another child of the parent have been involuntarily terminated.

IDAHO

- The parent has abandoned the child.
- The parent is unable to discharge his or her parental duties, and such inability will continue for a prolonged, indeterminate period.
- The parent has been incarcerated with no possibility of parole.

- The parent has abused or neglected the child.

- The parent has caused the child to be conceived as a result of rape, incest, lewd conduct with a minor under 16 years of age, or sexual abuse of a child under the age of 16 years.

- The parent has subjected the child to an aggravated circumstance, including, but not limited to, abandonment, torture, chronic abuse, or sexual abuse.

- Reasonable efforts to rehabilitate the parent have failed.

- The parent has been convicted of:
  - Murder or voluntary manslaughter of another child of the parent or the child's other parent
  - Aiding, abetting, attempting, or soliciting to commit murder or voluntary manslaughter of another child of the parent or the child's other parent
  - A felony assault that resulted in serious bodily injury to the child or another child of the parent

- The presumptive parent is not the natural parent of the child.

- The parent has failed to maintain a relationship with the child for a period of one year.

- Parental rights to another child of the parent have been involuntarily terminated.

ILLINOIS

- The parent has abandoned the child.

- The parent is unable to discharge his or parental duties due to:
  - Mental illness, mental deficiency, or developmental disability
  - A conviction and incarceration for a felony

- The parent has substantially and continuously or repeatedly neglected the child.

- The parent has been found, two or more times, to have physically abused any child, or to have caused the death of any child by physical child abuse.

- The parent has subjected the child to an aggravated circumstance, including, but not limited to, abandonment, torture, or chronic abuse.

- Reasonable efforts to rehabilitate the parent have failed.

- A child was born exposed to controlled substances, and a substance-exposed child was previously born to the same mother.

- The parent has been convicted of:
  - Murder or voluntary manslaughter of any child
  - Aiding, abetting, attempting, or soliciting to commit murder or voluntary manslaughter of any child
  - Aggravated battery or felony domestic battery that has resulted in serious bodily injury to any child
  - Aggravated criminal sexual assault

- The parent has repeatedly and continuously failed to provide the child with adequate food, clothing, and shelter, although financially able to do so.

- The parent has failed to maintain regular visitation, contact, or communication with the child for a period of 12 months.

- A putative father has failed to establish paternity.

- A child has been in foster care for 15 of the most recent 22 months.

- Parental rights to another child of the parent have been involuntarily terminated.

INDIANA

- The parent has abandoned the child.

- The parent has been convicted of:
  - Causing a suicide, involuntary manslaughter, rape, criminal deviate conduct, child molesting, exploitation, or incest, and the victim is a child of the parent or the parent of the child
  - Murder or voluntary manslaughter of another child of the parent or a parent of the child
  - Aiding, abetting, attempting, or soliciting to commit any of the above offenses
  - Battery, aggravated battery, criminal recklessness, or neglect of a dependent against the child or another child of the parent

- The child has been in foster care for 15 of the most recent 22 months.

- Parental rights to another child of the parent have been involuntarily terminated.

IOWA

- The parent has abandoned the child.

- The child is a newborn infant who was relinquished in accordance with chapter 232B.

- The child has been in foster care for 15 of the most recent 22 months.

- The parent is unable to discharge his or her parental duties due to:
  - Chronic mental illness
  - Severe, chronic substance abuse problems
  - A conviction and incarceration for a crime against a child and it is unlikely that the parent will be released for a period of five years or longer
  - A conviction and incarceration for physically or sexually abusing or neglecting the child or any child in the household

- The parent's conduct or omissions has resulted in the physical or sexual abuse or neglect of the child.

- The parent has been convicted of:
  - Child endangerment resulting in the death of the child's sibling
  - Three or more acts of child endangerment involving the child, a sibling, or another child in the household
  - Child endangerment resulting in serious injury to the child, a sibling, or another child in the household
  - Murder or voluntary manslaughter of another child of the parent
  - Aiding, abetting, attempting, or soliciting to commit murder or voluntary manslaughter of another child of the parent
  - A felony assault that results in serious bodily injury to the child or another child of the parent

- The parent has subjected the child to aggravated circumstances.

- Reasonable efforts to rehabilitate the parent have failed.

- The parent has failed to maintain significant and meaningful contact with the child for a period of six consecutive months.

- Parental rights to another child of the parent have been involuntarily terminated, and there is evidence that the parent continues to lack the ability or willingness to respond to services.

KANSAS

- The parent is unfit by reason of conduct or condition.

- The parent has abandoned the child.

- The parent is unable to discharge his or her parental duties due to:
  - Emotional illness, mental illness, mental deficiency, or physical disability
  - Excessive use of alcohol, narcotics, or dangerous drugs
  - A conviction and incarceration for a felony

- There has been an unexplained injury or death of another child or stepchild of the parent.

- The parent has physically, mentally, or emotionally neglected the child.

- The parent has subjected the child or another child to aggravated circumstances, including, but not limited to, abandonment, torture, chronic abuse, sexual abuse, or chronic, life-threatening neglect.

- Reasonable efforts to rehabilitate the parent have failed.

- The parent has been convicted of:
  - Murder or voluntary manslaughter of another child of the parent or the other parent of the child
  - Aiding, abetting, attempting, or soliciting to commit murder or voluntary manslaughter of another child of the parent or the other parent of the child
  - A felony assault that results in serious bodily injury to the child or another child of the parent

- The parent has failed to pay a reasonable portion of the cost of substitute care for the child when financially able to do so.

- The parent has failed to assume care of the child in the home when able to do so.

- The parent has failed to maintain regular visitation, contact, or communication with the child.

- Parental rights to another child of the parent have been involuntarily terminated.

KENTUCKY

- The parent has abandoned the child for a period of not less than 90 days.

- The parent is unable to discharge his or her parental duties due to:
  - Mental illness or mental retardation
  - Alcohol or other drug abuse

- The parent has inflicted or allowed to be inflicted upon the child, by other than accidental means, serious physical injury.

- The parent has continuously or repeatedly inflicted or allowed to be inflicted upon any child physical abuse, sexual abuse, neglect, or emotional injury, and such injury to the child named in the petition is likely to occur if parental rights are not terminated.

- The parent has subjected the child to aggravated circumstances, including one or more of the following:
  - The parent has not had or attempted contact with the child for a period of not less than 90 days.
  - The parent is incarcerated and will be unavailable to care for the child for at least one year.
  - The parent has sexually abused the child and refused available treatment.
  - The parent has engaged in abuse of the child that required removal from the home two or more times in the past two years.
  - The parent has caused serious physical injury.

- Reasonable efforts to rehabilitate the parent have failed.

- The parent has been convicted of:
  - In a criminal proceeding of having caused or contributed to the death of a child as a result of physical abuse, sexual abuse, or neglect
  - Committing a felony assault that resulted in serious bodily injury to the child or another child of the parent

- The parent has failed to provide essential food, clothing, shelter, medical care, or education to the child when financially able to do so.

- The child has been in foster care for 15 of the most recent 22 months.

- Parental rights to another child of the parent have been involuntarily terminated.

LOUISIANA

- The parent has abandoned the child.

- The parent has been incarcerated for an extended period of time and is unwilling or unable to provide care other than foster care for the child.

- The parent has subjected the child to abuse that is chronic, life threatening, or results in gravely disabling physical or psychological injury or disfigurement.

- The parent has subjected the child to sexual abuse.

- The parent has subjected the child or any other child in the household to egregious conduct or conditions, including but not limited to, extreme abuse, cruel and inhuman treatment, or grossly negligent behavior below a reasonable standard of human decency.

- Reasonable efforts to rehabilitate the parent have failed.

- The parent has been convicted of:
  - Murder or voluntary manslaughter of another child of the parent
  - Murder or unjustified intentional killing of the child's other parent
  - A felony that has resulted in serous bodily injury to the child or another child of the parent
  - Rape, sodomy, aggravated incest, torture, or starvation
  - Aiding, abetting, attempting, or soliciting to commit any of the above crimes

- The parent has failed to provide significant contributions to the care and support of the child for any period of six consecutive months.

- The parent has failed to maintain regular visitation, contact, or communication with the child for any period of six consecutive months.

- The parent has committed a felony rape that resulted in the conception of a child.

- The parent has relinquished a newborn infant in accordance with the law.

- Parental rights to another child of the parent have been involuntarily terminated.

MAINE

- The parent has abandoned the child.

- The parent is unable to discharge his or her parental duties due to a chronic substance abuse problem.

- The parent has subjected the child to aggravated circumstances, including but not limited to, rape, gross sexual conduct or assault, sexual abuse, incest, aggravated assault, kidnapping, promotion of prostitution, abandonment, torture, chronic abuse, or any other treatment that is heinous or abhorrent to society.

- Reasonable efforts to rehabilitate the parent have failed.

- The parent has been convicted of any of the following crimes, and the victim was any child in the parent's household:
  - Murder, felony murder, or manslaughter
  - Aiding, conspiring, or soliciting to commit murder or manslaughter
  - A felony assault that results in serious bodily injury

- The parent has failed to take responsibility for the child within a reasonable period of time.

- Parental rights to another child of the parent have been involuntarily terminated.

MARYLAND

- The parent has abandoned the child.

- The parent has a disability that renders the parent consistently unable to care for the child for long period of time.

- The parent has subjected the child to torture, chronic abuse, sexual abuse, or chronic and life-threatening neglect.

- The child was born exposed to cocaine, heroin, or a derivative thereof.

- The parent has committed acts of abuse or neglect toward any child in the family.

- Reasonable efforts to rehabilitate the parent have failed.

- The parent has been convicted of:
  - A crime of violence, as defined in § 14-101 of the Criminal Law article, against the child, another child of the family, or any person who resides in the household
  - Aiding, abetting, conspiring, or soliciting to a crime described above

- The child has been in foster care for 15 of the most recent 22 months.

MASSACHUSETTS

- The parent has abandoned the child.

- The parent is unable to discharge his or her parental duties due to:
  - Mental illness or deficiency
  - Alcohol or drug addiction
  - Incarceration for extended period of time

- The parent has subjected the child to aggravated circumstances, including, but not limited to, sexual abuse or exploitation, or severe or repetitive conduct of a physically or emotionally abusive nature.

- Reasonable efforts to rehabilitate the parent have failed.

- The parent has been convicted of:
  - Murder or voluntary manslaughter of another child of the parent
  - Aiding, abetting, attempting, or soliciting to commit murder or voluntary manslaughter of another child of the parent
  - A felony assault that results in serious bodily injury to the child or another child of the parent

- The parent has failed to support the child when financially able to do so.

- The parent has failed to maintain regular visitation, contact, or communication with the child.

- The child has been in foster care for 15 of the immediately preceding 22 months.

MICHIGAN

- The parent has abandoned the child.

- The parent is incarcerated for a period exceeding two years and has not provided for the child's care.

- The parent's conduct or neglect has resulted in physical injury or sexual abuse to the child or a sibling of the child.

- The parent has abused the child or a sibling of the child, and the abuse included one or more of the following:
  - Criminal sexual conduct involving penetration, attempted penetration, or assault with intent to penetrate
  - Battering, torture, or other severe physical abuse
  - Loss or serious impairment of an organ or limb
  - Life-threatening injury

- Murder or voluntary manslaughter
- Aiding, abetting, attempting, conspiring, or soliciting to commit murder or voluntary manslaughter
- Reasonable efforts to rehabilitate the parent have failed.
- The parent has failed to support the child when financially able to do so.
- The parent has failed to maintain regular visitation, contact, or communication with the child.
- Parental rights to another child of the parent have been involuntarily terminated, and attempts to rehabilitate the parents have been unsuccessful.

MINNESOTA

- The parent has abandoned the child.
- The parent has been diagnosed as chemically dependent and has failed to successfully complete a treatment plan.
- The parent has substantially, continuously, and repeatedly neglected the child.
- The parent has subjected the child to egregious harm of a nature, duration, or chronicity that indicates a lack of regard for the child's well-being.
- Reasonable efforts to rehabilitate the parent have failed.
- The parent has been convicted of:
  - Murder or voluntary manslaughter of another child of the parent
  - Aiding, abetting, attempting, or soliciting to commit murder or voluntary manslaughter of another child of the parent
  - An assault with a deadly weapon with the infliction of substantial bodily injury to the child or another child of the parent
  - Assault with a past pattern of child abuse
  - Assault with a victim under the age of four years
- The parent has failed to provide necessary support to the child when ordered to do so and financially able to do so.
- The parent has failed to maintain contact with the child for six months and has not demonstrated an interest in the child.

- A putative father has failed to register with the fathers' adoption registry.
- The child has been in foster placement for a cumulative period of 12 months within the preceding 22 months, and the parent has failed to correct the conditions that led to the placement.
- Parental rights to another child of the parent have been involuntarily terminated.

MISSISSIPPI

- The parent has abandoned the child.
- The parent is unable to discharge his or her parental duties due to:
  - Severe mental deficiencies, mental illness, or physical incapacitation
  - Alcohol or drug addiction
- The parent has been responsible for a serious of abusive incidents concerning one or more children.
- There is an extreme and deep-seated antipathy by the child toward the parent that was caused at least in part by the parent's serious neglect, abuse, or prolonged and unreasonable absence.
- The parent has subjected the child to an aggravated circumstance, including, but not limited to, abandonment, torture, chronic abuse, substance abuse, or sexual abuse.
- Reasonable efforts to rehabilitate the parent have failed.
- The parent has been convicted of:
  - Murder or voluntary manslaughter of another child of the parent
  - Aiding, abetting, attempting, or soliciting to commit murder or voluntary manslaughter of another child of the parent
  - A felony assault that results in serious bodily injury to the child or another child of the parent
- The parent has been convicted of any of the following offenses against any child:
  - Rape, sexual battery, exploitation, or touching of a child for lustful purposes
  - Felonious abuse or battery of a child
  - Carnal knowledge of a stepchild, an adopted child, or the child of cohabiting partner
- The parent has failed to exercise reasonable available visitation with the child.

- The parent has made no contact with a child under the age of three years for six months or a child three years of age or older for a period of one year.
- Parental rights to another child of the parent have been involuntarily terminated.

MISSOURI

- The child is an abandoned infant.
- The parent is unable to discharge his or her parental duties due to:
  - A mental condition
  - Chemical dependency
  - A conviction of a felony that would deprive the child of a stable home for a period of years
- The parent's conduct or neglect has subjected the child to a substantial risk of physical or mental harm.
- The parent has subjected any child in the family to a severe act or recurrent acts of physical, emotional, or sexual abuse, including an act of incest.
- The child was conceived and born as a result of an act of forcible rape.
- Reasonable efforts to rehabilitate the parent have failed.
- The parent has been convicted of:
  - Murder or voluntary manslaughter of another child of the parent
  - Aiding, abetting, attempting, or soliciting to commit murder or voluntary manslaughter of another child of the parent
  - A felony assault that results in serious bodily injury to the child or to another child of the parent
- The parent has failed to contribute to the cost of care and maintenance of this child when financially able to do so.
- The parent has failed to maintain regular visitation or other contact with the child.
- The child has been in foster care for 15 of the most recent 22 months.
- Parental rights to another child of the parent have been involuntarily terminated within or immediately preceding three years.

MONTANA

- The parent has abandoned the child.
- The parent is unable to discharge his or her parental duties due to:
  - Emotional illness, mental illness, or mental deficiency
  - A history of violent behavior by the parent
  - Use of intoxicating liquor or a narcotic or dangerous drug
  - A judicially ordered long-term confinement of the parent, including incarceration of more than one year.
- The parent's conduct or neglect has resulted in the death or serious physical injury of a child.
- The parent has subjected the child to aggravated circumstances, including, but not limited to, abandonment, torture, chronic abuse, sexual abuse, or chronic severe neglect.
- Reasonable efforts to rehabilitate the parent have failed.
- The parent has been convicted of:
  - Deliberate homicide of a child
  - Aiding, abetting, attempting or soliciting to commit deliberate homicide of a child
  - Aggravated assault against a child
  - Neglect of a child that resulted in serious bodily injury
- The parent is convicted of a felony in which sexual intercourse occurred and as a result, the child was born.
- A putative father as failed to contribute to the support of the child for an aggregate period of one year, to establish substantial relations with the child, or to register with the putative father registry.
- Parental rights to another child of the parent have been involuntarily terminated, and the circumstances related to the termination are relevant to the parent's ability to adequately care for the child at issue.

NEBRASKA

- The parent has abandoned the child for six months or more.
- The parent is unable to discharge his or her parental duties due to mental illness or mental

deficiency, and such condition will likely continue for a prolonged, indeterminate period.

- The parent has substantially and continuously or repeatedly neglected the child.

- The parent is unfit by reason of debauchery, habitual use of intoxicated liquor or narcotic drugs, or repeated lewd and lascivious behavior.

- The parent has inflicted, by other than accidental means, serious physical injury upon the child.

- The parent has subjected the child to aggravated circumstance, including, but not limited to, abandonment, torture, chronic abuse, or sexual abuse.

- Reasonable efforts to rehabilitate the parent have failed.

- The parent has been convicted of:
  - Murder or voluntary manslaughter of another child of the parent
  - Aiding, abetting, attempting, or soliciting to commit murder or voluntary manslaughter of another child of the parent
  - A felony assault that results in serious bodily injury to the child or another minor child of the parent

- The parent has failed to provide necessary care and subsistence for the child when financially able to do so.

- The child has been in out-of-home placement for 15 of the most recent 22 months.

- Parental rights to another child of the parent have been involuntarily terminated.

NEVADA

- The parent has abandoned the child for 60 days or more.

- The parent is unable to discharge his or her parental duties due to:
  - Emotional illness, mental illness, or mental deficiency
  - Excessive use of intoxicating liquors, controlled substances, or dangerous drugs
  - A conviction for a felony, if the facts of the crime are of such a nature to indicate the unfitness of the parent

- The parent has subjected the child to conduct of a physically or sexually cruel or abusive nature.

- The parent's conduct or neglect has resulted in substantial bodily injury to the child.

- Reasonable efforts to rehabilitate the parent have failed.

- The parent has committed, aided, abetted, attempted, or solicited to commit murder or voluntary manslaughter.

- The parent has failed, although physically and financially able, to provide the child with adequate food, clothing, shelter, education, or other necessary care.

- The parent has, for the previous six months, had the ability to contact the child and made no more than token efforts to do so.

- A putative father has failed to establish paternity.

- The child is less than one year of age and was delivered to a provider of emergency services pursuant to law.

- Parental rights to another child of the parent have been involuntarily terminated.

If the child has been placed outside his or her home, and has remained in that placement for 14 of any 20 consecutive months, the best interest of the child must be presumed to be served by termination of parental rights.

NEW HAMPSHIRE

- The parent has abandoned the child.

- The parent is unable to discharge his or her parental duties due to
  - Mental illness or mental deficiency
  - Incarceration for a felony offense

- The parent knowingly caused, or permitted another to cause, severe sexual, physical, mental, or emotional abuse of the child.

- Reasonable efforts to rehabilitate the parent have failed.

- The parent has been convicted of:
  - Murder or manslaughter of another child of the parent or the child's other parent
  - Attempting, soliciting, or conspiring to commit murder or manslaughter of another child of the parent or the child's other parent

- A felony assault that resulted in serious bodily injury to the child, another child of the parent, or the child's other parent

- The parent has substantially and continuously neglected to provide the child with necessary subsistence, education, and other necessary care when financially able to do so.

- The parent has failed to maintain regular communication with the child.

- The child has been in out-of-home placement for 12 of the most recent 22 months.

NEW JERSEY

- The parent has abandoned the child.

- The parent has subjected the child to aggravated circumstances of abuse, neglect, cruelty, or abandonment.

- Reasonable efforts to rehabilitate the parent have failed.

- The parent has been convicted of:
  - Murder, aggravated manslaughter, or manslaughter of another child of the parent
  - Aiding, abetting, attempting, or soliciting to commit the above murder, aggravated manslaughter, or manslaughter of the child or another child of the parent
  - Committing or attempting to commit an assault or similarly serious criminal act that resulted, or could have resulted, in the death or significant bodily injury to the child or another child of the parent

- Parental rights to another child of the parent have been involuntarily terminated.

NEW MEXICO

- The parent has abandoned the child.

- The parent has subjected the child to aggravated circumstances, including those circumstance in which the parent has:
  - Attempted, conspired to cause, or caused great bodily harm to the child or great bodily harm or death to the child's sibling
  - Attempted, conspired to cause, or caused great bodily harm or death to another parent, guardian, or custodian of the child

- Attempted, conspired to subject, or has subjected the child to torture, chronic abuse, or sexual abuse

- The child has been abused or neglected, and the conditions and causes of the abuse or neglect are unlikely to change in the near future.

- Reasonable efforts to rehabilitate the parent have failed or would be futile.

- Parental rights to another child of the parent have been involuntarily terminated.

NEW YORK

- The parent has abandoned the child for a period of six months.

- The parent is unable to discharge his or her parental duties due to:
  - Mental illness or mental retardation
  - Hospitalization or institutionalization for use of drugs or alcohol

- The parent has severely or repeatedly abused the child.

- The parent has substantially and repeatedly or continuously failed to maintain contact with or plan for the future of the child for a period of more than one year.

- An incarcerated parent has failed to cooperate with efforts to assist the parent to plan for the future of the child or to plan and arrange visits with the child.

- The parent has subjected the child to aggravated circumstances, where the child has been either severely or repeatedly abused.

- Reasonable efforts to rehabilitate the parent have failed.

- The parent has been convicted of:
  - Murder or manslaughter, or the attempt to commit such a crime, and the victim or intended victim was the child, another child of the parent, or a child who was the parent's legal responsibility
  - Criminal solicitation, conspiracy, or facilitation of murder or manslaughter, and the victim or intended victim was the child, another child of the parent, or a child who was the parent's legal responsibility

- Assault or aggravated assault upon a person less than 11 years old, or an attempt to commit any such crime, and the victim or intended victim was the child, another child of the parent, or a child who was the parent's legal responsibility
- Parental rights to another child of the parent have been involuntarily terminated.

NORTH CAROLINA

- The parent has willfully abandoned the child for six months.
- The parent is unable to discharge his or her parental duties due to:
  - Mental illness or mental retardation
  - Substance abuse
- The parent has abused or neglected the child.
- The parent has subjected the child to aggravated circumstances, including, but not limited to, abandonment, torture, chronic abuse, or sexual abuse.
- Reasonable efforts to rehabilitate the parent have failed.
- The parent has been convicted of:
  - Murder or voluntary manslaughter of another child of the parent or another child residing in the home
  - Aiding, abetting, attempting, or soliciting to commit murder or voluntary manslaughter of the child, another child of the parent, or another child residing in the home
  - A felony assault that results in serious bodily injury to the child, another child of the parent, or another child in the home
- The child is in foster care, and the parent, for a period of six months, has failed to pay a reasonable portion of the cost of the care when financially able to do so.
- The noncustodial parent has failed, for a period of one year, to pay for the care, support, and education of the child as required by the custody agreement.
- A putative father has failed to establish paternity or provide substantial financial support for the child.

- Parental rights to another child of the parent have been involuntarily terminated, and the parent lacks the ability or willingness to establish a safe home.

NORTH DAKOTA

- The parent has abandoned the child.
- The parent has subjected the child to aggravated circumstance, which means circumstances in which a parent:
  - Abandons, tortures, chronically abuses, or sexually abuses a child
  - Fails to make substantial, meaningful efforts to secure treatment for addiction, mental illness, behavior disorder, or any combination of those conditions
  - Engages in deviate sexual acts, sexual abuse, or sexual imposition in which a child is the victim or intended victim
  - Has been incarcerated under a sentence for which the release date is after the child reaches his or her majority or, for a child under the age of nine years, after the child is twice his or her current age
- The causes and conditions of a child's deprivation are likely to continue and for that reason the child is suffering or will probably suffer serious physical, mental, moral, or emotional harm.
- The parent has been convicted of:
  - Murder, voluntary manslaughter, negligently causing the death of another, or felony abuse or neglect of a child, and the victim is another child of the parent
  - Aiding, abetting, attempting, conspiring, or soliciting to commit any of the above crimes in which the victim is a child of the parent
  - Aggravated assault that results in serious bodily injury to a child of the parent
- The child has been in foster care for at least 450 of the previous 660 nights.
- Parental rights to another child of the parent have been involuntarily terminated.

OHIO

- The parent has abandoned the child.

- The parent is unable to discharge his or her parental duties due to:
  - Chronic mental or emotional illness
  - Mental retardation or physical disability
  - Chemical dependency
- The parent is incarcerated for an offense committed against the child or a sibling of the child.
- The parent is incarcerated and thereby will not be available to care for the child for at least 18 months, or the parent is repeatedly incarcerated, and the repeated incarceration prevents the parent from providing care for the child.
- The parent has committed any abuse against the child, or caused or allowed the child to suffer any neglect.
- Reasonable efforts to rehabilitate the parent have failed.
- The parent has been convicted of or pled guilty to:
  - Murder, aggravated murder, or voluntary manslaughter of another child of the parent or another child living in the household
  - Assault, aggravated assault, or felonious assault of the child, a sibling, or another child living in the household
  - Endangering children, rape, sexual battery, corruption of a minor, sexual imposition, or gross sexual imposition, and the victim was the child, a sibling, or another child in the household
  - A conspiracy or attempt to commit any of the offenses described above
- The parent has demonstrated a lack of commitment to the child by failing to regularly support, visit, or communicate with the child when able to do so.
- The parent, for any reason, is unwilling to provide food, clothing, shelter, and other basic necessities for the child or to prevent the child from suffering physical, emotional, or sexual abuse or physical, emotional, or mental neglect.
- The parent has placed the child at substantial risk of harm due to alcohol or drug abuse and has refused treatment.
- Parental rights to another child of the parent have been involuntarily terminated.

OKLAHOMA

- The parent has abandoned the child.
- The parent is unable to discharge his or her parental duties due to:
  - Mental illness or mental deficiency
  - Extensive, abusive, and chronic use of drugs or alcohol
  - Incarceration of a duration that would be detrimental to the parent-child relationship
- The parent has physically or sexually abused the child or a sibling of the child, or has failed to protect the child from physical or sexual abuse.
- The child has been adjudicated a deprived child as a result of a single incident of severe sexual abuse, severe neglect, or the infliction of serious bodily injury.
- The parent has inflicted chronic abuse, chronic neglect, or torture on the child, a sibling, or a child residing in the household.
- The child or a sibling has suffered severe harm or injury as a result of physical or sexual abuse.
- The child was conceived as a result of rape.
- Reasonable efforts to rehabilitate the parent have failed.
- The parent has been convicted of:
  - Causing the death of a child as a result of physical abuse, sexual abuse, or chronic abuse or neglect of such child
  - Murder or voluntary manslaughter of any child
  - Aiding, abetting, attempting, or soliciting to commit murder or voluntary manslaughter of any child
  - A felony assault that resulted in serious bodily injury to the child or another child of the parent
- The parent has willfully failed, refused, or neglected to contribute to the support of the child when financially able to do so.
- The parent has failed to maintain frequent and regular visitation, contact, or communication with the child.
- The child has been in foster care for 15 of the most recent 22 months.
- Parental rights to another child of the parent have been involuntarily terminated, and the

conditions that led to the termination have not been corrected.

OREGON

- The parent has abandoned the child.
- The parent is unable to discharge his or her parental duties due to:
  - Emotional illness, mental illness, or mental deficiency
  - Addictive or habitual use of intoxicating liquors or controlled substances
  - Criminal conduct that impairs the parent's ability to care for the child
- The parent has been found unfit by reason of a single or recurrent incident of extreme conduct toward any child. Such conduct can include:
  - Rape, sodomy, or sex abuse of any child of the parent
  - Intentional starvation or torture of any child of the parent
  - Abuse or neglect that results in death or serious physical injury
  - Conduct by the parent to aid or abet another person who, by abuse or neglect, caused the death of any child
  - Conduct by the parent to attempt, solicit, or conspire to cause the death of any child
  - Conduct by the parent that knowingly exposes any child of the parent to the storage or production of methamphetamines
- The parent has physically neglected the child.
- Reasonable efforts to rehabilitate the parent have failed.
- The parent has been convicted of:
  - Murder or manslaughter of another child of the parent
  - Aiding, abetting, attempting, or soliciting to commit murder or voluntary manslaughter of another child of the parent
  - A felony assault that resulted in serious bodily injury to the child or another child of the parent
- The parent has failed or neglected without reasonable or lawful cause to provide for the basic physical or psychological needs of the child for six months.

- The parent has failed to maintain regular visitation or other contact with the child.
- Parental rights to another child of the parent have been involuntarily terminated, and the conditions that led to the previous action have not been corrected.

PENNSYLVANIA

- The parent has abandoned the child.
- The parent has refused or failed to discharge parental duties.
- The repeated and continued incapacity, abuse, neglect, or refusal of the parent has caused the child to be without essential parental care, control, or subsistence.
- The parent is the presumptive, but not the natural, father of the child.
- The parent is the father of a child conceived as a result of rape or incest.
- The parent has subjected the child or another child of the parent to aggravated circumstances, including, but not limited to, physical abuse resulting in serious bodily injury, sexual abuse, or aggravated physical neglect.
- Reasonable efforts to rehabilitate the parent have failed.
- The parent has been convicted of any of the following offenses where the victim was a child:
  - Criminal homicide
  - Felony aggravated assault, rape, statutory sexual assault, involuntary deviate sexual intercourse, sexual assault, or aggravated indecent assault
  - Misdemeanor indecent assault
  - Attempt, solicitation, or conspiracy to commit any of the offenses listed above
- In the case of a newborn child, the parent has failed for a period of four months to maintain substantial and continuing contact and to provide substantial financial support for the child.
- The child has been removed from the home for 12 months or more, and the conditions that led to the removal continue to exist.
- Parental rights to another child of the parent have been involuntarily terminated.

RHODE ISLAND

- The parent has abandoned the child.
- The parent is unable to discharge his or her parental duties due to:
  - Institutionalization, including imprisonment, of such duration that the parent cannot care for the child for an extended period of time
  - A chronic substance abuse problem
- The parent has subjected the child to conduct of a cruel or abusive nature.
- The parent has subjected the child to aggravated circumstances, including, but not limited to, abandonment, torture, chronic abuse, or sexual abuse.
- The child has been in the custody of the department for at least 12 months, and reasonable efforts to rehabilitate the parent have failed.
- The parent has been convicted of:
  - Murder or voluntary manslaughter of another child of the parent
  - Aiding, abetting, attempting, or soliciting to commit murder or voluntary manslaughter of another child of the parent
  - A felony assault that results in serious bodily injury to the child or another child of the parent
- The parent has willfully neglected to provide proper care and maintenance for the child when financially able to do so.
- The parent has failed to communicate with the child.
- Parental rights to another child of the parent have been involuntarily terminated, and the parent continues to lack the ability to respond to services.

SOUTH CAROLINA

- The parent has abandoned the child.
- The parent is unable to discharge his or her parental duties due to:
  - Mental illness, mental deficiency, or extreme physical incapacity
  - Drug or alcohol addiction
- The parent has tortured, abused, or severely maltreated the child.
- The parent's physical abuse of the child has resulted in death or serious physical injury to the child requiring admission to a hospital.

- The parent has subjected the child to aggravated circumstances, including, but not limited to, abandonment, torture, severe or repeated abuse or neglect, or sexual abuse.
- Reasonable efforts to rehabilitate the parent have failed.
- The parent has been convicted of:
  - Murder or voluntary manslaughter of another child of the parent
  - Aiding, abetting, attempting, or soliciting to commit murder or voluntary manslaughter of another child of the parent
  - A felony assault that results in serious bodily injury to the child or another child of the parent
- The parent has been convicted of the murder of the child's other parent.
- The parent has willfully failed to support the child for a period of six months, when financially able to do so.
- The parent has willfully failed to visit the child for a period of six months.
- The presumptive legal father is not the biological father of the child.
- The child has been in foster care for 15 of the most recent 22 months.
- Parental rights to another child of the parent have been involuntarily terminated.

SOUTH DAKOTA

- The parent has abandoned the child for at least six months.
- The parent is incarcerated and unavailable to care for the child for a significant period of time.
- The parent has a documented history of abuse or neglect associated with chronic alcohol or drug abuse.
- The parent has subjected the child or another child to abandonment, torture, sexual abuse, chronic physical, mental, or emotional injury, or chronic neglect if the neglect was a serious threat to the safety of the child or another child.
- The parent has committed any of the following crimes:
  - Murder, felony murder, or manslaughter
  - Rape, incest, sexual exploitation of children, abuse of or cruelty to minors

- Aggravated assault against the child or another child of the parent
- The parent has exposed the child to or demonstrated an inability to protect the child from substantial harm or risk for substantial harm, and the child or another child:
  - Has been removed from the parents' custody on at least one previous occasion
  - Has been removed from the parent's custody on two separate occasions, and the Department of Social Services offered or provided services on each of those occasions
- Parental rights to another child of the parent have been involuntarily terminated.

TENNESSEE

- The parent has abandoned the child.
- The parent has been found to be mentally incompetent to adequately provide care for the child.
- The parent has committed severe child abuse against the child or any sibling or half-sibling.
- The parent has been incarcerated for a sentence of more than two years for conduct against the child.
- The parent has been incarcerated for a criminal act for a sentence of 10 or more years, and the child is under the age of eight years at the time the sentence is entered.
- The parent has been convicted of or found civilly liable for the intentional and wrongful death of the child's other parent or legal guardian.
- The parent has subjected the child to aggravated circumstances.
- Reasonable efforts to rehabilitate the parent have failed.
- The parent has committed:
  - Murder or voluntary manslaughter of sibling or half-sibling of the child
  - Aiding, abetting, attempting, or soliciting to commit murder or voluntary manslaughter of the child or any sibling or half-sibling
  - A felony assault that results in serious bodily injury to the child or any sibling or half-sibling
- The child has been in foster care for 15 of the most recent 22 months.

- The parent has failed to support the child in accordance with the child support guidelines.
- The parent has failed to seek reasonable visitation with the child, or when visitation has been granted, has failed to visit.
- A person has failed to establish paternity within 30 days after notice of alleged paternity.
- Parental rights to another child of the parent have been involuntarily terminated.

TEXAS

- The parent has abandoned the child.
- The parent is unable to discharge his or her parental duties due to:
  - Mental illness, emotional illness, or mental deficiency
  - Use of a controlled substance
  - Incarceration for not less than two years
- The parent knowingly placed or allowed the child to remain in conditions or surroundings or with persons who engaged in conduct that endangered the physical or emotional well-being of the child.
- Reasonable efforts to rehabilitate the parent have failed.
- The parent has been convicted of being criminally responsible for the death or serious injury of a child or any of the following crimes against a child:
  - Murder or capital murder
  - Indecency with a child, assault, sexual assault, aggravated assault, or aggravated sexual assault
  - Injury to a child, elderly individual, or disabled individual
  - Abandoning or endangering a child
  - Prohibited sexual conduct, sexual performance by a child, or possession or promotion of child pornography
- The parent is the father of a child conceived as a result of a sexual offense.
- The parent has failed to support the child in accordance with the parent's ability for one year.
- The parent abandoned the mother of the child during her pregnancy and failed to provide ade-

quate support or medical care for the mother, and failed to support the child since birth.

- An alleged father has failed to register with the paternity registry or to respond to notice.
- The parent has been the major cause of:
  - The child's failure to be enrolled in school as required by law
  - The child's absence from home without the consent of the parent or guardian for a substantial length of time or without the intent to return
- The parent has been the cause of the child being born addicted to alcohol or a controlled substance.
- The parent voluntarily delivered the child to a designated emergency infant care provider.
- The parent has failed to maintain regular visitation, contact, or communication with the child.
- Parental rights to another child of the parent have been involuntarily terminated.

UTAH

- The parent has abandoned the child.
- The parent is unable to discharge his or her parental duties due to:
  - Emotional illness, mental illness, or mental deficiency
  - Habitual or excessive use of intoxicating liquors, controlled substances, or dangerous drugs
  - A conviction and incarceration for a felony, and the sentence will deprive the child of a normal home for more than one year
  - A history of violent behavior
- The parent has subjected the child to conduct of a physically, emotionally, or sexually cruel or abusive nature.
- The parent's substantiated abuse or neglect has resulted in sexual abuse, injury, or death of a sibling of the child.
- The parent has subjected the child to a single incident of life-threatening or gravely disabling injury or disfigurement.
- Reasonable efforts to rehabilitate the parent have failed.
- The parent has committed, or aided, abetted, attempted, conspired, or solicited to commit murder or voluntary manslaughter of a child or child abuse homicide.

- The parent has repeatedly or continuously failed to provide the child with adequate food, clothing, shelter, education, or other care necessary for his or her physical, mental, and emotional health and development.
- The parent has failed to communicate with the child.
- The parent has met the terms and conditions of a safe relinquishment of a newborn child.
- Parental rights to another child of the parent have been involuntarily terminated.

VERMONT

- In the case of a child under the age of six months, the parent did not exercise parental responsibility once he or she knew or should have known of the child's birth or expected birth. In making a determination under this subdivision, the court shall consider all relevant factors, which may include the respondent's failure to:
  - Pay reasonable prenatal, natal, and postnatal expenses in accordance with his or her financial means
  - Make reasonable and consistent payments, in accordance with his or her financial means, for the support of the child
  - Regularly communicate or visit with the minor
  - Manifest an ability and willingness to assume legal and physical custody of the minor
- In the case of a child over the age of six months at the time the petition is filed, the respondent did not exercise parental responsibility for a period of at least six months immediately preceding the filing of the petition; in making a determination under this subdivision, the court shall consider all relevant factors, which may include the respondent's failure to:
  - Make reasonable and consistent payments, in accordance with his or her financial means, for the support of the child, although legally obligated to do so
  - Regularly communicate or visit with the minor
  - During any time the minor was not in the physical custody of the other parent, to manifest an ability and willingness to assume legal and physical custody of the minor
- The respondent has been convicted of a crime of violence or has been found by a court of compe-

tent jurisdiction to have committed an act of violence that violated a restraining or protective order, and the facts of the crime or violation indicate that the respondent is unfit to maintain a relationship of parent and child with the minor.

- An alleged father has failed to establish paternity.

VIRGINIA

- The parent has abandoned the child.
- The parent is unable to discharge his or her parental duties due to:
  - Emotional illness, mental illness, or mental deficiency
  - Habitual abuse or addiction to intoxicating liquors, narcotics, or other dangerous drugs
- The parent has subjected the child to aggravated circumstances, including, but not limited to, torture, chronic or severe abuse, or chronic or severe sexual abuse. It includes the failure to protect the child from such conduct.
- Reasonable efforts to rehabilitate the parent have failed.
- The parent has been convicted of:
  - Murder or voluntary manslaughter of a child of the parent, a child with whom the parent resided or the other parent of the child
  - Felony attempt, conspiracy, or solicitation to commit any such offense
  - A felony assault that results in serious bodily injury, felony bodily wounding, or felony sexual assault, and the victim was a child of the parent or a child residing with the parent
- The parent has failed to maintain continuing contact with the child for six months after the child has been placed in foster care.
- Parental rights to another child of the parent have been involuntarily terminated.

WASHINGTON

- The parent has abandoned the child.
- The parent is unable to discharge his or her parental duties due to:
  - Psychological incapacity or mental deficiency
  - Use of intoxicating or controlled substances
- The parent has subjected the child to aggravated circumstances, that may include one or more of the following:

- Conviction of the parent of rape, criminal mistreatment, or assault of the child
- Conviction of the parent of murder, manslaughter, or homicide by abuse of the child's other parent, a sibling, or another child
- Conviction of the parent of attempting, soliciting, or conspiring to commit any of the above crimes
- Commission of assault against a surviving child or another child of the parent
- A finding that the parent is a sexually violent predator
- Failure of the parent to complete available ordered treatment, and that failure has resulted in the termination of parental rights to another child
- Conviction of the parent of a sex offense or incest when a child is born of the offense
- The child has been found to be a dependent child, has been removed from the custody of the parent for at least six months, and there is little likelihood that conditions will be remedied so that the child can be returned to the parent in the near future.

WEST VIRGINIA

- The parent has abandoned the child.
- The parent is unable to discharge his or her parental duties due to:
  - Emotional illness, mental illness, or mental deficiency
  - Habitual abuse or addiction to alcohol, controlled substances, or drugs
- The parent has repeatedly or seriously injured the child physically or emotionally.
- The parent has sexually abused or exploited the child.
- The parent has subjected the child to an aggravated circumstance, including, but not limited to, abandonment, torture, chronic abuse, or sexual abuse.
- Reasonable efforts to rehabilitate the parent have failed.
- The parent has
  - Committed murder of voluntary manslaughter of another child of the parent
  - Attempted or conspired to commit murder or voluntary manslaughter of another child of the parent

- Committed a felonious assault that results in serous bodily injury to the child or another child of the parent
- Parental rights to another child of the parent have been involuntarily terminated.

WISCONSIN

- The parent has abandoned the child.
- The parent is unable to discharge his or her parental duties due to continuing parental disability due to mental illness or developmental disability.
- The parent has exhibited a pattern of physically or sexually abusive behavior that is a substantial threat to the health of child.
- The parent has caused death or injury to the child or children resulting in a felony conviction.
- The child was conceived as a result of sexual assault or incest.
- The parent has subjected the child to an aggravated circumstance, including, but not limited to, abandonment, torture, chronic abuse, or sexual abuse.
- Reasonable efforts to rehabilitate the parent have failed.
- The parent has committed a serious felony against one of the person's children, that may include:
  - Intentional homicide, reckless homicide, or felony murder
  - Aiding, abetting, attempting, conspiring, or soliciting to commit intentional homicide, reckless homicide, or felony murder
  - Battery, sexual assault, physical abuse, sexual exploitation or neglect of a child, incest with a child, or soliciting a child for prostitution
  - Neglect of a child that results in the death of the child
- The parent has committed homicide or solicitation to commit homicide of the child's other parent.
- The parent has failed to assume parental responsibility for the child.
- The parent has failed to visit or communicate with the child for three months or longer.

- The parent has relinquished the child when the child was 72 hours old or younger.
- Parental rights to another child of the parent have been involuntarily terminated.

WYOMING

- The parent has abandoned the child.
- The parent is incarcerated due to the conviction of a felony and a showing that the parent is unfit.
- The parent has subjected the child to aggravated circumstance, including, but not limited to, abandonment, torture, chronic abuse, or sexual abuse.
- The parent has abused or neglected the child, and reasonable efforts to rehabilitate the parent have failed.
- The child has been in foster care for 15 of the most recent 22 months, and there is a showing that the parent is unfit to have custody and control of the child.
- The child was relinquished to a safe haven provider, and neither parent has affirmatively sought the return of the child within three months.
- The parent has been convicted of:
  - Murder or voluntary manslaughter of another child of the parent
  - Aiding, abetting, attempting, conspiring, or soliciting to commit murder or voluntary manslaughter of another child of the parent
  - A felony assault that result in serious bodily injury to a child of the parent
- The child has been left in the care of another without provision for the child's support and without communication from the absent parent for at least one year.
- Parental rights to another child of the parent have been involuntarily terminated.

Source: Adapted from National Clearinghouse on Child Abuse and Neglect Information, Grounds for Involuntary Termination of Parental Rights. Available online at http://nccanch.acf.hhs.gov/general/legal/statutes/groundterminall.pdf. Downloaded on July 6, 2005.

APPENDIX VI

ADOPTIVE PARENT CHECKLIST: EVALUATING AND UNDERSTANDING YOUR FAMILY AND YOUR CHILD

* Authors' note: Some of the items in this list are not applicable to children who are being adopted from other countries. The list is drawn from information created for parents who are adopting children from foster care.

- Thoroughly research your child's social and emotional history.

- Ask to read the case file or a case summary prepared by the agency.

- Ask questions about the case file or summary if there are things written that you do not understand.

- Ask if it is possible to talk or meet with the child's current or previous foster parents.

- Ask if there are relatives, friends, or other significant individuals that your child should maintain contact with after placement. If there are, ask your social worker how best to maintain contact and keep them in your child's life.

- If this adoption will or may be an open adoption, talk to your social worker about the different types of open adoption. An open adoption is one in which the birth parent(s), adoptive parent(s), and child are known to one another and maintain some level of contact during the adoption process and throughout the child's life. Ask for resource information and materials on open adoption. Request legal information from the agency and a contact name to discuss the legal implications of an open adoption.

- Thoroughly research the medical history of your child. Ask your social worker to see all available medical records and ask who to contact for answers to your questions regarding diagnosis.

- Thoroughly research the medical history of your child's biological parents. Ask your social worker to see all available birth family medical records. Ask your agency what background health information is available under state and federal laws and regulations. Be aware that regulations issued as a result of the Health Insurance Portability and Accountability Act of 1996 (HIPAA), which went into effect in April 2003, may impact the ability of agencies to share birth family health information.

- Obtain your child's educational history. Seek information from your child's school(s) to determine if any special educational approaches have proven successful or unsuccessful for your child. Ask if your child is currently receiving special education services and whether s/he has an Individual Education Plan (IEP). Request a current assessment of your child's special educational need from your local school district if necessary. Research your child's rights to special education and related services under the Individuals with Disabilities Education Act (IDEA).

- Educate your family and your child to gain an understanding of the evolving issues in adoption of separation, grief and loss, and identity formation. Check with your agency to find out if they have a lending library or offer workshops and training and information on these subjects.

- If you're adopting transculturally or transracially, research the issues uniquely associated with these adoptions. Check with your state agency's adoption unit to find out if they have a lending library or offer workshops and training and information in the area of cultural, racial, and ethnic identity, awareness, and appreciation. Contact informational groups such as the New York State Citizen's Coalition for Children on their Web site at http://www.nysccc.org/T-Rarts/T-Rarts.html where links to articles, reports, books, videos, films, and informative Web sites are available.

- Evaluate your family resources. Discuss the estimated costs of increasing your family size with your social worker and other adoptive parents of children with special needs. Consider meeting with a financial consultant to plan your new family's finances. Remember that resources are not only financial. Include emotional and physical support resources such as local respite groups, adoptive parent support groups, and family members in your evaluation of resources that would help to more fully and successfully incorporate your child into your family.

- Check with your agency or other adoption professionals to find out if they have a lending library or offer workshops, training, and information on adoption sensitivity. You can research adoption sensitivity in your local library and use their computer to connection to adoption information. Web sites such as the Adoption Family Center's at http://www.adoptionfamilycenter.org offer articles to familiarize yourself with positive adoption language to prepare yourself to describe and discuss your child's adoption with your child, family members, friends, and school personnel.

- Talk to other adoptive parents about the joys and challenges of adopting a child with special needs. Meet adoptive parents through community and online adoptive parent support groups. Ask how to get connected to a parent support group in your area or contact AdoptUSKids.org. AdoptUSKids provides a parent support group section on its Web site. See the AdoptUSKids.org Web site at: http://www.adoptuskids.org.

- Fully discuss with agency staff your child's present and possible future needs as assessed by state child welfare professionals. If your child does not presently have physical, emotional, or psychological concerns, are they at risk of developing them? Ask for phone numbers, addresses, and contact names of agency professionals to contact if future need arise. Also consider contacting your child's doctor, teachers, or previous caregivers.

This information was taken from the "Adoptive Parent Checklist, Meeting Your Child's Special Needs," developed by the Association of Administrators of the Interstate Compact on Adoption and Medical Assistance (AAICAMA), secretariat services provided by the American Public Human Services Association (APHSA), with support from a federal grant awarded to AAICAMA by the U.S. Department of Health and Human Services.

APPENDIX VII
STATE LAWS ON ACCESS TO IDENTIFYING BIRTH FAMILY INFORMATION

Note that state laws are subject to change, and this appendix should be used as a general guide only.

Some states include "degrees" of kinship in their laws when defining the relationship of a child to a prospective caretaker relative, and may refer to first, second, third, and fourth degrees or even fifth degrees of kinship. In most cases, the relationship may be by "blood," (genetic/biological) or be formed by marriage or adoption.

A first degree relative of a child is the parent, while a second degree relative is a grandparent or sibling. (The sibling must be an adult in order to be a caretaker relative of a minor child.) Third degree relatives include great-grandparents, uncles and aunts, and nieces and nephews. Fourth degree relatives are great-great grandparents, great-uncles and great-aunts, and first cousins. Fifth degree relatives are great-great-great grandparents, great-great uncles and great-great aunts, or first cousins once removed. (A first cousin once removed is the child of a first cousin).

ALABAMA
Who May Access Information

- Adoptive parents
- Birthparents
- Adopted person, age 19 or older

Note: Only the adopted person may access identifying information.

Mutual Access to Identifying Information

Identifying information may be released if either birthparent gives consent in writing, or the adopted person may petition the court. The court will release the information after weighing the interest and rights of all the parties involved.

Access to Original Birth Certificate

- Available upon request to the adopted person age 19 or older. The noncertified copy may include other documents maintained with the record.
- The birthparent may file a contact preference form to accompany the original birth certificate.

Where the Information Can Be Located

- The State Department of Human Resources
- The licensed investigating agency appointed by the court per § 26-10-19(b),(c)

ALASKA
Who May Access Information

- Adopted person, age 18 or older
- Adoptive parent

Mutual Access to Identifying Information

- Upon request, the adopted person may have access to any change in the birthparent's name or address.
- Birthparents may access the most current name and address of an adopted person age 18 or older if consent is given.
- The information may include any documents provided by the birthparents for disclosure to the child, including photos, letters, etc.

Access to Original Birth Certificate

Provided upon request to an adopted person age 18 or older

Where the Information Can Be Located

State Registrar of Vital Statistics, Department of Health and Social Services

ARIZONA

Who May Access Information

- Adoptive parents or guardian
- Adopted person, age 18 or older
- Spouse or child of adopted person (if age 18 or older) if the adopted person is deceased
- Birthparents or other biological children of birthparents

Mutual Access to Identifying Information

- The court shall not release identifying information unless a compelling need for disclosure is established or consent was previously obtained from the birthparents.
- An adopted person, age 18 or older, may file at any time with the court and agency giving, withholding, or withdrawing consent to release confidential information to the birthparents.

Access to Original Birth Certificate

Only made available upon a court order as prescribed by rule

Where the Information Can Be Located

Arizona Confidential Intermediary Program, Arizona Supreme Court

ARKANSAS

Who May Access Information

- Adopted person
- Spouse or child of adopted person, if deceased
- Adoptive parents or guardian
- Birthparents
- Child welfare agency

Access contingent upon registration with Adoption Registry

Mutual Access to Identifying Information

- Identifying information may only be disclosed if each birthparent registers with the adoption registry by filing an affidavit.

- An adult adopted person may also voluntarily register with the adoption registry.
- Registry does not contain information regarding adoptive parents or siblings of an adopted person who are children of adoptive parents.

Access to Original Birth Certificate

Available only upon a court order

Where the Information Can Be Located

- Arkansas Department of Human Services, Division of Child and Family Services Mutual Consent Voluntary Adoption Registry
- The licensed agency involved in the adoption

CALIFORNIA

Who May Access Information

- Adopted person, age 21 or older
- Birthparent of an adopted person age 21 or older
- Adoptive parent of a child under age 21

Mutual Access to Identifying Information

- Identifying information such as name and current address of birthparents or an adopted person may be released upon request if consent in writing has been previously given.
- Information will only be released to adoptive parents if court finds that a medical necessity or other extraordinary circumstance justified disclosure.
- Information about a birth sibling may be released to another sibling provided both are age 21 or older and have provided a written waiver.
- Photos or letters, and other personal property should be released if requested, if the adopted person is age 18 or older and other conditions have been met.
- A reasonable fee may be charged for processing the request.

Access to Original Birth Certificate

Available by order of a court

Where the Information Can Be Located

- California Department of Social Services, Adoption Branch
- Licensed adoption agency

COLORADO

Who May Access Information

- Adult adopted person
- Birthparents
- Adoptive parent or legal guardian of a minor adopted person
- Adult descendant of adopted person
- Biological grandparent with consent of birthparent
- The legal representative of any the above listed persons

Mutual Access to Identifying Information

- Upon inquiry, identifying information may be released, if a consent form authorizing such release is present from the party about whom information is sought.
- For adoptions on or after 9/1/99, a birthparent shall have access to adoption records and contact with the adopted person or the adoptive family.
- Parties may also log consent with the Voluntary Adoption Registry, for which a reasonable fee may be charged.

Access to Original Birth Certificate

Available upon order of the court

Where the Information Can Be Located

- Colorado Voluntary Adoption Registry, Colorado Department of Public Health
- Colorado Confidential Intermediary Services
- Child placement agency involved in the adoption
- Colorado Adoption Family Resource Registry

CONNECTICUT

Who May Access Information

- Adult adopted person
- Adoptive parents or guardian
- Spouse or descendants of the adopted person, if the adopted person is deceased
- Legal representative of the adopted person

  Note: Only the adopted person may access identifying information.

Mutual Access to Identifying Information

Any authorized applicant may, by applying in person or in writing, release the request of identifying information. The information should be released unless:

- The consents required by § 45a-751b are not given.
- The release of the requested information would be seriously disruptive to or endanger the physical or emotional health of the applicant or the person whose identity is being requested.

Access to Original Birth Certificate

Available upon written order signed by a judge of the probate court

Where the Information Can Be Located

- The department and each child-placing agency involved in the adoption shall maintain registries.
- Connecticut Department of Children and Families, Office of Foster and Adoption Services

DELAWARE

Who May Access Information

- Adopted person, age 21 or older
- All other parties to an adoption

  Note: Only the adopted person may access identifying information.

Mutual Access to Identifying Information

Upon request, an adopted person, age 21 years or older, shall be notified of a birthparent or sibling's current name, address, and telephone unless a no-contact declaration is made either verbally or in writing and filed with the agency by the person being sought.

Access to Original Birth Certificate

The adopted person age 21 or older may request a copy unless the birthparent has filed an affidavit denying release.

Where the Information Can Be Located

- Delaware Adoption Registry
- The agency involved in the adoption

DISTRICT OF COLUMBIA

Who May Access Information
Not addressed by statutes reviewed

Mutual Access to Identifying Information
All records are sealed and may not be inspected except upon order of the court, and then only if the welfare of the child is promoted.

Access to Original Birth Certificate
The original birth certificate is a sealed record that cannot be opened without order of the court.

Where the Information Can Be Located
Contact the Child and Family Services Agency or the agency involved in the adoption.

FLORIDA

Who May Access Information
- Adopted person, age 18 or older
- Birthparents
- Adoptive parents

Mutual Access to Identifying Information
Identifying information about parties to an adoption may not be disclosed unless the respective party has authorized in writing the release of such information.

Access to Original Birth Certificate
Available only upon order of the court

Where the Information Can Be Located
Florida Adoption Reunion Registry

GEORGIA

Who May Access Information
- Adopted person
- Birthparents
- The child of the adopted person, if deceased
- Adoptive parents

The adoptive parents may access only nonidentifying information.

Mutual Access to Identifying Information
Upon written request of an adopted person age 21 or older, the name of the birthparents shall be released if:

- The birthparent submitted an unrevoked written permission for the release
- The identify of the birthparent has been verified
- The department or agency has the records

The adopted person also may petition the Superior Court of Fulton County to seek the release of such information. The court shall grant the petition if it finds that failure to release the identity of each parent would have an adverse impact upon the physical, mental, or emotional health of the adopted person.

Birthparents may also access information about an adopted person through the registry using the same process.

Access to Original Birth Certificate
Available by order of the court or as provided by statute

Where the Information Can Be Located
Georgia Adoption Reunion Registry

HAWAII

Who May Access Information
- Adopted person
- Adoptive parents

Mutual Access to Identifying Information
An adopted person, 18 years of age or older, may submit a written request to the family court for inspection of adoption records. Such records will be released unless the birthparents have filed a confidentiality affidavit. Such affidavits may be renewed every 10 years.

Access to Original Birth Certificate
Available only upon court order

Where the Information Can Be Located
Family Court Central Registry

IDAHO

Who May Access Information

- Adult adopted person
- Birthparents
- Adult birth siblings

Mutual Access to Identifying Information

- The registrar shall establish and maintain a list of adult adopted persons, birthparents, and adult birth siblings who consent to the release of identifying information.
- Consents may be revised.
- The registration fee is $10.

Access to Original Birth Certificate

Available upon a court order or in accordance with § 39-259A, which allows disclosure when all parties have consented through the State adoption registry.

Where the Information Can Be Located

Idaho Department of Health and Welfare, Voluntary Adoption Registry

ILLINOIS

Who May Access Information

- Birthparents and siblings
- Adoptive parents or legal guardians of an adopted person under age 21
- Adopted person age 21 or older

Mutual Access to Identifying Information

Identifying information, such as the name and last known address, may be obtained from the Registry upon a court order, an information exchange authorization form field by a registrant, or per § 18.3(h).

Access to Original Birth Certificate

- For adoptions finalized after January 1, 2000, provided through the adoption registry
- Otherwise, available upon a court order or as provided by regulation

Where the Information Can Be Located

Illinois Adoption Registry, Illinois Department of Public Health

INDIANA

Who May Access Information

- Adopted person, age 21 or older
- Birthparent or sibling
- Adoptive parent

- The spouse or relative of a deceased adopted person
- The spouse or relative of a deceased birthparent

Mutual Access to Identifying Information

Applies only to adoptions filed after 12/31/93

- An adopted person, age 21 or older, may request identifying information by submitting a written request to the State registrar.
- Birthparents may restrict access to such information by filing a written nonrelease form with the registry, which may be renewed or withdrawn at anytime.

Access to Original Birth Certificate

Withheld from inspection except for a child adopted by a stepparent or as provided in statutes pertaining to release of identifying information

Where the Information Can Be Located

Indiana Adoption History Registry

IOWA

Who May Access Information

- Adult adopted person
- Adult sibling
- Birthparents

Mutual Access to Identifying Information

The registrar may reveal identifying information to a party, if the person sought gives consent to the revelation of identity and the registrar has sufficient information to make the requested match.

Access to Original Birth Certificate

Available only upon court order

Where the Information Can Be Located

Iowa Mutual Consent Voluntary Adoption Registry, Department of Public Health, Bureau of Vital Records

KANSAS

Who May Access Information

- Adult adopted person
- Adoptive parents
- Birthparents

- Attorney or legal representative of any of the above persons

Mutual Access to Identifying Information

- Identifying information shall not be shared with the birthparent without the permission of the adoptive parents or the adopted person.
- The department may contact the birthparents at the request of the adopted person for any reason.

Access to Original Birth Certificate

May be opened:

- Upon demand of adopted adult
- By court order

Where the Information Can Be Located

Department of Social and Rehabilitative Services

KENTUCKY

Who May Access Information

- Adopted person, age 18 or older
- Birth sibling, age 18 or older
- A birthparent

Mutual Access to Identifying Information

When a written consent is on file, the records shall be available, upon request in writing.

Access to Original Birth Certificate

Available only upon court order

Where the Information Can Be Located

Program Specialist, Department for Social Services

LOUISIANA

Who May Access Information

- Adopted person, age 18 or older
- Birthparents
- Birth siblings, age 18 or older
- Adoptive parents

The access of adoptive parents is limited to non-identifying information.

Mutual Access to Identifying Information

The registry shall not release any information from the adoption records in violation of the privacy or confidentiality rights of a birthparent who has not authorized the release of any information. An exception is made if the parent is deceased.

Access to Original Birth Certificate

Available:

- Upon court order to the adopted person, or if deceased, the adopted person's descendants, or the adoptive parent
- To the agency that was a party to the adoption upon court order after a showing of compelling reasons

Where the Information Can Be Located

Louisiana Voluntary Adoption Registry

MAINE

Who May Access Information

- Adopted person, age 18 or older
- An adoptive parent or legal guardian
- A birthparent
- A birth sibling or half-sibling, if age 18 or older

Mutual Access to Identifying Information

Registrar will release identifying information if both parties have registered, thereby giving consent.

Access to Original Birth Certificate

Available only upon court order

Where the Information Can Be Located

Maine State Adoption Reunion Registry

MARYLAND

Who May Access Information

- Birthparents and siblings
- An adopted person age 21 or older, who does not have a birth sibling under the age of 21 with the same adoptive parents

Mutual Access to Identifying Information

- To register with the Registry, an individual shall submit a notarized affidavit containing identifying information, as outlined in the statute, such as the individual's current name, any previous name by which the individual was known, address, and telephone number.

- Information will be released when a match is made.
- A registrant may withdraw at any time by submitting an affidavit.

Access to Original Birth Certificate

An adopted adult, age 21 or older, and a birthparent of an adopted adult may apply to the Secretary of Health and Mental Hygiene for a copy.

Where the Information Can Be Located

Maryland Mutual Consent Voluntary Adoption Registry, Social Services Administration

MASSACHUSETTS

Who May Access Information

- Adopted person, age 18 or older
- Adoptive parents of an adopted person under age 18
- Birthparents

Mutual Access to Identifying Information

If written permission to release identity is present, the agency must comply with a request.

Access to Original Birth Certificate

Available only upon court order

Where the Information Can Be Located

Adoption Search Coordinator, Massachusetts Department of Social Services

MICHIGAN

Who May Access Information

- Adult adopted person
- Adoptive parents
- Birthparents and adult birth siblings

Adoptive parents may not access identifying information.

Mutual Access to Identifying Information

- For adoptions finalized before September 12, 1980, all identifying information, as described in § 710.27(3), shall be released to an adult adopted person, if both birthparents have on file with the central adoption registry a statement consenting to the release.

- For adoptions finalized on or after September 12, 1980, identifying information shall be released to the adult adopted person unless the birthparent has a statement on file with the central adoption registry denying consent to the release of identifying information.

Access to Original Birth Certificate

Can be provided to the adult adopted person upon request when accompanied by a copy of a central adoption registry clearance reply form, or by court order

Where the Information Can Be Located

- Central Adoption Registry
- Michigan Family Independence Agency

MINNESOTA

Who May Access Information

- Adopted persons age 19 years or older
- Adoptive parent—access to nonidentifying information only

Mutual Access to Identifying Information

- Each birthparent may file an affidavit objecting to release of identifying information.
- If no affidavit objecting to release of identifying information is on file, the information shall be released to the adopted person upon request.
- If an affidavit objecting to release is on file, the adopted person may petition the court for release of information.

Access to Original Birth Certificate

- Upon consent of the court and all interested parties
- Upon order of the court for good cause shown

Where the Information Can Be Located

Adoption Archive, Minnesota Department of Human Services

MISSISSIPPI

Who May Access Information

- Adopted person, age 18 or older
- Adoptive parent

- Legal guardian or custodian of an adopted person
- The offspring or blood sibling of an adopted person, if the requester is age 18 or older

Mutual Access to Identifying Information

- An adopted person age 21 or older may request identifying information regarding either or both of his or her birthparents, unless that birthparent has executed an affidavit prohibiting the release of such information.
- The adopted person must submit to counseling in connection with any release.

Access to Original Birth Certificate

- Upon order of the court, pursuant to §§ 93-17-201 through 93-17-233, in which identifying information may be obtained with the consent of the birthparents
- May also be provided through the Bureau upon an affidavit from birthparent authorizing it; affidavit may be revoked at anytime

Where the Information Can Be Located

- The Bureau of Vital Records, Mississippi State Board of Health
- Licensed adoption agency

MISSOURI

Who May Access Information

- Adoptive parents
- Legal guardians
- Adult adopted person

Mutual Access to Identifying Information

- A registry is maintained by which birthparents and adoptive adults may indicate their desire to be contacted by each other.
- If the birthparent fails, or refuses to file an affidavit authorizing the release of identifying information, it shall not be released. If rejected, a request may be made again in three years. Similar information about an adult birth sibling may be released for medical cause shown.

Access to Original Birth Certificate

Available only upon order of the court

Where the Information Can Be Located

Missouri Division of Family Services, Adoption Information Registry

MONTANA

Who May Access Information

- Adopted person
- Adoptive or birthparent
- An extended family member of an adopted person or birthparent
- Court-appointed confidential intermediary

Mutual Access to Identifying Information

- Information may be disclosed to any person who consents in writing to the release of confidential information to other persons who have also consented.
- Identifying information pertaining to minor adopted person may not be disclosed unless the adoptive parents consent.
- Specific information may also be released to assist an adopted person become a member of an Indian tribe.

Access to Original Birth Certificate

- For adoptions finalized prior to October 1, 1997, the department shall release a copy of the original birth certificate upon a court order.
- For adoptions finalized on or after October 1, 1997, an adopted person may be provided a copy of the original birth certificate upon written request unless the birthparent requests in writing that it not be released without a court order.
- The department may release a copy of the original birth certificate if it is required to assist the adopted person to become a member of an Indian tribe.

Where the Information Can Be Located

Office of Vital Statistics, Department of Public Health and Human Services

NEBRASKA

Who May Access Information

- Adopted person, age 21 or older
- An Indian adopted person, age 18 or older

Mutual Access to Identifying Information

- An adult adopted person may receive identifying information if a notice of nonconsent is not filed by the person being sought.
- An Indian adopted person shall be informed of the Tribal affiliation, if any, of the individual's birthparents and other information as may be necessary to protect any rights flowing from the adopted person's Tribal relationship.

Access to Original Birth Certificate

Adopted person age 25 years or older may file a written request. Both birthparents and adoptive parents may file nonconsent forms to bar release.

Where the Information Can Be Located

Nebraska Department of Health and Human Services

NEVADA

Who May Access Information

- Adopted person over age 18
- Birthparents
- Person related within the third degree to the adopted person

Mutual Access to Identifying Information

- Identifying information may be released about a person related within the third degree to an adopted person, or about an adopted person to a person related within the third degree, if the names and information about both persons are contained in the registry and written consent is given by the birthparents.
- An adopted person may restrict the release of any information concerning himself.

Access to Original Birth Certificate

Available only upon order of the court

Where the Information Can Be Located

Nevada Adoption Registry Services

NEW HAMPSHIRE

Who May Access Information

- Adult adopted person
- Birthparent
- Adoptive parent

Mutual Access to Identifying Information

Identifying information may be released to the adopted person:

- When an agency receives a request from the adult adopted person.
- A release of information has been signed by each birthparent, and has not been revoked or amended.
- The birthparents have been contacted to reaffirm desire to be contacted.

Access to Original Birth Certificate

Upon written application by an adult adopted person who was born in the State, the registrar shall issue a noncertified copy of the unaltered original birth certificate using the same procedures imposed on nonadopted citizens.

Where the Information Can Be Located

New Hampshire Department of Health and Human Services Office of Community and Public Health, Bureau of Vital Records

NEW JERSEY

Who May Access Information

Not addressed in statutes reviewed

Mutual Access to Identifying Information

Information available upon good cause shown to the court

Access to Original Birth Certificate

Available only upon order of the court

Where the Information Can Be Located

For public agency adoptions only: New Jersey Division of Youth and Family Services, Adoption Registry Coordinator

NEW MEXICO

Who May Access Information

- Adopted person, age 18 or older
- Adoptive parent of an adopted person under age 18
- An adopted person's birth sibling
- A guardian

Mutual Access to Identifying Information

- The identify of the birthparent and of the adopted person shall be kept confidential unless both have consented to the release of identity.

- If consent is absent, a party may file a motion with the court to obtain release for good cause shown. The court shall give primary consideration to the best interest of the adopted person.

- A confidential intermediary may be used to ascertain information.

Access to Original Birth Certificate

Available only upon order of the court

Where the Information Can Be Located

- New Mexico Adoption Registry

- Children, Youth, Family Department, Central Adoption Unit

NEW YORK

Who May Access Information

- Adopted person, age 18 or older

- A birth sibling, age 18 or older

- Adoptive parents of adopted person under age 18

Mutual Access to Identifying Information

Release of identifying information by the Registry is limited to names and address of registrants.

Access to Original Birth Certificate

Available only upon order of the court

Where the Information Can Be Located

Adoption Information Registry, New York State Department of Health

NORTH CAROLINA

Who May Access Information

- Adoptive parent

- Adult adopted person

- A minor adopted person who is a parent or an expectant parent

Mutual Access to Identifying Information

The consent to the release of identifying information shall be in written and signed.

Access to Original Birth Certificate

Available upon order of the court as authorized by § 48-9-105

Where the Information Can Be Located

State Registrar

NORTH DAKOTA

Who May Access Information

- The adoptive parents

- Adopted adult

- Birthparent

Mutual Access to Identifying Information

Identifying information about a birthparent or sibling may be released to an adopted person, age 18 or older, provided consent to such disclosure is present. A birthparent may request such information of an adopted person age 21 or older.

Access to Original Birth Certificate

Upon consent of the court and all interested persons, or in exceptional cases only, for good cause shown

Where the Information Can Be Located

Passive Registry, North Dakota Department of Human Services, Adoption Search/Disclosure

OHIO

Who May Access Information

- An adopted adult

- An adoptive parent of a minor adopted person

- Nonidentifying information by an adoptive family member of a deceased adopted person

- Nonidentifying information by a birthparent, or adult birth sibling if the birthparent is deceased

Mutual Access to Identifying Information

If there is no effective denial of release from the birthparents or siblings, and the fee required by § 3705.241 is paid, identifying information must be provided to the adopted person, age 21 or older, or an adoptive parent if the adopted person is at least age 18 but under age 21.

Access to Original Birth Certificate

Released upon order of the probate court

Where the Information Can Be Located

Ohio Adoption Registry, Ohio Department of Health-Vital Statistics

OKLAHOMA

Who May Access Information

- Adult adopted person
- Adult descendant of a deceased adopted person
- Birthparent
- Adult birth sibling or grandparent of an adult adopted person

Mutual Access to Identifying Information

- An eligible registrant may access information stating a registrant's current contact information and willingness to be identified to some or all eligible relatives.
- A confidential intermediary may arrange consent for exchange of identifying information.

Access to Original Birth Certificate

For adoptions finalized after November 1, 1997, an uncertified copy of the original birth certificate is available to an adopted person, age 18 or older, upon written request under the following conditions:

- He or she presents proof of identity.
- There are not biological siblings under age 18 who are currently in an adoptive family and whose whereabouts are known.
- The birthparents have not filed affidavits of nondisclosure.

Original birth certificates are also available upon order of the court for good cause shown, pursuant to § 7505-1.1

Where the Information Can Be Located

Adoption Reunion Registry, Oklahoma Department of Human Services

OREGON

Who May Access Information

- Adult adopted person
- Birthparents
- Putative fathers
- Any other specified person such as a birth sibling

Mutual Access to Identifying Information

- The Adoption Registry will disclose identifying information if the relevant parties have registered their consent to disclosure.
- Such information will also be disclosed to Indian Tribes or governmental agencies to establish an adopted person's eligibility for Tribal membership or for benefits or to the trustee of an estate that refers to the adopted person.

Access to Original Birth Certificate

Available upon order of the court or as provided by rule of the State registrar

Where the Information Can Be Located

Voluntary Adoption Registry, Oregon State Office for Services to Children and Families

PENNSYLVANIA

Who May Access Information

- Adopted person age 18 or older
- Adoptive parents, if adopted person is under age 18
- Legal guardian

Mutual Access to Identifying Information

In the event consent is not present, upon petition, the court may, through its designated agent, attempt to contact the birthparents, if known, to obtain their consent to release their identity and present place of residence to an adopted person.

Access to Original Birth Certificate

Available to the adopted person if age 18 or older or to the adoptive parent if the birthparent(s) have filed consent with the Department of Health.

Where the Information Can Be Located

Adoption Medical History Registry, Office of Children, Youth, and Families

RHODE ISLAND

Who May Access Information

- Birthparents and siblings
- Adult adopted person
- Surviving relatives of deceased birthparents and deceased adopted person

Mutual Access to Identifying Information

The listed parties may register their willingness with the court to the release of identifying information to each other, if requested.

Access to Original Birth Certificate

A noncertified copy can be obtained through the mutual consent registry to the adult adopted person when the birthparent(s) is/are registered and have given consent.

Where the Information Can Be Located

- State of Rhode Island and Providence Plantations Family Court, Juvenile Division
- The agency involved in the adoption

SOUTH CAROLINA
Who May Access Information

- Adopted person, age 21 or older
- Birthparents and siblings

Mutual Access to Identifying Information

A party may request, in writing, and receive identifying information about another party if an affidavit granting consent is present. Counseling concerning the effects of the disclosure is mandatory.

Access to Original Birth Certificate

- When an adoption is finalized, an amended birth certificate is issued in the name of the adopted person, free of any reference to the fact that the child was adopted.
- The amended certificate is filed in lieu of the original. The original is placed in a special sealed file by the State registrar.
- The statue does not specify a procedure for access to the original certificate. Presumably, access can be obtained through a court order.

Where the Information Can Be Located

Adoption Reunion Registry, South Carolina Department of Social Services

SOUTH DAKOTA
Who May Access Information

- Adoptive parent
- Adopted person, age 18 or older
- Birthparents

Mutual Access to Identifying Information

Consent to the release of identifying information shall indicate to whom the information may be released and whether the party desires release of the information after their death. A person who uses the registry may revoke consent at any time.

Access to Original Birth Certificate

Available upon order of the court

Where the Information Can Be Located

South Dakota Voluntary Registry

TENNESSEE
Who May Access Information

- Adopted person, age 18 or older
- Adoptive parents or guardian if adopted person is under age 18
- Birthparent or legal relatives
- The lineal descendants of an adopted person
- The legal representative of any of the above persons

Mutual Access to Identifying Information

The persons authorized by § 36-1-133, provided they are age 21 or older, may have their names entered in the registry stating either their willingness or unwillingness to be contacted and have identifying information disclosed.

Access to Original Birth Certificate

Available to parties who have established their eligibility to have access to adoption records

Where the Information Can Be Located

Advanced Notice Registry, Department of Children's Services, Post Adoption Services

TEXAS
Who May Access Information

- Adoptive parents
- Adult adopted person

Mutual Access to Identifying Information

- Access to identifying information is possible through the mutual adoption registry. A registrant is required to sign a written consent to disclosure form before a release may be completed.

- Such information shall be released without consent if the registrant is deceased, their registration was valid at the time of death, and they had authorized post-death disclosure.

Access to Original Birth Certificate
Only the court that granted the adoption may grant access.

Where the Information Can Be Located
Central Adoption Registry, Texas Department of Health, Bureau of Vital Statistics

UTAH
Who May Access Information
- Adoptive parents or legal guardian
- Adopted person
- Adopted person's spouse, or guardian of the adopted person's child, if the adopted person is deceased
- The adopted person's child or descendant
- The birthparent or adult birth sibling

Mutual Access to Identifying Information
The bureau may only release identifying information to an adult adopted person or birthparents and adult birth sibling when it receives requests from both the adopted person and the birth relative.

Access to Original Birth Certificate
Sealed except upon order of the court granting inspection

Where the Information Can Be Located
Mutual Consent Voluntary Adoption Registry, Utah Bureau of Vital statistics

VERMONT
Who May Access Information
- Adoptive parent or legal guardian of an adopted person
- Adopted person, age 18 or older
- Emancipated adopted person
- Deceased adopted person's direct descendant, age 18 or older, or his or her parent or guardian if the adopted person is under age 18

- The adopted person's birthparent, grandparent, or sibling

Mutual Access to Identifying Information
- For adoptions finalized before July 1, 1986, the registry shall disclose identifying information if the birthparent has filed in probate court or agency any document that consents to such disclosure.
- For adoptions finalized on or after July 1, 1986, the registry shall disclose identifying information unless a request for nondisclosure has been filed.
- An adult descendant of a deceased birthparent may consent to disclosure of information.
- If an adult adopted person consents, identifying information may be disclosed to a birthparent or adult birth siblings.
- A birthparent may prevent disclosure of identifying information about himself or herself by filing a request for nondisclosure with the registry as provided in § 6-105 of this title. A request for nondisclosure may be withdrawn at any time.

Access to Original Birth Certificate
- May be released upon request to an adopted person age 18 or older who has access to identifying information
- The original birth certificate is unsealed and becomes public record 99 years after the date of the adopted person's birth.

Where the Information Can Be Located
Vermont Adoption Registry

VIRGINIA
Who May Access Information
- Adopted person, age 18 or older
- Licensed or authorized child-placing agencies providing services to the child
- Adoptive parents

Mutual Access to Identifying Information
- For adoptions finalized after July 1, 1994, the adopted person, age 21 or older, the birthparents, and adult birth siblings can request identifying information.

- Upon the consideration of the effect of the disclosure on any party and a showing of good cause, identifying information from the adoption file will be disclosed to an adopted person, age 21 or older, the birthparent, and adult siblings.

Access to Original Birth Certificate
Available only upon order of the court

Where the Information Can Be Located
Department of Social Services, Vital Adoption Records

WASHINGTON
Who May Access Information
- An adoptive parent
- An adopted person
- A birthparent

Mutual Access to Identifying Information
A qualified party may petition the court to appoint a confidential intermediary to acquire consent to the release of identifying information. An adopted person must be age 21 or older, or, if under age 21, have the permission of the adoptive parents, in order to access such information.

Access to Original Birth Certificate
- A noncertified copy is available to the birthparent upon request.
- For adoptions finalized after October 1, 1993, a noncertified copy is available to the adopted person, age 18 or older unless the birthparent has filed an affidavit of nondisclosure.

Where the Information Can Be Located
State Adoption Department, Department of Social and Health Services

WEST VIRGINIA
Who May Access Information
- Adoptive parents
- An adult adopted person

Mutual Access to Identifying Information
The adult adopted person and each birthparent may voluntarily register to disclose identifying information by submitting a notarized affidavit to the appropriate registry stating his or her name, address, and telephone number and his or her willingness to be identified solely to the other relevant person who registers. A reasonable fee will be charged for this service.

Access to Original Birth Certificate
Original birth certificate is sealed from inspection, except upon order of the court.

Where the Information Can Be Located
West Virginia Mutual Consent Voluntary Adoption Registry, Department of Health and Human Resources

WISCONSIN
Who May Access Information
- Adopted person, age 21 or older
- A birthparent

Mutual Access to Identifying Information
Identifying information may be released to a requester if an unrevoked affidavit giving consent to such a release is present. If no consent is on file, the department or agency shall conduct a diligent search for the person, to be completed within six months.

Access to Original Birth Certificate
Available upon request to adopted person age 21 or older if the birthparents have filed affidavits authorizing disclosure

Where the Information Can Be Located
Adoption Records Search Program

WYOMING
Who May Access Information
- Adult adopted person
- Adoptive parent
- Birthparent, sibling, or grandparent

All parties must be age 18 or older.

Mutual Access to Identifying Information
Any qualified person may:

- File a motion in the court where the adoption took place or where the parental rights were terminated
- Request the appointment of one or more confidential intermediaries for the purpose of determining the whereabouts of an unknown birth relative or relatives in order to gain their consent to release identifying information

Costs related to the proceeding and investigation shall be the responsibility of the party filing the motion.

Access to Original Birth Certificate
Not subject to inspection except by court order

Where the Information Can Be Located
Wyoming Confidential Adoption Intermediary Services

Source: National Adoption Information Clearinghouse, "Access to Family Information by Adopted Persons: Summary of State Laws," U.S. Department of Health and Human Services, Administration for Children and Families, Children's Bureau, Washington, D.C., 2004.

BIBLIOGRAPHY

Acosta, Marie Teresa, M.D., Mauricio Arcos-Burgos, M.D., and Maximilian Muenke, M.D., "Attention Deficit/Hyperactivity Disorder (ADHD): Complex Phenotype, Simple Genotype," *Genetics in Medicine* 6, no. 1 (2004): 1–15.

Adamec, Christine. "Adoption and the Internet," *Adoption Factbook III*. Washington, D.C.: National Council for Adoption, 1999, 405–407.

———. *The Adoption Option Complete Handbook 2000–2001*. Rocklin, N.Y.: Prima Publishing, 1999.

———. *The Complete Idiot's Guide to Adoption*. New York: Alpha Books, 2005.

———. *Is Adoption for You? The Information You Need to Make the Right Choice*. New York: John Wiley & Sons, 1998.

———. *There ARE Babies to Adopt: A Resource Guide for Prospective Parents*. New York: Kensington, 2002.

Adesman, Andrew, M.D., with Christine Adamec. *Parenting the Adopted Child: A Basic Approach to Building a Strong Family*. New York: McGraw-Hill, 2004.

Administration for Children, Youth and Families, Department of Health and Human Services. *Child Maltreatment 2003*. Washington, D.C., 2005.

———. *National Survey of Child and Adolescent Well-Being: One Year in Foster Care Report*. Washington, D.C. (November 2003).

Altstein, Howard, and Rita J. Simon. *Intercountry Adoption: A Multinational Perspective*. New York: Praeger, 1991.

American Psychiatric Association. *Diagnostic and Statistical Manual of Mental Disorders*, 4th ed., text revision (DSM-IV-TR). Washington, D.C.: American Psychiatric Association, 2000.

Atwater, Martha W. "A Modern-Day Solomon's Dilemma: What of the Unwed Father's Rights?", *University of Detroit Law Review* 66 (1989): 267–296.

Austin, Lisette. "Mental Health Needs of Youth in Foster Care: Challenges and Strategies," *Connection* 20, no. 4 (winter 2004): 6–13.

Avery, Rosemary J., ed. *Adoption Policy and Special Needs*. Westport, Conn.: Auburn House, 1997.

Babb, L. Anne, and Rita Laws. *Adopting and Advocating for the Special Needs Child: A Guide for Parents and Professionals*. Westport, Conn.: Bergin & Garvey, 1997.

Baden, Amanda. "Psychological Adjustment of Transracial Adoptees: An Application of the Cultural-Racial Identity Model," *Journal of Social Distress and the Homeless* 11, no. 2 (April 2002): 167–191.

Barth, Richard P. "Disruption in Older Child Adoptions," *Public Welfare* 46 (winter 1988): 23–29.

———. "Educational Implications of Prenatally Drug Exposed Children," *Social Work in Education* 13 (1991): 130–136.

———. "Timing Is Everything: An Analysis of the Time to Adoption and Legalization," *Social Work Research* 18, no. 3 (September 1994): 139–148.

Barth, Richard P., and Marianne Berry. *Adoption and Disruption: Rates, Risks, and Responses*. New York: Aldine De Gruyter, 1988.

Barth, Richard P., et al. "Predicting Adoption Disruption," *Social Work* 33 (May–June 1988): 277–233.

Bartholet, Elizabeth. "International Adoption: Propriety, Prospects and Pragmatics," *Journal of the American Academy of Matrimonial Lawyers* 13, no. 2 (winter 1996): 181–210.

Bassuk, Ellen, M.D., and Lenore Rubin. "Homeless Children: A Neglected Population," *American Journal of Orthopsychiatry* 57 (April 1987): 279–285.

Beckett, Celia, et al. "Behavior Patterns Associated with Institutional Deprivation: A Study of Children Adopted from Romania," *Developmental and*

Behavioral Pediatrics 23, no. 5 (October 2002): 297–303.

Benson, Peter L., Anu Sharma, and Eugene C. Roehlkepantain. *Growing up Adopted: A Portrait of Adolescents and Their Families.* Minneapolis, Minn.: The Search Institute, 1994.

Berman, Michael D. "Unsealing Adoption Records," *Maryland Bar Journal* 22 (September/October 1989): 33–35.

Berry, Marianne, and Richard P. Barth. "A Study of Disrupted Adoptive Placements of Adolescents," *Child Welfare* 69, no. 3 (May/June 1990): 209–225.

Bierut, Laura Jean, M.D. "Defining Alcohol-Related Phenotypes in Humans: The Collaborative Study on the Genetics of Alcoholism," *Alcohol Research & Health* 26, no. 3 (2002): 208–213.

Blanton, Terril L., and Jeanne Deschner. "Biological Mothers' Grief: The Postadoptive Experience in Open Versus Confidential Adoption," *Child Welfare* 69, no. 6 (November–December 1990): 525–535.

Boccaccini, Marcus T., and Eleanor Willemson. "Contested Adoption and the Liberty Interest of the Child," *Thomas Law Review* 10, no. 2 (winter 1998): 211–228.

Boehner, John, and Mike Castle. *Individuals with Disabilities Education Act (IDEA): Guide to "Frequently Asked Questions."* Available online. URL: http://www.house.gov/ed_workforce/issues/109th/education/idea/ideafaq.pdf. Downloaded on April 3, 2005.

Bohman, Michael. *Adopted Children and Their Families.* Stockholm, Sweden: Proprius, 1970.

Boris, Neil W. "Attachment, Aggression and Holding: A Cautionary Tale," *Attachment & Human Development* 5, no. 3 (September 2003): 245–247.

Bouchard, Thomas J. Jr., and Matt McGue. "Genetic and Environmental Influences on Human Psychological Differences," *Journal of Neurobiology,* 54, no. 1 (2003): 4–45.

Brace, C. L. *The Best Method of Disposing of Our Pauper and Vagrant Children.* New York: Wynkoop, Hallenbeck & Thomas, 1859.

Branscomb, Robert. "Clinical Evaluation and the Role of the Laboratory in Diagnosing Pediatric Lead Poisoning," *Lab Medicine* 36, no. 3 (2005): 178–180.

Brinich, Paul M., and Evelin B. Brinich. "Adoption and Adaptation," *Journal of Nervous and Mental Disease* 170, no. 8 (1982): 489–493.

Brodzinsky, David M., and Marshall D. Schecter, eds. *The Psychology of Adoption.* New York: Oxford University Press, 1990.

Cadoret, Remi J., M.D. "Adoption Studies," *Alcohol Health & Research* 19, no. 3 (summer 1995): 193–200.

Cadoret, Remi J., M.D., Colleen A. Cain, and William M. Grove. "Development of Alcoholism in Adoptees Raised Apart from Alcoholic Biologic Relatives," *Archives of General Psychiatry* 37, no. 5 (May 1980): 561–563.

Carlson, Richard R. "Transnational Adoption of Children," *Tulsa Law Journal* 23 (spring 1988): 317–377.

Catholic Adoptive Parents Association. *Media Guidelines on Adoption Language.* Harrison, N.Y.: Catholic Adoptive Parents Association, 1988.

Centers for Disease Control and Prevention. "CDC Recommendations for Lead Poisoning Prevention in Newly Arrived Refugee Children." Available online. URL: http://www.cdc.gov/nceh/lead/Refugee%20Recommendations.pdf. Accessed on May 15, 2005.

———. *HIV/AIDS Surveillance Report,* 2003. Available online. URL: http://www.cdc.gov/hiv/stats/2003SurveillanceReport.htm. Downloaded on September 30, 2005.

———. *Preventing Lead Exposure in Young Children: A Housing-Based Approach to Primary Prevention of Lead Poisoning.* Available online. URL: http://www.cdc.gov/nceh/lead/Publications/Primary%20Prevention%20Document.pdf. Downloaded on September 30, 2005.

———. "Recommended Childhood and Adolescent Immunization Schedule, United States, 2005," Department of Health and Human Services. Available online. URL: http://www.cdc.gov/nip/recs/child-schedule-bw.pdf. Downloaded on April 15, 2005.

———. "Surveillance for Elevated Blood Levels Among Children—United States, 1997–2001," *Morbidity and Mortality Weekly Report* 52, no. SS-10 (September 12, 2003): 1–21.

Chandra, Anjani, et al. "Adoption, Adoption Seeking, and Relinquishment for Adoption in the United States," *Advance Data* 306 (May 11, 1999): 1–16.

Chen, Lin H., M.D., Elizabeth D. Barnett, and Mary E. Wilson, M.D. "Preventing Infectious Diseases during and after International Adoption," *Annals of Internal Medicine* 139, no. 5, Part I (2003): 371–378.

Cherian, Varghese I. "Birth Order and Academic Achievement of Children in Transkei," *Psychological Reports* 66 (1990): 19–24.

Chess, Stella, and Alexander Thomas. *Know Your Child: An Authoritative Guide for Today's Parents.* New York: Basic Books, 1989.

Ciccarelli, Janice C., and Linda J. Beckman. "Navigating Rough Waters: An Overview of Psychological Aspects of Surrogacy," *Journal of Social Issues* 61, no. 1 (2005): 21–43.

Ciccarelli, John K., and Janice C. Ciccarelli. "The Legal Aspects of Parental Rights in Assisted Reproductive Technology," *Journal of Social Issues* 61, no. 1 (2005): 127–137.

Clark, E. Audrey, and Jeanette Hanisee. "Intellectual and Adaptive Performance of Asian Children in Adoptive American Settings," *Development Psychology* 18 (1982): 595–599.

Clark, Natalie Loder. "New Wine in Old Skins: Using Paternity-Suit Settlements to Facilitate Surrogate Motherhood," *Journal of Family Law* 25, no. 3 (1986–87): 483–527.

Clark, Robin B., Judith Freeman Clark, and Christine Adamec. *The Encyclopedia of Child Abuse.* New York: Facts On File, 2001.

Clarke, Ann, and Alan Clarke. "Early Experience and the Life Path," *Psychologist* (September 1998): 433–436.

Clay Wright, Victoria, et al. "Assisted Reproductive Technology Surveillance, United States, 2002," *Morbidity & Mortality Weekly Report Surveillance Summaries* 54, no. SS02 (June 3, 2005): 1–24.

Cole, Elizabeth, and Kathryn Donley. "History, Values, and Placement Policy Issues in Adoption," in *The Psychology of Adoption.* New York: Oxford University Press, 1990.

Coleman, Loren, et al., eds. *Working with Older Adoptees: A Sourcebook of Innovative Models.* Portland: University of Southern Maine, Human Services Development Institute, 1988.

Combs, Claire Grandpre. "Wrongful Adoption: Adoption Agency Held Liable for Fraudulent Representations," *Cincinnati Law Review* 56 (1987): 343–359.

Costin, Lela B., et al. *Child Welfare, Policies and Practice.* White Plains, N.Y.: Longman, 1991.

Custer, Marcia. "Adoption as an Option for Unmarried Pregnant Teens," *Adolescence* 28, no. 112 (winter 1993).

Davidson, Howard A. "Protecting America's Children: A Challenge," *Trial* 35, no. 1 (January 1999): 22.

De Haymes, Maria Vidal, Shirley Simon, and Jerome Blakemore. *Children of Color in Foster Care and the Multiethnic Placement Act: The Experiences of Families Involved in Transracial and Same Race Adoptions in an Illinois Sample: Final Report.* Available online. URL: http://cfrcwww.social.uiuc. edu/pubs/pdf.files/childofcolor.pdf. Downloaded on August 5, 2005.

Depp, Carole H. "Placing Siblings Together," *Children Today* 12, no. 7 (March–April 1983): 14–19.

Derdeyn, Andrea P., and Charles L. Graves. "Clinical Vicissitudes of Adoption," *Child and Adolescent and Psychiatric Clinics of North America* 7, no. 2 (April 1998): 273–294.

Desetta, Al, ed. *The Heart Knows Something Different: Teenage Voices from the Foster Care System.* New York: Persea Books, 1996.

Donley, Kathryn. "Sibling Attachments and Adoption," Unpublished, National Resource Center for Special Needs Adoption, Chelsea, Michigan.

Eley, Thalia C., et al. "An Adoption Study of Depressive Symptoms in Middle Childhood," *Journal of Psychology and Psychiatry and Allied Disciplines* 39, no. 3 (March 1998): 337–345.

Eschelbach Hansen, Mary, and Rita J. Simon. "Transracial Placement in Adoptions with Public Agency Involvement: What Can We Learn from the AFCARS Data?" *Adoption Quarterly* 8, no. 2 (2004): 45–56.

Fanshel, David, Stephen J. Finch, and John F. Grundy. "Foster Children in Life-Course Perspective: The Casey Family Program Experience," *Child Welfare* 68, no. 5 (September–October 1989): 467–478.

Feigelman, William. "Adjustments of Transracially and Inracially Adopted Young Adults," *Child and Adolescent Social Work* 17, no. 3 (June 2000): 165–184.

Festinger, Trudy. *Necessary Risk: A Study of Adoptions and Disrupted Adoptive Placement.* Washington, D.C.: Child Welfare League of America, 1986.

Field, Tiffany. "Attachment and Separation in Young Children," *Annual Review of Psychology* 47 (1996): 541–561.

French, Anne Wiseman. "When Blood Isn't Thicker than Water: The Inheritance Rights of Adopted-Out Children in New York," *Brooklyn Law Review* 53 (winter 1988): 1,007–1,049.

Freundlich, Madelyn D. "The Case against Preadoption Genetic Testing," *Child Welfare* 77, no. 6 (November 1, 1998): 663–679.

Freundlich, Madelyn D., and Joy Kim Lieberthal. *The Gathering of the First Generation of Adult Korean Adoptees: Adoptees' Perceptions of International Adoption.* New York: Evan B. Donaldson Adoption Institute, June 2000.

Fulker, D. W., J. C. DeFries, and Robert Plomin. "Genetic Influence on General Mental Ability Increases between Infancy and Middle Childhood," *Nature* 336, no. 6201 (December 1988): 767–769.

General Accounting Office. "Intercountry Adoption: Procedures Are Reasonable, but Sometimes Inefficiently Administered: Report to the Honorable Arlen Specter, U.S. Senate." Available online. URL: http://arcive.gao/gov/t2pbat6/149161.pdf. Downloaded on August 2, 2005.

Gennaro, Susan. "Vulnerable Infants: Kinship Care and Health," *Pediatric Nursing* 24, no. 2 (March–April 1998): 119–125.

Gill, Owen, and Barbara Jackson. *Adoption and Race: Black, Asian and Mixed Race Children in White Families.* London: Batsford Academic and Educational, 1983.

Glenn, Norval D., and Sue Keir Hoppe. "Only Children as Adults," *Journal of Family Issues* 5 (September 1984): 363–382.

Glennen, Sharon. "Language Development and Delay in Internationally Adopted Infants and Toddlers: A Review," *American Journal of Speech-Language Pathology* 11, no. 4 (November 2002): 333–339.

Goldsmith, H. H. "Genetic Influences on Personality from Infancy to Adulthood," *Child Development* 54 (1983): 331–355.

Goldstein, J., A. Freud, and Albert Solnit. *Beyond the Best Interests of the Child.* New York: Free Press, 1973, 1979.

Grabe, Pamela V., ed. *Adoption Resources for Mental Health Professionals.* Butler, Pa.: Mental Health Adoption Therapy Project, September 1986.

Grant, Bridget F., et al. "The 12-month prevalence and trends in DSM-IV alcohol abuse and dependence: United States, 1991–1992 and 2001–2002," *Drug and Alcohol Dependence* 74 (2004): 223–234.

Gwinnell, Esther, M.D. "A Parent's Guide to Attachment Problems," *Adoption/Medical News* 5, no. 4 (April 1998): 1–6.

Gwinnell, Esther, M.D., and Christine Adamec. *The Encyclopedia of Addictive Behaviors and Addictions.* New York: Facts On File, 2005.

Harris Interactive Market Research. *National Adoption Attitudes Survey Research Report.* Available online. URL: http://www.adoptioninstitute.org/survey/Adoption_Attitudes_Survey.pdf. Downloaded on February 14, 2005.

Hartfield, Bernadette W. "The Role of the Interstate Compact on the Placement of Children in Interstate Adoption," *Nebraska Law Review* 68 (1989): 292–329.

Herman-Giddens, Marcia E., et al. "Newborns Killed or Left to Die by a Parent: A Population-Based Study," *Journal of the American Medical Association* 289, no. 11 (March 19, 2003): 1,425–1,429.

Heymann, S. Jody, M.D., and Jeffrey Starker, M.D. "Pediatric Tuberculosis: What Needs to Be Done to Decrease Morbidity and Mortality," *Pediatrics* 106, no. 1 (2000): 1.

Hilborn, Robin. "Adoption Tax Credit of up to $1,600," Adoption Council of Canada. Available online. URL: http://www.adoption.ca/news/050223.tax.htm. Downloaded on May 20, 2005.

———. "China Leads Adoption Statistics for 2004." Available online. URL: http://www.adoption.ca/news/050527stats04.htm. Downloaded on June 27, 2005.

———. *Canadian Guide to Intercountry Adoption.* 4th ed. Ontario, Canada: Family Helper Publishing, 2004.

———. *Waiting Kids in Canada: All about Domestic Adoption.* Ontario, Canada: Family Helper Publishing, 2004.

Hollenstein, Tom, et al. "Openness in Adoption, Knowledge of Birthparent Information and Adoptive Family Adjustment," *Adoption Quarterly* 7, no. 1 (2003): 43–52.

Hollinger, Joan H., editor in chief. *Adoption Law and Practice.* New York: Lexis Nexis, 2004.

Hollinger, Joan H. "Second Parent Adoptions Protect Children with Two Mothers or Two Fathers," in *Families by Law: An Adoption Reader*. New York: New York University Press, 2004.

Hoopes, Janet L. *Prediction in Child Development: A Longitudinal Study of Adoptive and Nonadoptive Families*. Washington, D.C.: Child Welfare League of America, 1982.

Horn, Joseph M. "The Texas Adoption Project: Adopted Children and Their Intellectual Resemblance to Biological and Adoptive Parents," *Child Development* 54 (1983): 268–275.

Horner, R. Don. "A Practitioner Looks at Adoption Research," *Family Relations* 49 (2000): 473–477.

Hostetter, Margaret K., M.D., et al. "Unsuspected Infectious Diseases and Other Medical Diagnoses in the Evaluation of Internationally Adopted Children," *Pediatrics* 83, no. 4 (April 1989): 559–564.

Howard, Jeanne A., and Susan Livingston Smith. *After Adoption: The Needs of Adopted Youth*. Washington, D.C.: CWLA Press, 2003.

Howe, David. "Attachment Disorders: Disinhibited Attachment Behaviours and Secure Base Distortions with Special Reference to Adopted Children," *Attachment & Human Development* 5, no. 3 (September 2003): 265–270.

Howe, David, and Sheila Fearnley. "Disorders of Attachment in Adopted and Fostered Children: Recognition and Treatment," *Clinical Child Psychology and Psychiatry* 8, no. 3 (2003): 369–387.

Hughes, Daniel A. "Psychological Interventions for the Spectrum of Attachment Disorders and Intrafamilial Trauma," *Attachment & Human Development* 5, no. 3 (September 2003): 271–277.

Hughes, Timothy. "Interstate Succession and Stepparent Adoptions: Should Inheritance Rights of an Adopted Child Be Determined by Blood or Law?" *Wisconsin Law Review* (1988): 321–351.

Internal Revenue Service. "Tax Benefits for Adoption." Available online. URL: http://www.irs.gov/pub/irs-pdf/p968.pdf. Downloaded on September 30, 2005.

James, Sigrid. "Why Do Foster Care Placements Disrupt? An Investigation of Reasons for Placement Changes in Foster Care," *Social Service Review* 78, no. 4 (December 2004): 601–627.

Jewett, Claudia. *Helping Children Cope with Separation and Loss*. Boston: Harvard Common Press, 1982.

Jewett, Claudia L. *Adopting the Older Child*. Boston: Harvard Common Press, 1978.

Juffer, Femmie, and Marinus H. van IJzendoorn. "Behavior Problems and Mental Health Referrals of International Adoptees: A Meta-analysis," *Journal of the American Medical Association* 293, no. 20 (May 25, 2005): 2,501–2,515.

Juffer, Femmie, Geert-Jan J.M. Stams, and Marinus H. van IJzendoorn. "Adopted Children's Problem Behavior Is Significantly Related to Their Ego Resiliency, Ego Control, and Sociometric Status," *Journal of Child Psychology and Psychiatry* 45, no. 4 (2004): 697–706.

Katz, Linda. "An Overview of Current Clinical Issues in Separation and Placement," *Child and Adolescent Social Work* 4:3, no. 4 (fall, winter 1987): 209–223.

Keck, Gregory C., and Regina M. Kupecky. *Adopting the Hurt Child: Hope for Families with Special-Needs Kids*. Colorado Springs, Colo.: Pinon Press, 1995.

Kelly, Mary Margaret, et al. "Adjustment and Identity Formation in Adopted and Nonadopted Young Adults: Contributions of Family Environment," *American Journal of Orthopsychiatry* 63, no. 3 (July 1998): 497–500.

Kemper, Alex R., M.D., et al. "Follow-up Testing Among Children with Elevated Screening Blood Lead Levels," *Journal of the American Medical Association* 293, no. 18 (May 11, 2005): 2,232–2,237.

Kim, Wun Jung, M.D., et al. "Psychiatric Disorder and Juvenile Delinquency in Adopted Children and Adolescents," *Journal of the American Academy of Child and Adolescent Psychiatry* 27, no. 1 (January 1988): 111–115.

Kirk, H. D. *Adoptive Kinship*. Port Angeles, Brentwood Bay, British Columbia: Ben-Simon, 1982.

Kowal, Katherine A., and Karen Maitland Schilling. "Adoption through the Eyes of Adult Adoptees," *American Journal of Orthopsychiatry* 55, no. 3 (July 1985): 354–362.

Kraft, Adrienne D., et al. "Some Theoretical Considerations on Confidential Adoption," Part 3: "The Adoptive Child." In *Child and Adolescent Social Work* 2 (1983): 139–153.

Kreider, Rose. *Adopted Children and Stepchildren: 2000, Census 2000 Special Reports*. Available online. URL: http://www.census.gov/prod/2003

pubs/censr-6.pdf. Downloaded on September 30, 2005.

Krementz, Jill. *How It Feels to Be Adopted.* New York: Knopf, 1988.

Lears, Mary Kathleen, et al. "International Adoption: A Primer for Pediatric Nurses," *Pediatric Nursing* 24, no. 6 (November–December 1998): 578.

Lee, Richard M. "The Transracial Adoption Paradox: History, Research, and Counseling Implications of Cultural Socialization," *Counseling Psychologist* 31, no. 6 (November 2003): 711–744.

Lehmann, Michelle L. "The Indian Child Welfare Act of 1978: Does It Apply to the Adoption of an Illegitimate Indian Child?" *Catholic University Law Review* 38 (1989): 511–541.

LeMay, Susan Kempf. "The Emergence of Wrongful Adoption as a Cause of Action," *Journal of Family Law* 27, no. 2 (1988/89): 475–488.

LePere, Dorothy W. *Large Sibling Groups: Adoption Experiences.* Washington, D.C.: Child Welfare League of America, 1986.

Li, Ting-Kai, M.D. "The Genetics of Alcoholism," *Alcohol Alert* 60 (July 2003): 1–4.

Lieberman, Alicia F. "The Treatment of Attachment Disorder in Infancy and Early Childhood: Reflections from Clinical Intervention with Later-Adopted Foster Care Children," *Attachment & Human Development* 5, no. 3 (September 2003): 279–282.

Lieberman, Florence, Thomas K. Kenemore, and Diane Yost. *The Foster Care Dilemma.* New York: Human Sciences Press, 1987.

Lifton, Betty Jean. *Lost & Found: The Adoption Experience.* New York: Harper & Row, 1988.

Lightburn, Anita, and Barbara A. Pine. "Supporting and Enhancing the Adoption of Children with Developmental Disabilities," *Children & Youth Services Review* 18, no. 2 (1996): 139–162.

Littrell, Jill. "The Swedish Studies of the Adopted Children of Alcoholics," *Journal of Studies on Alcohol* 49, no. 6 (1988): 491–498.

Loehlin, John C., Joseph M. Horn, and Lee Willerman. "Modeling IQ Change: Evidence from the Texas Adoption Project," *Child Development* 60 (1989): 993–1,004.

Luman, Elizabeth T., et al. "Timeliness of Childhood Vaccinations in the United States: Days Undervaccinated and Number of Vaccines Delayed," *Journal of the American Medical Association* 93, no. 10 (March 9, 2005): 1,204–1,211.

Luo, Nili, and Kathleen Ja Sook Bergquist. "Born in China: Birth Country Perspectives on International Adoption," *Adoption Quarterly* 8, no. 1 (2004): 21–39.

MacLean, Kim. "The Impact of Institutionalization on Child Development," *Development and Psychopathology* 15, no. 4 (2003): 853–884.

Mandalakas, Anna M., M.D., and Jeffrey Starke, M.D. "Tuberculosis Screening in Immigrant Children," *Pediatric Infectious Disease Journal* 23, no. 1 (2004): 71–72.

Marquis, Kathlyn S., and Richard A. Detweiler. "Does Adopted Mean Different? An Attributional Analysis," *Journal of Personality and Social Psychology* 48, no. 4 (1985): 1,054–1,066.

Mason, Patrick, M.D., and Christine Narad. "Growth and Pubertal Development in Internationally Adopted Children," *Current Opinion in Endocrinology & Diabetes* 9, no. 1 (2002): 26–31.

McDermott, Virginia Anne. "Life Planning Services: Helping Older Placed Children with Their Identity," *Child and Adolescent Social Work* 4:3, no. 4 (fall, winter 1987): 245–263.

McDonald, Thomas C., et al. *Assessing the Long-Term Effects of Foster Care: A Research Synthesis.* Washington, D.C.: CWLA Press 1996.

McGloin, Jean Marie, and Cathy Spatz Widom. "Resilience Among Abuse and Neglected Children Grown Up," *Development and Psychopathology* 13 (2001): 1,021–1,038.

McKay, Mary, Richard Stolley, and Bea Evans. *Guatemala Travel and Etiquette: A Guide for Adoptive Parents,* second edition, June 2005. Available online. URL: http://www.guatadopt.com/documents/travelguide.pdf. Downloaded on July 2, 2005.

McNamara, Joan, and Bernard H. McNamara, eds. *Adoption and the Sexually Abused Child.* Portland: University of Southern Maine, Human Services Development Institute, 1990.

McRoy, Ruth G., Harold D. Grotevant, and Kerry L. White. *Openness in Adoption: New Practices, New Issues.* New York: Praeger, 1988.

McRoy, Ruth G., and Louis Z. Zurcher Jr. *Transracial and Inracial Adoptees: The Adolescent Years.* Springfield, Ill.: Thomas, 1983.

McWhorter Sember, Brette. *The Complete Adoption & Infertility Legal Guide.* Naperville, Ill.: Sourcebooks, Inc., 2004.

Meezan, W., S. Katz, and E. Manoff-Russo. *Adoptions Without Agencies: A Study of Independent Adoptions.* New York: Child Welfare League of America, 1978.

Miall, Charlene E. "The Stigma of Adoptive Parent Status: Perceptions of Community Attitudes Toward Adoption and the Experience of Informal Social Sanctioning," *Family Relations* 36 (January 1987): 34–39.

Miall, Charlene E., and Karen March. "Open Adoption as a Family Form: Community Assessments and Social Support," *Journal of Family Issues* 26, no. 3 (April 2005): 380–410.

———. "Social Support for Adoption in Canada: Preliminary Findings of a Canada-Wide Survey." Available online. URL: http://www.carleton. ca/socanth/Faculty/News%20Release% 20Adoption%20Survey.pdf. Downloaded on March 3, 2004.

Midyett, L. Kurt, M.D., Wayne V. Moore, M.D., and Jill D. Jacobson, M.D. "Are Pubertal Changes in Girls Before Age 8 Benign?" *Pediatrics* 111, no. 1 (2003): 47–51.

Miller, Laurie C., M.D. "Initial Assessment of Growth, Development, and the Effects of Institutionalization in Internationally Adopted Children," *Pediatric Annals* 29, no. 4 (April 2000): 224–232.

———. "International Adoption: Infectious Diseases Issues," *Clinical Infectious Diseases* 40, no. 1 (January 15, 2005): 286–293.

———. "International Adoption, Behavior, and Mental Health," *Journal of the American Medical Association* 293, no. 20 (May 25, 2005): 2,533–2,535.

Miller, Laurie C., M.D., and Nancy W. Hendrie, M.D. "Health of Children Adopted from China," *Pediatrics* 105, no. 6 (June 2000).

Miller, Laurie C., et al. "Serologic Prevalence of Antibodies to *Helicobacter pylori* in Internationally Adopted Children," *Helicobacter* 8, no. 3 (2003): 173–178.

Miller Wrobel, Gretchen, Harold D. Grotevant, and Ruth G. McRoy. "Adolescent Search for Birthparents: Who Moves Forward?" *Journal of Adolescent Research* 19, no. 1 (January 2004): 132–151.

Minde, Klaus. "Attachment Problems as a Spectrum Disorder: Implications for Diagnosis and Treatment," *Attachment & Human Development* 5, no. 3 (September 2003): 289–296.

Minnis, Helen, and Gregory Keck. "A Clinical/ Research Dialogue on Reactive Attachment Disorder," *Attachment & Human Development* 5, no. 3 (September 2003): 297–303.

Minocha, Anil, M.D., and Christine Adamec. *The Encyclopedia of the Digestive System and Digestive Disorders.* New York: Facts On File, 2004.

Muller, Ulrich, Peter Gibbs, and Sumi Gupta Ariely. "Predictors of Psychological Functioning and Adoption Experience in Adults Searching for Their Birthparents," *Adoption Quarterly* 5, no. 3 (2002): 25–53.

National Adoption Information Clearinghouse. "Access to Family Information by Adopted Persons: Summary of State Laws," State Statutes Series 2004, U.D. Department of Health and Human Services, Administration for Children and Families, 2004.

———. "Interstate Inheritance Rights." Available online. URL: http://naif.acf.hhs.gov/general/ legal/statutes/inheritance.pdf. Downloaded on September 30, 2005.

National Center for Health Statistics, *Health, United States, 2004 with Chartbook on Trends in the Health of Americans.* Available online. URL: http://cdc. gov/nchs/hus.htm. Downloaded on September 30, 2005.

National Institute of Child Health & Human Development. "Facts about Down Syndrome." Available online. URL: http://www.nichd.nih.gov/ publications/pubs/downsyndrome/down.htm. Accessed on June 6, 2005.

National Institute of Mental Health. "Depression Gene May Weaken Mood-Regulating Circuit," National Institutes of Health. Available online. URL: http://www. nih.gov/news/pr/May2005/ nimh-08.htm. Downloaded on September 30, 2005.

National Task Force on Fetal Alcohol Syndrome and Fetal Alcohol Effect. *Fetal Alcohol Syndrome: Guidelines for Referral and Diagnosis.* Centers for Disease Control and Prevention. Available online. URL: http://www.cdc.gov/ncbddd/fas/ documents/FAS_guidelines_accessible.pdf. Downloaded on September 30, 2005.

Nelson, Katherine A. *On the Frontier of Adoption: A Study of Special-Needs Adoptive Families.* New York: Child Welfare League of America, 1985.

Newlin, David B., et al. "Environmental Transmission of DSM-IV Substance Use Disorders in Adoptive and Step Families," *Alcoholism: Clinical and Experimental Research* 24, no. 12 (December 2000): 1,785–1,794.

Newman, Tony. *Promoting Resilience: A Review of Effective Strategies for Child Care Services.* Available online. URL: http://www.cebss.org/files/Promoting_Resilience.pdf. Downloaded on January 10, 2005.

Nichol, A. R., ed. *Longitudinal Studies in Child Psychology and Psychiatry.* New York: Wiley, 1985.

Nicholson, Laura A. "Adoption Medicine and the Internationally Adopted Child," *American Journal of Law and Medicine* 28 (2002): 473–490.

O'Brien, Shari. "Race in Adoption Proceedings: The Pernicious Factor," *Tulsa Law Journal* (1986): 485–498.

O'Connor, Thomas G., and Charles H. Zeanah. "Attachment Disorders: Assessment Strategies and Treatment Approaches," *Attachment & Human Development* 5, no. 3 (September 2003): 223–244.

———. "Current Perspectives on Attachment Disorders: Rejoinder and Synthesis," *Attachment & Human Development* 5, no. 3 (September 2003): 321–326.

Oerter Klein, Karen, et al. "Increased Final Height in Precocious Puberty after Long-Term Treatment with LHRD Agonists: The National Institutes of Health Experience," *Journal of Clinical Endocrinology & Metabolism* 86, no. 10 (2001): 4,711–4,716.

Office of the Assistant Secretary for Planning and Evaluation. *"Understanding Adoption Subsidies: An Analysis of AFCARS Data."* Washington, D.C.: U.S. Department of Health and Human Services, 2005.

Oppenheim, Elizabeth. "Adoption Assistance," *Public Welfare* 54, no. 1 (winter 1996).

Pannor, Reuben, and Annette Baran. "Open Adoption a Standard Practice," *Child Welfare* 63 (May–June 1984): 245–250.

Partridge, Susan, Helaine Hornby, and Thomas McDonald. *Learning from Adoption Disruption: Insights for Practice.* Portland, Maine: Human Services Development Institute, 1986.

Pecora, Peter J., et al. *Improving Family Foster Care: Findings from the Northwest Foster Care Alumni Study.* Seattle, Wash.: Casey Family Services, revised March 14, 2005.

Pelton, Jennifer, and Rex Forehand. "Orphans of the AIDS Epidemic: An Examination of Clinical Level Problems of Children," *Journal of the American Academy of Child & Adolescent Psychiatry* 44, no. 6 (June 2005): 585–591.

Petit, William A., Jr., M.D., and Christine Adamec. *The Encyclopedia of Endocrine Diseases and Disorders.* New York: Facts On File, 2005.

Pickering, L. K., ed. "Section 3. Summaries of Infectious Diseases," in *Red Book: 2003 Report of the Committee on Infectious Diseases,* 26th ed. Elk Grove Village, Ill: American Academy of Pediatrics, 2003, 642–660.

Plomin, Robert, and J. C. DeFries. "The Colorado Adoption Project," *Child Development* 54 (1983): 276–289.

Plomin, Robert, John C. Loehlin, and J. C. DeFries, "Genetic and Environmental Components of 'Environmental' Influences," *Developmental Psychology* 21 (1985): 391–402.

Podell, Richard J. "The Role of the Guardian Ad Litem: Advocating the Best Interests of the Child," *Trial,* April 1989, 31–34.

Powers, Douglas, ed. *Adoption for Troubled Children: Prevention and Repair of Adoptive Failures through Residential Treatment.* New York: Haworth Press, 1984.

Prescott, Carol A. "Sex Differences in the Genetic Risk for Alcoholism," *Alcohol Research & Health* 26, no. 2 (2002): 264–273.

Ramsey, Sarah H., and Douglas E. Abrams. *Children and the Law.* St. Paul, Minn.: West Group, 2001.

Raynor, Lois. *The Adopted Child Comes of Age.* London: George Allen & Unwin, 1980.

Register, Cheri. *"Are Those Kids Yours?": American Families with Children Adopted from Other Countries.* New York: Free Press, 1990.

———. *Beyond Good Intentions: A Mother Reflects on Raising Internationally Adopted Children.* St. Paul, Minn.: Yeong & Yeong Book Company, 2005.

Rhee, Soo Hyun, et al. "Genetic and Environmental Influences on Substance Initiation, Use, and Problem Use in Adolescents," *Archives of General Psychiatry* 60 (December 2003): 1,256–1,264.

Robinson, Jane R. "Attachment Problems and Disorders in Infants and Young Children: Identification, Assessment, and Intervention," *Infants and Young Children* 14, no. 4 (2002): 6–18.

Rutter, Michael. "Family and School Influences on Behavioural Development," *Journal of Child Psychology and Psychiatry* 26, no. 3 (1985): 349–368.

Sandmaier, Marian. *When Love Is Not Enough: How Mental Health Professionals Can Help Special-Needs Adoptive Families.* Washington, D.C.: Child Welfare League of America, 1988.

Scarr, Sandra, and Richard Weinberg. "The Minnesota Adoption Studies: Genetic Differences and Malleability," *Child Development* 54 (1983): 260–267.

Scarr, Sandra, et al. "Personality Resemblance Among Adolescents and Their Parents in Biologically Related and Adoptive Families," *Journal of Personality and Social Psychology* 40 (1981): 885–898.

Schechter, Marshall D. "Observations on Adopted Children," *Archives of General Psychiatry* 3 (July 1960): 21–32.

Schechter, Marshall D., M.D., Paul V. Carlson, M.D., James Q. Simmons, III, M.D., and Henry H. Work, M.D. "Emotional Problems in the Adoptee," *Archives of General Psychiatry* 10 (February 1964): 109–118.

Schiffer, Michele. "Fraud in the Adoption Setting," *Arizona Law Review* 29 (1987): 707–723.

Searles, John S. "The Role of Genetics in the Pathogenesis of Alcoholism," *Journal of Abnormal Psychology* 97 (May 1988): 153–167.

Senior, Neil, M.D., and Elaine Himadi, M.D. "Emotionally Disturbed, Adopted, Inpatient Adolescents," *Child Psychiatry and Human Development* 15 (spring 1985): 189–197.

Sharma, Anu R., Matthew McGue, and Peter Benson. "The Emotional and Behavioral Adjustment of United States Adopted Adolescents, Part II: Age at Adoption," *Children and Youth Services Review* 18, no. 1/2 (1996): 83–100.

Shih, Regina A., Pamela L. Bemonte, and Peter P. Zandi. "A Review of the Evidence from Family, Twin and Adoption Studies for a Genetic Contribution to Adult Psychiatric Disorders," *International Review of Psychiatry* 16, no. 4 (2004): 260–283.

Shireman, Joan F., and Penny R. Johnson. "A Longitudinal Study of Black Adoptions: Single Parent, Transracial, and Traditional," *Social Work* 31 (May–June 1986): 172–176.

Silber, Kathleen, and Phylis Speedlin. *Dear Birthmother: Thank You for Our Baby.* San Antonio, Texas: Corona, 1982.

Silverstein, Deborah N. "Identity Issues in the Jewish Adopted Adolescent," *Journal of Jewish Communal Service* (summer 1985): 321–329.

Simmel, Cassandra, et al. "Externalizing Symptomatology Among Adoptive Youth: Prevalence and Preadoptive Risk Factors," *Journal of Abnormal Child Psychology* 29, no. 1 (2001): 57–69.

Simon, Rita James. *Transracial Adoption.* New York: Wiley, 1977.

Simon, Rita J., and Howard Altstein. *Adoption across Borders: Serving the Children in Transracial and Intercountry Adoption.* Lanham, Md.: Rowman and Littlefield, Publishers, 2000.

———. *Transracial Adoptees and Their Families: A Study of Identity and Commitment.* New York: Praeger, 1987.

Simon, Rita J., Howard Altstein, and Marygold S. Melli. *The Case for Transracial Adoption.* Washington, D.C.: American University Press, 1994.

Singer, Leslie M., et al. "Mother-Infant Attachment in Adoptive Families," *Child Development* 56 (1985): 1,543–1,551.

Skomsvoll, J. F. "Reversible Infertility from Nonsteroidal Anti-Inflammatory Drugs," *Tidsskr Nor Laegeforen* 125, no. 11 (June 2, 2005): 1,476–1,478.

Skotko, Brian G. "Prenatally Diagnosed Down Syndrome: Mothers Who Continued Their Pregnancies Evaluate Their Health Care Providers," *American Journal of Obstetrics and Gynecology* 192 (2005): 670–677.

Slama, Jo Lynn. "Adoption and the Putative Father's Rights: *Shoecraft v. Catholic Social Services Bureau,*" *Oklahoma City University Law Review* 13 (spring 1988): 231–255.

Smith, Dorothy W., and Laurie Nehls Sherwen. *Mothers and Their Adopted Children—The Bonding Process.* New York: Teresias Press, 1983.

Smith, Jeanne, M.D., et al. "Asthma and Allergic Rhinitis in Adoptees and Their Adoptive Parents," *Annals of Allergy, Asthma and Immunology* 8, no. 1 (1998): 135–139.

Smyer, Michael A., et al. "Childhood Adoption: Long-Term Effects in Adulthood," *Psychiatry* 61, no. 3 (fall 1998): 191–205.

Sokol, Robert J., M.D., Virginia Delaney-Black, M.D., and Beth Nordstrom. "Fetal Alcohol Spectrum Disorder," *Journal of the American Medical Association* 290, no. 22 (December 10, 2003): 2,996–2,999.

Steele, Howard. "Holding Therapy Is Not Attachment Therapy: Editor's Introduction to This Invited Special Issue," *Attachment & Human Development* 5, no. 3 (September 2003): 219.

Steinberg, Gail, and Beth Hall. *Inside Transracial Adoption.* Indianapolis, Ind.: Perspectives Press, 2000.

Streissguth, Ann. *Fetal Alcohol Syndrome: A Guide for Families and Communities.* Baltimore, Md.: Paul Brookes Publishing Co., 1997.

Streissguth, Ann P., et al. "Risk Factors for Adverse Life Outcomes in Fetal Alcohol Syndrome and Fetal Alcohol Effects," *Journal of Developmental and Behavioral Pediatrics* 25, no. 4 (2004): 228–238.

Sullivan, Sharon, M.D. "Cultural and Socio-Emotional Issues of Internationally Adopted Children," *International Pediatrics* 19, no. 4 (2004): 208–216.

Swanton, Patricia. "The Adopted Child at School," *Journal of Family Health* Care 12, no. 6 (2002): 155–157.

Takayama, John I., et al. "Relationship Between Reason for Placement and Medical Findings Among Children in Foster Care," *Pediatrics* 101, no. 2 (February 1998).

Teasdale, T. W., and T. I. A. Sorensen. "Educational Attainment and Social Class in Adoptees: Genetic and Environmental Contributions," *Journal of Biosocial Science* 15 (1983): 509–518.

Ternay, Marilyn R., Bobbie Wilbom, and H. D. Day. "Perceived Child-Parent Relationships and Child Adjustment in Families with Both Adopted and Natural Children," *Journal of Genetic Psychology* 146, no. 2 (1985): 261–272.

Terpstra, Jake, M.S.W. "The Rich and Exacting Role of the Social Worker in Family Foster Care," *Child and Adolescent Social Work* 4, nos. 3 and 4 (fall, winter 1987).

Tieman, Wendy, Jan van der Ende, and Frank C. Verhulst. "Psychiatric Disorders in Young Adult Intercountry Adoptees: An Epidemiological Study," *American Journal of Psychiatry* 162 (2005): 592–598.

U.S. Department of Health and Human Services. *How Many Children Were Adopted in 2000 and 2001?* Washington, D.C.: National Adoption Information Clearinghouse, 2004.

Van IJzendoorn, Marinus H., and Marian J. Bakermans-Kranenburg. "Attachment Disorders and Disorganized Attachment: Similar and Different," *Attachment & Human Development* 5, no. 3 (September 2003): 313–320.

Van IJzendoorn, Marinus H., Femmie Juffer, and Caroline W. Klein Poelhuis. "Adoption and Cognitive Development: A Meta-Analytic Comparison of Adopted and Nonadopted Children's IQ and School Performance," *Psychological Bulletin* 131, no. 2 (2005): 301–316.

Volkman, Toby Alice, ed. *Cultures of Transnational Adoption.* Durham, N.C.: Duke University Press, 2005.

Ward, Margaret, and John H. Lewko. "Problems Experienced by Adolescents Already in Families that Adopt Older Children," *Adolescence* 23 (spring 1988): 221–228.

Weinberg, Richard A., et al. "Minnesota Transracial Adoption Study: Reports of Psychosocial Adjustment at Late Adolescence," *Adoption Quarterly* 8, no. 2 (2004): 27–44.

Weiss, Andrea. "Symptomology of Adopted and Non-adopted Adolescents in a Psychiatric Hospital," *Adolescence* (winter 1985): 763–774.

Wiedemeier Bower, Jeanette, and Rita Laws. *Support for Families of Children with Special Needs: A Policy Analysis of Adoption Subsidy Programs in the United States.* St. Paul, Minn.: North American Council on Adoptable Children, July 2002.

Witmer, Helen L., et al. *Independent Adoptions: A Follow-up Study.* New York: Sage Foundation, 1963.

World Health Organization. *Antiretroviral Drugs for Treating Pregnant Women and Preventing HIV Infection in Infants: Guidelines on Care, Treatment and Support for Women Living with HIV/AIDS and Their Children in Resource-Constrained Settings.* Geneva, Switzerland: World Health Organization, 2004.

Wu, S. S., et al. "Risk Factors for Infant Maltreatment: A Population-Based Study," *Child Abuse and Neglect* 28, no. 12 (2004): 1,253–1,264.

Xing Tan, Tony, and Yi Yang. "Language Development of Chinese Adoptees 18–35 Months Old," *Early Childhood Research Quarterly* 20 (2005): 57–68.

Zabriskie, Ramon B., and Patti Freeman. "Contributions of Family Leisure to Family Functioning Among Transracial Adoptive Families," *Adoption Quarterly* 7, no. 3 (2004): 49–77.

INDEX

Note: Page numbers in **boldface** indicate extensive treatment of a topic. Page numbers followed by *f* and *t* indicate figures and tables, respectively.